T0295177

OPTIMUM VITAMIN NUTRITION

for More Sustainable Swine Farming

OPTIMUM VITAMIN NUTRITION

for More Sustainable Swine Farming

E.O. Oviedo-Rondon, C. López-Bote, G. Litta and J.M. Hernandez

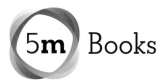 Books

Published by
5m Books Ltd,
Lings, Great Easton,
Essex CM6 2HH, UK,
Tel: +44 (0)330 1333 580
www.5mbooks.com

Follow us on
Twitter @5m_Books
Instagram 5m_books
Facebook @5mBooks
LinkedIn @5mbooks

A Catalogue record for this book is available from the British Library

ISBN 9781789182477
eISBN 9781789182538
DOI 10.52517/9781789182538

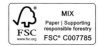

Book layout by Cheshire Typesetting Ltd, Cuddington, Cheshire
Printed by Bell & Bain Ltd, Glasgow
Photos by the authors unless otherwise indicated

CONTENTS

Authors and acknowledgements

Edgar O. Oviedo-Rondon
Prestage Department of Poultry Science, North Carolina State University

Clemente López-Bote
Department of Animal Production, Faculty of Veterinary Science, Complutense University Madrid

Gilberto Litta and José Maria Hernandez
dsm-firmenich, Animal Nutrition and Health

The authors are grateful to North Carolina State University Dr. Lina Maria Peñuela, Dr. Paula Lozano Cruz, Dr. John Nicolás Mejía from the University of Tolima, Ibague, Colombia, and Dr. Valmiro Aragão Neto (Nutrifeira, Brazil), who supported the work of Dr. Edgar O. Oviedo-Rondon at North Carolina State University, to Dr. Beatriz Isabel and Dr. Ana Isabel Rey who supported the work of Dr. López-Bote and to Dr. Thao Kiong Chung, Dr. John M. Reyes and Dr. Adsos Passos from dsm-firmenich Animal Nutrition & Health.

Abbreviations

AA	acetic acid
ACP	acyl groups carrier protein
ADFI	average daily feed intake
ADG	average daily gain
ADP	adenosine diphosphate
AMPK	AMP-activated protein kinase
ARC	Agriculture Research Council
ATP	adenosine triphosphate
AUC	area under the curve
BGP	bone Gla protein
BHMT	betaine homocysteine methyltransferase
CD	choline-deficient
CNS	central nervous system
CoA	coenzyme A
COP	cholesterol oxidation products
CRALBP	cellular retinaldehyde binding protein
CS	choline-sufficient
CSF	cerebrospinal fluid
DAG	diacylglycerol
DBP	D-binding protein
DBS	dried blood spots
DDGS	distillers dried grains with solubles
DFD	dry, firm, and dark
DTI	diffusion tensor imaging
ELISA	enzyme-linked immunosorbent assay
ELP	erythrocyte lipid peroxidation
ETKA	erythrocyte transketolase activity
FAD	flavin adenine dinucleotide
FAS	fatty acid synthase
FBP	folate-binding proteins
FCR	feed conversion ratio
FMN	flavin mono-nucleotide
FSV	fat-soluble vitamins
GABA	gamma-aminobutyric acid
GHG	greenhouse gas
GLO	L-Gulono-γ-lactone oxidase
GPX	glutathione peroxidase
HC	haptocorrin
HE	hematoxylin and eosin
HL	high level

HPLC	high-performance liquid chromatograph
IgA	immunoglobulin A
IgG	immunoglobulin G
IgM	immunoglobulin M
IU	international unit
IUGR	intrauterine growth retardation
KNN	K-nearest neighbor
LCA	life cycle assessment
LDL	low-density lipoproteins
LO	linseed and olive (oil)
LPS	lipopolysaccharide
LT	longissimus thoracic
MDA	malondialdehyde
MG	monoglutamate
MHD	mulberry heart disease
MK	menaquinone
MMA	mastitis-metritis-agalactia
MNB	menadione nicotinamide bisulfite
MPB	menadione dimethylpyrimidinol bisulfite
MRI	magnetic resonance imaging
MSB	menadione sodium bisulfite
MSBC	menadione sodium bisulfite complex
MSR	methionine sulfoxide reductase
MTHFR	N10-methylene-tetrahydrofolate reductase
MUFA	monounsaturated fatty acids
NAD	micotinamide adenine dinucleotide
NADH	nicotinamide adenine dinucleotide (reduced form)
NADP	nicotinamide adenine dinucleotide phosphate
NADPH	nicotinamide adenine dinucleotide phosphate
NL	normal (average) level
NN,nn	ryanodine receptor (RYR1) genotypes
NRC	National Research Council
OD	osteogenic disorder
OVN™	Optimum Vitamin Nutrition®
PABA	para-aminobenzoic acid
PAF	platelet-activating factor
PEDV	porcine epidemic diarrhea virus
PEM	polioencephalomalacia
PGC	primordial germ cells
PGZ	pioglitazone hydrochloride
PHA	phytohemagglutinin
PHS	periparturient hypogalactia syndrome
PIC	Pig Improvement Company
PL	pyridoxal
PLP	pyridoxal-5'-phosphate
PM	pectoralis major
PMP	pyridoxamine-5'-phosphate
PN	pyridoxol or pyridoxine

PNG   pyridoxine-5'-beta-D-glucoside
PNP   pyridoxine-5'-phosphate
PNS   peripheral nervous system
PPAR   peroxisome proliferators-activated receptor
PRV   porcine rotavirus
PSE   pale-soft and exudative
PTH   parathyroid hormone
PUFA   polyunsaturated fatty acids
RAR   retinoic acid receptors
RBP   retinol-binding protein
RIA   radioimmunoassays
RNA   ribonucleic acid
ROS   reactive oxygen species
RXR   retinoid X receptor
SCNT   somatic cell nuclear transfer
SD   standard deviation
SFA   saturated fatty acids
SOD   superoxide dismutase
SSP   shared socioeconomic pathways
SVS   single-voxel spectroscopy
TC   transcobalamin
TCA   tricarboxylic acid
TDP   thiamine diphosphate
THF   tetrahydrofolate
THFA   tetrahydrofolic acid
TMP   thiamine monophosphate
TPP   thiamine pyrophosphate
TTP   thiamine triphosphate
UPLC   ultra-performance liquid chromatography
USP   United States Pharmacopeia
UV   ultraviolet
UVB   ultraviolet B
VBP   vitamin D-binding protein
VDR   vitamin D receptor
VESD   vitamin E-selenium deficiency
VFI   voluntary feed intake
VLDL   very-low-density lipoproteins

Chapter 1

Contribution of vitamin nutrition to a more sustainable farming

ADDRESSING THE CHALLENGES OF TODAY AND TOMORROW

Today, well into the 21st century, the crucial issues relating to food production are changing. Key concepts such as productivity and efficiency continue to be of vital importance. Still, more and more, the emphasis is on the significance of terms such as sustainability, animal health and welfare, food quality from animal origin, and food waste.

Everything indicates that continuous development in the field of animal nutrition is becoming essential to meet current and future challenges. Challenges such as replacing antibiotics and coccidiostats, combatting higher incidences of more aggressive animal diseases, and responding to a growing focus on more sustainable farming, in which our industry has a critical role to play in shaping a better world in line with the Sustainable Development Goals of the United Nations. Specifically, our industry needs to:

- produce cost-effective animal protein production – for all
- provide high-quality food and feed – for a better life for all
- develop proper livelihoods – for the 30% of the world population working today in agriculture
- treat animals well until the end of their life – all of them
- eliminate the negative impact of food production – on us and the environment.

In parallel, as a player who aspires to be a leader in climate action, it is important for the feed industry to lead by example, constantly seeking to reduce carbon emissions and the environmental footprint of products and processes. That means closely managing absolute greenhouse gas (GHG) emissions and energy efficiency. A growing number of companies are setting long-term goals, validated by the Science Based Targets initiative (SBTi) aligned with the Paris Climate Agreement (COP 21) of 2015, to reach net-zero emissions before 2050. These are ambitious and long-term challenges in which the optimal use of vitamins in animal nutrition should be part of the solution.

COMMITMENT TO SUSTAINABILITY

Providing the right levels of high-quality and sustainably produced vitamins to feed mills, integrators, and farmers will help them improve animal health, well-being, and performance, while also protecting the environment, succeeding in a dynamic and ever-changing global market, and enhancing both profits and environmental sustainability. Optimizing the performance and improving the sustainability of feed additives and premixes plays an important role in reducing the environmental burden of animal protein production. Excipients such as rice hulls and calcium carbonate can make up to 50% of a premix composition, but little can be done to reduce their carbon footprint further. The critical products with potential to contribute to carbon footprint and environmental impact reductions in premixes are nutritional supplements such as vitamins. Reducing the impact of vitamins and other feed additive operations might enable feed mills and farmers to become more sustainable, reduce their risk profile, and potentially benefit from the value created from future carbon tax savings.

Some of the leading vitamin companies now share environmental impact information on their nutrient products, and their manufacturing processes and technology (including when possible comparisons to alternative products). This information is mainly based on life cycle assessment (LCA) standards.

Figure 1.1 shows an example of potential carbon dioxide savings available to a premixer or feed producer when selecting specific vitamin sources.

Carbon pricing – whether implemented as a tax or cap and trade system – seeks to reduce GHG emissions by putting a direct financial liability on industries and activities that are large GHG emitters. It is a policy intervention to encourage the reduction of harmful activities. The sustainability of mainstream animal production is increasingly questioned as demand rises. International bodies agree that animal protein production is one of the activities that need to reduce carbon emissions if we want to solve the climate crisis. The impact of agricultural and animal production processes can be reduced by greater use of sustainably produced nutritional solutions.

Additionally, governments may seek to impose low-carbon product standards, further environmental regulation, or tax schemes on animal protein production or products as an incentive to reduce emissions and steer consumer consumption. The groundwork for these interventions is already being laid. In Germany, value-added tax increases on meat and dairy products are being proposed. The New Zealand government has agreed to include farm-level emissions in its Emissions Trading Scheme by 2025, and the Dutch government has committed to studying 'fair meat prices' ahead of fiscal reforms in 2022.

The agricultural and animal protein product supply chain should prepare to minimize the risks posed by these changes or face severe financial penalties. The only way to do this is to significantly reduce animal production's impact on the climate and the environment. Equally, redesigning existing incentive systems (i.e., subsidies) and scaling up high-quality

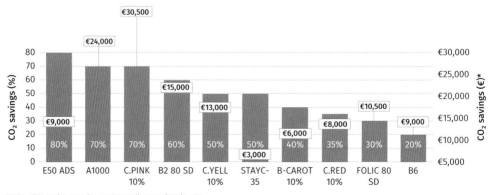

* Value of CO_2 saving assuming a carbon credit or tax of €50/ton CO_2

Figure 1.1 Carbon dioxide savings and potential value (carbon tax) per 10 t of feed additive: dsm-firmenich product *vs.* the main alternative (source: dsm-firmenich Animal Nutrition and Health, unpublished)

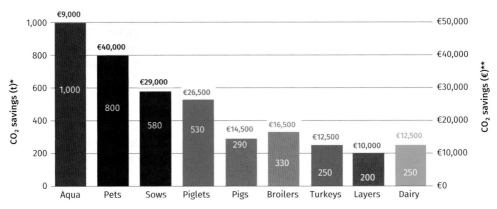

Figure 1.2 Carbon dioxide savings and potential value (carbon tax) of a more sustainable vitamin source for 100,000 t of feed produced (source: dsm-firmenich Animal Nutrition and Health, unpublished)

voluntary carbon credit systems to directly reward emission reductions can significantly accelerate the transition. This transition to a lower-carbon future for animal proteins can be facilitated by supplying nutritional ingredients, such as vitamins, with industry-leading performance to improve the efficiency of animal production systems while reducing the carbon footprint of these feed additives and those systems within which they are utilized. By considering the potential carbon dioxide savings when using certain sources of vitamins (as illustrated in Figure 1.1) and the average vitamin inclusion level in feed for different animal species, we can calculate the environmental benefits for those farmers interested in the sustainability of vitamins within their strategies to achieve more sustainable farming practices (Figure 1.2).

UPDATING THE NUTRITIONAL STANDARDS OF VITAMINS IN A CONSTANTLY EVOLVING WORLD

Vitamins play a decisive role in both human and animal nutrition. As organic catalysts present in small quantities in most foods, they are essential for the normal functioning of metabolic and physiological processes such as growth, development, health, and reproduction. The requirements for vitamins in animals are dynamic: they vary according to new genotypes, levels of yield, and production systems. Vitamin functions and requirements are becoming increasingly well known.

The concept of OVN Optimum Vitamin Nutrition® for animals is essential today. Its objective is to develop a new standard for vitamin supplementation in feed to improve animal health status and resilience to diseases and environmental stress, which will translate into better animal productivity and homogeneity. Moreover, the quality of food produced by those animals can be enhanced, improving human health and reducing food waste. The latter is critical in a global society in which, unfortunately, many people still do not have access to the correct quantity and quality of food. When we talk about optimum vitamin supplementation in the diet of animals, we refer to the provision of vitamin levels both over and above the established minimum requirements for avoiding deficiencies and adapted to the specific conditions of each animal species to achieve the objectives mentioned above.

Historically, the objective of the vitamin recommendations provided by various international scientific organs – such as the National Research Council (NRC USA), the Agriculture Research Council (ARC UK), and the National Research Institute for Agriculture, Food and Environment (Institut National de Recherche Agronomique et l'Environnement, INRAE, France) – was to prevent nutritional shortages or deficiencies. Some of the studies on which they are based are over 40 years old. We all know that the livestock industry today has little in common with the industry as it was at that time.

Table 1.1 shows the impressive performance improvement in the period 2016–2021 in the USA with a +1.3% annual increase in the number of live-born piglets per sow per year as well as a +1.5% per year increase in the number of weaned piglets per female and year. Close attention must be paid to the fact that this happens with a growing mortality in this 5 year period in pre-weaning piglets (+2.14%) as well as in sows and gilts (+48%!) with a culling rate higher than 46% in 2021.

Therefore, it is logical to assume that nutrition programs for farm animals, including vitamin supplements, need to be adjusted to be in line with improved animal management techniques and genetics. As indicated in Table 1.2, breeding companies performance goals for 2032 predict an additional annual improvement of +3.5% pigs/sow/year with a decrease in feed conversion of 1.4% per year.

Likewise, in recent times there have been important legislative changes around the world which limit the use of compounds such as antibiotics and growth promoters, substances that until recently had formed a regular part of animals' diets and the animal trials on which vitamins requirements were based. At the same time, many countries are developing new rules on animal welfare which, in the short to medium terms, will entail less "intensiveness" in the livestock industry, aiming to improve the animals' health and well-being. Meanwhile, our farmers need to be competitive enough regarding livestock productivity (weight gain, feed conversion ratio (FCR), the final weight of the animal, mortality, etc.) to survive strong international competition where free trade is a tangible reality. From the nutritional point of view, in these fast-changing circumstances, so different from those we have become accustomed to in recent years, it is essential to re-evaluate the vitamin requirements of animals with the aim of safely and efficiently producing healthy and nourishing food that meets consumer expectations, always under sustainable farming practices.

VITAMINS: ESSENTIAL MICRONUTRIENTS IN THE ANIMAL ORGANISM

Vitamins are unique and crucial nutrients in the diet of people and animals. They are important elements in the organism's vital functions: maintenance, growth, development, health, and reproduction. They also combine 2 characteristics.

- The daily requirement for each of the vitamins is very small, an aspect in which they differ from macronutrients such as carbohydrates, fats, and proteins.
- Vitamins are organic compounds, unlike other essential nutrients such as minerals (iron, iodine, zinc, etc.).

The discovery of vitamins and their function in preventing the classical deficiency diseases are milestones that stand among the most important achievements of the last century. Vitamins are particularly important because they allow optimum metabolism of other nutrients in the animal diet. In general, humans and animals need to derive them from their diet as they cannot produce the appropriate quantities by themselves. Vitamins are present in more

Table 1.1 Swine breeder and piglet performance summary (USA), 2016–2021

	2016 (416 farms)	2017 (340 farms)	2018 (375 farms)	2019 (365 farms)	2020 (305 farms)	2021 (292 farms)	% change 2021/ 2016	% change/year 2021/2016
Average pigs/litter (n)	13.95	14.22	14.43	14.71	14.99	15.2	8.96	1.8
Average born alive/litter (n)	12.58	12.71	12.9	13.2	13.46	13.54	7.63	1.5
Liveborn female/year (n)	27.74	28.53	28.62	29.74	29.38	29.54	6.49	1.3
Pre-weaning mortality (%)	15.37	14.69	14.85	14.55	15.42	15.7	2.14	0.4
Average age at weaning (day)	20.54	20.71	20.74	20.82	20.66	20.84	1.46	0.3
Average litter weaning weight (kg)	148.32	141	132.95	130.33	131.86	124.54	–16.03	–3.2
Pigs weaned per litter weaned (n)	11.03	11.16	11.23	11.48	11.77	11.85	7.43	1.5
Pigs weaned per female/year (n)	23.06	23.82	24.11	24.86	24.84	24.83	7.67	1.5
Sows and gilts death rate (%)	10	10.73	11.68	12.31	13.91	14.86	48.6	9.7
Culling rate (%)	44.51	42.31	45.06	45.69	48.79	46.29	3.99	0.8

Table 1.2 Swine productivity commercial performance 2022 and forecast for 2032 (PIC data, adapted from Saskia Bloemhof-Abma, AMVEC 2022, unpublished)

	2022	Annual change (unit)	Annual change (%)	2032
Pigs/sow/year (n)	33.5	1.2	3.5	45.5
Weaned/litter (n)	13.4	0.49	3.6	18.3
Weaned weight/sow year (kg)	201	8.5	4.2	286
Pigs weaned sow/lifetime (n)	60.9	2.2	3.6	82.9
Weight sold sow/year (kg)	4,058	198	4.9	6,039
% sold	93.2	0.38	0.4	97
Average market weight (kg)	130	1.1	0.9	141.4
Whole-system feed efficiency	2.5	0.036	1.4	2.14

than 30 reactions of the cellular metabolism and play, particularly in combination, a critical role in the Krebs or citric acid cycle (Figure 1.3).

Vitamins may only represent less than 1% of the cost of animal feed, but they are present in 100% of metabolic functions. This fact gives them the status of micronutrients of macro importance. Vitamins are found in minimal quantities in most feedstuffs. Their absence from the diet gives rise to specific deficiency diseases because of their significance for the normal functioning of the metabolism. While the need to provide additional vitamins in feed is unquestioned, the levels of supplementation needed to achieve an optimum economic return in field conditions are open to debate. As a general rule, the optimum economic supplementation level

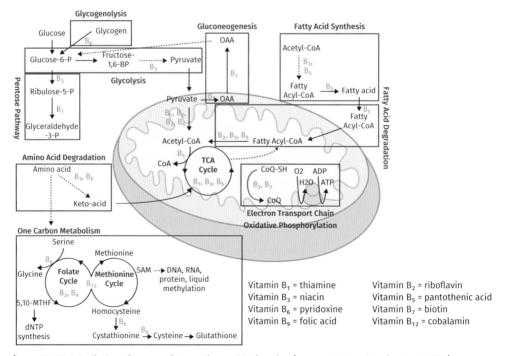

Vitamin B_1 = thiamine
Vitamin B_3 = niacin
Vitamin B_6 = pyridoxine
Vitamin B_9 = folic acid
Vitamin B_2 = riboflavin
Vitamin B_5 = pantothenic acid
Vitamin B_7 = biotin
Vitamin B_{12} = cobalamin

Figure 1.3 Metabolic functions and interactions of B vitamins (source: Godoy-Parejo et al., 2020)

is that which achieves the best index of growth, feed conversion, health status – including the immunocompetence – and which, in addition, provides the reserves appropriate for the organism. Nutrition is optimal when an animal efficiently utilizes the nutrients provided in the feed for survival, health, growth, and reproduction. Although all the nutrients, including proteins, fats, carbohydrates, minerals, and water, are essential for carrying out these vital functions, vitamins play a key role in basic functions, such as an appropriate immune response in animals.

As mentioned already, several factors – e.g., increased productivity driven by genetic improvement, intensive farming, and higher susceptibility to diseases – give rise to a growing vulnerability to vitamin deficiencies and a yield below the optimum. A great majority of nutritionists and investigators recognize that the minimum vitamin requirements needed to prevent clinical deficiency symptoms may not be sufficient to achieve an optimum state of health and yield. In Chapter 4 we will review the multiple metabolic functions specific to each of the vitamins in greater depth.

VITAMIN LEVELS IN ANIMAL DIET: THE NUTRITIONIST'S GREAT UNKNOWN QUANTITY

Establishing the vitamin supplementation level is something all nutritionists should concern themselves with. Economic cost and benefit must be a fundamental reason for revising and determining vitamin supplements in feed. The cost of supplementing feed with essential vitamins must be assessed considering the risk of suffering losses from deficiency symptoms and productive yields below the optimum. The great challenge for nutritionists is choosing a particular level from the numerous recommended tables. There are currently various sets of recommendations for vitamin levels in feed available from industries in the animal feed sector, research institutes, animal genetics companies, and vitamin manufacturers themselves (Table 1.3). In turn, fundamental differences can be seen in how the studies have been produced.

The ARC in the UK and the NRC in the USA periodically publish nutritional recommendations for different species, which generally constitute reference sources of limited value from the viewpoint of commercial feed formulation. The recommendations are based on establishment of the vitamin levels necessary to prevent clinical deficiency symptoms. NRC recommendations, for example, are revisions usually carried out based on studies done in experimental conditions that are perfectly controlled and therefore far removed from commercial conditions. For instance, they do not account for the stress factor, a frequent part of livestock rearing, which stress can drastically influence nutritional needs.

To make more efficient use of the NRC's vitamin recommendations, it is advisable to take into account the following considerations.

1   The indicated levels have been established to prevent deficiencies in the animal.
2   They do not include any kind of safety margin to prevent loss of vitamin activity stemming from usual feed storage conditions or feed processing. In other words, the recommended NRC levels must be those present in the animal's feed and when the animal is eating it.
3   They do not include safety margins for the eventuality that the animals are subjected to some sort of stress or subclinical disease.
4   They do not consider possible adverse environmental conditions, such as high temperatures, which may reduce the animal's food consumption.
5   In most cases, they are not specific to the new animal genotypes that are now being produced to optimize livestock farming.

Table 1.3 Vitamin inclusion levels (IU or mg/kg feed) for lactating sows according to 4 swine genetic companies

	Unit	Lactation					Breeder references
		Topigs, 2016	Hypor, 2017	PIC, 2021	Danbred, 2021	OVN™ (DSM, 2022)	
Vitamin A	IU	12,000	14,000	9,920	10,000	10,500–15,700	Lindeman et al. (2008): i.m. injections 250,000–500,000 IU gilts/sows, more born and weaned piglets
Vitamin D$_3$	IU	2,000	1,000	1,985	1,000	1,570–2,100	Industry practice and breeding companies recommendation
25OHD$_3$ (HyD®)	mg	–	–	–	–	0.05	Zhang et al. (2020): 0.05 mg improved immune and antioxidant response, bone strength, litter weight, piglet muscle development; Upadhaya et al., 2022 0.05 mg improved piglet performance
Vitamin E	mg	60	100	66	186.5	105–190	Industry practice and breeding companies recommendation; Wang et al. (2017): 250 mg better milk and sow colostrum, immune and antioxidant response, weaning weight, ADG
Vitamin K	mg	1	3	4.4	4.5	4.7–5.2	Industry practice and breeding companies recommendation
Vitamin B$_1$	mg	1–3	3	2.2	2.3	2.1–3	Audet et al. (2004): 20 mg improved sperm production and motility
Vitamin B$_2$	mg	5–7.5	7.5	10	5.7	6.3–10.5	Industry practice and breeding companies recommendation
Vitamin B$_6$	mg	2–4	4	3.3	3.4	3.7–5.7	Industry practice and breeding companies recommendation
Vitamin B$_{12}$	mg	0.030–0.1	0.01	0.037	0.03	0.032–0.052	Industry practice and breeding companies recommendation
Niacin	mg	15–100	100	44	23	40–100	Industry practice and breeding companies recommendation
D-pantothenic acid	mg	15–30	17.5	33	17	37–42	Wang et al. (2017): 100 mg milk production and quality, litter weight, ADG

Folic acid	mg	3–5	3	1.3	2	3.7–5.7	Wang et al. (2011) up to 100 mg/kg improved milk yield and quality, milk production efficiency and weaning performance; Matte and Girard (1999): 10 mg improved metabolism
Biotin	mg	0.3–0.5	0.5	0.22	0.5	0.52–0.84	Industry practice and breeding companies recommendation
Vitamin C	mg	–	–	–	Recommended	210–315	Lauridsen and Jensen (2005): 250 mg better immunity
Choline	mg	500–1,000	250	660	–	525–840	Industry practice and breeding companies recommendation
b-carotene	mg	–	–	–	–	300*	Industry practice and breeding companies recommendation

Note: For improved sow fertility the suggested level must be fed **per animal per day** immediately after weaning until confirmed conception.

Nutritionists usually consider stress and other economically important variables in their formulations. There is a great disparity between the levels of supplementation prescribed by the industry and those indicated by both NRC and ARC. While the industry continues to adjust vitamin supplementation in feed to achieve an optimum yield and state of health in the animal, the NRC has introduced only a few minor changes for most animal species in the last few decades. It is logical that the vitamin needs established some decades ago do not apply to today's animals. Most nutritionists agree on this aspect, and supplements of many vitamins are given at levels 5 or 10 times higher than those recommended by the NRC. The greatest differences are in the vitamins A, D_3, E, B_{12}, riboflavin and folic acid, while variations are lower with K_3, pantothenic acid, niacin and B_6.

BIOAVAILABILITY OF VITAMINS IN ANIMALS

Many feed materials used in animal nutrition contain variable quantities of vitamins. The amounts of vitamins available in the feed are limited by the nutritional requirements of these materials: hence, the vitamin levels in the diet obtained from feedstuffs tend to vary considerably. The overall content is low, and their presence in the feed does not guarantee their bioavailability or that the animal will indeed benefit from them.

It is well accepted that vitamin levels in feedstuffs vary significantly from one geographical region to another as well as depending on the time of harvesting and the climatic conditions at each harvest. Long storage periods and the use of preservatives, fungicides, etc., negatively affect the vitamin content. Some of the factors which most adversely affect the level of vitamins in the ingredients of feed are:

- origin of the harvest
- use of fertilizers
- genetic modifications which increase productive yield
- climate
- agricultural practices such as crop rotation
- harvesting conditions
- storage conditions and the use of preservatives
- bioavailability.

The real content of vitamins in feed is determined by complex chemical and microbiological analysis methods carried out in authorized laboratories, which provide the real value at a given time for a certain sample or batch of the respective ingredient. But given the great number of factors that affect the stability of vitamins (temperature, humidity, light, etc.), it would be necessary to undertake costly systematic analyses of the principal feed materials to be able to use those values reliably in the formulation – at minimum cost – of the feed, with the constant adaptation of the values to avoid possible variations of the desired level.

In many cases, vitamins derived from the feedstuffs are present in compound forms that are not bioavailable, hence, not available to be absorbed and participate in the animal's physiological and metabolic processes. At the practical level only the content of the vitamin in its free form is taken into account when calculating the total vitamin content in feed.

The term bioavailability refers exclusively to the vitamin content of an ingredient that is available to be absorbed and participate in the animal's different physiological and metabolic processes.

In commercial vitamin preparations, various substances protect them from harm during feed production processes and from aggressive environmental agents during storage. Therefore, it is essential to consider the bioavailability of these substances when determining the vitamin content of any feed ingredient.

In contrast, in nature, both in vegetable and animal products, substances can effectively destroy the vitamin activity or limit their bioavailability. These antinutritional agents can also be released by certain types of bacteria or fungi – e.g., mycotoxins – as by-products of their metabolic activity, as well as being present in the normal environment of the production facilities. Their most frequent mechanism of action consists of deactivating the free form of the vitamin or preventing its absorption. Among the most common scenarios are:

- deactivation of thiamine (B_1) by thiaminase
- formation of a compound with a metabolite, as in the case of the deactivation of biotin by avidin
- blocking the site of absorption or an independent chemical reaction, as in the case of dicumarol and vitamin K.

The addition of fats and oils as an energy source is common practice in the manufacture of feed. Attention should be paid to the total content of unsaturated fatty acids since they increase the likelihood that the oils and fats will become rancid. This would affect the absorption of fat-soluble vitamins such as A, E and D. Likewise, oxidation of the fats would also contribute to biotin deactivation.

STABILITY OF VITAMINS IN ANIMAL FEED

Diverse factors can affect the stability of substances as volatile as vitamins, whether in their pure commercial form, in vitamin-mineral premixes, or after the manufacture of compound feed and its subsequent storage. Some of these factors are connected with the catalytic activity of the molecules themselves, the handling of commercial forms and their premixes, the characteristics of the blend, the presence of various antagonistic substances, and the storage conditions. The vitamins present in primary materials are very susceptible to the adverse conditions mentioned above, and a heavy loss of vitamin activity is a common occurrence in these macroingredients. In contrast, the highest-quality commercial forms of vitamins are produced from industrial processes, which stabilize and protect the molecules of active substance during manufacture and storage, both in premixes and the feed.

Recent data from a European premix company shows large differences in vitamin A stability in pelleted feed at 90°C with 30, 60, or 120 seconds of holding time (up to 50%) when comparing 3 different vitamin A product forms (Figure 1.4).

However, it must again be emphasized that the stabilization of the vitamins must not compromise their bioavailability in the animal. Different methods are used to stabilize vitamins.

- Use of antioxidants – Antioxidants are included in the formulation of commercial vitamin products to prevent fat-soluble vitamins' oxidation and prolong these compounds' shelf life. In general, those commercial forms with an appropriate quantity of antioxidant substances have a longer effective shelf life. This period, during which vitamin content is guaranteed, will depend to a great extent on storage conditions. The ban of ethoxyquin in the EU and some other countries has put additional pressure on vitamin, premix, and feed manufacturers to adapt their product formulation technologies and

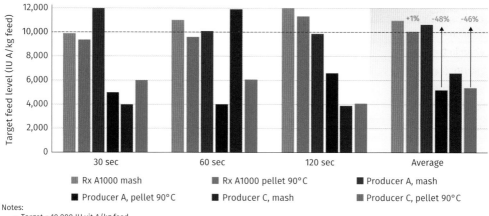

Notes:
- Target = 10,000 IU vit A/kg feed
- Premixes produced by large EU premixer with 3 different vitamin A products
- Feed corn/wheat/soy produced by Kolding Tech. Institute, Denmark
- Vitamin analyses carried out by LUFA Kiel lab, Germany (method REG(EC) 152/2009, IV, A)

Figure 1.4 Vitamin A stability in a 90°C pelleted feed at 30, 60, and 120 seconds holding time (source: elaboration by dsm-firmenich Animal Nutrition and Health based on data from a European premix company, 2020 unpublished)

sources to guarantee the right content of the active substance in the products they market.

- Mechanical methods – The process, in this case, covers the active substance with a stabilizing coat. This covering protects the vitamin molecule inside it from the adverse effect of aggressive external agents, such as the presence of oxygen, ultraviolet radiation, sunlight, humidity, different temperatures, etc. (Figure 1.5).

On a practical level, this method has proved highly effective in protecting these substances and, depending on their characteristics, can be combined with a process of spray drying, which provides a large number of active particles (all with the active form of the vitamin), which facilitates a subsequent homogenous mixture in the animal's food. This is particularly relevant for vitamins like biotin or B_{12} added into feed at very low levels (Figure 1.6).

At all events, the factors mentioned above affect vitamins in different ways:

- Vitamins A, D and carotenoids:
  - are prone to oxidation when exposed to air
  - are sensitive to oxidizing agents
  - isomerize in acid pH
  - are sensitive to prolonged heat
  - are sensitive to the catalytic effect of minerals.
- Vitamin E:
  - is prone to oxidation in the presence of air
  - is sensitive to alkaline mediums
  - the ester is relatively more stable.
- Vitamin K:
  - is sensitive to heat
  - is prone to oxidation in the presence of oxygen.

Additive	Temperature	Oxygen	Humidity	Light
Vitamin A	++	++	+	++
Vitamin D	+	++	+	+
25OHD$_3$ (calcifediol)	++	++	+	+
Vitamin E	0	+	0	+
Vitamin K$_3$	+	+	++	0
Vitamin B$_1$	+	+	+	0
Vitamin B$_2$	0	0	+	+
Vitamin B$_6$	++	0	+	+
Pantothenic acid	+	0	+	0
Nicotinates	0	0	0	0
Biotin	+	0	0	0
Folic acid	++	0	+	++
Vitamin C	++	++	++	0

++ Marked effect
+ Moderate effect
0 No effect

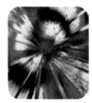
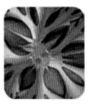

Figure 1.5 External factors influencing the stability of non-formulated vitamins (source: dsm-firmenich Animal Nutrition, dsm-firmenich Product Forms. Quality feed ingredients for more sustainable farming, 2022a)

Physical characteristics	ROVIMIX® Biotin 2% SD	ROVIMIX® Biotin HP 10% SD	Biotin 2% Triturate A
Soluble in water	yes	yes	no
Flowability (sec-100g)	medium	medium	low flow, tapping required
Average practical size (μm)	66	73	296
Mixability in feed, CV %	6%	5.7%	10.8%
Total particles per g product	>21 mio	>20 mio	>10 mio
Active particles per g product	100%	100%	2% (98% carrier)
Active Biotin particles per animal/day @ 0.2 mg biotin/Kg feed @ 10 g feed/day/chick	2000	400	20

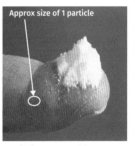

Approx size of 1 particle

*Biotin consumed by **1 sow** (or 20 birds, or 1 dog or 4 salmon) per year*

Figure 1.6 Confrontation of physical characteristics of biotin spray-dried form against biotin triturate (source: dsm-firmenich Animal Nutrition and Health, unpublished)

- Vitamin B$_1$ (thiamine):
  - is stable with low pH, loss of activity when pH of medium increases
  - is sensitive to the presence of oxygen and other oxidizing agents in neutral or alkaline solutions
  - splits on reacting with sulfites, with immediate separation at pH 6
  - is sensitive to metallic ions such as copper

- ○ the thiaminases present in some animal and vegetable products are known antagonists of this vitamin.
- Vitamin B_2 (riboflavin):
  - ○ is sensitive to light, especially in alkaline solutions
  - ○ is stable in acid and neutral mediums
  - ○ is unstable in alkaline solutions
  - ○ is sensitive to reducing agents.
- Vitamin B_6 (pyridoxine):
  - ○ is sensitive to light
  - ○ is relatively stable in acid solutions and dry mixes.
- Vitamin B_{12} (cobalamin):
  - ○ has little stability in alkaline or slightly acid mediums
  - ○ is sensitive to oxidizing reactions and reducing agents
  - ○ the metabolites of ascorbic acid, thiamine and nicotinamide accelerate this vitamin's decomposition
  - ○ is sensitive to light in very dilute solutions.
- Niacin:
  - ○ is relatively stable under practical conditions.
- Pantothenic acid:
  - ○ has little stability in alkaline or acid mediums
  - ○ is very hygroscopic, especially in its dl-calcium pantothenate form
  - ○ decomposes through hydrolysis, especially at low and high pH values.
- Biotin:
  - ○ is stable in air, acids and at neutral pH
  - ○ is slightly unstable in alkaline solutions.
- Folic acid:
  - ○ little stability in acid solutions below pH 5
  - ○ is sensitive to oxidizing reactions and reducing agents
  - ○ decomposes in sunlight
  - ○ little stability in hygroscopic environments and in the presence of minerals.
- Ascorbic acid:
  - ○ is sensitive to radiation
  - ○ oxidizes rapidly in all types of solution
  - ○ is catalyzed by metallic ions, such as copper and iron
  - ○ degrades rapidly at high temperatures.

OPTIMUM VITAMIN NUTRITION® IN PRACTICE

The objective of OVN™ is to supplement the diet of animals with the amounts of each vitamin considered most appropriate (the optimum) to optimize the state of health and the productivity of farm animals while guaranteeing the efficiency (desired effect at minimum cost) of the recommended levels. As already outlined, the levels of supplementation required for OVN™ are generally higher than those necessary to prevent clinical deficiency symptoms. These optimum supplementation levels should likewise compensate for the stress factors affecting the animal and its diet, thus guaranteeing these factors do not limit the animal's yield and health.

The following describes the concept of a cost-effective window for vitamin supplementation. This level must satisfy but not exceed the aim of achieving a state of optimum health and productivity. Below are some definitions of terms applicable to the OVN™ concept (Figure 1.7).

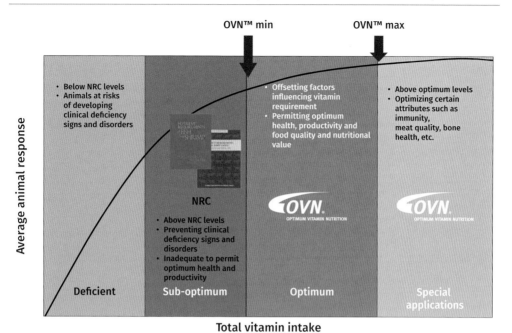

Figure 1.7 The OVN Optimum Vitamin Nutrition® concept (source: DSM Nutritional Products (2022b) OVN Optimum Vitamin Nutrition® guidelines)

1   **Average animal response** refers to productivity results – FCR, growth rate, reproductive status, level of immunity, the animal's health status, etc. – as a consequence of the ingestion of vitamins.

2   **Total vitamin intake** describes the total level of vitamins in the diet, feedstuff's bioavailable quantity, and supplementation.

3   **Deficient or minimum vitamin intake** refers to the vitamin level that puts the animal in danger of showing clinical deficiency symptoms and metabolic disorders and in which the level of vitamins falls short of the NRC supplementation level.

4   **A suboptimum intake** prevents the appearance of clinical deficiency symptoms. Its supplementation levels comply with or exceed the NRC's guidelines but are inadequate to permit an optimum state of health and productivity.

5   **An optimum intake** compensates for the negative factors which influence an animal's yield and therefore contributes to achieving an optimum state of well-being, health, and productivity.

6   **Special applications** are above optimum intake levels of vitamin supplementation for optimizing certain attributes such as immunity, meat quality, bone health, etc., or are directly used to produce vitamin-enriched meat or eggs. Concerning the safety of vitamins, only very large quantities (between 10 and 100 times the levels used in practice) of some vitamins such as A and D_3 in feed might occasionally cause some sort of disorder in animals. There is a growing demand for food with a greater added value, such as vitamin-rich eggs, meat, or milk, the occasional consumption of which contributes to a balanced human diet. This would necessitate such a higher vitamin content in the feed as described in item 6, the object of which would not only be to optimize the animal's productive response but to produce an "enriched" food with a greater added value for the final consumer.

There are various factors that affect an animal's vitamin requirements, and some may have an influence on the vitamin intake/supplement in the diet and its utilization. Among these factors are how we assess primary materials for their vitamin content, the process of harvesting these primary materials, as well as the processing and storage conditions of the ingredients in the feed, and the variability of the vitamins and their bioavailability.

Factors that influence vitamin requirements include the type and level of production, housing (especially whether or not animals are kept under cover), causes of stress, illnesses, other environmental conditions (for example, a warm environment or contamination by mycotoxins), vitamin antagonists, and the use of medicaments that may limit or even block the action of certain vitamins. Requirements will therefore vary depending on the severity of the above factors.

In summary, we can say that implementing a nutritional program with the most appropriate levels of all the vitamins in an animal's diet aims to offer the following benefits to the food chain.

1   **Optimum animal health and welfare** are a prerequisite for producing safe and healthy meat.
2   **Optimum productivity**, given better sanitary conditions and greater efficiency in animal farming within parameters such as FCR, final weight, weight gain, mortality, etc.
3   **Optimum food quality** offered to consumers provides them with whole food with balanced nutrient content.

1. Optimizing an animal's health and welfare

It is common knowledge that there is a close relationship between nutrition, health, and well-being. Improving the health and well-being of an animal nowadays constitutes a crucial aspect in the production of any food type of animal origin, so one essential objective regarding nutrition and management programs would be limiting the incidence of diseases and their debilitating effect on animals. Supplementing an animal's diet with optimum quantities of vitamins at times of greatest vulnerability to infection reduces the risk of contracting a disease.

Health and immunity

Vitamins, in sufficient quantities, play a fundamental role in the capacity of an animal's organism to develop an effective immune response to disease. Since the onset of an illness cannot be predicted, the immune system must be prepared to act before the disease attacks the organism.

Various studies have demonstrated a close relationship between low levels of vitamin E in the tissues and a decrease in immunocompetence (the immune system's response) long before any clinical signs of disease appear. Vitamins E and C are powerful antioxidants that protect cells from free radicals and other types of by-products harmful to an animal's metabolism.

The same studies proved that high levels of vitamin E in feed during the first 3 weeks produced:

• an improvement in the immune response to infection and vaccination
• improvement in batches affected by subclinical infections
• fewer relapses due to secondary infections.

More specifically, in pigs, the following effects were documented.

- Optimum levels of vitamin E in the diet significantly reduce mastitis-metritis-agalactia syndrome (MMA) in sows, as well as diarrhoeic processes in piglets.
- Providing an optimum level of vitamins in sow diets in gestation and lactation improves the nutritional value of colostrum and milk, augmenting the immune response and vitality of newborn piglets.
- Several studies have demonstrated beneficial effects in the health and development of recently weaned piglets which received a vitamin C supplement in their diet.

Reproduction
When breeding animals were fed diets rich in vitamin E during their periods of growth and production, the results were:

- an improved response in the production of antibodies during vaccination,
- a clear association between high levels of vitamin E in the liver and improved viability of newborn animals.

It is thus more effective to increase levels during embryogenesis, when the immune system is developing at a greater rate.

Welfare
Infections cause pain and suffering in animals. In general, farmers rearing businesses, and other people involved in their care have the greatest interest in them and will assume responsibility for ensuring satisfactory standards of well-being.

In the food sector, too, there are ever more retailers, wholesale distributors, and even fast food chains that have incorporated certain standards of animal welfare in their codes of best practice, with the aim of giving animals a healthy life which will contribute to guaranteeing healthier food to their consumers.

Optimum vitamin supplementation in an animal's diet will contribute to improving its welfare because:

- optimum vitamin levels contribute to improving the metabolism, nutrition and well-being of the animal
- improving immunity increases resistance to diseases
- some vitamins, such as biotin, contribute to reducing the incidence of digital dermatitis, thus preventing certain types of lameness, while others, such as vitamin C, alleviate the negative effects of stress on health and others like 25OHD$_3$, a more active D$_3$ metabolite, will improve bone health reducing lameness and other painful skeletal issues.

2. Optimizing productivity
In animals, advances have been achieved over decades through a process of natural genetic selection, accelerating growth rates and favoring certain genotypes to increase production of meat. These have changed the nutritional requirements of pigs because of improvements in the use of feed.

Data published recently have demonstrated that animals grow faster, under experimental and commercial conditions, when the supplementation of vitamins in the diet is increased

	Danish standard	OVN™	p value
Pens	101	102	
Pigs at trial start	1247	1259	
Pigs at trial end	1203	1231	
Start weight, kg	7.08	7.08	
Intermediate weight, kg	9.05	9.15	0.019
End weight, kg	32.59	32.82	0.101
Mortality, %	0.6	0.0	-
Dead and culled, %	3.3	2.1	0.056

	Danish standard	OVN™	p value
Feed intake, FUgp/pig/day	0.88	0.89	0.016c
Daily gain, g	551	566	<0.0001a
FCR, FUgp/kg gain	1.60	1.58	0.0003a
Production value	1.67	1.72	<0.0001a
Index	100	103.5	<0.0001a

Significant difference: a = 0.1% level; b = 1% level; c = 5% level
Least significant difference in indexes: 2,1 point

Vitamin levels (unit/kg feed)	Danish standard	OVN™
A, IU	6,250	15,000
D_3, IU	750	-
Hy-D, mg	-	0.050
C, mg	-	150
E, mg	150	150
B_1, mg	3	5
B_2, mg	6	15
B_6, mg	4.5	8
K_3, mg	4.8	6
Niacin, mg	30	55
Folicacid, mg	-	2.5
D-pantothenic acid, mg	15	45

Figure 1.8 Improving production value in feed for piglets (7–30 kg) with OVN (source: SEGES Denmark (Poulsen and Krogsdahl, 2018).

according to their requirements. From the economic viewpoint, the improvement in productive yield after optimizing the supply of vitamins in the feed gave rise to a significantly better cost to benefit ratio, in turn recompensing the farmer.

In the commercial sphere, stress represents a serious threat to achieving optimum yield. It reduces the intake of feed, necessitating an increase in the vitamin concentration to satisfy an animal's needs. Apart from anything else, stress alters an animal's metabolic needs, which will turn a nutritionally balanced meal into a diet with possible nutritional deficiencies. Recent investigations indicate that an appropriate supplement of vitamin C can alleviate the harmful effects of the stress caused by heat on the quality of semen, thus satisfying the nutritional requirements of boars in such demanding conditions.

Hyperprolific sows have been selected to produce large litters with the greatest possible number of healthy and viable piglets. Various studies have shown that optimum levels of biotin, folic acid, riboflavin, vitamin E, vitamin A and/or β-carotene in an animal's diet produce spectacular results in sow yield, such as a greater number of piglets born alive and weaned, and a decrease in the interval between weaning and covering.

SEGES (Agricultural Institute from Denmark) researchers researchers (Poulsen and Krogsdahl, 2018) carried out an ambitious trial with 2,500 piglets in 203 pens to evaluate the potential synergistic effect on the principal productive parameters of feeding animals with an optimum vitamin nutrition (OVN™) level.

OVN™ feed significantly improved all production traits and particularly increased by 3% the production value (growth value – feed cost) of piglets in the range 7–30 kg, compared to the Danish standards (Figure 1.8). No significant differences in health or mortality were observed although a numerical trend in favor of OVN™ was observed.

3. Optimizing the quality of food for the consumer

Meat is an essential source of protein in the human diet. A gradual and continuous increase in demand for processed meat products has been observed. This fact should be considered when defining the nutritional strategy that should be developed in animal diets. Lipid oxidation constitutes a problem for the conservation of meat since it can give rise to undesirable smells and flavors associated with rancidification, a fact of major relevance in processed meat particularly susceptible to this oxidation process.

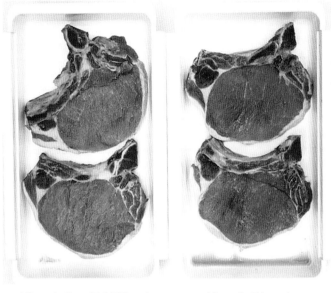

Vitamin E at OVN™ level   Vitamin E basal

Figure 1.9 Drip loss reduction in pork meat due to Vitamin E supplementation at OVN™ levels

Feeding animals a diet rich in unsaturated vegetable fats can considerably increase levels of monounsaturated and polyunsaturated fatty acids in meat. There is a series of polyunsaturated fatty acids that react with molecular oxygen until they are finally degraded to undesirable compounds with short chains, which cause the meat's organoleptic characteristics to deteriorate and, consequently, reduce acceptance of the meat by the consumer. Animals fed on diets with high levels of vitamin E can counteract this effect and so improve the final quality of the meat.

- by protecting the meat's lipids from oxidation and reducing the formation of undesirable smells and flavors
- by reducing the loss of exudates and improving the texture of the meat (Figure 1.9).

These findings have been confirmed by several researchers, such as Apple (2007) who concluded that 100, 200, or 400+ mg α-tocopherol/kg diet reduced pork drip losses by 10.1%, 30.5%, and 25.9%, respectively. More information is provided in Chapter 5.

OPTIMUM VITAMIN NUTRITION: A DYNAMIC PROCESS IN CONSTANT EVOLUTION

Optimum vitamin supplementation in an animal's diet, over and above the established minimum needs and adapted to the specific conditions of each animal species, will permit an improvement in the state of health and welfare of the animal, thus optimizing its productive potential at the same time as facilitating the production of high-quality food, which is nutritionally balanced.

These optimum levels are based on many studies carried out at university and industrial centers, on the requirements published by different associations and principal animal genetic producers and vitamin manufacturers, and on the continuous experience of the worldwide agricultural industry. These optimum levels guarantee farmers minimum impact of negative nutritional factors, such as variability in the natural content of feed ingredients, the existence of antinutritional factors, and different levels of stress.

Although the vitamin recommendations for feed also attempt to compensate for the majority of the factors mentioned that influence an animal's vitamin needs, in extreme conditions where the processing of premix or feed is very aggressive (e.g., the inclusion of trace minerals or choline chloride, the use of feed expanders or extruded feed) supplementary quantities of some vitamins may be necessary. The negative effect on the stability of vitamins can be reduced by using high-quality commercial vitamin forms where their covering and the bioavailability of the active substance they contain are key elements to be taken into account. And all this is considering the environmental impact of how vitamins are manufactured.

Chapter 5 reviews the impact of vitamins in swine nutrition as reported in the international research literature. These studies have endeavored to emphasize the beneficial effects that optimum vitamin levels have on an animal, both on the level of health and welfare and concerning productivity. The chapters also identify aspects on which there is currently insufficient information available, intending to address these gaps in future research and editions of this book.

Given that animal farming is a dynamic process levels of vitamin supplementation need to be reassessed more frequently – this is a change demanded, in the majority of cases, by society, for economic reasons related to the productivity of animals and by farming systems.

The concept of OVN™ always considers the costs of vitamin supplementation in an animal's diet (in many cases, less than 1% of the cost of feed, even less if we consider the impact on meat production cost) against the risk of suffering losses through vitamin deficiencies and through working with yield indices below the optimum.

Nutritionists who follow the recommended guidelines based on the OVN™ concept ensure that vitamins enable the development of an animal's genetic potential and contribute to a more sustainable animal farming.

Chapter 2

A brief history of vitamins

Vitamins were mostly discovered in the 20th century and were once regarded as "unknown growth factors" (Eggersdorfer *et al.*, 2012). The first phase of developing the concept of vitamins began many centuries ago and gradually led to the recognition that night blindness, xerophthalmia, scurvy, beriberi, and rickets are dietary diseases. These diseases had long plagued humankind and were mentioned in the earliest written records. Records of medical science from antiquity attest that researchers had already linked certain foods and diseases or infirmities, postulating that food constituents played a causal or a preventive role. These are considered the nebulous beginnings of essential nutrients (Eggersdorfer *et al.*, 2012).

Beriberi is probably the earliest documented deficiency disorder being recognized in China as early as 2697 BC. By 1500 BC, scurvy, night blindness, and xerophthalmia were described in Egyptian writings. Two books of the Bible contain accounts that point to vitamin A deficiency (McDowell, 2006). Jeremiah 14:6 states: "and the asses did stand in high places, their eyes did fail because there was no grass." In addition, the Bible mentions that fish bile was used to cure a blind man named Tobias.

In 400 BC, the Greek physician Hippocrates, known as the Father of Medicine, reported using raw ox liver dipped in honey to prevent night blindness. He also described soldiers afflicted with scurvy. Scurvy took a heavy toll on the Crusades of the Middles Ages because the soldiers traveled far from home, and their diet was deficient in vitamin C. During the long sea voyages between 1492 and 1600, scurvy posed a serious threat to the health of sailors and undermined world exploration. For example, while sailing worldwide, Magellan lost 80% of his crew to the disease. Vasco de Gama, another great explorer, lost 60% of his 160-man crew while mapping the coast of Africa. In 1536, during Jacques Cartier's expedition to Canada, 107 out of 110 men became sick with scurvy. However, the journey was saved when the Indians shared their knowledge of the curative value of pine needles and bark. In 1593, British Admiral Richard Hawkins wrote: "I have seen some 10,000 seamen die of scurvy; some sailors tried treating themselves by trimming the rotting, putrid black flesh from their gums and washing their teeth in urine."

In 1747, James Lind, a British naval surgeon, carried out the first controlled clinical experiment aboard a ship to find a cure for scurvy. Twelve patients with scurvy were divided into 6 treatment groups. Two sailors received a dietary supplement of oranges and lemons, while the other treatment groups were given nutmeg, garlic, vinegar, cider, and seawater, respectively. The 2 men who had received the citrus fruit were cured of scurvy. Where did Lind get the idea that scurvy was related to nutrition? He had been told a story of an English sailor with scurvy who was left to die on a lonely island with no food. Feeling hungry, the man nibbled a few blades of beach grass. The next day, he felt stronger and ate some more grass. After a few weeks on this "diet," he was completely well.

In the second half of the 19th century, there was another disease that killed thousands of sailors in the Japanese navy. In 1880, the Japanese navy recorded almost 5,000 deaths from beriberi in 3 years. Patients with beriberi became weak and eventually partially paralyzed, lost weight, and died. Doctors tried to find the germ that was causing beriberi. Finally, they listened to Japanese naval surgeon Kamekiro Takaki, who believed the sailors' diet was causing beriberi. Takaki noted a 60% incidence of beriberi on a ship returning from a 1-year voyage during which the sailors' diet had been mostly polished rice and some fish. He sent out a second ship under the same conditions but substituted barley, meat, milk, and fresh vegetables for some of the rice. The dietary change eliminated beriberi, but Takaki incorrectly concluded that the additional protein prevented the beriberi. Regardless, the Japanese knew they could avoid beriberi by not relying on polished rice as the only dietary staple.

Before the beginning of the 20th century, there was a growing body of evidence that nutritional factors, later known as vitamins, were implicated in certain diseases. Louis Pasteur was the chief opponent of the "vitamin theory," which held that certain illnesses resulted from a shortage of specific nutrients in foods. Pasteur believed there were only 3 classes of organic nutrients: carbohydrates, fats, and proteins. His research showed that microorganisms caused disease and made scientists with medical training reluctant to believe the vitamin theory. It has been said that the immensely successful "germ theory" of disease, coupled with toxin theory and the successful use of antisepsis and vaccination, convinced scientists of the day that only a positive agent could cause disease (Guggenheim, 1995). Until the mid-1930s, most US doctors still believed that pellagra was an infectious disease (McDowell, 2006).

VITAMIN THEORY TAKES SHAPE

Beginning in the mid-1850s, German scientists were recognized as leaders in the field of nutrition. In the late 1800s, Professor C. von Bunge, who worked at the German university in Dorpat, Estonia, and then at Basel, Switzerland, had some graduate students conduct experiments with purified diets for small animals (Wolf and Carpenter, 1997). In 1881, N. Lunin, a Russian student studying in von Bunge's laboratory, observed that some mice died after 16 to 36 days when fed a diet composed solely of purified fat, protein, carbohydrate, salts, and water. Lunin suggested that natural foods such as milk contain small quantities of "unknown substances essential to life."

Many great scientific advances have come about due to chance observations made by men and women of inspiration. In 1896, Dutch physician and bacteriologist Christiaan Eijkman made a historic finding concerning a cure for beriberi. Eijkman was researching in Indonesia to identify the causal pathogen of beriberi. He astutely observed that a polyneuritis condition in chickens produced clinical signs similar to those in humans with beriberi. This chance discovery was made when a new head cook at the hospital discontinued the supply of "military" rice (polished rice), and the chickens fed the wholegrain "civilian" rice recovered from the polyneuritis. After extensive experimentation, Eijkman proved that both polyneuritis and beriberi were caused by eating polished white rice. Both afflictions could be prevented or cured when the outer portions of the rice grain (e.g., rice bran) were consumed. Thus, Eijkman became the first to produce a vitamin deficiency disease in an experimental animal. He also noted that prisoners with beriberi eating polished rice tended to get well when fed a less milled product. In 1901, Grijns, one of Eijkman's colleagues in Indonesia, was the first to come up with a correct interpretation of the connection between the excessive consumption of polished rice and the etiology of beriberi. He concluded that rice contained "an essential nutrient" found in the grain's outer layers.

In 1902, a Norwegian scientist named Holst conducted some experiments on "ship-beriberi" (scurvy) using poultry, but the experiments failed. In 1907, Holst and Frolich produced experimental scurvy in guinea pigs. Later it was learned that poultry could synthesize vitamin C while guinea pigs could not.

In 1906, Frederick Hopkins, working with rats in England, reported that "no animal can live upon a mixture of pure protein, fat, and carbohydrate and even when the necessary inorganic material is supplied, the animal cannot flourish." Hopkins found that small amounts of milk added to purified diets allowed rats to live and thrive. He suggested that unknown nutrients were essential for animal life, calling them "accessory food factors." Hopkins' experiments were like those of Lunin; however, they were more in depth. He played an important role by recording his views in memorable terms that received wide recognition (McCollum, 1957). Hopkins also expressed that various disorders were caused by diets deficient in unidentified nutrients (e.g., scurvy and rickets). He was responsible for opening a new field of discovery that largely depended on experimental rats.

In 1907, Elmer McCollum (Figure 2.1) arrived in Wisconsin to work on a project to determine why cows fed wheat or oats (versus yellow corn) gave birth to blind or dead calves. The answer was found to be that wheat and oats lacked the vitamin A precursor carotene. Between 1913 and 1915, McCollum and Davis discovered 2 growth factors for rats, "fat-soluble A" and "water-soluble B." By 1922, McCollum had identified vitamin D as a substance independent of vitamin A. He bubbled oxygen through cod liver oil to destroy its vitamin A; the treated oil remained effective against rickets but not against xeropthalmia. Thus, "fat-soluble vitamin A" had to be 2 vitamins, not just one (DeLuca, 2014).

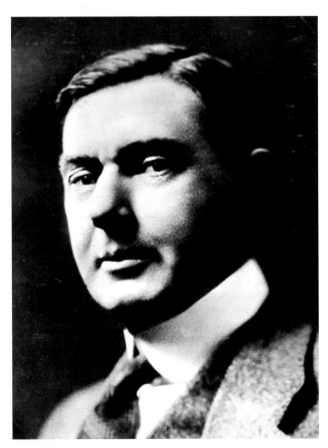

Figure 2.1 Elmer McCollum (source: Roche Historical Archive)

In 1912, Casimir Funk (Figure 2.2), a Polish biochemist working at the Lister Institute in London, proposed the "vitamin theory" (Funk and Dubin, 1922). He had reviewed the literature and made the important conclusion that beriberi could be prevented or cured by a protective factor present in natural food, which he successfully isolated from rice by-products. What he had isolated was named "beriberi vitamin" in 1912. This term "vitamin" denoted that the substance was vital to life and chemically an amine (vital + amine). In 1912, Funk proposed the theory that other "deficiency diseases" in addition to beriberi were caused by a lack of these essential substances, namely scurvy, rickets, sprue, and pellagra. He was the first to suggest that pellagra was a nutrient deficiency disease.

In 1923, Evans and Bishop discovered that vitamin E deficiency caused reproductive failure in rats. Steenbock (1924) showed that irradiation of foods as well as animals with ultraviolet light produced vitamin D. In 1928, Szent-Györgyi isolated hexuronic acid (later renamed "ascorbic acid") from foods such as orange juice. One year later, Moore proved that the animal body converts carotene to vitamin A. This experiment involved feeding 1 group of rats carotene and finding higher levels of vitamin A in their livers compared to controls. By 1928, Joseph Goldberger and Conrad Elvehjem had shown that vitamin B was more than one substance. After the "vitamin" was heated, it was no longer effective in preventing beriberi (B_1), but it was still good for rat growth (B_2). The 1930s and 1940s were the golden age of vitamin research.

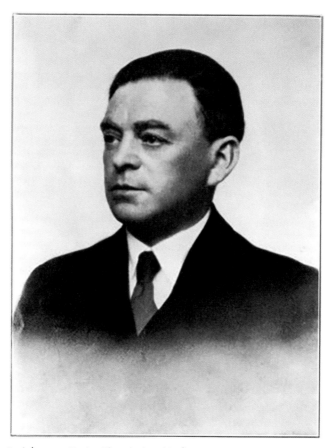

Figure 2.2 Casimir Funk (source: Roche Historical Archive)

During this period, the traditional approach was to (1) study the effects of a deficient diet, (2) find a food source that prevents the deficiency, and (3) gradually concentrate the nutrient (vitamin) in a food and test potency. Laboratory animals were used in these procedures.

Henrick Dam of Denmark discovered vitamin K in 1929 when he noted hemorrhages in chicks fed a fat-free diet. Ironically 1 year earlier, Herman Almquist, working in the United States, had discovered both forms of the vitamin (K_1 and K_2) in studies with chicks. Unfortunately, university administrators delayed the review of his paper, and when it was finally submitted to the journal *Science*, it was rejected. Therefore, only Henrick Dam received a Nobel prize for discovering vitamin K.

Vitamin B_{12} was the last traditional vitamin to be identified, in 1948. Shortly after that, it was discovered that cobalt was an essential component of the vitamin. Simple monogastric animals were found to require the vitamin, whereas ruminants and other species with large microbial populations (e.g., horses) require dietary cobalt rather than vitamin B_{12}.

Compared with the situation for night blindness, xeropthalmia, beriberi, scurvy, and rickets, there were no records from the ancient past of the disease of pellagra. The disease was caused by niacin deficiency in humans, a problem prevalent mainly in cultures where corn (maize) was a key dietary staple (Harris, 1919). Columbus took corn to Spain from America. Pellagra was not recognized until 1735, when Gaspar Casal, physician to King Philip V of Spain, identified it among peasants in northern Spain. The local people called it "mal de la rosa," and Casal associated the disease with poverty and spoiled corn. The popularity of corn spread eastward from Spain to southern France, Italy, Russia, and Egypt, and so did pellagra. James Woods Babcock of Columbia, South Carolina, who identified pellagra in the United States by establishing a link with the disease in Italy, studied the case records of the South Carolina State Hospital and concluded that the disease condition had occurred there as early as 1828. Most cases occurred in low-income groups, whose diet was limited to inexpensive foodstuffs. Diets characteristically associated with the disease were the 3 Ms, specifically meal (corn), meat (backfat), and molasses.

The word pellagra means rough skin, which relates to dermatitis. Other descriptive names for the condition were "mal de sol" (illness of the sun) and "corn bread fever." In the early 1900s in the United States, particularly in the South, it was common for 20,000 deaths to occur annually from pellagra. It was estimated that there were at least 35 cases of the disease for every death due to pellagra. Even as late as 1941, 5 years after the cause of pellagra was known, 2,000 deaths were still attributed to the disease. The clinical signs and mortality associated with pellagra are the 4 Ds: dermatitis (of areas exposed to the sun), diarrhea, dementia (mental problems), and death. Several mental institutions in the United States, Europe, and Egypt were primarily devoted to caring for pellagra sufferers or pellagrins.

In 1914, Joseph Goldberger, a bacteriologist with the US Public Health Service, was assigned to identify the cause of pellagra. His studies observed that the disease was associated with poor diet and poverty and that well-fed persons did not contract the disease (Carpenter, 1981). The therapeutic value of good diets was demonstrated in orphanages, prisons, and mental institutions in South Carolina, Georgia, and Mississippi. Goldberger, his wife, and 14 volunteers constituted a "filth squad" who ingested and injected various biological materials and excreta from pellagrins to prove that pellagra was not an infectious disease. These extreme measures did not result in pellagra, thus demonstrating the non-infectious nature of the disease. At the time, researchers and physicians did not want to believe that pellagra resulted from poor nutrition. They sought to link it to an infection in keeping with the popular "germ theory" of diseases (McDowell, 2006). An important step toward isolating the preventive factor for pellagra involved the discovery of a suitable laboratory animal for testing its potency in various concentrated preparations. It was found that a pellagra-like disease (black tongue) could be produced in dogs. Elvehjem and his colleagues (1974) isolated nicotinamide from the liver and identified it as the factor that could cure black tongue in dogs. Reports of niacin's dramatic therapeutic effects in human pellagra cases quickly followed from several clinics.

In 1824, James Scarth Combe first discovered fatal anemia (pernicious anemia) and suggested it was linked to a digestive disorder. George R. Minot and William Murphy reported in 1926 that large amounts of the raw liver would alleviate the symptoms of pernicious anemia. In 1948, E. L. Rickes and his colleagues in the United States and E. Lester Smith in England isolated vitamin B_{12} and identified it as the anti-pernicious anemia factor (McDowell, 2006). Much earlier, in 1929, W. B. Castle had shown that pernicious anemia resulted from the interaction between a dietary factor (extrinsic) and a mucoprotein substance produced by the stomach (intrinsic factor). Castle used an unusual but effective method to relieve the symptoms of pernicious anemia patients. He ate some beef, and after allowing enough time for the meat to mix with gastric juices, he regurgitated the food and mixed his vomit with the patients' food. With this treatment, the patients recovered because they received both the extrinsic (vitamin B_{12}) and intrinsic (a mucoprotein) factors from Castle's incompletely digested beef meal.

The importance of vitamins was well accepted in the first 3 decades of the 20th century. Table 2.1 provides an overview of the chronological evolution of the discovery, isolation, and assignment of the chemical structure and first production of the individual vitamins. The development of synthetic production of vitamins started in 1933 with ascorbic acid/vitamin C from Merck (Cebion®), which was isolated from plant leaves. However, the first industrial-scale chemical production of vitamin C was achieved by F. Hoffmann-La Roche in 1934 based on a combined fermentation and chemical process developed by Tadeus Reichstein. These scientific innovations were recognized with 12 Nobel Prizes and 20 laureates (Table 2.2). A complete description of the history of discovery, first syntheses, and current industrial processes used for producing each vitamin was described by Eggersdorfer *et al.* (2012) and McDowell (2013).

Table 2.1 Discovery, isolation, structural elucidation, and synthesis of vitamins (source: Eggersdorfer *et al.*, 2012)

Vitamin	Discovery	Isolation	Structural elucidation	First synthesis
Vitamin A	1916	1931	1931	1947
Vitamin D	1918	1932	1936	1959
Vitamin E	1922	1936	1938	1938
Vitamin B_1	1912	1926	1936	1936
Vitamin B_2	1920	1933	1935	1935
Niacin	1936	1936	1937	1837/1940*
Pantothenic acid	1931	1938	1940	1940
Vitamin B_6	1934	1938	1938	1939
Biotin	1931	1935	1942	1943
Folic acid	1941	1941	1946	1946
Vitamin B_{12}	1926	1948	1956	1972
Vitamin C	1912	1928	1933	1933

Note: *1837: synthesis of niacin used in photography before discovering its nutritional function; 1940: nicotinamide.

Table 2.2 Nobel prizes for vitamin research (source: Eggersdorfer *et al.*, 2012)

Year	Recipient	Field	Citation
1928	Adolf Windaus	Chemistry	Research into the constitution of steroids and connection with vitamins
1929	Christiaan Eijkman	Medicine, Physiology	Discovery of antineuritic vitamins
	Sir Frederick G. Hopkins	Medicine, Physiology	Discovery of growth-stimulating vitamin
1934	George R. Minot, William P. Murphy, George H. Whipple	Medicine, Physiology	Discoveries concerning liver therapy against anemias
1937	Sir Walter N. Haworth	Chemistry	Research into the constitution of carbohydrates and vitamin C
	Paul Karrer	Chemistry	Research into the constitution of carotenoids, flavins, and vitamins A and B_2
	Albert Szent-Györgyi	Medicine, Physiology	Discoveries in connection with biological combustion processes, with special reference to vitamin C and catalysis of fumaric acid
1938	Richard Kuhn	Chemistry	Work on carotenoids and vitamins
1943	Carl Peter Henrik Dam	Medicine, Physiology	Discovery of vitamin K
	Edward A. Doisy	Medicine, Physiology	Discovery of chemical nature of vitamin K
1953	Fritz A. Lipmann	Medicine, Physiology	Discovery of coenzyme A and its importance for intermediary metabolism
1964	Konrad E. Bloch, Feodor Lynen	Medicine, Physiology	Discoveries concerning mechanism and regulation of cholesterol and fatty acid metabolism
	Dorothy C. Hodgkin	Chemistry	Structural determination of vitamin B_{12}
1967	Ragnar A. Granit	Medicine, Physiology	Research which illuminated electrical properties of vision by studying wavelength discrimination by eye
	Halden K. Hartine	Medicine, Physiology	Research on mechanisms of sight
	George Wald	Medicine, Physiology	Research on chemical processes that allow pigments in the eye retina to convert light into vision

Vitamins became available in the following years through chemical synthesis, fermentation, or extraction from natural materials (Table 2.1). From 1930 to 1950, there was mainly small-scale production in several countries to reach local markets, but, as demand grew, larger plants became more common from 1950 to 1970. Still, it was not until 1987 that all the vitamins were accessible by industrial processes. Nowadays, chemical synthesis is still the dominant method of industrial production.

The large companies Hoffmann-La Roche (Figure 2.3) and BASF were market leaders, but numerous European and Japanese pharmaceutical companies produced and sold vitamins.

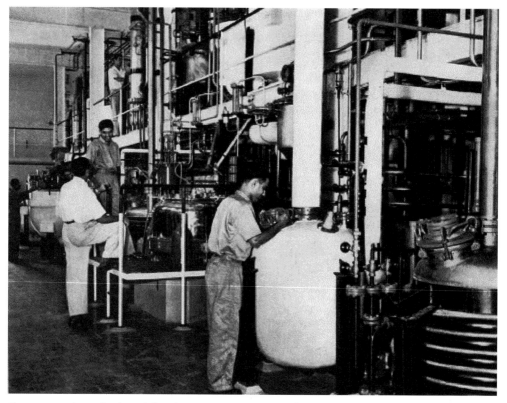

Figure 2.3 Early production of vitamin A at Roche Nutley, USA (source: Roche Historical Archive).

Between 1970 and 1990, production plants became even bigger and with global reach, and since 2000 China has become a larger producer. Fermentation technology started to gain importance, especially for vitamin B_{12} and B_2. New technologies have been emerging in the past 10 years, such as the overexpression of vitamins in plants by either using traditional breeding or genetically modified plants (Eggersdorfer *et al.*, 2012).

Chapter 3

Introduction to vitamins

VITAMIN DEFINITION AND CLASSIFICATION

A vitamin is an organic substance that is:

- a component of a natural compound but distinct from other nutrients such as carbohydrates, fats, proteins, minerals, and water
- present in most foods in a minute amount
- essential for normal metabolism in physiological functions such as growth, development, maintenance, and reproduction
- a cause of a specific deficiency disease or associated with a syndrome if absent from the diet or if improperly absorbed or utilized
- not (with very few exceptions) synthesized by the host in sufficient amounts to meet physiological demands and therefore must be obtained from the diet.

Vitamins are differentiated from trace elements, also present in the diet in small quantities, by their organic nature. Some vitamins deviate from the preceding definition in that they do not always need to be constituents of food (McDowell, 2000a; Combs and McClung, 2022). For example, companion animals and farm livestock can synthesize vitamin C (ascorbic acid) but not fish. Nevertheless, deficiencies have been reported in some species that synthesize vitamin C, and supplementation with this vitamin has been shown to have value for particular diseases or stress conditions (Feng *et al.*, 2018), toxicoses (Shi *et al.*, 2017; Su *et al.*, 2018), and to restore productivity or maximize performance (Solyanik *et al.*, 2021).

Likewise, for most species, niacin can be synthesized from the amino acid tryptophan (but not by the cat or fish species studied to date) and choline from the amino acid methionine. Nevertheless, dietary supplementation with niacin and choline is necessary for animal farming. Finally, vitamin D can also be synthesized in the skin under UV stimulation. Still, the diets of all farm animals are supplemented with this vitamin to provide the required quantity primarily for proper bone development.

The quantities of vitamins required are tiny, but they are essential for tissue integrity, normal development or physiological functions, and health maintenance. Their physiological and metabolic roles vary and are of great importance. They are involved in many biochemical reactions and participate in nutrient metabolism derived from the digestion of carbohydrates, lipids, and proteins.

A single vitamin may have several different functions, and many interactions between them are known. Classically, vitamins have been divided into 2 groups based on their solubilities in fat solvents or water. Thus, fat-soluble vitamins include A, D, E, and K, while B complex vitamins, vitamin C, and choline are water-soluble.

Fat-soluble vitamins are found in feedstuffs in association with lipids. The fat-soluble vitamins are absorbed along with dietary fats, apparently by mechanisms like those involved in fat absorption. The list of the 13 recognized vitamins with main functions and deficiency symptoms are listed in Table 3.1.

Conditions favorable to fat absorption, such as adequate bile flow and good micelle formation, also favor the absorption of fat-soluble vitamins (Harrison, 2012; Gonçalves et al., 2015; Maurya and Aggarwal, 2017). Water-soluble vitamins are not associated with fats, and alterations in fat absorption do not affect their absorption. The fat-soluble vitamins A, D, and, to a lesser extent, E are generally stored in appreciable amounts in the animal body (Rigotti, 2007). Water-soluble vitamins are not stored, and excesses are rapidly excreted, except for vitamin B_{12} and perhaps biotin. Table 3.2 lists the solubility characteristics of 16 vitamins classified as either fat or water-soluble.

Vitamins can seldom be regarded as nutrients in isolation because they display various interactions with each other and other nutrients (Calderón-Ospina and Nava-Mesa, 2020; Dalto and da Silva, 2020; Zhou et al., 2021b). For example, the fat-soluble vitamins compete for intestinal absorption, so an excess of one may cause deficiencies in the others (Hoppe et al., 1992; Gonçalves et al., 2015; Stacchiotti et al., 2021). The vitamins of the B group are regulators of intermediary metabolism. Some metabolic processes are interdependent: for example, choline, B_{12}, and folic acid interact in the methyl groups' metabolism, so a lack of one of them increases the requirement for the others (Matte et al., 2006). The same happens between B_{12} and pantothenic acid (Rucker and Bauerly, 2013). It may also occur that an excess of one vitamin induces a deficiency of others. Thus, biotin status deteriorates if the diet is supplemented with high levels of choline and other vitamins of the B group (Kopinski and Leibhilz, 1989; Kopinski et al., 1989a,b,c,d). High choline levels may similarly affect other vitamins during feed storage.

Vitamins are also known to interact in diverse ways with other nutrients, such as amino acids. For example, there is genetic variability in the conversion of tryptophan to nicotinic acid (Le Floc'h et al., 2017), so their requirements differ between pig breeds. Both methionine and choline can be a source of methyl groups, which are needed to synthesize both, and this relationship is of commercial importance because supplementation entails economic cost. Biotin, folic acid, and B_6 play a part in metabolic interconversions of amino acids, so their requirement increases if protein levels are high (Matte et al., 1997b, 2001, 2005). The same applies to those vitamins involved in the metabolism of carbohydrates (biotin, B_1), the requirements for which are higher with low-fat diets (Camporeale and Zempleni, 2006; Mock, 2013). Finally, there are also interactions between minerals and vitamins. The best-documented example is selenium and vitamin E (Sun et al., 2019). All these aspects will be treated in more detail in Chapters 4 and 5.

These interactions make it somewhat difficult to estimate the requirements for each vitamin precisely, and it is probably more appropriate to focus on the problem generally. Chapter 5 provides a detailed explanation of the situation. The classic evaluation of the dose-response curve, so widely used to estimate the requirements of other nutrients, is not an appropriate technique for vitamins, as their cost is generally low concerning the value of the response value and the potential consequences of inadequate levels. For these reasons, the usual practice is to define vitamin requirements by considering the maximum response obtained with the chosen evaluation criteria, traditionally weight gain or growth and FCR. However, growth is not a specific response: it may be affected by other factors associated with the feed (palatability, particle size, levels of other nutrients, etc.). This issue may explain the variability in response levels between studies on a particular vitamin, even if they are almost concurrent.

According to the extensive literature presented in this book, it would not be possible to establish precise mathematical relationships regarding vitamin requirements until all their interactions are known in detail, taking at the same time into account many factors like various diet types and changes in physical composition.

VITAMIN CONVERSION FACTORS

The recommended vitamin supplementation level is given in vitamin activity. Commercial products indicate the amount of vitamin activity: e.g., for vitamin A 1,000,000 international units (IU) per gram or for vitamin B_6 99% pyridoxine hydrochloride. In the latter case an additional correction must be applied when supplementing 1 mg vitamin B_6 (pyridoxine) it is advised 1.215 mg pyridoxine hydrochloride is required. Table 3.3 provides the conversion factors, the product forms, and their content. In some countries regulatory authorities may have stated different rules for vitamin declaration in premixes and feeds. It could be, for example, the case for vitamin E: usually the declaration is in milligrams whereas in some countries the declaration could be required in IUs. However, as indicated in the table, the international standard is that 1 mg all-rac-α-tocopheryl acetate is equal to 1 IU.

VITAMINS IN FEEDSTUFFS

The vitamin content of feedstuffs is highly variable, and current values have not been completely evaluated recently. There are severe limitations in relying on average tabular values of vitamins in feedstuffs. As an example, the vitamin E content of 42 varieties of corn varied from 11.1 to 36.4 mg/kg, a 3.3-fold difference (McDowell and Ward, 2008; Chen, Wang, Li *et al.*, 2019; Combs and McClung, 2022). As a reference, the average vitamin levels in some common feed ingredients are presented in Table 3.4 (Chen, Han, Guan *et al.*, 2019). Some sources of information (Combs and McClung, 2022) still rely on data published in the 1980s or before.

Generally, these average values are based on a limited number of assays published more than 50 to 70 years ago and were not adjusted for bioavailability and variations of vitamin levels within ingredients. Therefore, they may not reflect the changes in genetic characteristics, handling and storage of crops, cropping practices, and processing of feedstuffs over the years. Changing processing methods can significantly alter vitamin feed levels (Gadient, 1986; Ekanayake and Nelson, 1990; Emmert and Baker, 1997; Lewis *et al.*, 2015). For example, with changes in sugar technology, literature values for the pantothenic acid content of beet molasses have decreased from 50 to 110 mg/kg in the 1950s to about 1–4 mg/kg (Palagina *et al.*, 1990). Likewise, heat treatments in feed processing, like pelleting and extrusion, improve nutrient digestibility, reduce antinutritional factors and eventually control *Salmonella* and other pathogens, resulting in more significant vitamin destruction (Gadient, 1986; Svihus and Zimonja, 2011; Spasevski *et al.*, 2015; Yang *et al.*, 2020). In addition, values for some vitamins were not determined by current, more precise assay procedures. Additional information on the limitations of using average values of vitamins in feedstuffs when formulating animal rations have been reported (Kurnick *et al.*, 1972; Chen, Han, Guan *et al.*, 2019; Yang *et al.*, 2021b).

Vitamin levels from simple rations of feedstuff are generally lower than in complex rations. The currently used (e.g., corn-soybean meal diets) for animals exclude or contain lower amounts of the more costly vitamin-rich ingredients. The vitamin fortification levels in these simpler diets should be increased to "fill in the gaps" resulting from the reduced amounts of vitamins supplied by feedstuffs. Since ingredient changes are frequent

Table 3.1 Main functions of vitamins and symptoms of deficiency in swine

Vitamin	Basic function(s)	Deficiency disorder(s)/diseases
Vitamin A	• Essential for growth, health (immunity), reproduction (steroid synthesis), vision, development and integrity of skin, epithelia and mucosa	• Blindness or night-blindness (xeropthalmia) • Loss of appetite, poor absorption of nutrients, impaired growth and, in severe cases, death • Reduced immune response and increased risk of infections (respiratory and intestinal) • Reproduction defects such as failure of spermatogenesis in the male and fetal resorption or death in the female swine • Dry and scaly skin • Keratinization of epithelial tissues
Vitamin D_3	• Homeostasis of calcium and phosphorus (intestine, bones and kidney) • Regulation of bones calcification • Modulation of the immune system • Muscular cell growth	• Rickets, osteomalacia • Bone disorders (e.g., soft bones) and lameness • Stiff and hesitant gait • Reduced growth rate • Muscular weakness
$25OHD_3$	• Major serum metabolite of vitamin D_3 • More efficient absorption in the intestine • Faster response for calcium homeostasis • More efficient modulation of the immune system and muscular cells than vitamin D_3	• Rickets and osteomalacia • Bone disorders (e.g., soft bones) and lameness • Stiff and hesitant gait • Reduced growth rate • Muscular weakness
Vitamin E	• Most powerful fat-soluble antioxidant • Immune system modulation • Tissue protection • Fertility • Meat quality	• Muscular dystrophy and myopathy • Mulberry heart disease • Reduced immune response • Reduced fertility and Mastitis, Metritis and Agalactia (MMA) in sows • Meat quality defects: drip-loss, off-flavours
Vitamin K_3	• Blood clotting and coagulation • Coenzyme in metabolic process related to bone mineralization (Ca binding proteins) and protein formation	• Increased clotting time • Haemorrhages diseases, anemia and weakness • Bone disorders • Hematomas or blood swelling in the ears
Vitamin B_1	• Coenzyme in several enzymatic reactions • Carbohydrate metabolism (conversion of glucose into energy) • Involved in ATP, DNA and RNA production • Synthesis of acetylcholine, essential in transmission of nervous impulses	• Loss of appetite up to anorexia and vomiting • Reduced growth rate • Neuropathies (polioencephalomalacia-PEM), general muscle weakness, poor leg coordination • Fatty degeneration and necrosis of heart fibers (cardiac failure) • Mucosal inflammation with gastrointestinal malfunction
Vitamin B_2	• Fat and protein metabolism • Flavin coenzyme (FMN and FAD) synthesis, essentials for energy production (respiratory chain) • Involved in synthesis of steroids, red blood cells and glycogen • Integrity of mucosa membranes and antioxidant system within cells	• Reduced feed intake and growth • Reduced absorption of zinc, iron and calcium • Inflammation of the mucous membranes of the digestive tract • Scours and ulcerative colitis • Fertility impairments
Vitamin B_6	• Aminoacids, fats and carbohydrate metabolism • Essential for DNA and RNA synthesis • Involved in the synthesis of niacin from tryptophan	• Growth retardation, lesser feed intake and protein retention • Dermatitis, rough hair coat, scaly skin • Disorders of blood parameters

Vitamin	Functions	Deficiency symptoms
Vitamin B$_{12}$	• Synthesis of red blood cells and growth • Involved in methionine metabolism • Coenzyme in nucleic acids (DNA and RNA) and protein metabolism • Metabolism of fats and carbohydrates	• Brown exudate of the eyes • Anemia and ascites • Muscular convulsions, incoordination of movements and paralysis
Niacin or Vitamin B$_3$	• Coenzyme (active forms NAD and NADP) in amino acids, fats and carbohydrates metabolism • Required for optimum tissue integrity, particularly for the skin, the gastrointestinal tract and the nervous system	• Anemia • Growth retardation and lower feed conversion • Leg weakness • Embryo mortality, reduced piglet survival • Nervous system disorders • Inflammation and ulcers of mucous membranes • Reduced growth and feed efficiency • Dermatitis (pellagra), hair loss • Ulcerative necrotic lesions of the large intestine, diarrhoea • Reduced reproductive performance
Biotin or Vitamin B$_7$	• Coenzyme in protein, fat and carbohydrates metabolism • Normal blood glucose level • Synthesis of fatty acids, nucleic acids (DNA and RNA) and proteins (keratin)	• Reduced appetite, retarded growth • Fertility disorders • Skin ulcers, alopecia, hair loss and dermatitis • Inflammation of the hooves and hoof-sole lesions • Diarrhoea, eye inflammation and changes in oral mucosa
d-Pantothenic acid or Vitamin B$_5$	• Present in Coenzyme A (CoA) and Acyl Carrier Protein (ACP) involved in carbohydrate, fat and protein metabolism • Biosynthesis of long-chain fatty acids, phospholipids and steroid hormones	• Functional disorders of nervous system • Locomotive disorders • Scaly skin, dermatitis • Fatty degeneration of the liver • Reduced antibody formation • Reduced appetite, poor feed utilization and growth depression
Folic acid or Vitamin B$_9$	• Coenzyme in the synthesis of nucleic acids (DNA and RNA) and proteins (methyl groups) • Stimulates hematopoietic system • With vitamin B$_{12}$ it converts homocysteine into methionine	• Megaloblastic (macrocytic) anemia • Skin damages and hair loss • Retarded growth and reduced appetite • Compromised reproduction in sows • Embryonic mortality and smaller litter size
Vitamin C	• Intracellular (water-soluble) antioxidant • Immune system modulation: stimulation of phagocytosis • Collagen biosynthesis • Formation of connective tissues, cartilage and bones • Synthesis of corticosteroids and steroid metabolism • Conversion of vitamin D$_3$ to its active form 1,25(OH)$_2$D$_3$	• Weakness, fatigue and dyspnea • Bone pain • Haemorrhages of the skin, muscle and certain organs • Reduced fertility in both males (reduced sperm quality) and females (termination of corpus luteum)
Choline	• Membrane structural component (phosphatidylcholine) • Fat transport and metabolism in the liver • Support nervous system function (acetylcholine) • Source of methyl donors for methionine regeneration from homocysteine	• Fatty liver • Growth retardation
β-carotene	• Source of vitamin A • Stimulation of progesterone synthesis • Reproductive system function	• Poor reproductive performance e.g., prolonged estrus, retarded follicle maturation and ovulation • Increased susceptibility of young animals to infectious diseases

Table 3.2 Vitamin solubility characteristics (source: dsm-firmenich Animal Nutrition and Health, unpublished)

	Molecular weight	Water	Glycerol	Alcohol	Propylene glycol	Ethyl acetate	Ethanol
Vitamin A (retinol)	286.44	Practically insoluble	Practically insoluble	Insoluble	Practically insoluble	Practically insoluble	Practically insoluble
Vitamin D_3	384.62	Practically insoluble	Practically insoluble	Practically insoluble	Practically insoluble	Practically insoluble	Practically insoluble
Vitamin E (tocopherol)	430.69	Practically insoluble	Practically insoluble	Insoluble	Practically insoluble	Practically insoluble	Practically insoluble
Vitamin K_1	450.68	Slightly soluble	Practically insoluble	Practically insoluble	Practically insoluble	Practically insoluble	Slightly soluble
Vitamin K_2	580.9	Slightly soluble	Practically insoluble	Practically insoluble	Practically insoluble	Practically insoluble	Slightly soluble
Vitamin K_3	17.21	Slightly soluble	Practically insoluble	Slightly soluble	Practically insoluble	Practically insoluble	Practically insoluble
Vitamin B_1 (thiamine)	337.28	Insoluble	Insoluble	Insoluble	Insoluble	Practically insoluble	Practically insoluble
Vitamin B_2 (riboflavin)	376.36	Insoluble	Insoluble	Insoluble	Insoluble	Practically insoluble	Practically insoluble
Niacin	123.11	Practically insoluble	Practically insoluble	Insoluble	Practically insoluble	Practically insoluble	Practically insoluble
Pantothenic acid (vitamin B_5)	219.23	Insoluble	Practically insoluble	Practically insoluble	Practically insoluble	Insoluble	Practically insoluble
Vitamin B_6 (pyridoxine hydrochloride)	205.64	Insoluble	Practically insoluble	Insoluble	Insoluble	Practically insoluble	Practically insoluble
Biotin (vitamin B_7)	244.31	Insoluble	Practically insoluble	Insoluble	Insoluble	Practically insoluble	Practically insoluble
Folic acid (vitamin B_9)	441.4	Slightly soluble	Practically insoluble	Practically insoluble	Practically insoluble	Practically insoluble	Practically insoluble
Vitamin B_{12} (cyanocobalamin)	1355.42	Insoluble	Practically insoluble	Practically insoluble	Practically insoluble	Practically insoluble	Practically insoluble
Choline	121.18	Insoluble	Practically insoluble	Insoluble	Practically insoluble	Practically insoluble	Practically insoluble
Vitamin C (ascorbic acid)	176.12	Insoluble	Insoluble	Insoluble	Insoluble	Practically insoluble	Practically insoluble

Insoluble — Practically Insoluble — Slightly soluble

Methanol	Chloroform	Fats-oils	Organic solvents	Ether	Benzene	Acetone	Comments
							Freely soluble in dioxane and glacial acetic acid; moderately soluble in amyl alcohol
							Practically insoluble in butanol; Relatively soluble in acetic acid, phenol, pyridine, and solutions of alkali hydroxides and carbonates

Soluble   Not mentioned

Table 3.3 Vitamin conversion factors (source: dsm-firmenich Animal Nutrition and Health, unpublished)

Vitamin (active substance)	Unit	Conversion factor active substance form to vitamin form	Product form
Vitamin A (retinol)	IU	1 IU Vitamin A = 0.344 µg Vitamin A acetate (retinyl acetate)	ROVIMIX® A 1000
			ROVIMIX® A 500 WS
			ROVIMIX® A Palmitate 1.6
			ROVIMIX® AD3 1000/200
Vitamin D_3 (cholecalciferol)	IU	1 IU Vitamin D_3 = 0.025 µg Vitamin D_3	ROVIMIX® D_3-500
			ROVIMIX® AD3 1000/200
25OHD3 (25 hydroxy-cholecalciferol)	mg	1 µg 25OHD3 = 40 IU Vitamin D_3	ROVIMIX® Hy–D™ 1.25%
Vitamin E (tocopherol)	mg	1 mg Vitamin E = 1 IU Vitamin E = 1 mg all-rac-α-tocopheryl acetate	ROVIMIX® E-50 Adsorbate
			ROVIMIX® E 50 SD
Vitamin K_3 (menadione)	mg	1 mg of Vitamin K_3 = 2 mg of Menadione Sodium Bisulfite (MSB)	K_3 MSB
		1 mg of Vitamin K_3 = 2.3 mg of Menadione Nicotinamide Bisulfite (MNB)	ROVIMIX® K_3 MNB
Vitamin B_1 (thiamine)	mg	1 mg of Vitamin B_1 = 1.233 mg of Thiamine mononitrate	ROVIMIX® B_1
Vitamin B_2 (riboflavin)	mg		ROVIMIX® B2 80-SD
Vitamin B_6 (pyridoxine)	mg	1 mg Vitamin B_6 = 1.215 mg Pyridoxine hydrochloride	ROVIMIX® B_6
Vitamin B_{12} (cyanocobalamin)	mg		Vitamin B_{12} 1% Feed Grade
			ROVIMIX® B_{12} 1% Feed Grade
Vitamin B_3 (Niacin; nicotinic acid and nicotinamide)	mg	1 mg Nicotinic acid = 1 mg Niacin	ROVIMIX® Niacin
		1 mg Nicotinamide (or Niacinamide) = 1 mg Niacin	ROVIMIX® Niacinamide
Vitamin B_7 (d-Biotin)	mg	1 mg of Biotin = 1 mg D-Biotin	ROVIMIX® Biotin ROVIMIX® Biotin HP
Vitamin B_5 (d-Pantothenic acid)	mg	1 mg d-Pantothenic acid = 1.087 mg Calcium d-pantothenate or 2.174 mg Calcium dl-pantothenate	ROVIMIX® Calpan
Vitamin B_9 (Folic acid)	mg		ROVIMIX® Folic 80 SD
Vitamin C	mg	1 mg Vitamin C = 1 mg L-Ascorbic acid	STAY-C® 35
			STAY-C® 50
			ROVIMIX® C-EC
			Ascorbic acid
β-Carotene	mg		ROVIMIX® β-Carotene 10%
			ROVIMIX® β-Carotene 10% P

* M: Mash; P: Pellet; EXP: Expansion; EXT: Extrusion; W: Water
For more information about further dsm-firmenich products and product forms please ask your local dsm-firmenich representative

...ontent (min.)	Formulation technology	Application*
...000,000 IU/g	Beadlet	M, P, EXP, EXT
...00,000 IU/g	Spray-dried powder, water dispersible	W/MR
...500,000 IU/g	Oily liquid, may crystalize on storage	Oily solution
...tamin A 1,000,000 IU/g ...tamin D$_3$ 200,000 IU/g	Beadlet	M, P, EXP, EXT
...00,000 IU/g	Spray-dried powder, water dispersible	M, P, EXP, EXT, W/MR
...tamin A 1,000,000 IU/g ...tamin D$_3$ 200,000 IU/g	Beadlet	M, P, EXP, EXT
...25% 25OHD$_3$ (12.5 g/kg)	Spray-dried powder, water dispersible	M, P, EXP, EXT, W/MR
...% (500 g/kg)	Adsorbate on silicic acid	M, P, EXP, EXT
...% (500 g/kg)	Spray-dried powder, water dispersible	M, P, EXP, EXT, W/MR
...enadione: 51.5% (515 g/kg)	Fine crystalline powder	M, P, EXP, EXT, W/MR
...enadione: 43% (430 g/kg) ...cotinamide: 30.5% (305 g/kg)	Fine crystalline powder	M, P, EXP, EXT
...% (980 g/kg)	Fine crystalline powder	M, P, EXP, EXT
...% (800 g/kg)	Spray-dried powder	M, P, EXP, EXT, W/MR
...% (990 g/kg)	Fine crystalline powder	M, P, EXP, EXT, W/MR
...(10 g/kg)	Fine powder	M, P, EXP, EXT
...(10 g/kg)	Spray-dried powder	M, P, EXP, EXT
...5% (995 g/kg)	Fine crystalline powder	M, P, EXP, EXT
...5% (995 g/kg)	Fine crystalline powder	M, P, EXP, EXT, W/MR
...(20 g/kg) ...% (100 g/kg)	Spray-dried powder, water dispersible	M, P, EXP, EXT, W/MR
...% Calcium d-pantothenate (980 g/kg) ...lcium 8.2 – 8.6% (82 – 86 g/kg)	Spray-dried powder, water dispersible	M, P, EXP, EXT, W/MR
...% (800 g/kg)	Spray-dried powder, water dispersible	M, P, EXP, EXT, W/MR
...% of total phosphorylated ascorbic acid ...tivity (350 g/kg)	Spray-dried powder	M, P, EXP, EXT
...% of total phosphorylated sodium salt ascorbic ...id activity (500 g/kg)	Spray-dried powder	M, P, EXP, EXT, W/MR
...5% (975 g/kg)	Ethyl-cellulose coated powder	M, P, W/MR
...– 100% (990 – 1000 g/kg)	Crystalline powder	W/MR
...% (100 g/kg)	Encapsulated beadlet	M, P, EXP, EXT
...% (100 g/kg)	Cross linked beadlet	M, P, EXP, EXT

Table 3.4 Vitamin concentrations of feedstuffs, mean (SD) (source: adapted from Chen, Han, Guan et al., 2019)

Feed ingredients	Vitamins, mg/kg – mean (standard deviation)								
	β-carotene	Vitamin E	Vitamin B$_6$	Folic acid	Niacin	Pantothenic acid	Vitamin B$_2$ (riboflavin)	Vitamin B$_1$ (thiamine)	Choline
Corn	1.62 (0.44)	18.67 (9.48)	3.05 (1.19)	0.08 (0.07)	3.68 (1.73)	3.98 (1.20)	1.30 (0.20)	0.61 (0.17)	292.82 (80.55)
Corn DDGS	2.16 (0.58)	39.24 (9.97)	0.99 (0.47)	0.57 (0.31)	23.23 (13.13)	15.55 (3.02)	3.73 (0.66)	2.14 (0.54)	337.36 (173.38)
Corn germ meal	0.36 (0.09)	19.31 (5.89)	4.44 (1.80)	0.72 (0.49)	29.42 (5.73)	5.35 (2.98)	3.95 (2.28)	4.14 (2.34)	818.00 (513.98)
Corn gluten meal	11.10 (4.05)	7.00 (1.51)	2.13 (0.93)	0.02 (0.02)	36.46 (5.90)	3.93 (2.06)	0.72 (0.36)	0.37 (0.13)	80.04 (13.16)
Corn gluten feed	0.56 (0.11)	9.89 (2.62)	4.15 (1.01)	1.30 (0.46)	52.65 (11.94)	12.56 (3.14)	1.89 (0.80)	5.11 (1.04)	1525.18 (242.75)
Wheat	–	7.27 (1.73)	2.23 (1.33)	0.40 (0.18)	32.86 (8.63)	7.36 (3.60)	0.57 (0.19)	2.12 (1.09)	234.29 (81.65)
Wheat bran	–	19.79 (5.86)	6.52 (1.19)	0.40 (0.18)	102.53 (14.81)	12.35 (4.02)	0.96 (0.26)	2.52 (0.58)	931.59 (121.89)
Wheat shorts	–	9.03 (4.28)	3.93 (1.23)	0.62 (0.27)	4.54 (1.31)	8.18 (0.96)	1.18 (0.12)	3.69 (1.26)	830.48 (226.78)
Soybean meal	–	2.42 (0.85)	6.43 (1.07)	0.51 (0.11)	62.03 (6.21)	3.63 (0.85)	1.77 (0.37)	9.13 (1.51)	1686.54 (144.07)
Rapeseed meal	–	8.66 (2.40)	3.46 (1.80)	0.65 (0.47)	72.82 (10.53)	6.73 (2.75)	1.53 (0.41)	2.14 (0.90)	2276.32 (193.22)
Peanut meal	–	0.67 (0.27)	5.44 (1.11)	104.96 (13.40)	104.96 (14.07)	18.27 (3.46)	1.65 (0.41)	4.22 (1.47)	1527.60 (130.54)
Cottonseed meal	–	10.57 (7.83)	6.30 (1.64)	9.15 (1.87)	9.15 (1.87)	6.75 (1.92)	2.19 (0.32)	1.63 (0.48)	1546.24 (272.49)
Sunflower seed meal	–	1.04 (0.30)	7.57 (0.49)	183.91 (14.60)	183.91 (14.60)	27.25 (1.52)	3.65 (0.16)	1.78 (0.34)	399.96 (69.15)

Table 3.5 Sensitivity of vitamins to physical stress factors (source: dsm-firmenich Animal Nutrition and Health, unpublished)

Additive	Temperature	Oxygen	Humidity	Light
Vitamin A	Marked	Marked	Marked	Marked
Vitamin D	Marked	Marked	Marked	Marked
25OHD$_3$ (calcifediol)	Marked	Marked	Marked	Marked
Vitamin E	No effect	Marked	No effect	No effect
Vitamin K$_3$	Marked	Marked	Marked	No effect
Vitamin B$_1$	Marked	Marked	Marked	No effect
Vitamin B$_2$	No effect	Marked	No effect	Marked
Vitamin B$_6$	Marked	No effect	Marked	Marked
Vitamin B$_{12}$	Marked	No effect	Marked	Marked
Pantothenic acid	Marked	No effect	No effect	No effect
Nicotinates	No effect	No effect	No effect	No effect
Biotin	Marked	No effect	No effect	No effect
Folic acid	Marked	No effect	No effect	Marked
Vitamin C	Marked	Marked	Moderate	No effect
Carotenoids	Marked	Marked	Marked	Marked

Legend: **Marked effect** | **Moderate effect** | No effect

and unpredictable in computerized least-cost diet formulation, the low levels of vitamins likely to be supplied by feedstuffs should be disregarded, and adequate dietary vitamin fortification provided.

Vitamins, as pure substances, are almost all sensitive to various physical stress factors. Table 3.5 provides a simple qualitative overview of the sensitivity of each vitamin to these factors, which explains the importance, for industrial application, of properly formulating each vitamin to make it more stable and ensuring that the calculated amount per kilogram of feed reaches the animal.

FACTORS AFFECTING VITAMIN REQUIREMENTS AND UTILIZATION

1. Physiological makeup, genetics, and production function

Vitamin requirements of animals and humans depend significantly on their physiological makeup related to the traits given by decades of genetic selection, age, health, and nutritional status and function, such as producing meat, milk, eggs, hair or wool, or carrying a fetus (Roche, 1979; Stahly and Lutz, 2001; Stahly et al., 2007). For example, pig breeds with higher lean growth have higher vitamin B requirements than those with moderate muscle growth. Higher levels of vitamins A, D$_3$, and E are needed by sows in gestation and lactation than for finishing pigs.

Selection for a faster growth may allow animals to reach much higher weights at much younger ages with less feed consumption. This rapid growth may influence pigs' ability to develop their skeleton accordingly (Crenshaw, 2000). Leg problems in pigs and sows are still observed in commercial production. Vitamin supplementation can partly minimize some of these health and welfare issues through higher levels of biotin, folacin, niacin, and choline (Bryant et al., 1985a,c), ascorbic acid (Denis et al., 1997), vitamin K (Cashman and O'Connor, 2008; Monegue, 2013), and more available vitamin D (Lauridsen et al., 2010; Regassa et al., 2015; Zhou et al., 2017; Duffy et al., 2018a; Zhang et al., 2019a).

The recent data discussed in Chapter 5 from diverse sources and industry applications in primary swine-producing countries indicates that current genetic potential has improved growth rate, FCR, litter size, and milk production. Consequently, vitamin requirements determined several decades ago might not apply to today's swine.

2. Confined production versus access to pasture

The complete confinement of swine has been common for many decades, and consequently, vitamin nutrition has played an essential role in the success of intensive swine production (Kornegay and Meacham, 1973; Bryant et al., 1985c; Daza et al., 2005). The new trends are to give access to pasture in free-range systems. Since young, lush, green grasses or legumes are good vitamin sources, these production systems could provide significant quantities of most vitamins. More available vitamins A and E are present in pastures and green forage, which contain ample amounts of β-carotene, α-tocopherol, and flavonoids, compared to those found in grains, which are lower in bioavailability (Mutetikka and Mahan, 1993). The outdoor system has been proven to improve polyunsaturated omega-3 and the ratio between omega-6 and omega-3 fatty acids (Daza et al., 2005; Rey et al., 2006). However, adverse effects on oxidative stability have been observed.

The effect of foraging in swine is complex, depending on the balance between anti- and pro-oxidant compounds and on the kinetic activity of the animal, which drives oxidation. Oxidation may be low with grass intake because green forage has high levels of tocopherols, tocotrienols, carotenoids, vitamin C, and polyphenols. Consequently, free-range swine could also benefit from vitamin supplementation (Daza et al., 2005).

3. Antioxidants and immunological role of vitamins

Immunological response and disease conditions are intimately related to the requirements of specific vitamins (Surai and Dvorska, 2005; Konowalchuk et al., 2013; Feng et al., 2021; Liu et al., 2021). Disease conditions influence the antioxidant vitamins (vitamins E, C, and β-carotene) (Bacou et al., 2021; Lauridsen et al., 2021b). These nutrients play essential roles in animal health by inactivating harmful free radicals from various stressors produced through regular cellular activity. Free radicals can damage biological systems (Bacou et al., 2021). Free radicals, including hydroxy, hypochlorite, peroxyl, alkoxy, superoxide, hydrogen peroxide, and singlet oxygen, are generated by autoxidation, radiation, or some oxidases, dehydrogenases, and peroxidases. Also, phagocytic granulocytes undergo respiratory bursts to produce oxygen radicals to destroy pathogens. However, these oxidative products can, in turn, damage healthy cells if they are not eliminated. Antioxidants stabilize these highly reactive free radicals, maintaining cells' structural and functional integrity (McCay, 1985; Eichenberger et al., 2004; Zhou et al., 2022). Therefore, antioxidants are vital to swine's immune defense and health (Bacou et al., 2021; Lauridsen et al., 2021b).

Tissue defense mechanisms against free-radical damage generally include vitamin C, E, and β-carotene as significant vitamin antioxidant sources. In addition, several metalloenzymes, which include glutathione peroxidase (selenium), catalase (iron), superoxide dismutase (copper, zinc, and manganese), and even pyridoxine (Dalto and Matte, 2017) are also critical in protecting the internal cellular constituents from oxidative damage. These nutrients' dietary and tissue balance protects tissues against free-radical damage (Combs and McClung, 2022).

A compromised immune system will reduce animal production efficiency through increased susceptibility to disease, leading to animal morbidity and mortality. Both *in vitro* and *in vivo* studies show that antioxidant vitamins enhance cellular and noncellular immunity. The antioxidant function of these vitamins could, at least in part, enhance immunity by maintaining the function and structural integrity of critical immune cells.

Vitamin C is the most crucial antioxidant in extracellular fluids. It can protect biomembranes against lipid peroxidation damage by eliminating peroxyl radicals in the aqueous phase before the latter can initiate peroxidation (Johnston *et al.*, 2013; Bleilevens *et al.*, 2019). Data from several animal species indicate that vitamin C is required for an adequate immune and antiviral response in limiting lung pathology after influenza virus infection (Li *et al.*, 2006; Colunga Biancatelli *et al.*, 2020). One of the protective effects of vitamin C may partly be mediated through its ability to reduce circulating glucocorticoids (Degkwitz, 1987). In addition, ascorbate can regenerate the reduced form of α-tocopherol, perhaps accounting for the observed sparing effect of these vitamins (Jacob, 1995; Tanaka *et al.*, 1997). In the process of sparing fatty acid oxidation, tocopherol is oxidized to the tocopheryl free-radical. Ascorbic acid can donate an electron to the tocopheryl free radical, regenerating the reduced antioxidant form of tocopherol (Min *et al.*, 2018).

Vitamin C and E supplementation resulted in a 78% decrease in the susceptibility of lipoproteins to mononuclear cell-mediated oxidation. As an effective scavenger of reactive oxygen species, ascorbic acid minimizes the oxidative stress associated with activated phagocytic leukocytes' respiratory burst, thereby controlling the inflammation and tissue damage associated with immune responses (Chien *et al.*, 2004). Ascorbic acid is very high in phagocytic cells, which use free radicals and other highly reactive oxygen-containing molecules to help kill pathogens that invade the body. However, these reactive species may damage cells and tissues in the process. Ascorbic acid helps to protect these cells from oxidative damage (Min *et al.*, 2018; Combs and McClung, 2022).

Vitamin A strongly influences the immunological response, although it has less antioxidant potential than β-carotene. Animals deficient in vitamin A will show increased frequency and severity of bacterial, protozoal, and viral infections and other disease conditions (Fachinello *et al.*, 2018). As a function of vitamin A, part of the disease resistance is related to maintaining mucous membranes and normal adrenal gland functioning to produce corticosteroids needed to combat disease. An animal's ability to resist illness depends on a responsive immune system, and a vitamin A deficiency causes a reduced immune response (Hu *et al.*, 2020; Combs and McClung, 2022).

Vitamin A deficiency affects several cells of the immune system. Vitamin A deficiency affects immune functions, particularly the antibody response to T-cell-dependent antigens (Hu *et al.*, 2020). The RAR-alpha mRNA expression and antigen-specific proliferative response of T-lymphocytes are influenced by vitamin A status *in vivo* and directly modulated by retinoic acid. Repletion with retinoic acid effectively re-establishes the number of circulating lymphocytes (Zhao and Ross, 1995) and can even have transgenerational effects on the progeny when supplemented to sows (Amavizca-Nazar *et al.*, 2019; Langel *et al.*, 2019).

A diminished primary antibody response could also increase the severity and duration of an episode of infection. In contrast, a diminished secondary reaction could increase the risk of developing a second disease episode. Vitamin A deficiency causes decreases in phagocytic activity in macrophages and neutrophils. The secretory immunoglobulin A (IgA) system is an essential first line of defense against infections of mucosal surfaces (McGhee *et al.*, 1992). Several studies in pigs have shown that the intestinal IgA response is impaired by vitamin A suboptimal levels, reducing response against rotavirus or infections during the weaning period (Kandasamy *et al.*, 2014; Hu *et al.*, 2020; Zhou *et al.*, 2021a,b).

An optimal vitamin A range enhances vitamin A responses because both deficient and excessive levels suppress immune function. In many experiments with laboratory and domestic animals, including pigs, the effects of both clinical and subclinical deficiencies of vitamin A on the production of antibodies and the resistance of different tissues to microbial infection or parasitic infestation (*Trichuris suis*) have frequently been demonstrated (Pedersen *et al.*, 2001). Vitamin A deficiency may alter the functional integrity of the mucosal intestinal epithelium, disrupting the ordinarily delicate attachment of *T. suis* and leading to rapid termination of infection (Pedersen *et al.*, 2001).

Vitamin A supplementation improves the antioxidant capacity, immune status, intestinal cells, and growth performance of weanling piglets (Surai and Fisinin, 2015; Hu *et al.*, 2020; Wang *et al.*, 2020). Supplementation of vitamin A can also inhibit the harmful action of lipopolysaccharides on the intestinal barrier function, contributing to maintaining gut health (He *et al.*, 2019). However, levels above 40,000 IU/kg can decrease serum levels of vitamin E and inhibit vitamin K_2 synthesis and liver metabolism.

Animal studies indicate that specific carotenoids like canthaxanthin, retinoic acid, and lycopene, with antioxidant capacities but without vitamin A activity, can enhance many aspects of immune functions and act directly as antimutagens and anticarcinogens (Chew and Park, 2004; Fachinello *et al.*, 2018). They can protect against radiation damage and block photosensitizers' damaging effects. Also, carotenoids can directly affect gene expression, and this mechanism may enable carotenoids to modulate the interaction between B-cells and T-cells, thus regulating humoral and cell-mediated immunity (Wiedermann *et al.*, 1993; Zhao and Ross, 1995).

Vitamin E is perhaps the most studied nutrient related to the immune response (Jensen *et al.*, 1988; Meydani and Han, 2006). Evidence accumulated over the years and in many species indicates that vitamin E is an essential nutrient for the normal function of the immune system (Wuryastuti *et al.*, 1993). Furthermore, studies suggest that the beneficial effects of certain nutrients, such as vitamin E, on reducing disease risk can affect the immune response. Deficiency in vitamin E impairs B- and T-cell-mediated immunity. Vitamin E partially reduces prostaglandin synthesis and prevents the oxidation of polyunsaturated fatty acids (PUFAs) in cell membranes (Shanker, 2006).

Considerable attention is being directed to vitamin E and selenium's role in protecting leukocytes and macrophages during phagocytosis, the mechanism whereby animals immunologically kill invading bacteria and viruses (Beck, 2007). Both vitamin E and selenium may help these cells survive the toxic products produced to effectively kill ingested bacteria (Badwey and Karnovsky, 1980). Most of the benefits of this combination depend on the excellent synergistic antioxidant effect of these 2 nutrients (Chen *et al.*, 2016). Vitamin and selenium can also improve immunoglobulin transfer from the sow to piglets (Hayek *et al.*, 1989).

Since vitamin E acts as a tissue antioxidant and aids in quenching free radicals produced in the body, any infection or other stress factor may exacerbate the depletion of the limited vitamin E stores in various tissues. Regarding immunocompetency, dietary requirements may be adequate for average growth and production; however, higher levels have improved cellular and humoral immune status (Chew, 1995; Ching *et al.*, 2002; Johnson *et al.*, 2019; Johnson and Popoola, 2020). The former 2 responses are generally used as criteria for determining the requirements of a nutrient. There is an increase in glucocorticoids, epinephrine, eicosanoids, and phagocytic activity during stress and disease. Eicosanoid and corticoid synthesis and phagocytic respiratory bursts are prominent producers of free radicals that challenge the antioxidant systems. Vitamin E has been implicated in stimulating serum antibody synthesis, particularly IgG antibodies (Tengerdy, 1980). The productive effects of vitamin E on animal health may reduce immunosuppressive glucocorticoids (Golub and Gershwin, 1985). Vitamin E also most likely has an immuno-enhancing impact by altering arachidonic acid metabolism and subsequent prostaglandin synthesis, thromboxanes, and leukotrienes. Under stress conditions, increased levels of these compounds by endogenous synthesis or exogenous entry may adversely affect immune cell function (Hadden, 1987). These results suggest that the criteria for establishing requirements based on overt deficiencies or growth do not consider optimal health.

4. Stress, disease, or adverse environmental conditions

Intensified production increases stress and subclinical disease-level conditions because of the higher densities of animals in confined areas. Animal stress and disease conditions may increase the essential requirement for specific vitamins. Several studies indicated that nutrient levels adequate for growth, feed efficiency, gestation, and lactation might not be sufficient for normal immunity and maximizing the animal's resistance to disease (Cunha, 1985; Nockels, 1988; Lauridsen et al., 2021a; Matte and Lauridsen, 2022).

The adverse effect of environmental stress on a pig's health, welfare, and performance cannot be underemphasized. Environmental stressors can cause an upsurge in stress hormone secretion, negatively affecting growth and leading to severe mortality. However, effective management techniques are crucial to raising healthy pigs and profit maximization in the swine industry. To enhance pigs' adaptability under stress conditions, it is essential to understand the functions of different vitamins and the appropriate dosage in pig diets to alleviate stress. The synergistic effects of various vitamins and minerals could promote growth performance and reduce environmental stress in pigs (Feng et al., 2017; Surai and Fisinin, 2015; Liu et al., 2016).

Diseases or parasites affecting the gastrointestinal tract will reduce the intestinal absorption of vitamins from dietary sources and those synthesized by microorganisms. If they cause diarrhea or vomiting, they decrease intestinal absorption and increase vitamin needs. Vitamin A deficiency is often seen in heavily parasitized animals that supposedly receive adequate vitamins (Bebravicius et al., 1987).

Any disease that includes bleeding of the intestinal wall increases both vitamin loss and vitamin requirements for tissue regeneration. Likewise, a condition that causes a loss in appetite and feed intake increases the need for vitamins per unit of feed consumed to meet daily body needs. Diseases that adversely affect the integrity of the intestinal wall may interfere with vitamin A conversion from β-carotene and increase the animal's vitamin A needs. Cunha (1987) suggested that the transformation of vitamin D to its functional forms in the liver and kidney would be affected by diseases of these organs (Arnold et al., 2015).

Mycotoxins are known to cause a digestive disturbance, such as vomiting, diarrhea, and internal bleeding, and to interfere with the absorption of dietary vitamins A, D, E, and K (Surai and Dvorska, 2005). Moldy corn containing mycotoxins has been associated with deficiencies of vitamin D (rickets) and vitamin E, even though these vitamins were supplemented at levels regarded as satisfactory (Van Heugten, 2000).

Vitamin C has been found to promote vitamin D metabolism and is also known to counter the effects of multiple stresses (Cantatore et al., 1991; DeLuca, 2014). Heat stress depresses feed intake, immunity, sow livability, and reproductive performance in pigs (Horký et al., 2016; Feng et al., 2021). Ascorbic acid supplementation has improved these factors (Sosnowska *et al.*, 2011). Ascorbic acid (250 mg/kg) can also alleviate environmental stress. Adenkola *et al.* (2009) showed that ascorbic acid modulates the body temperature of pigs by decreasing the maximum rectal temperature value and may alleviate the adverse effects of thermal or transportation stress on the health and productivity of pigs during the cold, dry season or hot, dry season (Asala *et al.*, 2010).

Although vitamin C is commonly associated with alleviating the effects of heat stress in pigs (Feng *et al.*, 2021), there is evidence that combination with vitamin E can also play a vital role in minimizing the adverse effects of stress in growth as well as in sow and boar reproductive ability (Sahin *et al.*, 2001; Horký *et al.*, 2016; Liu *et al.*, 2016). Selenium supplementation can also be combined with these antioxidant vitamins to improve their efficacy in coping with stress (Oldfield, 2003).

In recent years, several research reports have confirmed that almost all vitamins may directly improve the gut health of pigs during stressful periods, like weaning. Positive results have been observed when supplementing piglet or sow diets with β-carotene (Li *et al.*, 2021), lycopene (Meng *et al.*, 2022; Liu *et al.*, 2022), vitamin D (Zhang *et al.*, 2020, 2022; Zhao *et al.*, 2022), ascorbic acid (Trawińska *et al.*, 2012), niacin (Liu *et al.*, 2021; Feng *et al.*, 2021), folic acid (Wang *et al.*, 2021b), and choline (Qiu *et al.*, 2021; Zhong *et al.*, 2021). All these vitamins can improve intestinal immunity, enhance gut antioxidant status (Xu *et al.*, 2014), modulate gut microbial communities, and stimulate mucosa development and intestinal barrier functions in weaned piglets or sows.

The direct effect of vitamins on gut microbiome had not received much attention until recently. The now enlarging body of scientific evidence supports the statement that vitamins are essential for health (Lauridsen *et al.*, 2021b; Matte and Lauridsen, 2022). Vitamins can enhance animal host and gut microbiota metabolism to obtain favorable outcomes for the health and growth of pigs (Stacchiotti *et al.*, 2021). In pigs, weaning could be the most critical period in life and is when most of the genetic growth potential is at risk. Vitamins can support a more manageable transition during weaning.

5. Vitamin antagonists

Vitamin antagonists (anti-metabolites) interfere with the activity of various vitamins. Oldfield (1987) summarized the action of antagonists, which:

- could cleave the vitamin molecule and render it inactive, as occurs with thiaminase, found in raw fish and some feedstuffs, and thiamine (pyrithiamine is another thiamine antagonist)
- could bind with the metabolite, with similar results, as happens between avidin, found in raw egg white, and streptavidin, from *Streptomyces* mold and biotin
- could, because of structural similarity, occupy reaction sites and deny them to the vitamin, as with dicumarol, found in certain plants, and vitamin K
- inactivate, through rancid fats, biotin and destroy vitamins A, D, E, and possibly others.

These effects were also reviewed by Woolley (2012).

The presence of vitamin antagonists in animal and human diets should be considered when adjusting vitamin allowances, as most vitamins have antagonists that reduce their utilization. Mycotoxins are antagonists in the feed that can substantially decrease antioxidant nutrient assimilation and increase their requirements to prevent the damaging effects of free radicals and toxic products. It is now increasingly recognized that at least 25% of the world's grains are contaminated with mycotoxins (Surai and Dvorska, 2005). Mycotoxins cause digestive disturbances such as vomiting and diarrhea, and internal bleeding and interfere with the absorption of dietary vitamins A and vitamins D, E, and K (Surai and Dvorska, 2005; McDowell, 2006). Vitamin C can reduce the toxicity of certain mycotoxins (Su et al., 2018).

Toxic minerals may be antagonists and will likewise increase vitamin requirements. Vitamin E protects against the toxicity of certain heavy metals (e.g., cadmium, mercury, and lead), which increases the need for the vitamin (McDowell, 2000a). Rothe et al. (1994) reported that dietary vitamin C (1000 mg) reduced by 35–40% the elevated levels of cadmium in pig kidneys and liver induced by high supplementation of copper (175 mg Cu/kg feed).

Specific vitamins can likewise be antagonistic to other vitamins. Excess vitamin A (40,000–60,000 IU/kg) can affect the metabolism (e.g., absorption) of other fat-soluble vitamins (Olivares et al., 2009b). Large excesses of vitamin E have been shown to result in hemorrhages in some species, apparently by reducing vitamin K absorption. The problem can be eliminated with additional dietary vitamin K.

6. Use of antimicrobial drugs

Some antimicrobial drugs will increase the vitamin needs of animals by altering intestinal microflora and inhibiting the synthesis of specific vitamins. Certain sulfonamides may increase the requirements for biotin, folic acid, vitamin K, and possibly others when intestinal synthesis is reduced. These gut health issues may be insignificant except when antagonistic drugs toward a particular vitamin are added in excess, i.e., sulfaquinoxaline versus vitamin K and sulfonamide potentiators versus folic acid (Perry, 1978).

7. Levels of other nutrients in the diet

The fat level in the diet may affect the absorption of the fat-soluble vitamins A, D, E, and K and the requirements for vitamin E and possibly other vitamins. Fat-soluble vitamins may fail to be absorbed if fat digestion is impaired by liver damage or when the enterohepatic recirculation of bile acids is interrupted. Type (e.g., animal fats, vegetable oils, and blends) and quality (e.g., cis versus trans, saturated versus PUFAs, and oxidized sources) of fats can influence individual vitamin allowances (Ellis and Madsen, 1944; Thode Jensen et al., 1983; Astrup and Langebrekke, 1985; Hidiroglou et al., 1993; Gebert et al., 1999a; Babinszky et al., 1991a,b; Cerolini et al., 2000).

For example, a precise vitamin E : PUFA ratio may not apply to all diet and health status types. Therefore, there has been no consensus on the exact vitamin E : PUFA ratio to determine the vitamin requirement. However, the published human data for a diet with an average concentration of PUFA and containing mainly linoleic acid indicates that the additional vitamin E requirement ranges from 0.4 to 0.6 mg RRR-α-tocopherol/g of PUFA in the diet. A ratio of 0.5 mg RRR-α-tocopherol/g of linoleic acid was used in the diet, and the degree of unsaturation of the dietary fatty acids was also considered to evaluate the required vitamin E. Thus, using the proposed equation, humans' estimated requirement for vitamin E varied from 12 to 20 mg/day for a typical range of dietary PUFA intake (Raederstorff et al., 2015). Calculations in animal diets indicate that high dietary PUFA increases the vitamin E requirement by 3 mg/g PUFA (Bieber-Wlaschny, 1988). Many interrelationships of vitamins with other nutrients exist and affect requirements. For example, prominent interrelationships exist for vitamin E with selenium, vitamin D with calcium and phosphorus, choline with methionine, and niacin with tryptophan.

8. Body vitamin reserves

The fat-soluble vitamins A, D, and E but not vitamin K, are more inclined to remain in the body. This is especially true of vitamin A and carotene, which may be stored by an animal in its liver and fatty tissue in sufficient quantities to meet its requirements for varying periods (Heying *et al.*, 2013). Body storage of B group vitamins, except for vitamin B$_{12}$, is irrelevant (Blair and Newsome, 1985; Dove and Cook, 2000; Said, 2012). Overall, a daily supplementation at the proper levels typical of each species and growth stage is generally recommended in animal husbandry in industrial conditions.

Chapter 4

Vitamin description

FAT-SOLUBLE VITAMINS

Vitamin A

Chemical structure and properties

Vitamin A is used as a generic term for all the non-carotenoid β-ionone derivatives possessing the biological activity of all-*trans*-retinol (Combs and McClung, 2022). Retinol is the alcohol form of vitamin A. Replacement of the alcohol group (-OH) by an aldehyde group (-CHO) yields retinal, and replacement by an acid group (-COOH) gives retinoic acid (Ross and Harrison, 2013). Vitamin A products for feed use include retinyl acetate, propionate, and palmitate esters (Figure 4.1). Other vitamin A compounds in the body include retinoyl β-glucuronide in bile and retinyl phosphate, an intermediate in glycoprotein synthesis.

Vitamin A alcohol (retinol) is a nearly colorless, fat-soluble, long-chain, unsaturated compound with 5 bonds. Since it contains double bonds, vitamin A can exist in different isomeric forms. Vitamin A and its precursors, carotenoids, are rapidly destroyed by oxygen, heat, light, and acids. Carotenoids are usually found in nature in the all-*trans* form; however, they are easily isomerized to form *cis*-isomers following exposure to heat and/or light (Lindshield and Erdman, 2006). Moisture and trace minerals reduce vitamin A activity in feeds (Olson, 1984).

Swine diets are supplemented with synthetic retinol as the contribution of carotenoids from the feed in the formation of vitamin A is minimal (Darroch, 2000; Surles *et al.*, 2007). The combined potency in a feed, represented by its vitamin A and carotene content, is referred to as its vitamin A value. In animal tissues, they exist predominantly as retinal, retinol, retinaldehyde, retinoic, and retinyl esters (Ross and Harrison, 2013).

Vegetables contain a variety of carotenoids. Over 600 forms of carotenoids have been isolated, which differ in molecular structure and biological function (Goodwin, 1984; Ross and Harrison, 2013). Only 80 carotenoids have provitamin A activity. The carotenes are orange-yellow pigments, found mainly in green leaves and, to a lesser extent, in corn. Six carotenoids are the focus of nutritional research: α-carotene, lutein, lycopene, β-carotene (the most active provitamin A carotenoid), γ-carotene, and β-cryptoxanthin, one of the main carotenoids of corn, possessing the β-ionone ring (C15=C15), are critical because of their provitamin A activity. In corn and corn by-products, β-carotene, β-zeacarotene, and β-cryptoxanthin are present in a ratio of 25 : 25 : 50.

Lycopene, an important carotenoid for its antioxidant function, does not possess the β-ionone ring structure. It is not considered a precursor of vitamin A and is frequently listed as a food colorant (Johnson *et al.*, 1997; Cao *et al.*, 2021). However, recently it has been observed that pigs are very sensitive to lycopene. Positive effects of lycopene have been observed in the cellular and humoral immune responses of finishing pigs. The highest anti-bovine serum albumin IgG production was achieved by supplementing 20.06 mg lycopene/kg diet (Fachinello *et al.*, 2018). Dietary lycopene supplementation (200 mg/kg) can also improve

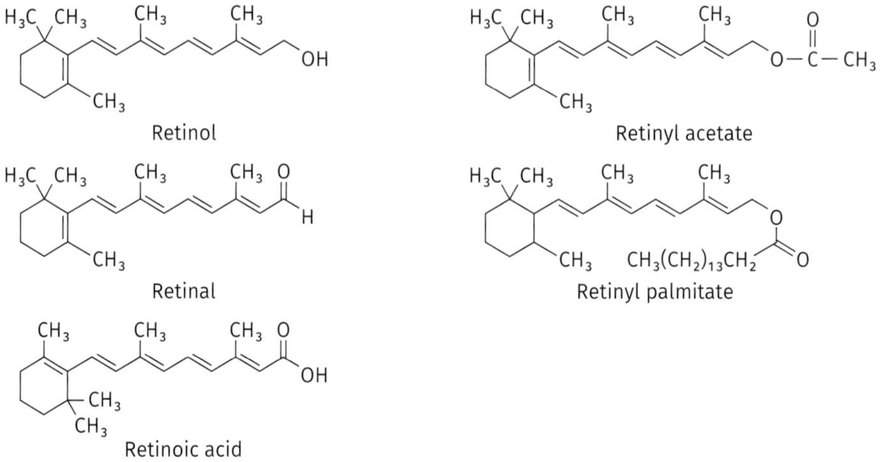

Figure 4.1 Vitamin A chemical structure of some natural and synthetic forms

intestinal morphology and barrier function, enhancing tight junction function, antioxidant capability, inhibiting inflammatory response, and gut microbiota of weaned piglets (Liu et al., 2022; Meng et al., 2022).

Dietary lycopene supplementation improved meat quality, antioxidant capacity, and skeletal muscle fiber type transformation in finishing pigs (Liu et al., 2022; Wen et al., 2022). Improvements in pork quality have been reported recently (An et al., 2019; Fachinello et al., 2020a,b; Wen et al., 2022). Dietary lycopene supplementation causes molecular changes in muscle fibers. It activated 5' AMP-activated protein kinase (AMPK) through the NRF1/CaMKKβ axis (nuclear respiratory factor 1/calcium calmodulin-dependent protein kinase kinase-β), activating Sirtuin 1 and PGC-1α (peroxisome proliferator-activated receptor-γ coactivator-1α) and inducing skeletal muscle fiber transformation from fast-twitch to slow-twitch. Skeletal muscle, rich in slow-twitch fiber, has a red appearance, better taste and flavor, and stronger aerobic metabolism (Zhang et al., 2019c). Lycopene can also improve maternal reproductive performance and in vitro development of porcine embryos by reducing oxidative stress and apoptosis, placental and immune status, and modulating milk composition (Kang et al., 2021; Sun et al., 2021). Lycopene can also alleviate the cytotoxicity caused by mycotoxins such as zearalenone in piglet Sertoli cells (Cao et al., 2021).

Vitamin A activity of β-carotene is substantially greater than other carotenoids (Ross and Harrison, 2013). For example, both α-carotene and cryptoxanthin have about one-half the conversion rate of β-carotene (Tanumihardjo and Howe, 2005). Theoretically, 2 molecules of vitamin A could be formed from one molecule of β-carotene. However, biological tests have consistently shown that pure vitamin A has twice the potency of β-carotene on a weight-to-weight basis. Early researchers (Parrish et al., 1951) recognized that unit-for-unit carotene is less effective than preformed vitamin A as a swine supplement during early gestation and early lactation. In addition, Myers et al. (1959) reported that vitamin A provided a greater rate of change per unit of intake than a corresponding increase in carotene intake.

Pigs are less efficient than poultry in converting β-carotene to vitamin A (Hendricks et al., 1967; Ullrey, 1972). Based on liver storage, the biopotency of 1 mg of carotene in corn fed to weanling pigs is 261–267 IU vitamin A (Hentges et al., 1952b; Wellenreiter et al., 1969, NRC, 1988). This is less than 16% of the conversion efficiency for vitamin A in rats or poultry. The activity of β-carotene decreases further with increasing intake. At higher levels of all-*trans*-carotene intake from corn gluten meal, 1 mg β-carotene had a vitamin A potency of only 123–174 IU. Ullrey *et al.* (1965) reported that 1 mg of β-carotene from a fermentation process equaled 192 IU of all-*trans*-vitamin A palmitate.

Schweigert *et al.* (2001) detected 1–8 ng/ml of β-carotene in plasma of gilts supplemented with a 100 mg/kg diet of β-carotene and 4,000 IU/kg vitamin A and estimated a conversion rate of β-carotene to vitamin A of 40 to 1 on a weight basis. In this same study, the authors observed an accumulation of β-carotene in tissues associated with reproduction, quantitatively not high, but that might explain some of the effects of β-carotene observed in porcine reproduction. Biologically, the retinal is active in vision and plays a role in reproduction, whereas retinoic acid is essential for cells' average growth and differentiation.

Natural sources

In its active form, vitamin A is scarce in nature, as it is found as an ester only in fish oil, meat meal (liver tissue representing the major source), and oilseeds. Green plants contain almost 100 molecules with provitamin A activity. β-carotene is the most abundant and active precursor of vitamin A, although the content varies significantly according to the species, state of maturity, and preservation. Maize and its derivatives contain significant quantities of pigmenting carotenoids, with much lower provitamin activity (cryptoxanthin) or lacking provitamin activity, such as lutein and zeaxanthin.

The potency of yellow corn is only about one-eighth that of good roughage. There is evidence that yellow corn may lose carotene rapidly during storage. For instance, a hybrid corn high in carotene lost one-half of its carotene in 8 months of storage at 25°C and about three-quarters in 3 years. Less carotene was lost during storage at 7°C (Quackenbush, 1963). The bioavailability of natural β-carotene was less than chemically synthesized forms (White *et al.*, 1993). Aside from yellow corn and its by-products, practically all concentrates used in feeding animals are devoid of vitamin A value, or are nearly so.

Commercial forms

The vitamin A activity contained in the ingredients of typical swine diets is very unpredictable. Therefore, the provision of vitamin A in swine diets is achieved mainly through synthetic forms. The most convenient and effective means of providing vitamin A is the inclusion in premixes added to feed.

The major sources of supplemental vitamin A used in animal diets are trans-retinyl acetate and trans-retinyl palmitate (Schoenbeck *et al.*, 1994). The propionate ester is much less common (McGinnis, 1988). These are available in gelatin beadlet product forms for protection against oxidative destruction in premixes, mash, and pelleted and extruded feeds. Carbohydrates, gelatin, and antioxidants are generally included inside the beadlet to stabilize the vitamin A to provide physical and chemical protection against factors either ordinarily present in the feed or due to feeding treatment and storage that are destructive to vitamin A. Unprotected vitamin A oxidizes rapidly in feedstuffs when moisture levels exceed 12%.

The vitamin A acetate products most frequently used in swine feeds contain 500,000 and 1,000,000 IU or United States Pharmacopeia (USP) units per gram of product. The values of 1 IU or 1 USP are the same and equal the activity of the 0.3 µg of all-*trans*-retinol (1 mg retinol = 3,333 IU vitamin A), or 0.344 µg of all-*trans* retinyl acetate, 0.359 µg propionate or 0.55 µg of palmitate, or 0.6 µg of β-carotene, that is to say, 1 mg of β-carotene is equivalent to 1,667 IU of vitamin A. Other forms included in the generic denomination of vitamin A are the aldehyde or retinal form, which plays an essential role in the development of vision and reproduction, and the acid form (retinoic acid), essential in cellular growth and differentiation.

Several factors can influence the loss of vitamin A from feedstuffs during storage. The trace minerals in feeds and supplements, particularly copper, are detrimental to vitamin A stability (Yang *et al.*, 2021a,d). Dash and Mitchell (1976) reported the vitamin A content of 1,293 commercial feeds over 3 years, and the loss of vitamin A was over 50% in 1 year. Vitamin A loss in commercial feeds was evident even if the commercial feeds contained stabilized vitamin A supplements.

It is therefore important to carefully assess the quality of the commercial product. The gelatin beadlet, in which the vitamin A ester is emulsified into a gelatin-antioxidant viscous liquid formulation and spray-dried into discrete dry particles, results in products with good chemical stability, physical stability, and excellent biologic availability (Shields *et al.*, 1982). The reaction between gelatin and sugar makes the beadlet insoluble in water and gives it a more resistant coating that can sustain higher pressure, friction, temperature, and humidity (Frye, 1994).

Vitamin A supplements should not be stored for prolonged periods before feeding. Chen (1990) measured the stability of 3 commercial cross-linked vitamin A beadlets on the market in trace mineral premixes and feeds. After 3 months of storage at high temperatures and humidity, vitamin A retention varied from 30% to 80%, depending on the antioxidant present in the beadlet.

Vitamin A (and carotene) destruction also occurs when feed is processed with steam and pressure. Pelleting effects of vitamin A in the feed are determined by die thickness and hole size, which produce frictional heat and a shearing effect that can break supplemental vitamin A beadlets and expose the vitamin. In addition, steam application exposes feed to heat and moisture. In a 30% concentrate pelleted at 93°C, after 3 months of storage at high temperature and humidity, retention varied from 57% to 62%. Running fines back through the pellet mill exposes vitamin A to the same factors a second time. Between 14% and 40% of vitamin A present at mixing may be destroyed during pelleting of swine feed (Kostadinović *et al.*, 2014; Spasevski *et al.*, 2015). In feeds, PUFA and peroxides also contribute to vitamin A oxidation. One gram of PUFA can destroy 3,000 IU of vitamin A. In practical situations, vitamin A in swine feeds and premixes is moderately stable, and losses may vary between 0.5% and 11% per month.

Metabolism
Absorption and transport
Dietary carotenoids and retinyl esters (e.g., acetate) are released by pepsin in the stomach. Vitamin A and β-carotene become dispersed in micelles before absorption through the intestine (O'Byrne and Blaner, 2013). These molecules are hydrolyzed to retinol in the intestine (duodenum) by pancreatic retinyl ester hydrolase, absorbed as free alcohol retinol, and then re-esterified in the mucosa, primarily to palmitate. β-carotene in feed is cleaved in the intestinal mucosa by dioxygenase, an enzyme, to retinal, which is then reduced to retinol (vitamin A), as described by Harrison (2012). Early researchers, including Hentges *et al.* (1952b) and Fidge *et al.* (1969), compared the properties of the rat and hog mucosal cleavage enzymes and found similar mechanisms of catalyzing β-carotene to retinal.

The leading site of vitamin A and carotenoid absorption is the mucosa of the proximal jejunum. These micelles are composed of mixtures of bile salts, monoglycerides, and long-chain fatty acids, together with vitamins D, E, and K, all of which influence the transfer of vitamin A and β-carotene to the intestinal cell. Pigs do not appear to absorb or store significant quantities of intact β-carotene (Harrison, 2012). For the pig, almost all the β-carotene is converted to vitamin A in the small intestine, which is converted to various esters. Either dietary retinol or retinol resulting from the conversion of carotenoids is then esterified with a long-chain fatty acid, usually palmitate, in the enterocytes (Poor *et al.*, 1987; Debier and Larondelle, 2005; Harrison, 2012; Ross and Harrison, 2013).

β-carotene present in feed is converted to retinal in the intestinal mucosa by an enzyme. The retinal is then reduced to retinol (vitamin A). However, extensive evidence exists also for random (excentric) cleavage, resulting in retinoic acid and retinal, with a preponderance of apocarotenals formed as intermediates (Wolf, 1995). The main site of vitamin A and carotenoid absorption is the mucosa of the proximal jejunum. Although carotenoids are typically converted to retinol in the intestinal mucosa, they may also be converted in the liver and other organs (McGinnis, 1988).

Intestinal absorption of vitamin A is believed to be 80–90%, while that of β-carotene is about 50–60% (Olson, 1984). Many factors may modify it, either positively, such as the inclusion of fats in the diet, the addition of antioxidants, and the use of moderate levels of vitamin E or other synthetic antioxidants (Noel and Brinkhaus, 1998) or negatively, such as high levels of vitamin E, the presence of aflatoxins (Harvey *et al.*, 1995; Cabassi *et al.*, 2004) or enteric infections (Lauridsen *et al.*, 2021a). The efficiency of vitamin A absorption decreases somewhat with very high doses. Thus, intestinal diseases reduce their levels of plasma and hepatic reserves, which increases the requirements for vitamin A because of poor absorption and oxidation induced by the cellular immune response. Vitamin A deficiencies reduce resistance to intestinal challenges (Lauridsen *et al.*, 2021b).

Several factors affect the absorption of carotenoids. *Cis-trans* isomerism of the carotenoids is important in determining their absorbability, with the *trans* forms being more efficiently absorbed (Stahl *et al.*, 1995). Dietary fat is important in the absorption process (Fichter and Mitchell, 1997). Dietary antioxidants (e.g., vitamin E) also affect carotenoid utilization and absorption. Interactions between different fat-soluble compounds competing for the same absorption mechanism have been identified. In pigs, there is evidence of the inhibition of retinyl acetate over tocopherol acetate *in vitro* (Lauridsen *et al.*, 2002) or *in vivo* (Johnson *et al.*, 2019). It is uncertain whether the antioxidants contribute directly to the efficient absorption or whether they protect both carotene and vitamin A from oxidative breakdown. Protein deficiency reduces the absorption of carotene from the intestine.

The retinyl esters, triglycerides, phospholipids, and cholesteryl esters are transported mainly by lymph chylomicrons to the liver (Riabroy and Tanumihardjo, 2014). Chylomicrons, through exocytosis, pass from enterocytes into the lymph and eventually enter the general blood circulation (Darroch, 2000). Hydrolysis of the ester storage form mobilizes vitamin A from the liver as free retinol. Retinol is released from the hepatocyte as a complex with retinol-binding protein (RBP) and transported to peripheral tissues (Figure 4.2). The liver takes up the majority of dietary vitamin A that is absorbed into the body within 4 to 6 hours.

In pigs, liver storage levels of vitamin A increased from 56 nmol/g to 89 nmol/g liver when dietary vitamin A levels increased from the NRC (1988) recommended levels to 1.6 times the NRC requirement. In lipocytes, which represent only 7% of total liver cells, the storage form of vitamin A represents a lipoglycoprotein complex consisting of 96% retinyl esters and 4% unesterified retinol (Darroch, 2000; O'Byrne and Blaner, 2013).

Retinol, associated with RBP, circulates in peripheral tissues complexed to a thyroxine-binding protein, transthyretin (Chew *et al.*, 1991; Blomhoff *et al.*, 1991; Ross and Harrison, 2013). In most species, 90% of serum RBP is saturated with retinol. The half-life of the *holo*-RBP-transthyretin complex in plasma is approximately 11–16 hours. Unbound *holo*-RBP and *apo*-RBP are turned over in about 4 hours. Dever *et al.* (2011) reported that chylomicron-derived retinyl esters, rather than RBP-bound retinol, are likely to be the significant source of retinol

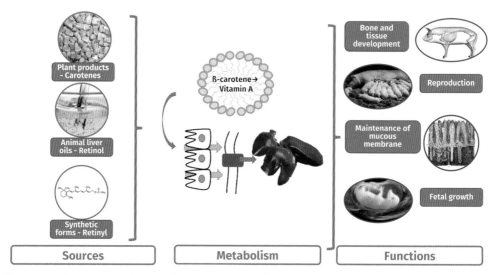

Figure 4.2 Main sources and types of the precursors of vitamin A. Schematic illustration of the absorption, the purpose of the metabolites, and the main functions developed

in the milk of vitamin A-deficient lactating sows. Also, uterine RBP helps to transfer retinol and retinoic acid from the maternal blood supply to the areolae in the placenta.

The retinol-transthyretin complex is transported to target tissues, where the complex binds to a cell-surface receptor. The receptor was found in all tissues known to require retinol for their function, particularly the pigment epithelium of the eye (Wolf, 2007). Once the retinoids are transferred into the cell, they are quickly bound by specific RBP in the cell cytosol. These intracellular RBP show high specificity and affinity for particular retinoids and seem to control retinoid metabolism both qualitatively and quantitatively. They protect retinoids from nonspecific interactions, and on the quantitative side, they have been stated to "chaperone" access of metabolic enzymes to retinoids. (Solomons, 2006). The intracellular RBP binds retinol, retinal, and retinoic acid to protect against decomposition, solubilize them in an aqueous medium, render them nontoxic, and transport them within cells to their site of action (Ross and Harrison, 2013). These intracellular RBP also present the retinoids to the appropriate enzymes for metabolism (Wolf, 1991, 1993).

In target cells, retinol can be either reconverted to retinyl esters or oxidized to retinal and, in a second step, to retinoic acid. The pathway selected is influenced by the presence of specific cytoplasmic RBP. Conversion of retinol to retinyl esters occurs by lecithin: retinol acyltransferase and acyl-CoA : retinol acyl transferase. The NADH retinol dehydrogenase mediates the oxidation of retinol to retinoic acid. Retinoic acid is formed from the irreversible oxidation of the retinal (O'Byrne and Blaner, 2013).

The final key mediators of vitamin A function in the cells are the all-*trans* retinoic acid and 11-*cis* retinal. The all-*trans* retinoic acid is a regulator of gene transcription for all biological roles in cell growth, differentiation, organogenesis, immunity, bone development, and other functions. In contrast, 11-*cis* retinal acts as a chromophore for visual functions.

Some of the principal forms of intracellular or cytoplasmic RBP are CRBP (I and II), cellular retinoic acid-binding proteins (CRABP, I and II), cellular retinaldehyde binding protein (CRALBP), and 6 nuclear retinoic acid receptors – retinoic acid receptor (RAR) and retinoid X receptor (RXR) – with α, β and γ forms. There are 2 classes of nuclear receptors with all-*trans* retinoic acid, the ligand for RAR; 9-*cis*-retinoic acid is the ligand for RXR (Kastner *et al.*, 1994; Kliewer *et al.*, 1994). Vitamin A also contributes to maintaining lysozyme stability inside the cells.

Storage and excretion

The liver typically contains about 90% of the body's total vitamin A. The remainder is stored in the kidneys, lungs, adrenals, and blood, with small amounts found in other organs and tissues. Serum retinol is not always sensitive to vitamin A status (Debier and Larondelle, 2005). In contrast to gastrointestinal tract absorption, some tissues, such as the eyes, prefer *cis*-isomers of carotenoids (Darroch, 2000; O'Byrne and Blaner, 2013).

Carotenoid interactions can affect uptake from the gastrointestinal tract and tissues and lead to differences in tissue storage levels. Non-provitamin A carotenoids such as lutein, lycopene, and xanthophylls can reduce β-carotene cleavage to retinal through competitive inhibition of β-carotene-15–15′-dioxygenase (Darroch, 2000).

Early investigations by Grummer *et al.* (1948) profiled the concentrations of vitamin A in plasma from birth through weaning compared to those in mature pregnant sows. Vitamin A blood values for mature pregnant sows were similar to those of weanling pigs but quite different from the blood values of newborns. The researchers could not detect any measurable amount of carotene in swine blood. Christensen *et al.* (1958) reported early on that administration of vitamin A caused rapid storage and sharp increases in vitamin A content in the liver. Several studies have shown that the liver can store enough vitamin A to protect the animal from long periods of dietary scarcity. This large storage capacity must be considered in studies of vitamin A requirements to ensure that intakes that appear adequate for a given function are not being supplemented by reserves stored before the observation period. Wemheuer *et al.* (1996) reported that serum retinol of the lowest vitamin A-treated boars began to decrease only after 3 months because of the high retinol reserve capacity of the liver.

The main excretory pathway for vitamin A is elimination as glucuronide conjugates in the bile before fecal excretion, but elimination can also occur in the urine. Oxidized, polar metabolites of retinol, retinal, and retinoic acid that retain intact chains in their structures are converted into β-glucuronides, which pass into the bile. Once in the bile, these glucuronides can be lost in the feces or recycled in the enterohepatic circulation. Oxidized, chain-shortened metabolites of retinoic acid display little or no biological activity and are predominantly excreted in the urine. Esterification of retinol in tissues also represents a recycling mechanism and, together with enterohepatic recycling, influences the vitamin A status of the pig. The conversion of retinol to a retinyl-phosphomannose metabolite relates to vitamin A role in cell communication and differentiation. The regulation of vitamin A metabolism and expression of RBP depends on vitamin status or all-*trans* retinoic acid production (Darroch, 2000; O'Byrne and Blaner, 2013).

Biochemical functions

Vitamin A is necessary to support growth, immunity, health, and life in all major animal species (Debier and Larondelle, 2005; Nabi *et al.*, 2020). Without vitamin A, animals will cease to grow and eventually die. Vitamin A and its derivatives, the retinoids, profoundly influence organ development, cell proliferation, and cell differentiation, and their deficiency originates or predisposes several disabilities (McDowell, 2000a; Esteban-Pretel *et al.*, 2010). During embryogenesis, retinoic acid has been shown to influence processes governing the patterning of neural tissue and craniofacial, eye, and olfactory system development; retinoic acid affects the outcome, regeneration, and well-being of neurons (Debier and Larondelle, 2005; Asson-Batres *et al.*, 2009).

Recent discoveries have revealed that most, if not all, actions of vitamin A in development, differentiation, and metabolism are mediated by nuclear receptor proteins that bind retinoic acid, the active form of vitamin A (Iskakova *et al.*, 2015). A group of retinoic acid-binding proteins (receptors) function in the nucleus by attaching to promoter regions in several specific genes to stimulate their transcription and thus affect growth, development, and differentiation. RAR in cell nuclei are structurally homologous and functionally analogous to the known receptors for steroid hormones, thyroid hormone (triiodothyronine), and vitamin D 1,25(OH)$_2$D$_3$. Very early, it was recognized that vitamin A sources affected ergocalciferol requirement (Hendricks *et al.*, 1967). Thus, retinoic acid is now recognized as a hormone regulating many genes' transcription activity (Ross, 1993; Shin and McGrane, 1997). Vitamin A can also inhibit the action of lipopolysaccharides (LPS) on the intestinal epithelial barrier function and tight junction proteins (He *et al.*, 2019).

Vision

Retinol is utilized in the aldehyde form (all-*trans*-retinaldehyde) and transformed to 11-*cis*-retinaldehyde in the retina of the eye. It forms part of the prosthetic group (opsin) in rhodopsin for dim light vision (rods) and as the prosthetic group in iodopsin for bright light and color vision (cones). When light falls on the retina, rhodopsin breaks down into opsin and all-*cis*-retinaldehyde, which reverts to all-*trans*-retinaldehyde, initiating an action potential that travels up the optic nerve. In the dark, the all-*trans*-retinaldehyde is isomerized back to all-*cis*-retinaldehyde, and the latter recombines with opsin to regenerate rhodopsin, resensitizing the retina to light. Rhodopsin is vital for sight, especially in swine adapting to low-intensity light in intensive production. Retinoic acid has been found to support growth and tissue differentiation but not vision or all aspects of reproduction (McDowell, 2000a; Solomons, 2006; O'Byrne and Blaner, 2013).

Tissue differentiation

Retinoic acid regulates the differentiation of epithelial, connective, adipose, and hematopoietic tissues (Safonova *et al.*, 1994; O'Byrne and Blaner, 2013). The nature of the growth and differentiation response elicited by retinoic acid depends upon cell type. Retinoic acid can inhibit many cell types, reducing adipose tissues in meat-producing animals (Suryawan and Hu, 1997; Brandebourg and Hu, 2005; O'Byrne and Blaner, 2013; Ayuso *et al.*, 2015b). Proliferation and cellular aggregation are both critical features for the survival and self-renewal of primordial germ cells (PGCs).

The activities of retinoic acid are crucial in early embryonic development (Kam *et al.*, 2012). During gastrulation, retinoic acid signaling exerts its function in the regionalization of all 3 germ layers along the anteroposterior axis, especially in the mesoderm. Vitamin A-deficient rats fed retinoic acid were healthy in every respect, with normal estrus and conception, but failed to give birth and resorbed their fetuses (Chew *et al.*, 1984; Chew, 1993). When retinol was given even at a late stage in pregnancy, fetuses were saved, which can be related to proteins in uterine secretions induced by progesterone that are affected by retinol (Clawitter *et al.*, 1990).

Early reports indicated that male rats on retinoic acid were healthy but produced no sperm, and without vitamin A, both sexes were blind. However, without affecting sight, suboptimal vitamin levels can affect the reproduction of domestic mammals (Kolb and Seehawer, 1997; Kumar *et al.*, 2010), and effects have been observed in sows (Schoenbeck *et al.*, 1994;

Pusateri *et al.*, 1996; Washington *et al.*, 1997; Whaley *et al.*, 1997, 2000; Lindemann *et al.*, 2008) and boars (Wemheuer *et al.*, 1996).

Keratinization of epithelial tissues results in loss of function in the alimentary, genital, reproductive, respiratory, and urinary tracts. Such altered characteristics increase the susceptibility of the affected tissue to infection. Thus, diarrhea and pneumonia are typical secondary effects of vitamin A deficiency. It has been suggested that retinoic acid is an effective antidiabetic agent that could be considered in treating type 2 diabetes (Manolescu *et al.*, 2010; Wolf, 2010).

Immunity
Adequate dietary vitamin A is necessary to help maintain resilience to stress and disease (Chew and Park, 2004) and wound healing (Polcz and Barbul, 2019). Disease resistance is a function of vitamin A, which is required to maintain mucous membranes and the normal function of the adrenal gland (Nabi *et al.*, 2020). Vitamin A deficiency can impair the regeneration of normal mucosal epithelium damaged by infection or inflammation (Ahmed *et al.*, 1990; Stephensen *et al.*, 1996) and thus could increase the severity of an infectious episode and prolong recovery from that episode. An animal's ability to resist infectious disease depends on a responsive immune system; a vitamin A deficiency causes a reduced immune response. Many experiments with laboratory and domestic animals have frequently demonstrated the effects of both clinical and subclinical deficiencies of vitamin A on the production of antibodies, the number of lymphocytes, and the resistance of different tissues against microbial infection or parasitic infestation (Bebravicius *et al.*, 1987; Kelley and Easter, 1987; Vlasova *et al.*, 2013; Kandasamy *et al.*, 2014; Zhou *et al.*, 2021a).

Several studies indicate that specific carotenoids without vitamin A activity have antioxidant capacities. Such carotenoids can enhance many aspects of immune functions, act directly as antimutagens and anticarcinogens, protect against radiation damage, and block the damaging effects of photosensitizers (Chew, 1995; Lindshield and Erdman, Jr., 2006). β-carotene can function as a chain-breaking antioxidant and aid healing after injuries (Polcz and Barbul, 2019). It deactivates reactive chemical species such as singlet oxygen, triplet photochemical sensitizers, and free radicals, which would otherwise induce potentially harmful processes like lipid peroxidation (McDowell, 2004; Nabi *et al.*, 2020). Vitamin A can also protect against LPS's toxic effects in the gut (He *et al.*, 2019).

Bone development
Vitamin A plays a role in normal bone development by controlling the activity of osteoclasts of the epithelial cartilage, the cells responsible for bone resorption (Blair *et al.*, 1992; Tanumihardjo, 2013). In vitamin A deficiency, the activity of osteoclasts is reduced with excessive deposition of periosteal bone due to stimulation of osteoblasts (depositing bone cells) and joint irritation. However, hypervitaminosis A also causes bone lesions (Wolke *et al.*, 1968).

Reproduction
Chew *et al.* (1982) and Brief and Chew (1985) suggested that β-carotene is independent of vitamin A in swine reproduction. Their research indicated that maternal plasma vitamin A or β-carotene elevation improves embryonic survival because more uterine-specific proteins are secreted. One protein with a great affinity for retinol has been identified in the endometrium, the ovary, the testicle, and the embryo. Talavera and Chew (1988) found that β-carotene was more effective in stimulating progesterone secretion by pig *corpus luteum in vitro* than either retinol or retinoic acid and the preparation of uterine mucosa. Previous studies of the effects

of injections of vitamin A or supplementation of the ration had demonstrated a positive impact on reproductive yield in primiparous sows with deficiencies (Brief and Chew, 1985) or in the number of piglets born alive when it was administered in concentrations of 11,000 IU/kg feed (Coffey and Britt, 1993).

The functions of vitamin A in reproduction have not been sufficiently investigated, but there is sufficient evidence of its influence on reproductive success (Chew, 1993; Preś et al., 1993; Whaley et al., 1997, 2000; Debier and Larondelle, 2005; Lindemann et al., 2008; Kumar et al., 2010). Still, the vitamin A functions on reproduction could be related to the intracellular transport of vitamin A and its passage to the embryo, where it is probably needed to regulate cellular differentiation and proliferation, steroid production (Talavera and Chew, 1988), immune response (Thomas et al., 1947; Hoskinson et al., 1989; 1992), and transcription of specific genes. Secretion of porcine uterine RBP increases 390-fold between days 10 and 13 of gestation (Mahan and Vallet, 1997), a critical period in embryo development and survival. The increase in RBP may ensure the delivery of retinol and other compounds to the conceptus and protect fetal tissues against oxidative reactions enhancing early embryonic survival. In this respect, it has also been demonstrated in pigs that mutations in the retinol-binding protein 4 (RBP4) gene are directly related to the number of piglets born and weaned (Terman et al., 2007; Omelka et al., 2008; Mencik et al., 2019).

Whaley et al. (1997) presented data leading them to conclude that retinol palmitate treatment may influence the follicular environment and thus would synchronize the resumption of meiosis and enhance early embryonic survival in pigs. This study injected retinol palmitate (1,000,000 IU) 6 days before estrus to gilts fed high-energy diets. Gilts had restored embryo survival if vitamin A was injected, possibly due to decreased variation in embryo size. Whaley et al. (1997) indicated that vitamin A also increased serum concentrations of progesterone and slightly advanced the embryo's development. Whaley et al. (1997) concluded that the improvement in litter size is not due to an increased ovulation rate but to effects on embryonic survival. The lack of vitamin A impact on ovulation rate reported supported earlier findings by Coffey and Britt (1993). A later report by Whaley et al. (2000) concluded that treatment with vitamin A might alter the pattern of follicular hormone production and stimulate the earlier resumption of meiosis, causing more oocytes to reach an advanced meiotic stage by the time of ovulation. Vitamin A may promote more uniform and advanced oocytes, and early embryos can have a higher survival rate in utero.

Da Silveira et al. (1998) reported similar positive results of vitamin A (450,000 IU retinol palmitate) injection at weaning or mating on the number of piglets born alive, total number born, and litter weight. Darroch et al. (1998) reported a cooperative regional study combining 417 litters from 4 universities. Intramuscular injections of 250,000 IU or 500,000 IU of vitamin A were given at weaning and breeding. The researchers reported that vitamin A injections increased the number of pigs weaned per litter but did not influence the number of pigs born alive.

In contrast to the numerous studies reporting positive effects associated with vitamin A injections, Pusateri et al. (1996) found no effect of vitamin A injection (1,000,000 IU) on total or live litter size. Injections were given at weaning or on the following days: 0, 2, 6, 10, 13, 19, 30, 70, or 110 post-breeding. These authors suggested that multiple injections or a sustained-release form of vitamin A or β-carotene were required to elicit a response.

Likewise, Washington et al. (1997) reported no effect on the number of embryos or embryo survival in gilts induced to ovulate. The study involved a minimal number of gilts with an injection of 1,000,000 IU of vitamin A before breeding. In disagreement with the numerous positive responses reported with β-carotene injections, Stender et al. (1999) observed no benefits of β-carotene injection on litter parameters. Still, they did not report the levels or stages when the injection was given. Kolb and Seehawer (1997) reviewed the significance of carotenes and vitamin A for the reproduction of cattle, horses, and pigs. It was found that retinoic acid is necessary for the function of the germ cell epithelial, Sertoli cells, and interstitial cells. The promoted synthesis of proteins, estrogens, and progesterone was included in the actions credited to *cis*- and all-*trans*-retinoic acid. During embryogenesis, retinoic acid has been shown to influence processes governing the patterning of neural tissue and craniofacial, eye, and olfactory system development. Retinoic acid influences neuron development, regeneration, and well-being (Asson-Batres *et al.*, 2009). Retinoic acid also regulates the differentiation of epithelial, connective, and hematopoietic tissues (Safonova *et al.*, 1994).

Meat quality
Vitamin A has also been associated with certain characteristics related to meat quality attributed to the possible action of vitamin A in controlling the differentiation of adipocytes, such as intramuscular fat content (D'Souza *et al.*, 2003) or the percentage of certain fatty acids deposited in different tissues (Gregoire *et al.*, 1998; Brandebourg and Hu, 2005; O'Byrne and Blaner, 2013; Ayuso *et al.*, 2015b) and in the activity of certain desaturating enzymes (Suryawan and Hu, 1997; Olivares *et al.*, 2009b).

However, responses vary among genetic lines, age, length, and level of vitamin A supplementation. D'Souza *et al.* (2003) reported that crossbred (Large White × Landrace × Duroc) female pigs, fed grower and finisher diets without vitamin A, improved intramuscular fat without detrimental effect on growth and carcass quality. Olivares *et al.* (2009a) reported that Duroc × (Large White × Landrace) castrated male pigs fed with diets enriched with vitamin A (100,000 IU/kg *vs.* 7,500 IU/kg) showed a higher C16:0 and total saturated fatty acid levels in liver lipids, and reduced C18:1 n-9 and total monounsaturated fatty acid levels in subcutaneous backfat without affecting main fatty acids of intramuscular lipids.

In contrast, Tous *et al.* (2014), comparing the effects of diets with 0, 1,250, and 5,000 IU vitamin A/kg feed fed to barrows, found that omitting dietary vitamin A does not affect performance, decreases perirenal fat and possibly overall fat deposition without a significant reduction on intramuscular fat. But Ayuso *et al.* (2015b) observed that suppression of vitamin A during the growing phase increased the preadipocyte number in longissimus thoracic muscle in the early growth period and the neutral lipid content and composition with higher monounsaturated fatty acids and lower saturated fatty acid content at the end of the finishing period of Iberian pigs, comparing with pigs fed 10,000 IU of vitamin A/kg feed.

In most cases, the mechanism of vitamin A action is similar to that of steroid hormones. It is carried out by binding to specific receptors located in the cellular cytoplasm of target tissues. When the active form (retinoic acid) is bound to the receptor, the receptor translocates to the nucleus, where it attaches to chromatin acceptors and causes the production of a messenger ribonucleic acid (RNA) and, consequently, of a specific cytoplasmic protein (Shin and McGrane, 1997).

Nutritional assessment
Retinol and its fatty acid esters are the compounds relevant to the determination of vitamin A status. Serum retinol is not always sensitive to vitamin A status. Surles *et al.* (2011) suggested that the vitamin A form 3,4-didehydroretinol in lactating swine serum is a good indicator of vitamin A status and milk, 4-didehydroretinol : retinol may replace serum measurements during lactation. Plasma retinol has been used as a general indicator of vitamin A status primarily for determining a vitamin A deficiency defined in humans as a plasma retinol level <0.7 µmol/l or 196 µg/l (Höller *et al.*, 2018). However, plasma level is not a good

indicator since the plasma concentration is under strict homeostatic control (Tanumihardjo, 2011) and can be influenced by health status, e.g., depression in case of infection or inflammation (Tanumihardjo *et al.*, 2016). Liver reserves are the gold standard because the liver contains most total body vitamin A stores unless the overall status is deficient.

In blood and tissues, retinol can be determined using a reversed-phase high-performance liquid chromatograph (HPLC). Retinol can be measured using dried blood spots (DBS), providing the ability to collect small blood samples under field conditions with limited infrastructure. Stability issues have limited widespread practical application. Still, some improvements have been made, indicating its validity for assessing a low (or a high) retinol status and not a broader evaluation of its nutritional status (Gannon *et al.*, 2020). The provitamin A carotenoids and primarily β-carotene could be used as an indirect measurement of vitamin A status by considering, as discussed in previous paragraphs, that the biological activity of these compounds relative to retinol is estimated to be in the order of 50% for β-carotene and 25% for carotenoids with only one β-ionone end group. Carotenoids are mainly assessed from plasma using HPLC coupled with visible spectrophotometry. The feed industry has used spectrophotometric and chemical (Carr–Price) methods to determine the biopotency of vitamin A, but accuracy, sensitivity, and specificity have been variable, limiting their use. These methods have been replaced mainly by growth, microbiological, or analytical assays with assay variations for vitamin A and β-carotene ranging from 10% to 25% and 5% to 20%, respectively (Darroch, 2000).

Deficiency signs
Factors causing vitamin A deficiency
Vitamin A deficiency is unlikely in practice (Darroch, 2000), and marginal deficiencies may result when working with minimum levels in feed or vitamin premixes stored for a long time (Yang *et al.*, 2021a). Under stressful conditions, such as abnormal temperatures or exposure to mycotoxins and disease conditions, requirements and the probability of deficiency are higher. The efficiency of conversion of ß-carotene to vitamin A is reduced under these conditions.

For example, coccidiosis destroys the gut's vitamin A and injures the intestinal wall's microvilli (Joachim and Shrestha, 2019). Mycotoxins cause digestive disturbances such as vomiting, diarrhea, and internal bleeding, in piglets. They can also interfere with the absorption of dietary vitamins A, D_3, E, and K (van Heugten, 2000; Surai and Dvorska, 2005; Joachim and Shrestha, 2019). Nitrates and nitrites can affect the utilization of carotenes in growing pigs (Wood *et al.*, 1967). After studying the effects of nitrates and nitrites in feed, Hutagalung *et al.* (1968) reported that serum vitamin A values were reduced when potassium nitrite (0.3%) was included in the diet. However, nitrate treatments did not affect liver, serum, or methemoglobin levels.

Signs of vitamin A deficiency
In pigs, deficiency symptoms appear when serum vitamin A levels fall below 0.35 µmol/l (Cooper *et al.*, 1997). Marginal deficiencies are characterized by the following:

- night blindness or hemeralopia
- infertility in breeding animals
- abortion or the birth of dead, weak, or blind young (Heaney *et al.*, 1963; O'Byrne and Blaner, 2013)
- reduced appetite and delayed growth rate
- changes in skeletal development (Darroch, 2000)
- a fall in the number of antibodies and a reduction in cellular immunity (Kandasamy *et al.*, 2014; Hu *et al.*, 2020; Zhou *et al.*, 2021a)

- rapid depletion of hepatic reserves (Surles *et al.*, 2007; Tanumihardjo, 2011)
- a drop in muscle glycogen reserves (Sundeen *et al.*, 1980).

More pronounced deficiencies and severe disruptions occur in respiratory and intestinal epithelia (Chew and Park, 2004; Tanumihardjo, 2011; Wang *et al.*, 2020; Zhou *et al.*, 2021b) and, in extreme cases, blindness and death (Darroch, 2000).

A stratified squamous, keratinizing epithelium replaces the mucous epithelium. The mucous membranes of the nasal passage, mouth, esophagus, and pharynx are affected and develop white pustules (Darroch, 2000). The kidneys may be distended with uric acid deposits, and the epithelium of the eye is affected, producing exudates and, eventually, xerophthalmia (Figures 4.3).

Rahman *et al.* (1996) recorded signs associated with vitamin A deficiency on a commercial hog farm and found agreement with observations reported by earlier researchers (Hughes *et al.*, 1928). Goodwin and Jennings (1958) and Palludan (1961) described the aborted fetuses, stillbirths, debilitation, and congenital malformations associated with vitamin A deficiency in pregnant sows (Heaney *et al.*, 1963). In pigs, the absence of vitamin A results principally in nervous system symptoms, such as unsteady gait, incoordination, trembling of the legs, spasms, and paralysis of the hind limbs (Hentges *et al.*, 1952a; Sheffy *et al.*, 1954; Frape *et al.*, 1959a; Darroch, 2000) (Figure 4.3). Eye lesions are less common (Hale, 1935). Reduced growth is a sign of vitamin A deficiency in all species. Insufficient vitamin A in rats reduces the efficiency of the urea synthesis pathway, thus accounting for the increased amino nitrogen excretion seen with the deficiency (John and Sivakumar, 1989). The effect of vitamin A deficiency in swine on appetite or rate of gain often does not occur until eventual paralysis and weakness prohibit movement to the feeder (Cunha, 1977). Increased cerebrospinal fluid (CSF) pressure is often associated with vitamin A deficiency. Nelson *et al.* (1962) reported that 18–35 mg of vitamin A per kilogram of body weight per day could lower CSF pressure. Nelson *et al.* (1964) reported CSF fluid pressure as a very sensitive criterion for establishing the vitamin A status of pigs fed vitamin A or vitamin A acid.

Hjarde *et al.* (1961) reported that the influence of vitamin A deficiency depends on the animal's age at the time of depletion. During reproduction and lactation, vitamin A deficiency in the sow produces the following clinical signs: failure of estrus; resorption of young; wobbly gait; weaving and crossing of the hind legs while walking; dropping of the ears; curved posture

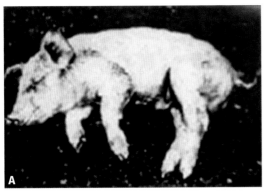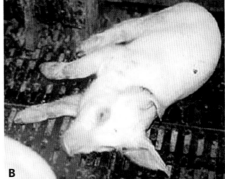

Figure 4.3 Vitamin A deficiency: (A) pig exhibiting partial paralysis and seborrhea. The pig is in the initial stages of spasms (source: courtesy of J.F. Hentges, R.H. Grummer, and the University of Wisconsin); (B) pig exhibiting partial paralysis (source: courtesy of Done)

with head down to one side; spasms; loss of control of hindquarters and forequarters, hence the inability to stand up; and impaired vision (Cunha, 1977; Heaney *et al.*, 1963).

Depending on the degree of severity of vitamin A deficiency, fetuses were resorbed, born dead, or carried to term. Fetuses carried to term showed a variety of defects, including various stages of arrested formation of the eyes (sometimes complete lack of eyeballs), harelips, cleft palate, misplaced kidneys, accessory ear-like growths, some with one eye, some with one large and one small eye and bilateral cryptorchidism (Hale, 1935; Guilbert *et al.*, 1937; Sheffy *et al.*, 1954; Cunha, 1977) (Figure 4.4). Hjarde *et al.* (1961) reported that vitamin A deficiency at breeding age led to impaired spermiogenesis, metaplasia of the oviduct, cervix, and vagina, and brain compression.

Epithelial tissue disorders

Since the 1930s, vitamin A supplementation has been used to protect the epithelial tissues and mucous membranes, which are natural barriers to pathogens and prevent infections (Latshaw, 1991, Eggersdorfer *et al.*, 2012; Kandasamy *et al.*, 2014), and to assist wound healing (Polcz and Barbul, 2019).

Respiratory problems in vitamin A-deficient animals may relate to altered enzyme regulation and activity. In vitamin A-deficient guinea pigs, superoxide dismutase, glutathione peroxidase activities, and glutathione levels were reduced. These compounds protect the lung from toxic oxygen free radicals. In addition, cytochrome P-450 enzymes involved in the microsomal detoxification of inhaled xenobiotics were increased, and this could have contributed to the pool of reactive free radicals in damaged lung tissue (Darroch, 2000).

Severe vitamin A deficiency causes increased intestinal mucosal cell numbers (hyperplasia), reduced intestinal mucosal cell size, the loss of mucosal protein, reduced villus height and crypt depth, and diminished gut disaccharidases, transpeptidase, and alkaline phosphatase activity (Wang *et al.*, 2020; Zhou *et al.*, 2021b). Vitamin A deficiency leads to a breakdown of the epithelium of many systems in the body. Loss of membrane integrity, in turn, alters water retention and impairs resistance to infection (Lauridsen *et al.*, 2021b). Bacteria and other pathogenic microorganisms may invade tissues and enter the body, producing infections secondary to the original vitamin A deficiency signs (Kandasamy *et al.*, 2014).

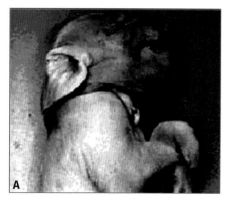 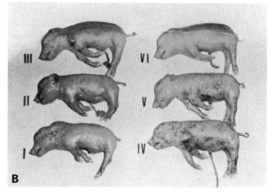

Figure 4.4 Vitamin A deficiency: (A) malformations in newborn piglets due to deficiency of vitamin A in the sow's diet; (B) malformations: microphthalmia, hypotrichosis, contracture of the limbs, and general edema (Source: Palludan, 1961)

Impairment of the immune function
Low dietary vitamin A has been shown to cause reduced antibody production, depressed T-cell responses, distributed immunoglobulin (Ig) metabolism, reduced neutrophil chemot- axis, phagocytosis, and decreased resistance to infection by bacterial and viral pathogens and protozoan enteropathogens (Vlasova *et al.*, 2013; Kandasamy *et al.*, 2014; Patel and Vajdy, 2015).

Vitamin A deficiency affects the immune function related to the antibody response to T-cell-dependent antigens (Ross, 1992; Nabi *et al.*, 2020). The RAR-alpha mRNA expression and antigen-specific proliferative responses to T-lymphocytes are influenced by vitamin A status *in vivo* and directly modulated by retinoic acid (Patel and Vajdy, 2015). Vitamin A deficiency affects several immune system cells, and repletion with retinoic acid effectively re-establishes the number of circulating lymphocytes (Zhao and Ross, 1995; Patel and Vajdy, 2015).

A diminished primary antibody response could also increase the severity and duration of an episode of infection. In contrast, a diminished secondary response could increase the risk of developing a second episode of illness. Vitamin A deficiency causes decreased phagocytic activity in macrophages and neutrophils. The secretory immunoglobulin A (IgA) system is an essential first line of defense against infections of mucosal surfaces (McGhee *et al.*, 1992). Several studies in animal models have shown that the intestinal IgA response is impaired by vitamin A deficiency (Wiedermann *et al.*, 1993; Stephensen *et al.*, 1996). Vitamin A is needed for the proper functioning of such important lymphoid organs.

Defects in bone growth
Vitamin A deficiency can cause alterations in bone growth, which creates several areas of compression in the central nervous system with loss of mobility (Palludan, 1961). For example, vitamin A appears to be required for growth hormone secretion and thyroid hormone secretion and action (Frape *et al.*, 1959b; De Luca *et al.*, 2000; Tanumihardjo, 2013).

Defects in reproduction
Vitamin A deficiency has significant detrimental effects on reproductive function directly and indirectly. Deficiency can affect steroidogenesis, epithelium of reproductive organs, oocyst, spermatozoa, and conceptus development (Palludan, 1966; Selke *et al.*, 1967; Chew, 1993; Skliarov *et al.*, 2020). Consequently, it can affect maturity, sexual function, pregnancy, parturition, and postpartum. In gilts, deficiency signs are more evident near maturity and include pneumonia, enteritis, anorexia, unsteady gait, anestrus, and poor conception rates; few pigs are farrowed usually, and many young were stillborn.

Retinoic acid given to pregnant retinol-deficient gilts prevented some symptoms, but parturition was impaired. In deficient gestating sows, defects in embryos can occur as early as 20 days after conception. These defects in the ocular area of embryos included defective closure of the fetal fissure, eversion of the retinal nerve, and cysts in the ocular bulb. The testes had narrower tubules in vitamin A-deficient boars with abnormal or absent spermatogenesis. The interstitial tissue was thicker, with desquamated Sertoli cells.

Safety
In general, the possibility of vitamin A toxicity in swine is remote. However, of all vitamins, vitamins A and D_3 have the greatest chance of being provided in toxic concentrations to swine. Excess vitamin A has been demonstrated to have harmful effects in most species studied. Presumed upper safe levels are 4 to 10 times the nutritional requirements for non-ruminant animals, including swine (NRC, 1998). Thus, small excesses of vitamin A for short periods should not exert any harmful effects. Recommended safe upper levels of vitamin A for swine

are 20,000 IU per kilogram diet for growing pigs and 40,000 IU per kilogram diet for breeding animals. Most of the harmful effects have followed feeding over 100 times the daily requirements for a sustained period of time. Thus, small excesses of vitamin A should not be harmful for short periods.

The amount of vitamin A added to swine diets is usually more than the NRC requirements because no safety factors were built into these values (Olson, 1984). Additional vitamin A is added to allow for activity loss due to oxidative destruction of the vitamin A ester during feed processing and storage, variability of carotenes in feedstuffs, changes in feed consumption, genetic differences in animals, and stress due to disease and other environmental factors. Stahly et al. (1997) reported that requirements for one or more antioxidant vitamins, i.e., vitamins A, E, and C, are greater than NRC (1988) estimates when pigs are exposed to a high level of antigens.

The most characteristic signs of hypervitaminosis A are skeletal malformations, spontaneous fractures, and internal hemorrhage (Anderson et al., 1966; Wolke et al., 1968; NRC, 1998). Gross toxicity signs also include a roughened hair coat, scaly skin, hyperirritability and sensitivity to touch, bleeding from cracks that appear in the skin about the hooves, blood in urine and feces, loss of control of legs accompanied by the inability to rise, and periodic tremors, (NRC, 1998). Other signs include loss of appetite, slow growth, loss of weight, skin thickening, suppressed keratinization, increased blood-clotting time, reduced erythrocyte count, enteritis, congenital abnormalities, and conjunctivitis. Degenerative atrophy, fatty infiltration, and reduced liver and kidney function are also typical. A variety of effects of chronic hypervitaminosis A in weanling pigs were reported by Hurt et al. (1966). Dobson (1969) documented the impact of massive-induced hypervitaminosis A on newborn pigs.

In addition to reduced growth and high plasma, liver, and kidney vitamin A levels, as well as a characteristic gait, Pryor et al. (1969) reported pathologic changes in the bones of pigs subjected to levels of vitamin A sufficient to produce hypervitaminosis A. Bone abnormalities might include extensive bone resorption and narrowing of the bone shaft, bone fragility, and short bones because of retarded growth. Wolke et al. (1968) reported the effects of excessive vitamin A on the pig's endochondral and intramembranous bone formation. Abnormalities in bone modeling are the fundamental causes of fractures, and the cartilage matrix of bone may be destroyed. Since the advent of high-dose treatment with systemic retinoic acid for leukemia and other malignant conditions, a condition known as "retinoic acid syndrome" has been identified (Solomons, 2006). It is characterized by reduced weight gain, hypotension, kidney failure, and respiratory distress. High doses of retinoid analogs can also increase intracranial pressure (Friedman, 2005).

The effects of supplementing the diets of weanling pigs with up to 100 times the NRC (1988) estimated requirements for vitamin A have been investigated (Blair et al., 1989, 1992). Blair et al. (1989) indicated that a level of only 10 times the requirement, even after just over 4 weeks, may induce osteochondrosis. The allowable vitamin A range set out in the Canadian Feeds Regulations (1983) was appropriate for practical pig production (Blair et al., 1992). Hidiroglu (1996) reported that an intramuscular dose of 2.5×10^6 IU vitamin A resulted livers with high vitamin A levels considered hazardous to health.

Another area of attention has focused on whether or not excessive vitamin A can affect vitamin E status or vice versa. Vitamin A has been reported to affect vitamin E significantly (Ching et al., 2002). Blair et al. (1996) indicated that a tolerable dietary range of vitamin A for young pigs in the range of 10 to 30 kg is up to 10 times the requirement. Ching et al. (2002) fed weanling pigs 6 times the vitamin A requirement (13,200 IU/kg feed). As dietary vitamin A levels increased, serum and liver α-tocopherol concentrations declined, suggesting a reduced absorption and retention of α-tocopherol when weaned pigs were fed high dietary vitamin A concentrations. Fuhrmann *et al.* (1997) reported that 20,000 IU/kg diet vitamin A reduced plasma and tissue vitamin E levels, which in turn led to an increase of lipid peroxidation as indicated by higher production of hydrocarbons. Blair *et al.* (1996) considered this raised concern about further increases in vitamin A supplementation in early weaned pigs.

In breeding pigs, Preś *et al.* (1993) studying carotene, vitamin A, and E supplementation, reported that while synthetic β-carotene and vitamin A increased the number of viable embryos and yellow bodies in the sows slaughtered on day 28 of gestation, vitamin E had a harmful influence on β-carotene action. Moreover, β-carotene subsequently improved the fertility of sows in the next reproductive cycle. In contrast, Anderson *et al.* (1997) concluded that during early gestation, the vitamin E status of gilts was not detrimentally influenced by 3 350,000 IU injections of vitamin A shortly before, at, and shortly after breeding.

Weaver *et al.* (1989) reported a significant interaction between vitamin A and vitamin E for plasma tocopherol. Higher levels of vitamin A, when supplied with a high level of vitamin E, lowered plasma tocopherol concentrations. Hoppe *et al.* (1992) indicated that dietary retinol at up to 10,000 IU per kilogram of diet does not affect α-tocopherol concentrations in plasma or tissues selected except for cardiac muscle. α-tocopherol levels in the heart and liver displayed an inverse relationship with dietary retinol levels of 5,000, 10,000, 20,000, or 40,000 IU/kg.

Anderson *et al.* (1995a) reported that feeding a high level of retinyl acetate (20,000 IU/kg) did not influence animal performance, blood serum, or tissue α-tocopherol concentrations in growing-finishing pigs. In contrast, dietary retinol did not affect α-tocopherol levels in the *Longissimus* muscle or backfat. Zomborszky-Kovács *et al.* (1998) reported a numeric decrease in plasma vitamin E concentration in unsupplemented versus carotene-supplemented weaned pigs. Beginning 1 week before weaning, the supplemented group received 855 mg β-carotene per kilogram diet (10 times the NRC (1988) recommendation). The carotene-supplemented and control pigs had vitamin E concentrations in plasma of 2.12 mg/dl and 5.58 mg/dl, respectively.

Vitamin D
Chemical structure and properties
The term vitamin D covers a group of closely related compounds possessing antirachitic activity. This includes ergosterol, ergocalciferol, and cholecalciferol. Provitamin D_2 ergosterol is a sterol found in green plants, fungi, and yeasts that undergoes a photochemical reaction caused by ultraviolet (UV) radiation from sunlight to form vitamin D_2 or ergocalciferol.

Vitamin D_3 or cholecalciferol is produced only in animals via UV radiation of provitamin D_3 or 7-dehydrocholesterol present in the skin. The provitamin 7-dehydrocholesterol, derived from cholesterol or squalene, is synthesized in the body and present in large amounts in the skin, the intestinal wall, and other tissues (DeLuca, 2014; Combs and McClung, 2022). Sterols with vitamin D activity have a common steroid nucleus and differ like the lateral chain attached to carbon 17 (Figure 4.5). Vitamin D precursors have no antirachitic activity.

In its pure form, vitamin D is a colorless crystal, insoluble in water but readily soluble in alcohol and other organic solvents. Vitamin D can be destroyed by over-treatment with UV light and by peroxidation in the presence of rancidifying PUFA. Like vitamins A and E, it is destroyed by oxidation unless vitamin D_3 is stabilized. Its oxidative destruction is increased by heat, moisture, and trace minerals. There is negligible loss of crystalline cholecalciferol during storage for 1 year or crystalline ergocalciferol for 9 months in amber-evacuated capsules at refrigerator temperatures (Zheng and Teegarden, 2013; Combs and McClung, 2022).

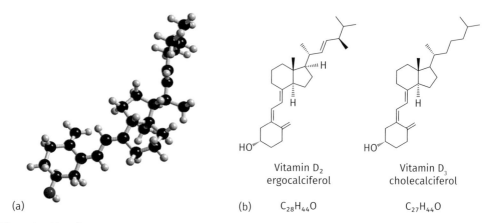

(a)　　　　　　(b)　　　C_{28}H_{44}O

Vitamin D$_2$
ergocalciferol

Vitamin D$_3$
cholecalciferol

C$_{28}$H$_{44}$O　　　　　C$_{27}$H$_{44}$O

Figure 4.5 Vitamin D structure

Natural sources

Sources of vitamin D are natural foods, irradiated sebaceous material licked from skin or hair, and directly absorbed products or irradiation formed on or in the skin. In the great majority of tables comprising the nutritional value of feedstuffs, the vitamin D content is calculated based on the equivalent bioactivity of vitamin D$_2$ plus D$_3$. However, vitamin D$_2$ is a poor source of vitamin D for swine due to its low bioavailability. Besides fish oil and meal, vitamin D$_3$ is scarce in feed ingredients, so supplementation is required. Ergocalciferol occurs naturally in some mushrooms, and cholecalciferol occurs naturally in fish (Johnson and Kimlin, 2006).

A source of the antirachitic factor in the diets of farm animals is the action of radiant energy upon ergosterol in forages. Legume hay cured to preserve most of its leaves and green color contains considerable vitamin D activity. Alfalfa, for example, will range 650–2,200 IU/kg (Maynard et al., 1979). Swine that received sun-cured alfalfa leaf meal in their diet would receive a limited amount of vitamin D from this source. However, fewer commercial swine operations now use alfalfa leaf meals than in the past. For non-forage-consuming species, the natural vitamin D in unfortified food is generally derived from animal products. There is less destruction of vitamin D$_3$ in freeze-dried fish meals during drying, possibly because of decreased atmospheric oxygen.

Commercial forms

The majority of vitamin D$_3$ used for fortifying animal feeds comes in the form of a spray-dried formulation containing 500,000 IU/g. A combination of vitamin A and D$_3$, usually in a 5 : 1 ratio – i.e., vitamin A 1,000,000 IU/g and vitamin D$_3$ 200,000 IU/g is also used in feed fortification.

Three commercial metabolites of vitamin D are used for animal feed supplementation. These metabolites are 25OHD$_3$, 1-α-hydroxycholecalciferol, and 1,25(OH)$_2$D$_3$-glycoside. For over 25 years, the first metabolite, 25OHD$_3$ has been largely used as a feed additive (tradename Rovimix® HyD) in spray-dried form for poultry (Soares et al., 1995) and more recently for swine.

Alfacalcidol, or 1-α hydroxycholecalciferol or 1-α-hydroxyvitamin D$_3$, is a synthetic, non-endogenous analog of vitamin D. Alfacalcidol is activated by the enzyme 25-hydroxylase in the liver to mediate its effects in the body, or most importantly, the kidneys and bones. An initial evaluation in young pigs showed no positive effects (Biehl and Baker, 1996). However, recent evaluations (Lee and Stein, 2022) indicated the high efficacy of 1-α-hydroxyvitamin D$_3$ in increasing digestibility, calcium and phosphorus retention, and digestible and metabolizable energy. Finally, a form of calcitriol as $1,25(OH)_2D_3$ – glycoside is also available as feed material. This metabolite is extracted from the plant *Solanum glaucophyllum* (Bachman *et al.*, 2013). This metabolite was evaluated by Cromwell *et al.* (1996, 1997) with variable results on phosphorus utilization.

Synthetic D_2, D_3, and metabolites are stable when stored at room temperature. In complete feeds and mineral-vitamin premixes, Schneider (1986) reported activity losses of 10% to 30% after either 4 or 6 months of storage at 22°C. However, pure vitamin D_3 crystals or vitamin D_3 resin are susceptible to degradation upon exposure to heat or contact with mineral elements. The resin is stored under refrigeration with nitrogen gas. Dry, stabilized supplements retain potency much longer and can be used in high-mineral supplements. It has been shown that vitamin D_3 is much more stable than D_2 in feeds containing minerals.

Stabilization of the vitamin can be achieved by (1) rapid compression of the mixed feed, for example, into pellets so that air is excluded; (2) storing feed under cool, dry, dark conditions; (3) preventing close contact between the vitamin and potent metallic oxidation catalysts (e.g., manganese); (4) including natural or synthetic antioxidants in the mix. The vitamin can also be protected by enclosing it in durable gelatin beadlets.

The stability of dry vitamin D supplements is affected most by high temperature, high moisture content, and contact with trace minerals, such as ferrous sulfate, manganese oxide, and others. Hirsch (1982) reports the results of a "conventional" or non-stabilized vitamin D_3 product being mixed into a trace mineral premix or animal feed and stored at ambient room temperature (20–25°C) for up to 12 weeks. The feed had lost 31% of its vitamin D activity after 12 weeks, and the trace mineral premix had lost 66% of its activity after only 6 weeks in storage.

Metabolism
Absorption, conversion to active forms, and transport
Vitamin D requirements can be met in 2 ways: by ingestion and via the endogenous synthesis of vitamin D_3 from cholesterol, a process that requires the animals to be exposed to sunlight (Wahlstrom and Stolte, 1958). Four important variables selectively determine the amount of vitamin D_3 that will be photochemically produced by skin exposure to sunlight (Norman and Henry, 2007).

The 2 principal determinants are the quantity and intensity of UV light and the appropriate wavelength of the UV light (290 and 315 nm). A third important variable determining skin vitamin D synthesis is the concentration of 7-dehydrocholesterol present in the skin. A fourth determinant of vitamin D_3 production is the concentration of melanin in the skin (skin color). The darker the skin, the longer time required to convert 7-dehydrocholesterol to vitamin D_3 (Zheng and Teegarden, 2013; Combs and McClung, 2022).

On average, only 50% of an oral dose of vitamin D is absorbed. However, considering sufficient vitamin D is usually produced by daily exposure to sunlight, it is not surprising that the body has not evolved a more efficient mechanism for dietary vitamin D absorption (Horst *et al.*, 1982; Norman and Henry, 2007). Effective treatment of rickets by rubbing cod liver oil on the skin indicates that vitamin D can also be absorbed through the skin (DeLuca, 2014).

The presence of the provitamin 7-dehydrocholesterol in the skin's epidermis and sebaceous secretions is well recognized, and vitamin D is synthesized in the skin of many herbivores and omnivores. The cholecalciferol formed by the UV irradiation of 7-dehydrocholesterol is removed from the skin into the circulatory system by the blood transport protein for vitamin D, the vitamin D-binding protein (DBP) (Norman and Henry, 2007). This mechanism is of little significance when animals are kept indoors, so vitamin D_3 must be provided in the feed.

Dietary vitamin D is absorbed by passive diffusion from the ileal portion of the intestinal tract in association with fats, as are all the fat-soluble vitamins. Like others, it requires the presence of bile salts for absorption (Braun, 1986) and is absorbed with other neutral lipids via chylomicron into the lymphatic system (Norman and Henry, 2007; Zheng and Teegarden, 2013; DeLuca, 2014; Combs and McClung, 2022; Maurya and Aggarwal, 2017; Yang and Ma, 2021).

Following its absorption, vitamin D and its metabolites circulate in the plasma, like other steroids, bound to the vitamin D-binding protein (VBP or DBP). Regardless of origin (conversion in the skin or absorption), the vitamin is carried by the blood to the liver to start an activation process. By itself, vitamin D cholecalciferol is biologically inactive and must be converted to the active form through 2 hydroxylations.

This first hydroxylation occurs in the liver and is catalyzed by the hepatic microsomal enzyme of the cytochrome P450 (CYP) family 25-hydroxylase (CYP2R1 and CYP27A1) with the transformation of cholecalciferol to 25-hydroxy-cholecalciferol ($25OHD_3$, or calcidiol or calcifediol), which is the circulating and storage form of vitamin D. This conversion step is not metabolically regulated. The concentration of $25OHD_3$ in circulation is considered a good indicator of vitamin D status in general, able to indicate adequacy, deficiency, or toxicity of vitamin D (McDowell, 2000a; DeLuca, 2014).

$25OHD_3$ is then transported to the kidney, on the VBP, where it can be converted, in the proximal convoluted cells, to a variety of compounds, of which the most important is 1,25 dihydroxy-cholecalciferol ($1,25(OH)_2D_3$ or calcitriol) by the action of 1α-hydroxylase (CYP27B1) (DeLuca, 2008; DeLuca, 2014). Vitamin C is involved in this stage. The parathyroid hormone (PTH) regulates this second hydroxylation according to the concentrations of calcium and phosphorus. The $1,25(OH)_2D_3$ is more active but is in a much lower concentration (pg/ml vs. ng/ml) and has a much shorter half-life than $25OHD_3$ (4 to 6 hours vs. 2 to 3 weeks). Moreover, as its production is under strict regulation its presence in the blood does not provide an indication of vitamin D status.

Subsequently, the $1,25(OH)_2D_3$ is transported to the intestine, the bones, or another part of the kidney, which participates in calcium and phosphorus metabolism (Figure 4.6). VBP has the greatest affinity for $25OHD_3$, the main circulating form, then for cholecalciferol, and finally for $1,25(OH)_2D_3$. Another important enzyme is the renal 24-hydroxylase (CYP24A1), catalyzing the first step of its inactivation from $25OHD_3$ to $24,25(OH)_2D_3$. The physiological role of this metabolite is less clear. It was considered only one of the primary metabolites destined for excretion, however, research (Seo et al., 1997) has identified a potential role in bone mineralization.

Although the kidney is the main site of 1-α-hydroxylation, other cells and organs, such as the intestinal cells, immune cells, endothelial cells, brain, mammary glands, pancreatic islets, parathyroid glands, placenta, prostate, and skin, express active 1α-hydroxylase (Johnson and Kimlin 2006; DeLuca, 2008; Shanmugasundaram and Selvaraj, 2012). Hence, a local production of calcitriol occurs in these cells and is not regulated as for kidney production.

$1,25(OH)_2D_3$ acts metabolically as a hormone. Under conditions of low calcium, PTH activates renal mitochondrial 1α-hydroxylase, which converts $25OHD_3$ to $1,25(OH)_2D_3$, and inactivates renal and extrarenal 24- and 23-hydroxylases (Goff et al., 1991).

In contrast, under conditions of low calcium stress (when little PTH is secreted), the 1-α-hydroxylase can also be directly stimulated by low blood calcium or phosphorus concentrations. High plasma $1,25(OH)_2D_3$ concentration has an inhibitory effect on renal 1-α-hydroxylase and a stimulatory effect on tissue 24-hydroxylase (Engstrom et al., 1987). Thus, the production and catabolism of the hormone $1,25(OH)_2D_3$ are tightly regulated. It is now known that the most critical point of regulation of the vitamin D endocrine system

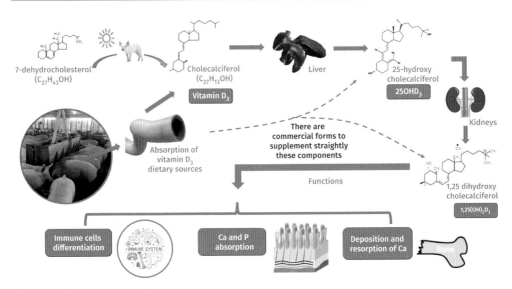

Figure 4.6 Vitamin D metabolism

occurs through stringent control of the renal 1-α-hydroxylase activity. In this way, the production of the hormone 1,25(OH)$_2$D$_3$ can be modulated according to the calcium needs of the organism (Zheng and Teegarden, 2013; DeLuca, 2014; Yang and Ma, 2021).

Storage and excretion

For most mammals, vitamin D, 25(OH)D$_3$, and possibly 24,25(OH)$_2$D$_3$ and 1,25(OH)$_2$D are all transported on the same protein (transcalciferin DBP). This protein is essential in maintaining an adequate vitamin D level in the organism. DBP has a greater affinity for 25(OH)D$_3$, the main circulating form, then for cholecalciferol, and finally for 1,25(OH)$_2$D$_3$.

Horst *et al.* (1982) determined that the mean (±SD) ratios of plasma cholecalciferol to ergocalciferol concentration in pigs were 1.5±0.1, while in chickens were 6.3±1.2. The mean ratios of plasma 25-hydroxycholecalciferol to 25-hydroxyergocalciferol concentration were 4.0±0.1 in pigs and 10.7±3.4 in chickens. The mean plasma cholecalciferol/ergocalciferol ratios for the 24,25-dihydroxy-, 25,26-dihydroxy- and 1,25-dihydroxy-derivatives in the pig were 2.6±0.6, 5.8±1.3 and 5.8±0.8, respectively.

In contrast to aquatic species, which store significant amounts of vitamin D in the liver, land animals do not store appreciable amounts of the vitamin. The body can store vitamin D, although to a much lesser extent than vitamin A. Principal stores of vitamin D occur in fat, blood (as 25OHD$_3$), and the liver. It is also found in the lungs, kidneys, and elsewhere in the body. During times of deprivation, vitamin D is released slowly, especially in the skin and adipose, thus meeting the vitamin D needs of the animal over a longer period (Norman and Henry, 2007).

In addition to the regulation of 1,25(OH)$_2$D$_3$ synthesis, degradation of this potent hormone is also regulated by apparently separate but highly specific cytochrome P-450 enzymes. In degradation, 1,25(OH)$_2$D$_3$ is hydroxylated in the target tissue (bone and intestine) and the liver and kidney to an inert, water-soluble calcitroic acid. Both 25OHD$_3$ and 1,25(OH)$_2$D$_3$ undergo a 24-hydroxylation to form 24,25-dihydroxyvitamin D$_3$ (24,25-(OH)$_2$D$_3$) and 1,24,25-trihydroxyvitamin D$_3$, respectively.

The 24-hydroxylated derivatives are considered to be inert, first-step products of biodegradation. But, some observations imply possible, yet undefined, roles for 24,25-$(OH)_2D_3$ in bone formation, fracture healing, and embryonic development (Seo et al., 1997). Excretion of absorbed vitamin D and its metabolites occurs primarily through the feces with the aid of bile salts (Zheng and Teegarden, 2013; DeLuca, 2014).

Biochemical functions
Classical functions
The classical function of vitamin D is to regulate the absorption, transport, deposition, and mobilization of calcium and phosphorus. The active form is 1,25$(OH)_2D_3$, which acts together with PTH, calcitonin, and FGF23 (Fibroblast Growth Factor), similarly to steroid hormones. PTH, calcitonin, and FGF23 function in a delicate relationship with 1,25$(OH)_2D_3$ to control blood calcium and phosphorus levels (Engstrom and Littledike, 1986). The production rate of 1,25$(OH)_2D_3$ is under physiological control. When blood calcium is below the normal range, PTH upregulates the production of calcitriol, elevating plasma calcium and stimulating specific ion pump mechanisms in the intestine, bone, and kidney (Deluca, 2014). FGF23 responds similarly in relationship to phosphorus level and interacts with the mechanism regulating calcium level.

These 3 sources of calcium and phosphorus provide reservoirs that enable vitamin D to elevate calcium and phosphorus in blood to levels necessary for normal bone mineralization and other functions ascribed to calcium. Contrary to the other 2, Calcitonin regulates high serum calcium levels by depressing gut absorption, halting bone demineralization, and depressing reabsorption in the kidney.

The hormone enters the cell in the target tissue and binds to a cytosolic receptor or a nuclear receptor. 1,25$(OH)_2D_3$ regulates gene expression by binding to tissue-specific receptors and subsequent interaction between the bound receptor and the DNA (Norman, 2006). The receptor-hormone complex moves to the nucleus. It attaches to the chromatin and stimulates the transcription of particular genes to produce specific mRNAs, which code for synthesizing particular proteins. Evidence for transcription regulation of a specific gene typically includes 1,25$(OH)_2D_3$-induced modulation in mRNA levels.

Additionally, evidence may consist of measurements of transcription and a vitamin D responsive element within the promoter region of the gene (Hannah and Norman, 1994). Several studies (Kliewer et al., 1992; Whitfield et al., 1995) have identified a heterodimer of the vitamin D receptor (VDR) and a vitamin A receptor (RXR) within the nucleus of the cell as the active complex for mediating positive transcriptional effects of 1,25$(OH)_2D_3$. This classical function is driven by the effects of vitamin D at intestinal, bone, and kidney levels (Yang and Ma, 2021). The 2 receptors (vitamins D and A) selectively interact with specific hormone response elements composed of direct repeats of specific nucleotides located in the promoter of regulated genes. The complex that binds to these elements consists of 3 distinct elements: the 1,25$(OH)_2D_3$ hormonal ligand, the VDR, and one of the vitamins A (retinoid) X receptors (RXR) (Kliewer et al., 1992; Whitfield et al., 1995).

Intestinal effects
Vitamin D stimulates the active transport of calcium and phosphorus across the intestinal epithelium. This stimulation does not involve PTH directly but affects the active form of vitamin D (Zheng and Teegarden, 2013). PTH indirectly stimulates intestinal calcium absorption by stimulating the production of 1,25$(OH)_2D_3$ under conditions of hypocalcemia.

Vitamin D promotes calcium and phosphorus absorption, but the mechanism is still not completely understood. Current evidence (Wasserman, 1981; Zheng and Teegarden, 2013; Combs and McClung, 2022) indicates that $1,25(OH)_2D_3$ is transferred to the nucleus of the intestinal cell, where it interacts with the chromatin material. In response to the $1,25(OH)_2D_3$, specific RNAs are elaborated by the nucleus. When these are translated into particular proteins by ribosomes, the events leading to calcium and phosphorus absorption enhancement occur (Adeola et al., 1998). In the intestine, calcitriol promotes the synthesis of calbindin (Ca-binding protein, CaBP) and other proteins and stimulates calcium and phosphorus absorption.

Initially, it was felt that vitamin D did not regulate phosphorus absorption and transport. In 1963, through an *in vitro* inverted sac technique, it was demonstrated that vitamin D plays such a role (Harrison and Harrison, 1963). The more recently discovered phosphaturic hormone FGF23, primarily produced in osteoblast and osteocyte cells, is responsible for phosphorus homeostasis through a pathway that involves feedback regulation between FGF23, vitamin D, phosphorus, and calcium (Sitara et al., 2006; David et al., 2013).

Bone effects

Vitamin D_3 plays an essential role in the metabolism and development of the skeleton in pigs, maintaining complex balances with calcium and phosphorus. Increasing the dosage of vitamin D_3 increases the plasma concentration of ionized and total calcium and reduces the concentration of phosphorus and sodium. It also improves phosphorus absorption and retention and utilization of phytic phosphorus (Adeola et al., 1998; Crenshaw, 2000; Lee et al., 2022) and intervenes in the differentiation and maturation of chondrocytes.

It must be noticed that other vitamins (B_6, folic acid, C, and K) and mineral trace elements (copper, zinc, magnesium, boron, fluorine, and aluminum) are also involved in the ossification process. Minerals are deposited on the protein matrix (Zheng and Teegarden, 2013; Combs and McClung, 2022). This is accompanied by an invasion of blood vessels that gives rise to trabecular bone. This process causes bones to elongate. This organic matrix fails to mineralize during a vitamin D deficiency, causing rickets in the young and osteomalacia in adults. The active metabolite calcitriol brings about the mineralization of the bone matrix.

Vitamin D has another function in bone: mobilizing calcium from bone to the extracellular fluid compartment. PTH shares this function. It requires metabolic energy and presumably transports calcium and phosphorus across the bone membrane by acting on osteocytes and osteoclasts. Rapid, acute plasma calcium regulation is due to the interaction of plasma calcium with calcium-binding sites in bone material as blood comes in contact with bone. Changes in plasma calcium are brought about by a difference in the proportion of high- and low-affinity calcium-binding sites, access to which is regulated by osteoclasts and osteoblasts, respectively (Snow et al., 1986; Bronner and Stein, 1995). Another role of vitamin D is in bone collagen biosynthesis in preparation for mineralization (Zhou et al., 2017; Duffy et al., 2018a; Zhao et al., 2022; Combs and McClung, 2022). $25OHD_3$ is more potent than vitamin D_3 (2.5–4 times more) in improving calcium and phosphorus metabolism.

Kidney effects

There is evidence that vitamin D functions in the distal renal tubules to improve calcium reabsorption and is mediated by the Ca-binding protein calbindin (Bronner and Stein, 1995). It is known that 99% of renal-filtered calcium is reabsorbed without vitamin D and PTH. Although it is unknown whether they work in concert, the remaining 1% is controlled by these 2 hormonal agents. It has been shown that $1,25(OH)_2D_3$ improves renal calcium reabsorption (Sutton and Dirks, 1978).

Non-classical functions (beyond bone mineralization)

Other functions that we can call non-classical are connected with the discovery of the presence of 1α-hydroxylase and the receptor of the active metabolite in several tissues like the pancreas, bone marrow, cells of the ovary, cells of the brain, breast, and epithelial cells, suggesting a role in many other aspects like immune system modulation, muscle cells differentiation and reproduction (Machlin and Sauberlich, 1994; DeLuca, 2014; Yang and Ma, 2021). More than 50 genes have been reported to be transcriptionally regulated by $1,25(OH)_2D_3$ (Hannah and Norman, 1994; Zheng and Teegarden, 2013; Combs and McClung, 2022).

Immune system modulation

The actions of $1,25(OH)_2D_3$ are recognized as being involved in regulating the growth and differentiation of various cell types, including those of the hematopoietic and immune systems (Reinhardt and Hustmyer, 1987; Lemire, 1992; Yang and Ma, 2021). Recent studies have suggested $1,25(OH)_2D_3$ as an immunoregulatory hormone (both innate and adaptive immune system), and $25OHD_3$ appears more efficient than vitamin D in modulating immune response (Shanmugasundaram and Selvaraj, 2012; Konowalchuk et al., 2013; Yang et al., 2019a,b; Yang and Ma, 2021).

Elevated $1,25(OH)_2D_3$ was also associated with a significant 70% enhancement of lymphocyte proliferation in cells treated with pokeweed mitogen (Hustmyer et al., 1994). Calcitriol or its metabolites have also been credited with functions regulating the cells of the immune system (Reinhardt and Hustmyer, 1987; Zhao et al., 2014; Yang et al., 2019a,b; Yang and Ma, 2021; Zhou et al., 2022).

Muscle cells differentiation and meat tenderization

It has been shown that feeding $25OHD_3$ affects pig vitamin D status and could stimulate satellite cell-mediated muscle hypertrophy response (Hines et al., 2013). Satellite cells are muscle stem cells giving rise, when activated, to a skeletal muscle cell precursors pool, they are able to differentiate and fuse to increase the nuclei accretion into existing muscle fibers or to form new fibers. These adult stem cells are involved in the normal growth of skeletal muscle and regeneration following injury or disease.

Very high levels of vitamin D_3 have been fed to pigs for short periods before slaughter to increase meat quality (Wilborn et al., 2004). Enright et al. (1998) fed diets with 331, 55,031, or 176,000 IU/kg vitamin D_3. The higher levels reduced feed intake and average daily gains while increasing serum calcium concentration. This high blood calcium reduced drip loss and meat color values (Hunter L* measurement), improving subjective color and firmness scores. With the same objective, Sparks et al. (1998) determined that the optimal dosage of vitamin D_3 was 500,000 IU daily for 3 days before slaughter to maximize blood calcium concentration. However, in this initial study, pork tenderness and other measures of pork quality were not improved. However, Wiegand et al. (2002), using the same dose (500,000 IU daily) 3 days before slaughter, improved Hunter's color values at 14 days of storage. However, meat quality characteristics, measured by subjective scores, or tenderness measured with Warner-Bratzler shear force test were not improved.

Reproduction

Parenteral cholecalciferol (vitamin D_3) treatment of sows before parturition proved an effective means of supplementing young piglets with cholecalciferol (via the sow's milk) and its more polar metabolites via placental transport (Goff et al., 1984). Parental transfer has been shown to be required for the embryonic development of the chick or the pig embryo (Yang and Ma, 2021). Experimental evidence suggests that vitamin D may play a role in the maternal-conceptus cross-talk (Viganò et al., 2003; Yang and Ma, 2021). However, irrespective of the dietary dose and form of vitamin D (D_3 or $25OHD_3$) provided to sows, little vitamin D was transferred to the progeny (Lauridsen et al., 2010; Matte and Audet, 2020).

One question that remained unanswered is whether the hormone form $1,25(OH)_2D_3$ acts alone or if there is some response from a second vitamin D metabolite or hormone (e.g., $24,25(OH)_2D_3$) (Feldman et al., 2003). This question has possibly been answered in a study where the 24-position of 25-$(OH)D_3$ was blocked with fluoro groups to prevent 24-hydroxylation (DeLuca, 2008). For 2 generations, all systems were normal, indicating a need for only $1,25(OH)_2D_3$. Therefore, research suggests that $1,25(OH)_2D_3$ appears to be the only functional form of vitamin D in biology (DeLuca, 2008; Yang and Ma, 2021).

For mammals, $1,25(OH)_2D_3$ is a critical factor in maintaining sufficient maternal calcium for transport to the fetus. It may play a role in the normal skeletal development of the neonate (Lester, 1986). A liberal vitamin D intake during gestation provides sufficient storage in newborns to help prevent early rickets. For example, newborn lambs can be provided enough to meet their needs for 6 weeks.

Nutritional assessment

As previously discussed, in the body, vitamin D undergoes successive metabolic hydroxylation into $25OHD_3$ and $1,25(OH)_2D_3$ in the liver and kidney, respectively. The first hydroxylation product $25OHD_3$ is recognized as the best status marker for humans and other mammals (Höller et al., 2018). Very briefly, vitamin D cannot be used as a reliable marker as it is transformed quickly through the 25-hydroxylation, and the production of $1,25(OH)_2D_3$ is strictly regulated according to calcium and phosphorus plasma levels.

Since the body does not store $25OHD_3$, the concentration in circulation (plasma or serum) can be used for status determination. Both competitive chemiluminescence immunoassays and HPLC coupled with tandem mass spectrometry (HPLC-MS/MS) assays are used in clinical practice. The pros and cons of both technologies have been reviewed in depth (Van den Ouweland, 2016).

The varying selectivity of the antibodies for $25OHD_3$ (and $25OHD_2$) and the potential for cross-reactivity with related metabolites such as $24,25(OH)_2D_3$ impact the repeatability between different immune-based assays. This aspect is critical when using immune assays with animal plasma. Most commercial immune kits are based on human antibodies, and few are "optimized" for use in poultry or other animal species.

HPLC-MS/MS has been referred to as the gold standard. However, in common with several delicate analyses, the result can also be erroneous as this technique requires the skills of an experienced analyst (Atef, 2018). Vitamin D is stable at room temperature on DBS and was one of the first vitamins analyzed with this sampling method (Eyles et al., 2009).

Experts still debate about the human adequate $25OHD_3$ plasma level. A 75 nmol/l or 30 ng/ml (conversion factor 2.5) is a cut-off between adequate and inadequate vitamin D nutritional status (Holick, 2007). However, some authors and health bodies have placed this threshold at 50 nmol/l (Cashman, 2018), while others consider such values to be the low-end of adequacy (Heaney and Holick, 2011). Levels above 150 nmol/l or 60 ng/ml are considered excessive in humans, although these figures are also a matter of debate. One point of discussion is the fact that vitamin D nutritional status is typically assessed using calcium and phosphorus metabolism and bone status as an endpoint. Research has progressively indicated that besides the endocrine function, vitamin D has broader autocrine and paracrine functions like immune system modulation and muscle cell development. These functionalities seem to require higher $25OHD_3$ circulating levels to be activated.

A direct transposition of human data to animals is impossible, and the establishment of clinical ranges upon which to adjust dietary supplementation is underway. As a general reference, the human cut-off value of 30 ng/ml can be used for swine (Arnold *et al.*, 2015). Finally, the dietary administration of 25OHD$_3$ has been shown in different studies carried out in humans and animal species to increase more efficiently than vitamin D$_3$ the 25OHD$_3$ plasma level (see, for example, Upadhaya *et al.*, 2022).

Deficiency signs

The primary vitamin D deficiency sign is a bone disorder called rickets in young animals or osteomalacia in older pigs. It is generally characterized by a decreased concentration of calcium and phosphorus in the organic matrices of cartilage and bone (Combs *et al.*, 1966a,b). Vitamin D deficiency results in clinical signs like those indicating a lack of calcium, phosphorus, or both, as all 3 are concerned with proper bone formation (Miller *et al.*, 1964).

For mammals, 1,25(OH)$_2$D$_3$ is a critical factor in maintaining sufficient maternal calcium for transport to the fetus. It may play a role in the normal skeletal development of the neonate (Lester, 1986). Deleting vitamin D$_3$ supplementation in diets fed to sows during gestation and lactation significantly compromised skeletal bone mineral content in offspring at 13 weeks of age and decreased the age at which pigs displayed kyphosis (backward curvature of the spinal column) (Crenshaw, 2010).

In the adult, osteomalacia is the counterpart of rickets and, since cartilage growth has ceased, is characterized by a decreased concentration of calcium and phosphorus in the bone matrix (Wang *et al.*, 2022a). Outward signs of rickets include the following skeletal changes, varying somewhat with species depending on anatomy and severity:

1   weak bones causing curving and bending of bones (Figure 4.7a)
2   rickets, hypertrophied chondrocytes, extensive osteoclastic activity, and diaphyseal fractures (Figure 4.7b)
3   beaded ribs, with coastal rosary (Figure 4.7c) and deformed thorax
4   lordosis, kyphosis or humped-back (Figure 4.7d)
5   enlarged hock and knee joints (Figure 4.7e)
6   tendency to drag hind legs (Figure 4.7f).

In severe vitamin D deficiency, pigs may exhibit calcium and magnesium deficiency, including tetany (Wahlstrom and Stolte, 1958; NRC, 2012). It takes 4–6 months for pigs fed a vitamin D-deficient diet to develop signs of a deficiency (Johnson and Palmer, 1939; Quarterman *et al.*, 1964). Reproductive performance concerning stillborn pigs was influenced by vitamin D supplementation (Lauridsen *et al.*, 2010). There were fewer stillborn piglets with larger doses of vitamin D (1,400 and 2,000 IU per kilogram of vitamin D in feed resulting in 1.17 and 1.13 stillborn piglets per litter, respectively) compared with 200 and 800 IU of vitamin D per kilogram of feed, resulting in 1.98 and 1.99 stillborn piglets per litter, respectively.

The trend toward confinement of swine in completely closed houses through their life cycle increases the importance of adequate dietary vitamin D fortification. Goff *et al.* (1984) concluded that subclinical rickets might become more of a problem as swine producers convert to confinement operations, which deprive sows and piglets of the UV irradiation needed for the endogenous production of cholecalciferol. Research has shown that sunshine cannot always be depended on to meet vitamin D requirements of growing or finishing pigs during winter in northern latitudes. Of all vitamins provided in swine feeds, vitamin D is one of 2 (the other being vitamin B$_{12}$) that is most likely to be deficient. Typical grain- and soybean-based

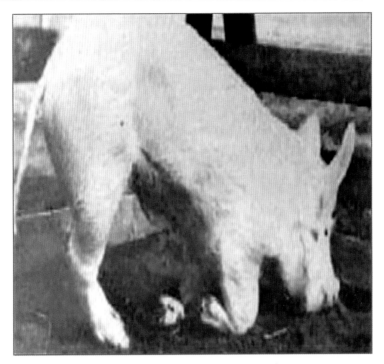

Figure 4.7(a) Vitamin D deficiency (source: Dr H. Weiser, dsm-firmenich)

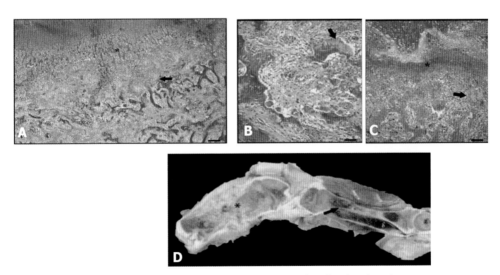

Figure 4.7(b) Rickets: case series and diagnostic review of hypovitaminosis D in swine. Bone photomicrographs. (A) Distal rib growth plate with hypertrophied chondrocytes (*), retained cartilage tongues (arrow), and medullary spaces containing abundant fibrous connective tissue; fibrous osteodystrophy. Hematoxylin and eosin (HE). Bar = 200 μm. (B) Distal rib with extensive osteoclastic activity, fibrous osteodystrophy, and widened osteoid seams (arrow). HE. Bar = 50 μm. (C) Proximal tibial infraction with hemorrhage (*) and retained cartilaginous tongues (arrow). HE. Bar = 100 μm. (D) Pig; femur and tibia. A chronic diaphyseal fracture with callus formation in the femur (*) on the left. Note misalignment of cortical bone. An acute proximal diaphyseal fracture (arrow) with adjacent soft tissue bleeding is present in the tibia (source: Madson *et al.*, 2012)

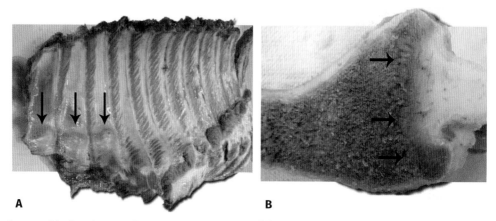

A   **B**

Figure 4.7(c) Vitamin D deficiency syndromes in swine: (A) flared costochondral junction, rachitic rosary, with (B) irregular and elongated growth cartilage (arrows) (source: Madson and Goff, 2012)

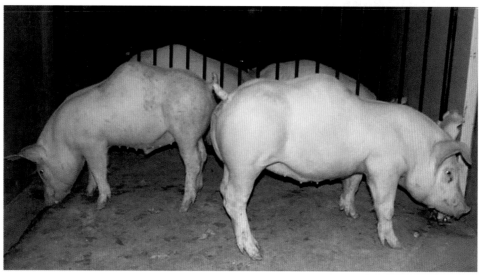

Figure 4.7(d) Vitamin D deficiency: kyphosis or humpback (source: University of Wisconsin, Swine Research and Teaching Center)

diets contain virtually no vitamin D. Miller *et al.* (1965a,b) determined that the vitamin D_2 level needed to obtain optimal growth rate in piglets fed diets with soybean protein was 500 IU/kg. In comparison, piglets fed casein diets only needed 100 IU/kg (Miller *et al.*, 1964). Therefore, supplemental vitamin D must be provided for all swine operations where growing and breeding animals remain confined.

Safety
After vitamin A, vitamin D is the next most likely to be consumed in concentrations toxic to animals (Fraser, 2021). Although vitamin D is toxic at high concentrations, short-term administration of as much as 100 times the required level may be tolerated. For most species, the presumed maximal safe level of vitamin D_3 for long-term feeding conditions (more than

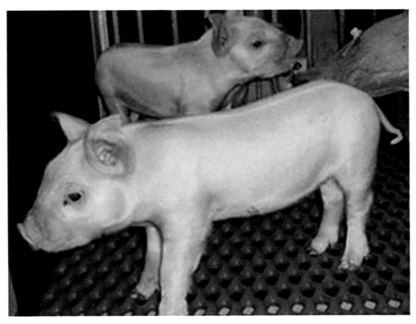

Figure 4.7(e) Vitamin D deficiency: rickets in piglets with enlarged hocks and knees (source: http://marphavet.com/en/news/Disease-Treatment/Rickets-in-pigs-60/)

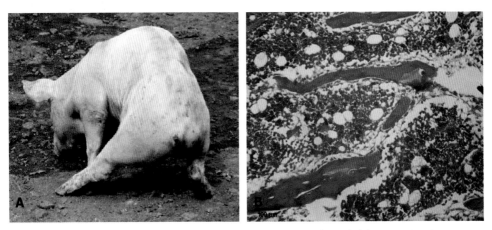

Figure 4.7(f) Outbreak of rickets in pigs from west of Santa Catarina (Brazil). (A) Swine with rickets showing signs of ataxia due to posterior paralysis. (B) Microscopic view of trabecular bone from swine with rickets. Haversian systems are filled with pale pink, unmineralized osteoid [HE; 100×] (source: Gris *et al.*, 2020)

60 days) is 4 to 10 times the dietary requirement. Studies in a number of species indicate that vitamin D_3 is 10 to 20 times more toxic than vitamin D_2 when provided in excessive amounts (NRC, 1987).

For swine, the upper safe dietary level for an exposure below 60 days is 33,000 IU per kg diet (NRC, 1998). In practical conditions, vitamin D toxicosis for swine would only be expected due to feeding mixing errors and then over a relatively long period. Excessive vitamin D intake produces various effects, all associated with abnormal elevation of blood Ca. Elevated blood calcium is caused by greatly stimulated bone resorption and increased intestinal calcium absorption.

Von Rosenberg et al. (2016) studied the tolerance of piglets to 25OHD$_3$. Forty-eight crossbred piglets were used in a 42-day tolerance trial. The control group received 50 µg/kg feed (or 2,000 IU) of vitamin D$_3$ (recommended dose), and the experiment groups received 25OHD$_3$ at the recommended dose of 50 µg/kg, at 250 µg/kg (5 times the recommended dose) and 500 µg/kg (10 times the recommended dose). The results of this study demonstrated that feeding piglets with 25OHD$_3$ at 5 or 10 times the recommended level had no adverse effects on any of the biological parameters measured. It was concluded that 25OHD$_3$ could be regarded as a supplement with a very high safety margin when used at the recommended level.

The primary pathologic effect of ingestion of massive doses of vitamin D is the widespread calcification of soft tissues. In pigs, signs of toxicity are anorexia, stiffness, lameness, back-arching, polyuria, and aphonia. Death was reported in 4 days when young pigs received 473,000 IU per kilogram in the diet (Long, 1984). Hancock et al. (1986) suggested reduced gains and feed efficiency when young pigs received 22,000–44,000 IU per kilogram of diet.

The potential for vitamin D toxicosis, that is, hypercalcemia and soft tissue calcification, is much higher when animals have access to formulations of 1,25(OH)$_2$D$_3$ since this hormone form of vitamin D has bypassed the stringent physiological point of the vitamin D endocrine system, namely the hydroxylation of 25OHD$_3$ by 1α-hydroxylase of the kidney (Norman and Henry, 2007).

Vitamin E
Chemical structure and properties

The term vitamin E includes all tocopherol and tocotrienol derivatives that qualitatively have α-tocopherol activity. This definition was given by the International Union of Pure and Applied Chemistry-International Union of Biochemistry (IUPAC-IUB, 1973) Commission on Biochemical Nomenclature. Both the tocopherols and the tocotrienols consist of a hydroquinone nucleus or chromanol ring and an isoprenoid side chain (4 carbon atoms in a straight chain and a side chain of a single carbon). Tocopherols have a saturated side chain, whereas tocotrienols have an unsaturated side chain containing 3 double bonds (Brigelius-Flohé, 2021).

There are 4 principal compounds of each of these 2 sources of vitamin E activity (α, β, γ and δ), differentiated by the presence of methyl (-CH$_3$) groups at positions 5, 7, or 8 of the chroman ring (Figure 4.8). α-tocopherol, the most biologically active of these compounds, is the predominant vitamin E active compound in feedstuffs and the form used commercially to supplement animal diets. The biological activity of the other tocopherols is limited, but other functions have been found for non-α-tocopherol forms of vitamin E (Schaffer et al., 2005; Freiser and Jiang, 2009; Traber, 2013). The differences between the different forms are due to the position and number of methyl groups in the chromanol ring. The other position of the methyl groups gives rise to the different racemic forms of tocopherols and tocotrienols. If the methyl groups are located on the same plane, they are called R forms, but if they are located on different planes, they are called S forms.

The tocopherol molecule has 3 asymmetric carbon atoms (methyl groups) located at the 2', 4', and 8' positions. These 3 asymmetric carbon atoms generate 8 possible forms or isomers RRR-, RSR-, RRS-, RSS-, SRR-, SSR-, SRS-, and SSS-α-tocopherol. The D-form of α-tocopherol (D-α-tocopherol) has all of the methyl groups in these positions facing in one direction and is referred to as the RRR-form, which is the form found in plants and is considered the natural product. The all-rac (all racemic), or chemically synthesized form of DL-α-tocopherol, has an equal mixture of the R and S configurations at each of the 3 positions and contains the racemic mixture of all 8 stereoisomers (Mahan et al., 2000; Mahan, 2000; Traber, 2013).

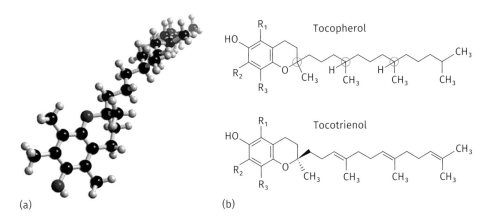

Figure 4.8 Vitamin E structure

Approximately 99% of what is found in tissues consists of R isomers in position 2, probably because of differences in the affinity of the α-tocopherol transporting hepatic protein. Of the total tocopherol retained in the tissues, the RRR-form predominates (more than 30%), followed by the RRS and RSR (around 27%) and the RSS (around 17%). The 4 isomers SSS, SRR, SSR, and SRS together comprise less than 1%, even if the animals have a high supplementation of all-*rac*-α-tocopherol (Lauridsen and Jensen, 2005).

Mahan *et al.* (2000) observed a greater absorption of the natural forms in breeding sows, and Wilburn *et al.* (2008) later observed the same effect. Rey and López-Bote (2014) reported that a higher presence of RRR-stereoisomers in pig fat indicated a greater consumption of the natural form of tocopherol provided by acorns and grass. In contrast, a higher proportion of S forms were related to a higher mixed diet intake. Analysis of the RRR-stereoisomer with γ- and α-tocopherol determination can be considered a potent tool with 90% success in sample classification for distinguishing fat from pigs fed under free-range conditions or exclusively with acorns and grass from those receiving a supplemented diet at any time of their fattening phase.

D-α-tocopherol is a yellow oil insoluble in water but soluble in organic solvents, resistant to heat, but readily oxidized. Natural and synthetic forms of vitamin E are degraded by oxidation and accelerated by heat, moisture, rancid fat, copper, and iron. The insertion of an acetate or succinate moiety on carbon 6 of the chromanol ring of either the natural or synthetic source stabilizes the compound. When acetate is inserted, the commercial names DL-α-tocopheryl acetate (all-*rac*-α-tocopheryl acetate) and D-α-tocopheryl acetate (RRR-α-tocopheryl acetate) are for the synthetic and naturally derived vitamin E products, respectively. The succinate form is less biologically active than the acetate form (Mahan, 2000). D-α-tocopherol is an excellent natural antioxidant that protects carotene and other oxidizable materials in feed and in the body. However, in the process of acting as an antioxidant, it is destroyed. The relative biological activity of vitamin E is expressed in International Units (IU), 1 IU corresponding to the activity of 1 mg of (all-rac)-α-tocopheryl acetate.

Natural sources
Vitamin E is widespread in nature. The synthesis of vitamin E is a function of plants: thus, their products are the principal sources. The richest sources are vegetable oils, cereal products containing these oils, eggs, liver, legumes, and green plants, especially leaves, and buds. Tender grass contains around 200 mg/kg (Rey *et al.*, 2006).

It is abundant in whole cereal grains (10–40 mg/kg), particularly in germ, and thus in by-products containing the germ (McDowell, 2000a; Traber, 2006, 2013). Rice bran, wheat germ, and some by-products of corn usually have larger quantities (50–70 mg/kg), although the remaining content is very variable depending on the technological treatment applied. Feed table averages are often of little value in predicting the individual content of feedstuffs or the bioavailability of vitamins. Barley (35–40 mg/kg) and oats (20–25 mg/kg) are the cereals that contain the largest quantity (Madsen *et al.*, 1973). There is wide variation in the vitamin content of feeds, with many feeds having a 3- to 10-fold range in reported α-tocopherol values. Vitamin E content of 42 varieties of corn varied from 11.1 to 36.4 IU/kg, a 3.3-fold difference (McDowell and Ward, 2008).

Legumes generally have a moderate α-tocopherol content (around 10 mg/kg). Oleaginous feeds have very variable content depending on whether or not the oil has been extracted and the extraction procedure itself. For example, the α-tocopherol content of whole soy seed is around 50 mg/kg. The cake obtained by mechanical extraction, however, contains approximately 7–10 mg/kg, and the cake obtained from solvent extraction has a value of around 3 mg/kg. In general, products of animal origin have insufficient quantities because, in live animals, the concentration rarely exceeds 2–4 mg/kg of tissue. The processing methods are usually very aggressive to tocopherols.

Naturally occurring vitamin E activity of feedstuffs cannot be accurately estimated from earlier published vitamin E or tocopherol values. α-tocopherol is exceptionally high in wheat germ oil and sunflower oil. Corn and soybean oil contain predominantly γ-tocopherol and some tocotrienols (McDowell, 2000a; Traber, 2006, 2013). Cottonseed oil contains both α- and γ-tocopherols in equal proportions. In practice, supplements are added in the more stable form of DL-α-tocopherol acetate.

The stability of all naturally occurring tocopherols is poor. Substantial losses (up to 90%) of vitamin E activity occur in feedstuffs after a few days or weeks when processed (drying, dehydration) and stored and during manufacturing (milling) and storage of finished feeds (Gadient, 1986; Dove and Ewan, 1991; McDowell 1996). For this reason, the vitamin E content of products, like dried alfalfa, can vary considerably depending on the production process (from 30 mg/kg or below up to a value of around 180 mg/kg). Vitamin E sources in these ingredients are unstable under conditions that promote oxidation of feedstuffs – heat, oxygen, moisture, oxidizing fats, and trace minerals. Vegetable oils that usually are excellent sources of vitamin E can be deficient in the vitamin if oxidation has been promoted. Oxidized oil has little or no vitamin E, destroying the vitamin E in other feed ingredients and depleting animal tissue stores of vitamin E.

Oxidation of vitamin E increases after grinding, mixing with minerals, adding fat, and pelleting for balanced feed. When feeds are pelleted, the destruction of vitamins E and A may occur if the diet does not contain sufficient antioxidants to prevent their accelerated oxidation under moisture and high-temperature conditions.

Iron salts (i.e., ferric chloride) can destroy vitamin E. Dove and Ewan (1987, 1991) investigated the effect of numerous trace minerals (18% crude protein soybean meal diets with no trace minerals, standard trace mineral levels, or with common trace minerals plus either 250 ppm copper, 1,000 ppm iron, 1,000 ppm zinc, or 100 ppm manganese) on the stability of vitamin E in swine grower diets. They concluded that the oxidation rate of natural tocopherols is increased in diets containing increased levels of copper, iron, zinc, or manganese. The authors also indicated that corn-soybean meal diets containing high levels of copper might require α-tocopheryl acetate to maintain recommended levels of vitamin E in diets during storage, especially when additional unsaturated fat is included (D'Arrigo *et al.*, 2002; Daza *et al.*, 2005). Dove and Ewan (1990) had previously reported that the addition of growth-promoting levels of copper increased the loss of natural tocopherols from feed and that supplemental tocopherol may be required to maintain serum tocopherol levels of pigs fed diets containing 250 ppm copper.

Artificial drying of corn results in a much lower vitamin E content. Studies testing vitamin E stability reported that artificial corn drying for 40 minutes at 87°C produced an average 10% loss of α-tocopherol and 12% loss of other tocopherols (Adams, 1973; Adams *et al.*, 1975). When corn was dried for 54 minutes at 93°C, the α-tocopherol loss averaged 41%. Young *et al.* (1975) reported concentrations of 9.3 and 20 mg/kg α-tocopherol in artificially dried corn versus undried, respectively.

Further decomposition of α-tocopherol occurs over an extended time until the grain eventually has α-tocopherol levels of less than 1 mg/kg, commonly found in propionic acid-treated barley (Madsen *et al.*, 1973). In alfalfa stored at 33°C for 12 weeks, vitamin E losses of 54–73% have been observed, and losses of 5–33% have been found with commercial dehydration of alfalfa. Apparently, the damage is not due to moisture alone but to the combined propionic acid/moisture effect (McMurray *et al.*, 1980).

Commercial forms

Vitamin E is usually incorporated into feeds as DL-α-tocopherol acetate (Chen, Wang, Li *et al.*, 2019). Other vitamin E esters are produced, like propionate or succinate, but the acetate form has been shown to be the one providing the best bioavailability. All-*rac*-α-tocopheryl acetate is manufactured by condensing trimethyl hydroquinone and isophytol and conducting ultra-vacuum molecular distillation, producing a highly purified form of α-tocopherol. This material may then be acetylated. As previously stated, all-*rac*-α-tocopherol is a mixture of α-tocopheryl acetate's 8 stereoisomers (4 enantiomeric pairs). The enantiomeric pairs, racemates, are present in equimolar amounts (Van Vleet *et al.*, 1973; Van Vleet, 1982; Cohen *et al.*, 1981; Amazan *et al.*, 2014). This finding indicates that the manufacturing processes lead to all-*rac*-α-tocopheryl acetate with similar proportions to all 8 stereoisomers (Weiser and Vecchi, 1982).

The vitamin E acetate product form, primarily used in animal feeding, is an adsorbate that provides good stability to storage and physical treatments applied in feed manufacturing, like pelleting or extrusion with the use of temperature and steam. Vitamin E acetate is also available in the spray-dried form, water-soluble, for application in drinking water or milk replacers. The spray-dried formulation is also indicated when stability may be critical, like aggressive premixes with very high pH or canned pet food.

Commercially there is no truly "natural" tocopherol product available since the D-form, or RRR-form of α-tocopherol commercial products, are obtained from the original raw material only after several chemical processing steps. Hence, it should be referred to as "natural-derived" and not natural. In addition, the International Unit (IU) is the standard of vitamin E activity; consequently, it is the same regardless of the source.

However, some studies undertaken in several species comparing the naturally derived RRR to the synthetic all-*rac*-α-tocopheryl acetate have shown the former to be more effective in elevating plasma and tissue concentrations when administered on an equal IU basis (Jensen *et al.*, 2006). Research in humans, poultry, sheep, pigs, guinea pigs, fish, and horses, in which the elevation of plasma concentrations was measured, indicated that the biopotency of RRR-α-tocopherol compared to all-*rac*-α-tocopherol can vary from the "official" figure of 1.36 : 1 up to closer to 2 : 1 (Traber, 2013), with differences among species. Considering the 1.36 : 1 ratio 1 mg of all-*rac*-α-tocopheryl acetate can be replaced by 0.74 mg RRR-α-tocopheryl acetate. In Figure 4.9, the vitamin E activity of different forms is reported relative to DL-α-tocopheryl acetate or all-*rac*-tocopheryl acetate set at 1.

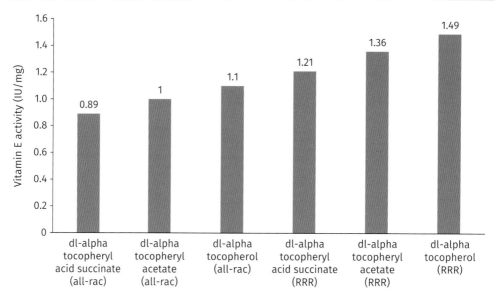

Figure 4.9 Vitamin E Activity of different chemical forms (IU/mg) relative to dl-α-tocopheryl acetate or all-*rac*-tocopheryl acetate set at 1 (source: United States Pharmacopeia, 1980)

As indicated previously, the acetate forms of α-tocopherol are commercially available from 2 primary sources: (1) D-α-tocopherol vegetable oil refining by-products, molecular distillation to obtain the α-form, and then acetylation to form the acetate ester; and (2) DL-α-tocopheryl acetate is made by complete chemical synthesis, producing a racemic mixture of equal proportions of 8 stereoisomers. Feeding a higher dietary level of DL-α-tocopheryl acetate could circumvent the lower bioavailability of the DL-α-form-tocopheryl acetate. The requirements of an animal and the level in the feed can be found expressed in IU of vitamin E (1 IU is equivalent to 1 mg DL-α-tocopherol acetate) or are expressed in mg of α-tocopherol equivalents (α-TE), which corresponds to the activity of D-α-tocopherol, the most active form (1 mg α-TE = 1 mg D-α-tocopherol =1.49 mg DL-α-tocopherol acetate).

Anderson *et al.* (1995b) evaluated the bioavailability of various vitamin E compounds by supplementing the diets of finishing swine for 28 days and comparing the concentration of α-tocopherol in blood serum and tissue. They indicated that both the acetate ester and alcohol forms of vitamin E resulted in rapid increases in serum concentration of vitamin E in finishing pigs. However, the serum concentrations remained higher longer, and the tissue concentrations of α-tocopherol were higher when supplementation was with the acetate ester forms. This difference was likely due to the greater stability of acetate forms in mixed feed. The most significant relative bioavailability in this swine trial was found when D-α-tocopheryl acetate was supplemented based on serum and tissue tocopherol concentrations. Furthermore, the authors concluded that the bioavailability of this form seems to be greater for finishing swine than the predicted values from traditional rat bioassays. The RRR-α-tocopherol potency is underestimated compared to all-*rac*-α-tocopherol in bioavailability for weanling pigs (Wilburn *et al.*, 2008), finishing swine (Yang *et al.*, 2009), and sows and suckling piglets (Mahan *et al.*, 2000; Lauridsen *et al.*, 2002).

Huang *et al.* (1995) evaluated the effectiveness of individual tocopherols and mixtures of these tocopherols in inhibiting the formation and decomposition of hydroperoxides in bulk corn oil, which had been stripped of natural tocopherols. Based on hydroperoxide formation, the concentrations required for maximum antioxidant activity of 1 : 1 mixtures of α- and γ-tocopherol or natural soybean tocopherol mixtures (α : γ: δ = 13 : 64 : 21) were 250 and 500 ppm, respectively.

Microencapsulation has emerged as a protection option for vitamin E. It allows its incorporation and controlled delivery into functional products. The procedure can be performed using different techniques and materials, which should be selected according to suitability with the delivery system's final purpose (Ribeiro *et al.*, 2021).

Metabolism

Absorption and transport

Early researchers investigated the effect of dietary fat on the intestinal absorption of tocopherol (Duncan *et al.*, 1960; Brigelius-Flohé, 2021). Vitamin E absorption is related to fat digestion and is facilitated by bile and pancreatic lipase (Sitrin *et al.*, 1987). Jensen *et al.* (1997) found that the ileal digestibilities of tocopherols vary based on the dietary fat source.

Tocopheryl acetate, the naturally occurring tocopherol form, is almost wholly hydrolyzed before absorption by duodenal pancreatic esterase, the enzyme which releases free fatty acids from dietary triacyl glycerides (Gallo-Torres, 1980; Gallo-Torres *et al.*, 1980; Hidiroglou *et al.*, 1995). Tocopherol absorption occurs predominantly in the median portion of the small intestine through the portal vein to the liver. The ester bond, which increases stability, is hydrolyzed, and the resulting alcohol form is absorbed in the formation of bile salt micelles and lipids from the ration.

Vitamin E is thus passively transferred into the micelle and absorbed through the brush border cells. The enterocytes of the upper and middle third of the small intestine absorb these micelles and transport them in the portomicrons and lipoproteins via lymph to the general circulation. Like all fat-soluble vitamins, carotenoids, and other fat-soluble dietary components, vitamin E is incorporated into chylomicrons. In healthy conditions, the efficiency of vitamin E absorption varies from 35% to 50%, lower than that of vitamin A. Digestibility may be even less in some cases, such as that in piglets. In studies carried out with rats, Gallo-Torres *et al.* (1980) found that absorption of α-tocopherol and/or its esters, when ingested orally, was 20–40%. Similar data have been described in swine.

As the dietary vitamin E level increases, the total amount of vitamin E absorbed will increase, but the relative amount absorbed will decline. Of the natural vitamin E compounds, approximately 32% of the α-, 18% of the β-, 30% of the γ-, and <2% of the δ-tocopherol forms are absorbed. Approximately 20–30% of orally ingested vitamin E is absorbed (Mahan, 2000; Debier and Larondelle, 2005; Rigotti, 2007).

Any ester form, i.e., tocopheryl acetate, succinate, or propionate, to be absorbed into the body is converted to the alcohol form, and an α-tocopherol transfer protein has been identified (Traber, 2006, 2013). In piglets, the lower efficiency of the esterase can limit digestion and absorption. The young pig consumes sow colostrum and milk, high in fat and α-tocopherol concentrations. Milk fat is considered highly digestible (>95%) by the young pig. Consequently, α-tocopherol and γ-tocopherol are both in sow milk and are highly available, as reflected by their high serum α-tocopherol concentration in the nursing pig. Serum α-tocopherol, however, has been found to decline rapidly upon weaning but subsequently increases within 3 to 4 weeks post-weaning (Mahan, 2000).

When comparing feeds with or without added fat, a higher concentration of α-tocopherol (between 10% and 15%) is generally observed in pigs given fatty feeds. This may be due partially to the high content of tocopherols in vegetable oils, although not exclusively so, because the same phenomenon is observed (to a lesser extent) when they are given animal fats (with very low vitamin E content), so tocopherol absorption is likely helped by the inclusion of fat in the feed. Initial work has concluded that PUFAs reduce the apparent absorption of vitamin E (Gallo-Torres, 1980). However, Tijburg *et al.* (1997) concluded that levels of these fatty acids might not affect vitamin E absorption. Medium-chain triglycerides enhance vitamin E absorption, whereas ferric ions could destroy vitamin E. In a study by Amazan *et al.* (2014), it was proven that oral supplementation given to sows of 30 mg/kg of micellized D-α-tocopherol could result in similar concentrations of tocopherol in piglets comparable with those resulting from the synthetic form. A ratio of 1 : 2 doses of micellized α-tocopherol is needed to optimize the immune response in piglets.

The simultaneous digestion and absorption of dietary fats enhance the absorption of vitamin E. Most vitamin E is absorbed as alcohol, whether presented as free alcohol or as esters. Esters are hydrolyzed mainly in the intestinal wall, and the free alcohol enters the intestinal lacteals and is transported via the lymph to the general circulation. An α-tocopherol transfer protein has been identified (Traber, 2006, 2013).

The animal appears to prefer tocopherol versus other tocols. Rates and amounts of absorption of the various tocopherols and tocotrienols are in the same general order of magnitude as their biological potencies. α-tocopherol is absorbed best, with γ-tocopherol absorption slightly less than α-forms but with a more rapid excretion. Generally, most of the vitamin E activity within plasma and other animal tissues is α-tocopherol (Ullrey, 1981). The mechanisms for the uptake of vitamin E absorption into enterocytes are not well understood. According to Reboul and Borel (2011), nonvitamin E-specific transporters like cholesterol and lipid transporters should be involved (Rigotti, 2007).

No plasma-specific vitamin E transport proteins have been identified. Vitamin E in plasma is attached mainly to lipoproteins in the globulin fraction within cells and occurs mainly in mitochondria and microsomes. The liver takes the vitamin, which is released in combination with low-density and very-low-density lipoproteins (LDL and VLDL) (Rigotti, 2007; Traber, 2013).

Plasma vitamin E concentrations depend on α-tocopherol secretion from the liver (Kaempf-Rotzoll *et al.*, 2003). Additionally, the newly absorbed vitamin E, rather than that returning from the periphery, appears to be preferentially secreted into the plasma from the liver (Traber *et al.*, 1998). Thus, the liver, not the intestine, discriminates between tocopherols (Traber, 2013). In contrast to α-tocopherol, the 7 other vitamers are not recognized by the α-tocopherol transfer protein (α-TTP) in the liver.

After hepatic uptake, the α-tocopherol form of vitamin E is preferentially resecreted into the circulation. The α-tocopherol transfer protein (α-TTP) is a critical regulator of vitamin E status, which stimulates the movement of vitamin E between membrane vesicles *in vitro* and facilitates the secretion of tocopherol from hepatocytes. Recent studies have shown that the liver has a critical role in the biodiscrimination of stereoisomers because of the presence of α-TTP, which preferentially transfers α-tocopherol, compared with other dietary vitamin E forms (Panagabko *et al.*, 2002). This protein preferentially selects RRR and 2R α-tocopherol for secretion into plasma (Leonard *et al.*, 2002). Some authors suggested that the metabolism of 2S stereoisomers in the liver may be faster than that of 2R ST: thereby, the reduced presence of 2S stereoisomers in the liver and other tissues could be caused by faster metabolism rather than the lower affinity of the α-TTP (Kiyose *et al.*, 1995; Kaneko *et al.*, 2000). Specific receptors explain tissue distribution in tissues for lipoprotein carriers, passive diffusion from membrane lipoproteins to tissues, or lipoprotein lipase acting as a carrier protein (Parker, 1989; Rigotti, 2007). It has also been established that there is a negative interaction between vitamin E and vitamin A or β-carotene, as they interfere with each other in their absorption and deposition processes (Preś *et al.*, 1993; Gonçalves *et al.*, 2015).

Lindberg (1973) reported that average values for tocopherol in plasma from pigs are much lower than those measured in plasma from dogs. Tocopherol levels are higher in pigs approaching slaughter weight than in newly weaned pigs. Froseth (1978) reviewed various studies to evaluate the effects of dietary additions of selenium, vitamin E, and different inorganic elements on selenium and vitamin E metabolism, including serum tocopherol levels and tissue selenium.

The sow's diet influences stores in the young pig at birth and the amount obtained from the mother's milk. However, vitamin E is ineffective in passing through swine placental membranes (Whiting and Loosli, 1948; Whiting et al., 1949; Mahan, 1990; Lauridsen et al., 2002; Hidiroglou et al., 2003). Thus, the vitamin E reserves of pigs at farrowing are low (Urbanova and Toulova, 1975; Hakkarainen et al., 1978b). As the placental transfer of tocopherol from the dam to the fetus is minimal, milk's importance for enhancing the newborn's vitamin E status is greater (Lauridsen et al., 2002; Debier and Larondelle, 2005; Matte and Audet, 2020). However, Hidiroglou et al. (2003) reported a substantial transfer of 2H-labelled α-tocopherol across the placenta and through the mammary gland in guinea pigs. The relative bioavailability (d3:d6) across fetal and neonatal tissues was, on average, 1.81:1.00, with a range from 1.62:1.00 to 2.01:1.00. Maternal tissues had a mean ratio of 1.77:1.00. A higher relative bioavailability ($p \leq 0.05$) was observed with natural compared with synthetic α-tocopherol, as shown by a higher d3:d6 ratio in all tissues examined. Vitamin E was highest in colostrum on day 2 and then declined by day 5. Results from this present experiment further question the accepted biological potencies of natural: synthetic α-tocopheryl acetate of 1.36:1.00.

Storage and excretion

Vitamin E is stored throughout all body tissues, with the greatest concentrations in the liver and the fat (Mahan, 2000; Traber, 2013; Brigelius-Flohé, 2021). However, vitamin E is not accumulated in the liver as it contains only a tiny fraction of total body stores, in contrast to vitamin A, for which about 95% of the body reserves are in the liver. Hoppe et al. (1993) indicated that adipose tissue contained the highest concentrations of vitamin E, followed by liver, cardiac muscle, and musculus longissimus in decreasing order. Hoppe et al. (1993) suggested the discrepancy might be due to whether or not the pigs were sacrificed with or without fasting. The authors noted in their study that the pigs were slaughtered after 24 hours of fasting, which likely caused partial depletion of liver vitamin E.

Subcellular fractions (endoplasmic reticulum or the nuclear membrane) from different tissues vary considerably in their tocopherol content, with the highest levels found in membranous organelles, such as microsomes and mitochondria, which contain highly active oxidation-reduction systems (McCay et al., 1981; Rigotti, 2007; Traber, 2013; Brigelius-Flohé, 2021). Nevertheless, this distribution is not homogeneous in all animal cells.

Marked differences have been observed in α-tocopherol deposition depending on the oxidative capacity of muscle fiber. Oxidative muscles present a greater concentration of vitamin E associated with a greater phospholipid content, increased vascular development, and greater activity of mitochondrial enzymes (Jensen et al., 1990). Small amounts of vitamin E will persist tenaciously in the body for a long time. However, stores are exhausted rapidly by PUFA in the tissues. The rate of disappearance is proportional to the intake of PUFA.

Plasma α-tocopherol levels in swine seem to be lower than in other species. Blood and serum α-tocopherol were associated with lipoproteins, but the correlation of α-tocopherol to blood triglyceride or cholesterol was not high in the young weanling pig (Mahan, 2000).

The major excretion routes of absorbed vitamin E are feces and bile, in which toco-pherol appears mainly in the free form (McDowell, 2000a). The tocopherols that pass through the intestinal tract occur from incomplete absorption, secretion from the mucosal cells into the lumen, desquamation of intestinal epithelial cells, and biliary excretion. Of the absorbed tocopherols, some are converted to quinone and excreted. The biliary route can excrete tocopheryl acetates and tocopherol, but the amount is relatively small (~2.4%) (Mahan, 2000; Traber, 2013).

Biochemical functions

Vitamin E is essential for the reproductive, circulatory, nervous, immune, and muscular sys-tems (Figure 4.10) (Hoekstra, 1975; Sheffy and Schultz, 1979; Bendich, 1987; Hoffmann-La Roche, 1991; McDowell, 2000a; Traber, 2013; Brigelius-Flohé, 2021). In fact, it is one of the vitamins to which the greatest investigative efforts have been dedicated for discovering its mechanism of action and requirements (Mahan, 2000; Pinelli-Saavedra, 2003).

Vitamin E:

- is the primary antioxidant in blood and, on a cellular level, it maintains the integrity of the cellular and vascular membranes
- it acts as a detoxifier and takes part in many other biochemical reactions
- is essential for fertility
- it promotes the activity of immune system cells
- it can alleviate stress and increase immunocompetence (Jensen *et al.*, 1988; Bonnette *et al.*, 1990a,b; Pinelli-Saavedra, 2003)
- is also involved in the prevention of cardiovascular and carcinogenic diseases.

Classical α-tocopherol functions of Vitamin E
Antioxidant

Numerous studies have established the relationship between vitamin E consumed and the prevention of oxidation or oxidative distress in biological systems (Meyer *et al.*, 1981;

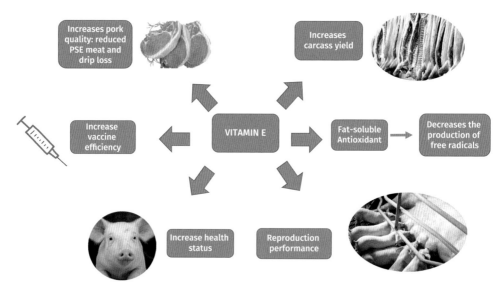

Figure 4.10 Vitamin E functions (source: adapted from Nawab *et al.*, 2019 and Shojadoost *et al.*, 2021)

Buckley *et al.*, 1995; Singh *et al.*, 2005; Cardenia *et al.*, 2011; Lima *et al.*, 2012; Amazan *et al.*, 2014; Buchet *et al.*, 2017; Bacou *et al.*, 2021; Brigelius-Flohé, 2021). Under physiological conditions, cells maintain redox homeostasis by producing oxidants, i.e., reactive oxygen species (ROS) and other free radicals, and their elimination by an antioxidant system. When the balance favors oxidants, we have oxidative distress (Dunnett, 2003; Surai *et al.*, 2019; Bacou *et al.*, 2021).

Free-radical reactions are ubiquitous in biological systems and are associated with energy metabolism, biosynthetic reactions, natural defense mechanisms, detoxification, and intra- and intercellular signaling pathways. Redox homeostasis is an essential mechanism for aerobic organisms (bacteria, plants, animals, and humans). Highly ROS such as the superoxide anion radical (O_2-), hydroxyl radical (OH), hydrogen peroxide (H_2O_2), and singlet oxygen (O_2-) are continuously produced in the course of normal aerobic cellular metabolism. Also, phagocytic granulocytes undergo respiratory bursts to produce oxygen radicals to destroy intracellular pathogens. However, these oxidative products can, in turn, damage healthy cells if they are not eliminated. Antioxidants serve to stabilize these highly reactive free radicals, thereby maintaining the structural and functional integrity of cells (Chew, 1995; Singh *et al.*, 2005; Brigelius-Flohé, 2021).

Vitamin E is a quenching agent for free-radical molecules with single, highly reactive electrons in their outer shells. Free radicals attract a hydrogen atom, along with its electron, away from the chain structure, satisfying the electron needs of the original free radical but leaving the PUFA short one electron. Thus, a fatty acid-free radical is formed that joins with molecular oxygen to form a peroxyl radical that steals a hydrogen-electron unit from yet another PUFA. This reaction can continue in a chain, destroying thousands of PUFA molecules (Gardner, 1989). Free radicals can be highly damaging to biological systems (McCay, 1985).

Vitamin E has a crucial role within the cellular defense system in the face of oxidation at both intracellular and extracellular levels. α-tocopherol is integrated within the cellular membrane and protects lipids from oxidation, preventing them from being attacked by reactive oxygen and free radicals (Surai and Fisinin, 2015; Brigelius-Flohé, 2021). Tocopherols remove the peroxyl radical, donating a hydrogen atom and converting it to peroxide. Support for the antioxidant role of vitamin E *in vivo* also comes from observations that synthetic antioxidants can either prevent or alleviate certain clinical signs of vitamin E deficiency diseases. Therefore, antioxidants are vital to humans' and animals' immune defense and health (Singh *et al.*, 2005).

Most vitamin E deficiency symptoms are related to disorders of the cellular membrane due to the oxidative degradation of PUFAs and phospholipids (Chow, 1979) and critical sulfhydryl groups (Tollersrud, 1973; Brownlee *et al.*, 1977). The orientation of vitamin E within cell membranes appears to be essential to its functionality (Surai and Fisinin, 2015). It has been demonstrated how the deposition of α-tocopherol in animal tissues increases in direct proportion to its supply in the diet and is accompanied by greater oxidative stability (Buckley *et al.*, 1995; Jensen *et al.*, 1997; Cardenia *et al.*, 2011; Sobotka *et al.*, 2012). Conversely, it is known that susceptibility to oxidation increases as the number of double bonds of fatty acids increases (Gardner, 1989).

As the profile of fatty acids in the ration is reflected in the fatty acid composition of the different tissues of the animal, increasing the degree of unsaturation in the feed increases susceptibility to oxidation and reduces the quantity of α-tocopherol deposited in the tissues (Malm *et al.*, 1976a; Astrup and Langebrekke, 1985; Rammell *et al.*, 1988; Rice and Kennedy, 1989; Grela and Jakobsen, 1994; Muggli, 1994; Gebert *et al.*, 1999a,b). The type of fatty acid and tocopherol levels also vary between organs and can be modified by the diet (Berlin *et al.*, 1994). Hence, high levels of PUFA in the diet cause an increase in the susceptibility of tissues to lipid oxidation, increasing the requirements for vitamin E (Dutta-Roy *et al.*, 1994; Muggli, 1994). Vitamin E reserves become depleted when acting as an antioxidant, which explains the frequent observation that the presence of dietary unsaturated fats (susceptible to peroxidation) increases or precipitates a vitamin E deficiency. Consequently, vitamin E supplementation should increase in parallel to the amount of unsaturated fatty acids and the degree of oxidation of the fat added to the feed (Grela and Jakobsen, 1994; D'Arrigo *et al.*, 2002; Daza *et al.*, 2005).

Farm livestock require 2.5–3.0 mg dl-α-tocopheryl acetate for each gram of PUFA in the diet. Using blended fats with an 18% PUFA, 5 mg of vitamin E should be added for every 1% blended fat. Requirements also depend on the presence or absence of other compounds that intervene in the tissue oxidation defense system, such as selenium. It should be borne in mind that depending on the feed ingredients and hence the content of tocopherols, carotenoids, and other antioxidants, there will be a variation in the oxidative state of the animal and, therefore, the requirements of antioxidants and specifically of vitamin E (Bacou *et al.*, 2021). Interruption of fat peroxidation by tocopherol explains that dietary tocopherols protect or spare body supplies such oxidizable materials as vitamin A, vitamin C, and carotenes.

Relationship with selenium in tissue protection

Vitamin E and selenium share several molecular functions in regulating many genes encoding for proteins with potent antioxidant activity (Yen *et al.*, 1985). Consequently, both have been included in the study of the selenogenome (Sun *et al.*, 2019). Tissue breakdown occurs in most species receiving diets deficient in vitamin E and selenium, mainly through peroxidation. Peroxides and hydroperoxides are highly destructive to tissue integrity and lead to disease development.

Selenium has been shown to act in aqueous cell media (cytosol and mitochondrial matrix) by destroying hydrogen peroxide and hydroperoxides via the enzyme glutathione peroxidase (GSH-Px), which is a cofactor (Meyer *et al.*, 1981; Sun *et al.*, 2019). This capacity prevents the oxidation of unsaturated lipid materials within cells, thus protecting fats within the cell membrane from breakdown. The various GSH-Px enzymes are characterized by different tissue specificities and are expressed from other genes. Different forms of GSH-Px perform their protective functions in concert, each providing antioxidant protection at various body sites.

Therefore, selenium has a sparing effect on vitamin E and delays the onset of deficiency signs. Likewise, vitamin E and sulfur amino acids partially protect against or delay the onset of several forms of selenium deficiency syndromes (Surai *et al.*, 2019). Vitamin E in cellular and subcellular membranes appears to be the first line of defense against the peroxidation of vital phospholipids. Still, even with adequate vitamin E, some peroxides are formed. As part of the enzyme GSH-Px, selenium is a second line of defense that destroys these peroxides before they can cause damage to membranes.

Therefore, through different biochemical mechanisms, selenium, vitamin E, and sulfur-containing amino acids can prevent some of the same nutritional diseases. Vitamin E prevents fatty acid hydroperoxide formation, sulfur amino acids are precursors of GSH-Px, and selenium is a component of GSH-Px, which has been evaluated in weanling pigs (Tollersrud, 1973; Smith *et al.*, 1974; Meyer *et al.*, 1981).

Membrane structure and prostaglandin synthesis

α-tocopherol may be involved in forming structural components of biological membranes, thus exerting a unique influence on the architecture of membrane phospholipids (Ullrey, 1981;

Surai *et al.*, 2019). It is reported that α-tocopherol stimulated the incorporation of 14C from linoleic acid into arachidonic acid in fibroblast phospholipids. Also, it was found that α-tocopherol exerted a pronounced stimulatory influence on the formation of prostaglandins and thromboxanes from arachidonic acid, while a chemical antioxidant had no effect (Traber, 2013).

Meat quality

To improve oxidative stability and thus increase the shelf life of meat, antioxidants have been successfully added to animal feeds (Hvidsten and Astrup, 1973; Gray *et al.*, 1989). Several compounds, such as carotenoids, vitamin E, vitamin C, and selenium, are known to have potent antioxidant effects on pork meat. Of them, α-tocopherol has demonstrated the highest biological efficiency in preventing lipid oxidation *in vivo* (Marusich, 1978; Van Heugten, 1999; Trefan *et al.*, 2011).

Myodystrophic tissue is common in cases of vitamin E-selenium deficiency, with leakage of cellular compounds such as creatinine and various transaminases through affected membranes into plasma. The more active the cell (e.g., the cells of skeletal and involuntary muscles), the greater the inflow of lipids for energy supply. The greater the risk of tissue damage if vitamin E is limited. For example, Hoz *et al.* (2003) analyzed pork tenderloin muscles (psoas major) from pigs fed diets that only vary on the oil source sunflower (C), linseed (L), and linseed and olive (1/1, w/w) (LO), and α-tocopherol supplementation at 20 or 200 mg/kg diet in a factorial arrangement of treatments. The n-6/n-3 ratio in pork tenderloin was markedly modified by dietary linseed oil administration, which was due to the increase in the C18 : 3 n-3 (and total n-3 fatty acids) and the decrease in the C18 : 2 n-6 (and total n-6 fatty acids) contents ($p<0.05$). The α-tocopherol content of tenderloin from pigs fed 20 mg/kg was about 2.8 mg/kg of muscle, significantly greater ($p<0.05$) than about 0.7 mg/kg muscle found in tenderloin from pigs receiving diets with C, L, and LO. These authors observed that dietary supplementation with α-tocopheryl acetate markedly reduced tenderloin lipid oxidation from animals fed diets enriched in n-3 fatty acids.

Certain consequences of vitamin E deficiency (i.e., dietary muscular dystrophy) can be prevented by diet supplementation with other antioxidant nutrients, which help validate the antioxidant role of tocopherols (Orstadius *et al.*, 1963; Mahan *et al.*, 1973). Chemical antioxidants are stored at shallow levels and thus are not as effective as tocopherol. To improve oxidative stability and thus increase the shelf life of meat, antioxidants have been successfully added to animal feeds. In the last few years, besides vitamin E, different compounds such as carotenoids, vitamin C, selenium, and plant extracts have been tested in various experiments to verify their potential antioxidant effect on pork quality (Gray, 1990; Osborne *et al.*, 1998; Corino *et al.*, 1999; Kerth *et al.*, 2001; Hasty *et al.*, 2002; Peeters *et al.*, 2005; Guo *et al.*, 2006a, 2006b; Morel *et al.*, 2008). Of them all, α-tocopherol demonstrated the highest biological efficiency in preventing lipid oxidation *in vivo* (Hoving-Bolink *et al.*, 1998).

Immune response

Vitamin E is perhaps the most studied nutrient related to the immune response (Meydani and Han, 2006). Evidence accumulated over the years and in many species indicates that vitamin E is an essential nutrient for the normal function of the immune system. Furthermore, studies suggest that disease-reducing beneficial effects of certain nutrients, such as vitamin E, can affect the immune response of pigs (Riedel-Caspari *et al.*, 1986; Jensen *et al.*, 1988; Bonnette *et al.*, 1990b; Babinszky *et al.*, 1991a; Nemec *et al.*, 1994; Pinelli-Saavedra, 2003; Amazan *et al.*, 2014).

Considerable attention is presently being directed to vitamin E and selenium's role in protecting leukocytes and macrophages during phagocytosis, the mechanism whereby animals immunologically kill invading bacteria. Vitamin E and selenium may help these cells survive the toxic products produced to effectively kill ingested bacteria (Badwey and Karnovsky, 1980). Macrophages and neutrophils from vitamin E-deficient animals have decreased phagocytic activity (Khan *et al.*, 2012).

Since vitamin E acts as a tissue antioxidant and aids in quenching free radicals produced in the body, any infection or other stress factor may exacerbate the depletion of the limited vitamin E stores in various tissues. The former 2 responses are generally used to determine a nutrient requirement.

During stress and disease, there is an increase in the production of glucocorticoids, epinephrine, eicosanoids, and phagocytic activity. Eicosanoid and corticoid synthesis and phagocytic respiratory bursts are prominent producers of free radicals, which challenge the animal's antioxidant systems. In 1987, Duthie *et al.* proposed that stress-susceptibility syndrome may be associated with abnormal vitamin E metabolism. Subsequently, Duthie *et al.* (1989) reported that the results of their study indicated that stress-susceptible pigs have antioxidant abnormalities, which can be partially compensated for by increasing dietary vitamin E supplementation. Therefore, vitamin E supplementation may reduce the number of stress-related deaths among stress-susceptible pigs. In a related study, Hoppe *et al.* (1989) evaluated the effects of adding ascorbic acid (vitamin C) in addition to vitamin E to increase the antioxidant content of the ration. These authors reported that antioxidant supplementation significantly protected cell membrane integrity in stress-susceptible pigs.

Vitamin E also most likely has an immunoenhancing effect by virtue of altering arachidonic acid metabolism and subsequent synthesis of prostaglandins, thromboxanes, and leukotrienes. Under increased stress conditions, levels of these compounds by endogenous synthesis or exogenous entry may adversely affect immune cell function (Hadden, 1987; Khan *et al.*, 2012). Vitamin E has been implicated in stimulating serum antibody synthesis, particularly IgG antibodies (Tengerdy, 1980). The protective effects of vitamin E on animal health may reduce glucocorticoids, which are known to be immunosuppressive (Golub and Gershwin, 1985).

Vitamin E and selenium enhance host defenses against infections by improving phagocytic cell function. Both vitamin E and GSH-Px are antioxidants that protect phagocytic cells and surrounding tissues from oxidative attack by free radicals produced by the respiratory burst of neutrophils and macrophages during phagocytosis (Baker and Cohen, 1983; Babior, 1984; Surai *et al.*, 2019). Hogan *et al.* (1990, 1992, 1996) reported that dietary vitamin E supplementation increased the intracellular kill of *Staphylococcus aureus* and *Escherichia coli* by neutrophils.

Likewise, Morrow *et al.* (1987) reported that vitamin E improved the health status of pigs from sows housed in confinement and that it was possible to enhance the cellular and humoral immune responses of these young pigs with vitamin E as compared to pigs from sows that were kept on alfalfa pasture during gestation. These authors also indicated that pigs injected at birth and 10 days of age with 400 IU of vitamin E were heavier than controls at 28 days of age.

Babinszky *et al.* (1991a) investigated the effects of dietary vitamin E in pregnant and lactating sow diets on serum vitamin E concentration and cell-mediated and humoral immune response in suckling and weaned piglets. Not only did vitamin E in the sow's diet increase serum vitamin E concentrations in the 1 week-old piglets, but the phagocytic cell activity of the piglets was also increased. Furthermore, the immune response against ovalbumin increased 1 week after immunization for weaned pigs from litters fed high levels (136 mg α-tocopherol/kg feed) of vitamin E.

In a subsequent study, Babinszky et al. (1991b) indicated that the humoral immune system of lactating sows may be affected by the combinations of α-tocopherol and fat that are included in gestation and lactation diets. They did not find evidence that the cell-mediated immunity of sows was affected by either α-tocopherol or fat addition to their diets. Mudron et al. (1996) reported that T-lymphocyte percentages and the metabolic activity of phagocytes were more significant after injection of vitamin E (20 mg tocopheryl acetate per kg body weight).

Teige et al. (1982) reported that when pigs were fed minced colon from swine with dysentery or with a pure culture of *Treponema hyodysenteriae*, vitamin E and selenium supplementation in a deficient diet increased resistance to the disease. In a separate study, Teige et al. (1982) indicated that the effect of selenium on *T. hyodysenteriae* was greater than the effect of vitamin E. Larsen and Tollersrud (1981) noted that dietary vitamin E or selenium increased the phytohemagglutinin (PHA) response of peripheral pig lymphocytes. Furthermore, adding vitamin E increased the PHA response regardless of selenium levels. Peplowski et al. (1980) found an additive effect of vitamin E and Se, which increased hemagglutination titers when these nutrients were provided through dietary sources or injections. Jensen et al. (1988) reported that lymphocyte response to pokeweed mitogen was at least twice as high in pigs with serum vitamin E values above 3 mg per liter compared with lymphocytes from animals with lower concentrations of serum vitamin E.

Data from Wuryastuti et al. (1993) implied that if gestating sows do not obtain sufficient vitamin E and (or) selenium, the sows and their piglets will be more susceptible to disease in the peripartum period. Selenium restriction impaired neutrophil function, while vitamin E affected lymphocytes and neutrophils. The authors concluded that maintaining a 0.3 mg of selenium per kilogram diet for swine is justified and that the immune response should be considered when the NRC reevaluates vitamin E requirements. Bonnette et al. (1990a) evaluated the influence of supplemental dietary vitamin E (11 or 220 IU/kg diet) on performance, humoral antibody production, and serum cortisol levels of young pigs. The higher level of supplemental vitamin E increased serum vitamin E concentration. Still, performance, cortisol levels, immune response, and antibody titers in red blood cells were not affected as measured under the conditions of this experiment. The authors concluded that pigs nursed by sows fed NRC-estimated nutrient requirements for vitamin E and selenium have sufficient stores of vitamin E at weaning so that providing the young pigs 220 versus 11 IU vitamin E per kilogram of diet offers no advantage. These results confirm the findings obtained in a separate study by Bonnette et al. (1990b). Goss and Bilkei (1994) could not detect a significant influence of dietary vitamin E supplementation on pregnant sows on periparturient hypogalactia syndrome (PHS) or postnatal piglet losses. However, these authors did observe that supplementing the sow rations with vitamin E during gestation resulted in a significant weaning litter weight improvement. The authors suggested that a subclinical manifestation of PHS in the sows fed the unsupplemented diet might have resulted in less milk production, contributing to the lowered weight gain in these piglets.

The administration of LPS is a well-documented model for evaluating disease stress (Wyns et al., 2015). The response to LPS can be attributed to events that include cytokine synthesis and release (Dinarello, 1996; Webel et al., 1997). Cytokines are released from activated macrophages in response to immunologic challenges and are primarily responsible for the subsequent metabolic effects (Webel et al., 1997). Webel et al. (1998) investigated whether or not vitamin E might affect pro-inflammatory cytokine production. In their *in vivo* study, the effects of intramuscular injection of vitamin E (d-α-tocopherol) on plasma interleukin-6 (IL-6) and cortisol in pigs subjected to a challenge dose of LPS were evaluated. Pigs that received vitamin E before the LPS challenge had substantially lower peak levels of IL-6 and cortisol than pigs not provided with vitamin E injections. The authors suggested that the improved survival and growth performance of pigs after weaning noted by other authors, who provided pigs with vitamin E injections, might be partially due to the reduction of excess pro-inflammatory cytokines during the stressful post-weaning period (Van Vleet *et al.*, 1973, 1975; Weaver *et al.*, 1991).

Antioxidants, including vitamin E, play a role in resistance to viral infection. Vitamin E deficiency allows a usually benign virus to cause disease (Beck *et al.*, 1994). In mice, enhanced virulence of a virus resulted in a myocardial injury that was prevented with adequate vitamin E. A selenium or vitamin E deficiency leads to a change in viral phenotype, such that a non-virulent strain of a virus becomes virulent, and a virulent strain becomes more virulent (Beck, 1997, 2007; Sheridan and Beck, 2008). Thus, host nutritional status should be considered a driving force for the emergence of new viral strains or newly pathogenic strains of known viruses.

Reproduction

The semen quality of boars was improved with selenium and vitamin E supplementation, with vitamin E playing a role in maintaining sperm integrity in combination with selenium (Marin-Guzman *et al.*, 1989). In 1995, Brzezinska-Slebodzinska *et al.* evaluated the antioxidant effect of vitamin E and glutathione on lipid peroxidation in boar semen plasma. 7 weeks of oral DL-α-tocopheryl acetate (1,000 IU/day/boar) caused a decrease in semen plasma thiobarbituric acid reactive substances. The measurement is chosen to reflect lipid peroxidation. Furthermore, vitamin E supplementation significantly increased the number of spermatozoa per cubic centimeter of ejaculate. The authors indicated that vitamin E protects boar semen against fatty acid peroxidation and positively influences semen quality. These antioxidant effects on erythrocyte hemolysis, testicular fatty acids, and selenium status had been observed by McDowell *et al.* (1974, 1977) when boars were fed diets with oxidized cottonseed oil.

Marin-Guzman *et al.* (1997) confirmed that dietary vitamin E and selenium could affect boar semen quality but reported that the more significant effect seemed to be from selenium. These authors also suggested that selenium and vitamin E might act separately, perhaps maintaining semen and sperm quality through their antioxidant properties. In a later study (Marin-Guzman *et al.*, 2000), this research group observed that low selenium-diets fed to boars resulted in abnormal spermatozoan mitochondria, a lower adenosine triphosphate (ATP) concentration in the spermatozoa, and a loose apposition of the plasma membrane to the helical coil of the tail midpiece. Adding sodium selenite to the semen extender reduced sperm cell motility. Still, no effect from inadequate vitamin E was demonstrated.

Gilts supplemented with vitamin E (DL-α-tocopherol acetate 50 or 100 mg/kg) had 16% lower anestrus (Grandhi *et al.*, 1993). Injection with vitamin E (Myer, 1992; Pardo, 1995) or diet fortification (Piatkowski *et al.*, 1979; Mutetikka and Mahan, 1993) together with selenium before breeding, gestation (11 IU/kg diet) or lactation (22 IU/kg diet) has been shown to improve reproductive performance of gilts and sows and positively affect piglets. The supplementation of sow diets with vitamin E and vitamin C (Sosnowska *et al.*, 2011) or selenium has shown positive effects on sow livability and piglet antioxidant status. In a more recent study, Chen *et al.* (2016) concluded that vitamin E supplementation (30 or 90 IU/kg) did not improve the reproductive performance of sows during gestation and lactation. Still, levels of α-tocopherol increased in serum, colostrum, and milk. In contrast, organic selenium (0.30 mg Se/kg feed) improved antioxidant capacity, milk composition, and the number of pigs weaned compared with sow-fed inorganic selenium.

Blood clotting

Vitamin E is an inhibitor of platelet aggregation (McIntosh et al., 1985). It may play a role by inhibiting the peroxidation of arachidonic acid, which is required to form prostaglandins involved in platelet aggregation (Panganamala and Cornwell, 1982; Machlin, 1991; Traber, 2013). The antioxidant property of vitamin E also ensures erythrocyte stability and capillary blood vessel integrity maintenance.

Cellular respiration, electron transport, and deoxyribonucleic acid

Vitamin E is involved in biological oxidation-reduction reactions (Traber, 2013). Vitamin E also appears to regulate the biosynthesis of deoxyribonucleic acid (DNA) within cells. Vitamin E seems to be of particular importance in the cellular respiration of the heart and skeletal muscles (Berlin et al., 1994; Rey et al., 1997).

Relationship to toxic elements or substances

Both vitamin E and selenium protect against the toxicity of various heavy metals (Whanger, 1981). Vitamin E is highly effective in reducing the toxicity of metals such as silver, arsenic, and lead and shows slight effects against cadmium and mercury toxicity. Vitamin E can be effective against other toxic substances (Cabassi et al., 2004).

Vitamin E but not selenium was found to be effective in preventing the development of lesions induced by silver supplementation in weanling pigs' diets (Van Vleet, 1976). Miller (1971) reported that supplemental vitamin E partially prevented copper toxicity. Based on the results of their study, Van Vleet et al. (1981) suggested that increased amounts of selenium and vitamin E might be needed to prevent the development of selenium-vitamin E deficiency in animals fed rations containing large concentrations of several trace elements (silver, tellurium, cobalt, zinc, cadmium or vanadium). Hitchcock et al. (1978), in a feeding trial and 2 balance studies with vitamin E (6 or 28 IU/kg), selenium from corn or sodium selenite at 0.1 ppm, and arsanilic acid (99 ppm), observed that vitamin E supplementation increased selenium retention from seleniferous corn by decreasing urinary and fecal selenium loss. Arsanilic acid decreased selenium excretion and, consequently, increased selenium retention.

Tollerz (1973) indicated that certain pigs have an abnormally high sensitivity to iron and that vitamin E or selenium supplementation raised the tolerance level to iron in piglets and other species. Nielsen et al. (1979) reported that iron toxicity was observed in piglets that were not supplied with adequate dietary vitamin E. Vitamin E can be effective against other toxic substances. For example, treatment with vitamin E gave protection to weanling pigs against monensin-induced skeletal muscle damage (Van Vleet et al., 1987).

Non-α-tocopherol functions of Vitamin E

Although α-tocopherol has been the most widely studied form of vitamin E, other tocopherols and tocotrienols have been shown to have biological significance (Qureshi et al., 2001; Eder et al., 2002; McCormick and Parker, 2004; Schaffer et al., 2005; Nakagawa et al., 2007; Sun and Alkon, 2008; Freiser and Jiang, 2009; Traber, 2013; Surai et al., 2019). The greater emphasis on α-tocopherol undoubtedly arises from observations that γ-tocopherol and δ-tocopherol are only 10% and 1% as effective as α-tocopherol, respectively, in experimental animal models of vitamin E deficiency.

Research with tocotrienols and non-α-tocopherols has been conducted with laboratory animals and in vitro studies. In humans, it has been well studied the use of supplemental vitamin E in chronic diseases such as ischemic heart disease, atherosclerosis, diabetes, cataracts, Parkinson's disease, and Alzheimer's disease (Traber and Sies, 1996). γ-tocopherol has beneficial properties as an anti-inflammatory and possibly anti-atherogenic and anti-cancer agent (Wolf, 2006). Tocotrienols have been shown to possess excellent antioxidant activity *in vitro* and have been suggested to suppress reactive oxygen substances more efficiently than tocopherols (Schaffer *et al.*, 2005; Khan *et al.*, 2012). Studies have shown that tocotrienols exert more significant neuroprotective, anti-cancer, and cholesterol-lowering properties than tocopherols (Qureshi *et al.*, 2001; Sun and Alkon, 2008).

Other functions
Additional functions of vitamin E that have been reported (Traber, 2013) include (1) normal phosphorylation reactions, especially of high-energy phosphate compounds, such as creatine phosphate and adenosine triphosphate (ATP); (2) a role in the synthesis of vitamin C (ascorbic acid); (3) a role in the synthesis of ubiquinone; and (4) a role in sulfur amino acid metabolism.

Pappu *et al.* (1978) have reported vitamin E plays a role in vitamin B_{12} metabolism. A vitamin E deficiency interfered with converting vitamin B_{12} to its coenzyme 5′ deoxy-adenosyl-cobalamin and, concomitantly, the metabolism of methylmalonyl-CoA to succinyl-CoA. In humans, Turley and Brewster (1993) suggested that cellular deficiency of adenosyl cobalamin may be one mechanism by which vitamin E deficiency leads to neurologic injury. In piglets, Van Heugten *et al.* (1997) reported that water supplementation of vitamin E and selenium can increase blood levels of vitamin E. In one experiment, they observed gain-to-feed ratios higher for piglets after 5 weeks of supplementation. Recently, Chen, Wang, Li *et al.* (2019) demonstrated the effects on small intestinal histomorphology, digestive enzyme activity, and the expression of nutrient transporters.

In rats, vitamin E deficiency has been reported to inhibit vitamin D metabolism in the liver and kidneys by interfering with forming active metabolites and decreasing the concentration of the hormone-receptor complexes in the target tissue. Liver vitamin D hydroxylase activity decreased by 39%, 1-α-hydroxylase activity in the kidneys decreased by 22%, and 24-hydroxylase activity by 52% (Sergeev *et al.*, 1990).

Nutritional assessment
Vitamin E has been assessed based on α-tocopherol concentrations in erythrocytes, lymphocytes, platelets, lipoproteins, adipose tissue, buccal mucosal cells, and LDL, and on α-tocopherol: γ-tocopherol in serum or plasma. Erythrocyte susceptibility to hemolysis or lipid oxidation, breath hydrocarbon exhalation, oxidative resistance of LDL, and α-tocopheryl quinone concentrations in cerebrospinal fluid have been used as functional markers of vitamin E status in humans. However, many of these tests tend to be nonspecific and poorly standardized.

The recognition that vitamin E has essential roles in platelet, vascular, and immune function, and its antioxidant properties may lead to the identification of more specific biomarkers of vitamin E status (Morrissey and Sheehy, 1999). Vitamin E analyses encompass 8 naturally occurring vitamers, 4 tocopherols, and 4 tocotrienols. Still, only α-tocopherol is routinely measured and used for status determination since this form is preferably maintained in circulation.

α-tocopherol concentrations in plasma allow quantification by HPLC with fluorescence or UV detection. Using normal-phase HPLC, tocopherols, and tocotrienols can also be separated. A recently introduced fast and sensitive reversed-phase HPLC method resolves the challenging separation of β- and γ-tocopherol, while the separation and quantification of the 8 stereoisomers of α-tocopherol are much more challenging (Höller *et al.*, 2018).

Further research into functional markers of vitamin E status (e.g., products of lipid peroxidation) or assay systems would have more potential for point-of-care applications. Cell activity assays based on measuring hemolysis of erythrocytes under oxidative stress are another possible functional marker for α-tocopherol (Sauberlich, 1999; Bacou *et al.*, 2021).

There is a relatively high correlation between plasma and liver levels of α-tocopherol and also between the amount of dietary α-tocopherol administered and plasma levels. This has been observed in rats, chicks, pigs, lambs, and calves within relatively wide intake ranges. However, plasma tocopherol levels can be affected by blood lipid transport capacity.

Plasma α-tocopherol concentration of 3.5 mg/l (8 μmol/l) is considered deficient in humans, with values of 9 mg/l (20 μmol/l) referred to as acceptable. Similar reference values can be regarded as indicative for assessing vitamin E nutritional status in pigs. Jensen *et al.* (1988) observed that impaired lymphocyte function could be expected when serum vitamin E levels fall below 3 mg/l. Therefore, when examining problem herds, this serum value could be a helpful indicator of suboptimal lymphocyte function due to vitamin E deficiency.

Deficiency signs
Specific vitamin E deficiency signs
Nafstad and Tollersrud (1970), Wastell *et al.* (1972), and Nafstad (1973) reviewed some of the experimental work and reports available at that time concerning vitamin E-selenium deficiency in swine. In 1976, MacDonald *et al.* reviewed various aspects of the etiology, pathogenesis, and biochemistry of vitamin E-selenium-responsive diseases. Van Vleet (1989) reviewed selenium-vitamin E deficiency in swine, including its effects on the liver, heart, and skeletal muscle, diagnosis, differential diagnosis, and control and prophylactic measures. Mahan (2000) and Oldfield (2003) also reviewed similar effects of deficiencies and included impacts on reproduction and immunity.

Mortimer (1983) discussed various factors that may contribute to the deficiency. Deficiency is reported in commercial swine operations where the largest, fastest-growing animals seem more prone to sudden death. This death generally occurs within 2 to 4 weeks post-weaning but is also reported with growing-finishing pigs at a lower frequency.

Numerous authors have studied relationships between levels of alanine aminotransferase and aspartate aminotransferase activities and vitamin E deficiency. The findings have not been of consistent diagnostic value (Simesen *et al.*, 1979; Tollersrud and Nafstad, 1970). Young *et al.* (1976) found correlations between percent peroxide hemolysis and vitamin E intake or serum vitamin E. Fontaine and Valli (1977) concluded that red cell lipid peroxide measurement was a reliable test for vitamin E deficiency in swine. Red cell lipid peroxides were found to be increased in vitamin E-deficient pigs but not in selenium-deficient pigs.

Thode Jensen *et al.* (1979) reported that glutathione peroxidase activity and resistance against erythrocyte lipid peroxidation (ELP) measurement were valuable methods for assessing vitamin E or selenium status in growing pigs. Simesen *et al.* (1982) stated that although blood and liver selenium and blood vitamin E were regarded as the best indicators for selenium-vitamin E deficiencies, determination of glutathione peroxidase activity and ELP may be suitable alternatives. Thode Jensen *et al.* (1983) determined that ELP was a more sensitive index of vitamin E status than were vitamin E levels in young pigs. Malm *et al.* (1976b) reported that providing 0.5 ppm of supplemental selenium to sows' diets prevented the serum enzyme changes commonly associated with vitamin E-selenium deficiency.

Rammell *et al.* (1988) suggested that rather than analyzing for one analyte, monitoring multiple factors such as feed and tissue vitamin E, selenium, and PUFAs would provide a more accurate diagnosis. These authors indicated that liver vitamin E concentration of greater than 10 mmol/kg appeared to be adequate, while less than 2.5 mmol/kg could indicate vitamin E deficiency. The selenium and PUFA measurements would help determine deficiencies when vitamin E concentrations fell to intermediate levels. Ewan (1971) reported that calcium levels were increased in the livers of pigs fed diets deficient in selenium and vitamin E and that sodium levels were increased in muscle tissue from this same group. Vitamin E displays the greatest range of deficiency signs of all vitamins. Deficiency signs differ among species and even within the same species.

Vitamin E deficiency in blood parameters

Nafstad (1965) and Nafstad and Nafstad (1968) reported that vitamin E-deficient pigs had nuclear abnormalities in erythroid precursors within their bone marrow, inadequate erythroid produc-tion, and increased destruction of erythroid cells and irregularities in the formation of myeloid cells. In 1972, Baustad and Nafstad indicated that piglets born to vitamin E-deficient mothers had morphological abnormalities of blood and bone marrow cells similar to those reported in growing pigs following vitamin E deficiency. The authors suggested that vitamin E might be regarded as a hemopoietic factor in the newborn piglet. However, Fontaine et al. (1977b) indi-cated that vitamin E is not a limiting factor for normal erythropoiesis in young, growing pigs. Most vitamin E deficiency signs for the pig have been associated with selenium deficiency.

Scientists usually refer to vitamin E and (or) selenium deficiency since it is not clear which is involved. Generally, dietary levels of both must be low to bring about deficiency signs and lesions. Since the early 1950s, reports in the European literature have revealed tissue degen-eration signs in swine under field conditions associated with vitamin E deficiency. The signifi-cance of selenium deficiency was not realized until 1957.

Fontaine et al. (1977a,b) summarized their studies concerning vitamin E-selenium deficiency concerning hematological and biochemical changes in young pigs. They reported that serum creatine phosphokinase activities were associated with vitamin E and selenium deficiency and that the interaction was also significant. They concluded that these increases reflect the occur-rence of subclinical dietary muscular dystrophy and that selenium and vitamin E deficiencies have additive effects in the induction of skeletal muscular dystrophy.

Nutritional muscular dystrophy and hepatosis

Blaxter (1962) reported that nutritional muscular dystrophy seemed to be the one syndrome commonly encountered in vitamin E deficiency in all species (Figure 4.11a). This dystrophy is fundamentally Zenker's degeneration of skeletal and cardiac muscle fibers (Figure 4.11b). Connective tissue replacement that follows is observed grossly as white striations in the muscle bundles (Orstadius et al., 1963).

Nutritional muscular dystrophy is observed worldwide, but its incidence or diagnosis varies widely in different countries and regions, particularly in a mild or subclinical form (McDowell et al., 1983). Considerable research has revealed the positive relationship between selenium content in soil and the geographical occurrence of vitamin E-selenium-responsive muscu-lar dystrophy (Mahan et al., 1973). Numerous authors have described ultrastructural altera-tions in the cardiac tissue (Sweeny and Brown, 1972; Piper et al., 1975; Van Vleet et al., 1977a,b) and skeletal muscle (Mahan et al., 1973; Piper et al., 1975; Van Vleet et al., 1976) of pigs with selenium-vitamin E deficiency that had been experimentally induced. Ruth and Van Vleet (1974) reported that selective destruction of type I skeletal muscle fibers and a lack of phosphorylase activity in type II fibers were evident in experimentally induced selenium-vitamin E deficiency in growing swine.

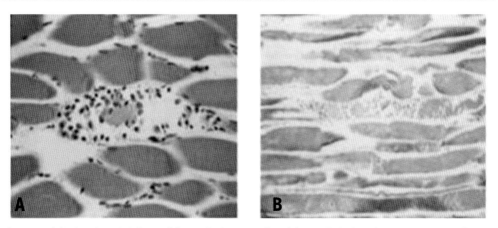

Figure 4.11(a) Vitamin E deficiency: (A) muscle degeneration; (B) muscle lesions (source: Courtesy of L.R. McDowell, University of Florida)

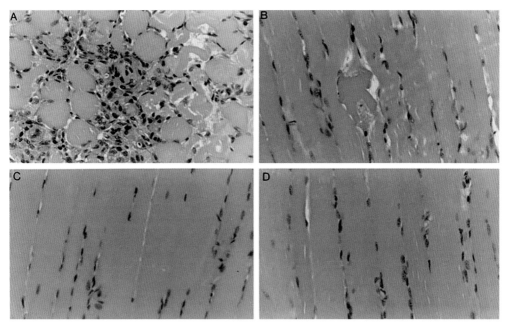

Figure 4.11(b) Combined selenium and vitamin E deficiency cause fatal myopathy in guinea pigs. Photomicrographs of quadriceps muscle from guinea pigs fed the diets differing in selenium and vitamin E concentrations for 37 days. (A) 0 Se-0 E diet; (B) 0 E diet; (C) 0 selenium diet; (D) C diet. The original magnification was 400× (source: Hill *et al.*, 2001)

Nutritional muscular dystrophy and dietetic hepatosis (toxic liver dystrophy) were widespread in Sweden's swine industry. Hepatosis dietetic is characterized by extensive necrosis of the liver. Obel (1953) reported that records from the State Veterinary Medical Institute of Stockholm from 1947 to 1952 revealed that of 4,382 pigs autopsied, more than 10% suffered from hepatosis dietetic. The description of and experimental induction of hepatosis dietetic reported by Obel (1953) was confirmed shortly after that by Hove and Seibold (1955).

Selenium-vitamin E deficiencies have been readily produced in swine diets through highly unsaturated fats (i.e., cod liver oil, as in Lannek *et al.*, 1961) and rancid fats. However, naturally occurring vitamin E-selenium deficiencies were not reported in the United States until the late 1960s (Orstadius *et al.*, 1963; Michel *et al.*, 1969), and in the 1970s, they became widespread.

The high incidence of vitamin E-selenium deficiencies in swine was believed to be due to several factors (Trapp *et al.*, 1970), including:

1   swine raised in complete confinement, without access to pasture
2   low selenium content in the midwestern US feeds
3   solvent-extracted protein supplements low in vitamin E
4   limited feeding programs for sows, or low tocopherol and selenium dietary levels
5   loss of vitamin E and selenium from corn due to oxidation as a result of air and heat drying or storing high-moisture grains (Young *et al.*, 1977, 1978; Whitehair *et al.*, 1983a)
6   selection for leaner pigs that require more selenium (evidence also suggests that moldy feed-in bulk-holding bins may produce mycotoxins that either inhibit the uptake of vitamin E in the small intestine or affect the antioxidant balance of cells)
7   higher dietary levels of some trace minerals (copper and iron) that can destroy natural α-tocopherols
8   early weaning with lower tissue storage reserves.

A decrease in the utilization of pasture and forages accompanied the confinement rearing of swine on concrete floors or slats. Such crops are excellent sources of vitamin E and provide the more highly available form of the vitamin, α-versus γ-tocopherol. Vitamin E-selenium deficiency in swine is often associated with sudden death (Piper *et al.*, 1975; Rice and Kennedy, 1989). In most cases, clinical signs of the condition were not observed before death (Michel *et al.*, 1969; Trapp *et al.*, 1970), although occasionally, pigs were followed with clinical signs of icterus, difficult locomotion, reluctance to move, and weakness. Clinical signs also include peripheral cyanosis (particularly the ears), dyspnea (abdominal respiration), and a weak pulse, all occurring shortly before death. In many cases, the faster-growing, more thrifty-appearing pigs died suddenly.

Many pathological reports of vitamin E-selenium deficiency note that the most striking lesion was liver necrosis (Trapp *et al.*, 1970). The most common pathologic lesions include massive hepatic necrosis (hepatosis dietetic) (Figures 4.12a, 4.12b, and 4.12c), degenerative myopathy of cardiac (Figures 4.12d and 4.12e) and skeletal muscles, edema, esophagogastric ulceration, icterus, nephrosis, hemoglobinuria, acute congestion, skin lesions and hemorrhaging in various tissues (Figures 4.12f and 4.12g) (Ewan *et al.*, 1969; Trapp *et al.*, 1970; Piper *et al.*, 1975) and yellowish discoloration of adipose tissue ("yellow fat"). Still, bilateral paleness of skeletal muscle was the gross lesion most commonly found.

At an early age, vitamin E-selenium deficiency is characterized by myocardial damage, also known as nutritional microangiopathy or Mulberry heart disease (MHD), which may cause substantial losses within a litter. This is the most serious of the disorders since when heart muscle tissue has been damaged, the result is usually sudden death. There may be hemorrhagic lesions within the heart that give the characteristic "mulberry" appearance of MHD (for a case description, see Tutt and Gale, 1957). Harding (1960) reported histopathological observations associated with the disease, including bleeding with parenchymal degeneration and mild perivascular mononuclear infiltration. Grant (1961) thoroughly reviewed the morphological and etiological findings associated with mulberry hearts during the early 1960s.

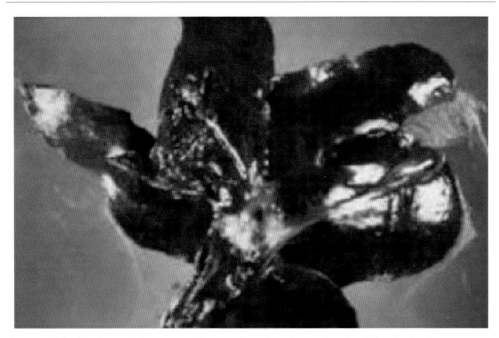

Figure 4.12(a) Vitamin E deficiency: hepatic necrosis. Lesions in growing pigs fed a diet low in vitamin E (7.0 IU α-tocopherol/kg diet) and selenium (0.061 ppm). The liver with severe acute lesions is characteristic of a hepatosis dietetic, consisting of a mosaic pattern of deep red and yellow lobules of massive coagulation necrosis (source: McDowell L.R. and Piper R.C., Washington State University)

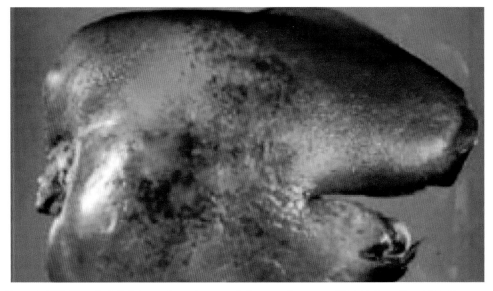

Figure 4.12(b) Vitamin E deficiency: hepatic necrosis (source: Courtesy of L.R. McDowell and R.C. Piper, Washington State University)

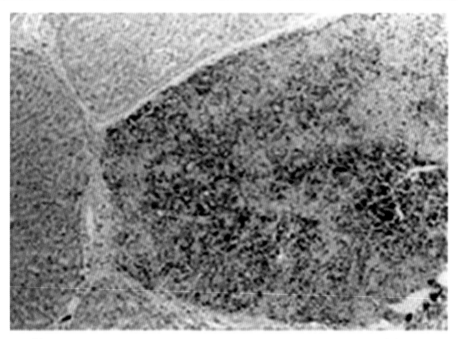

Figure 4.12(c) Vitamin E deficiency: hepatic necrosis lesions in the liver of growing pigs fed a diet low in vitamin E (7.0 IU α-tocopherol/kg diet) and selenium (0.061 ppm). Shown is an individual hepatic lobule that has undergone acute massive coagulation necrosis; the necrosis cells are replaced by blood (source: Courtesy of L.R. McDowell and R.C. Piper, Washington State University)

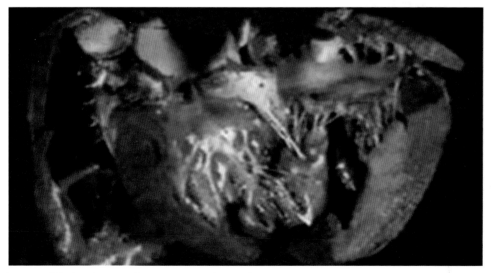

Figure 4.12(d) Vitamin E deficiency: degenerative cardiac myopathy. The lesion in the heart of the growing pig was fed a diet low in vitamin E (7.0 IU α-tocopherol/kg diet) and selenium (0.061 ppm). Note the degenerative cardiac myopathy and the large pale areas due to degeneration and necrosis of myocardial fibers that are most severe along the inner border of the left ventricle (source: Courtesy of L.R. McDowell and R.C. Piper, Washington State University)

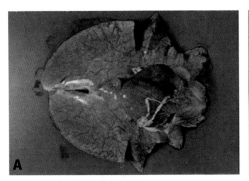
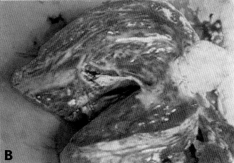

Figure 4.12(e) The vitamin E deficiency syndrome in pigs. Gross changes in the heart. (A) Subepicardial hemorrhages and right ventricular dilatation. The pericardia sac, which was distended by transudate, has been opened. Fibrin strands have been left on the epicardium. Interstitial lung edema is visible. (B) Subendocardial hemorrhages and mottling of the myocardium ("Mulberry heart") (source: Nafstad and Tollersrud, 1970)

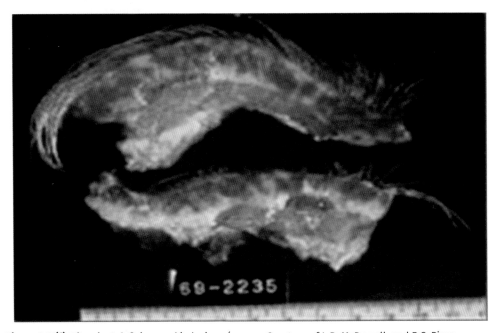

Figure 4.12(f) Vitamin E deficiency: skin lesions (source: Courtesy of L.R. McDowell, and R.C. Piper, Washington State University)

In some pigs, microscopic lesions in the liver were either absent or minimal, whereas changes in skeletal muscles were extensive. In other cases, the reverse was true. Bengtsson *et al.* (1978) reported various vitamin E and selenium deficiency symptoms, including lesions such as hepatosis dietetic, mulberry heart, muscular degeneration, and microangiopathy in weaned pigs fed a selenium-deficient diet. Only the highest vitamin E supplementation level utilized in their study could overcome the symptoms. Numerous authors have also studied dietary induction of mulberry heart and hepatosis dietetic, including Sharp *et al.* (1970a,b,c) and Moir and Masters (1979). Sharp *et al.* (1972b) reported that dietary selenium (0.5 ppm) and

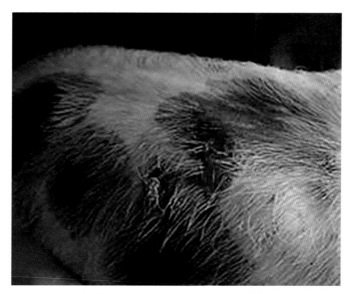

Figure 4.12(g) Exudative epidermitis in nursery piglets (source: https://www.3tres3.com/latam/articulos/carencia-de-vitamina-e-y-selenio_10231/)

(or) vitamin E (25 IU/kg diet) prevented skeletal muscular dystrophy and exudative diathesis. Hakkarainen *et al.* (1978a) investigated whether providing dietary vitamin E and selenium could reverse vitamin E-selenium deficiency (VESD) once the syndrome had been allowed to develop. Using the same combination (5 mg α-tocopheryl acetate and 135 mg selenium per kg diet) shown previously to prevent the onset of VESD, the therapy was found to result in recovery from VESD syndrome. However, with less supplementation (5 mg α-tocopherol acetate and 45 mg selenium per kg diet), the VESD syndrome was not reversed.

Vitamin E deficiency in reproduction and young piglets
Other conditions reported in swine breeding herds with VESD include MMA syndrome in sows (today more often referred as postpartum dysgalactia syndrome or PDS), spraddled rear legs in newborn pigs, gastric ulcers, infertility, susceptibility to swine dysentery, and poor skin condition. These conditions were believed initially to be unrelated to pig deaths from a VESD. However, a noticeable reduction in these conditions occurred after supplementation with dietary vitamin E or injections of selenium and vitamin E (Trapp *et al.*, 1970).

Whitehair *et al.* (1983b, 1984) provided evidence that the MMA syndrome may be alleviated by supplementing the gestation-lactation diet with vitamin E and selenium. In one experiment, vitamin E was shown to help reduce the incidence of MMA from 50% to 14% (Ullrey, 1969; Piatkowski *et al.*, 1979). MMA occurrence decreased from 39% to 24% in 2 studies involving 191 farrowing (Ullrey *et al.*, 1971). High dietary fat during gestation may affect vitamin E content in the colostrum and sow's milk yield (Nielsen *et al.*, 1973). Maximum incidence of death due to VESD generally occurs at 6 to 8 weeks of age, with the incidence declining up to the 16th week of life; however, conceptuses can be adversely affected before parturition resulting in stillborn pigs (Putnam, 1984).

Data from Dvorak (1974a) confirmed that the post-weaning period of low plasma vitamin E levels presents a health hazard to young piglets if vitamin E supplementation is not provided. The vitamin E-selenium syndromes (nutrition-related microangiopathy; nutritional hepatic dystrophy; muscle degeneration in the back, pelvis, and upper thigh) can also be found in the fattening and reproductive stage of pig production (Bostedt, 1980). Clinical conditions characterized by cellular damage often occur after stress, such as changing feed or housing, transportation, or weaning (Mackenzie et al., 1997). A Michigan survey diagnosed vitamin E-selenium deficiencies in swine herds with mortality ranging from 3% to 10% (Michel et al., 1969; Trapp et al., 1970). One producer, however, lost approximately 300 of 800 pigs weaned. Cline et al. (1974) evaluated the effect of supplemental vitamin E (0, 44, or 220 IU/kg) for sows during gestation and lactation on the incidence of VESD syndrome in sows and their progeny. In their diets, the sows receiving 0, 44, and 220 IU supplemental vitamin E had progeny deaths of 53, 33, and 7%, respectively. Thus, vitamin E in sow diets was found to be partly effective in preventing death and other VESD symptoms in their progeny.

It has been recognized for many years that vitamin E-deficient animals are more subject to the effects of "stress" than normal animals. The concept of stress is, in itself, difficult to define. Still, experience has shown that dietary and environmental abnormalities of various kinds can lead to clinical signs of disease and death in animals deprived of vitamin E. Death is often associated with unaccustomed muscular activity. The incidence of death in baby pigs is significantly increased because of fighting when animals are weaned and mixed with different litters. Castration is additional stress that has been implicated in the early death of selenium- and vitamin E-deficient pigs (Piper et al., 1975).

In 1989, Nielsen et al. suggested that the development of MHD in Denmark may not always be due to deficiencies of selenium or vitamin E but might be associated with an individual disposition related to rapid growth. Some researchers have demonstrated a low tolerance of vitamin E- and selenium-deficient baby pigs to intramuscular injections of iron-dextran to prevent anemia. At 2 or 3 days, piglets die from iron shock if given routine treatment with iron, with death resulting from iron-induced lipid peroxidation in tissues. Pretreatment with vitamin E, selenium, or ethoxyquin was protective against the toxic effects of injectable iron (Tollerz and Lannek, 1964). Dvorak (1974a) reported that injection of the iron-dextran complex at 4 or 2 days of age did not negatively affect plasma vitamin E levels in suckling piglets.

Gut health issues related to vitamin E deficiency

Concerning gastric ulcers associated with vitamin E deficiency, Bebiak (1977) conducted a preliminary investigation of how an absence of vitamin E could indirectly influence ulcerogenesis. They determined that microvascular endothelial peroxidative disruption of vessels perfusing the non-glandular region of the gastric mucosa was the principal mechanism by which vitamin E was involved in the development of gastric ulcers.

Dobson (1967) could not detect a beneficial effect of selenium and vitamin E on preventing gastric ulceration or improving growth rate. In their study, pigs were given intramuscular injections of selenium and vitamin E for 3 days (0.25 mg Se + 68 IU vitamin E), 2 weeks (0.20 mg Se + 13.6 IU vitamin E), and 8 weeks (0.75 mg Se + 51 IU vitamin E). The pigs were slaughtered for evaluation between 6 and 6.5 months.

Studies by Teige et al. (1982) have shown that susceptibility to dysentery resulting from exposure to the spirochete *Treponema hyodysenteriae* was greatly increased by the combined dietary deficiencies of vitamin E and selenium. Teige and Nafstad (1978) reported ultrastructural changes in colonic epithelial cells in vitamin E-selenium-deficient pigs and observed changes that would decrease the resistance to spirochetes and other intestinal factors in swine dysentery.

Safety

Compared with vitamins A and D, in both acute and chronic studies with animals, vitamin E is relatively nontoxic but not entirely devoid of undesirable effects. Hypervitaminosis E studies in rats, chicks, and humans indicate maximum tolerable levels in the range of 1,000–2,000 IU/kg diet (NRC, 1998).

Vitamin E toxicity due to dietary supplementation has not been demonstrated in swine (Weaver *et al.*, 1991). Levels as high as 550 mg/kg diet have been fed to growing pigs without toxic effects (Bonnette *et al.*, 1990b). The toxicity of vitamin E has been reported when it has been injected in high doses and for several days (Weaver *et al.*, 1991). Batra *et al.* (1995) indicated that 1 to 2 days following injection of 3 to 5 times the manufacturer's recommended dose of vitamin E in pigs, lambs, or calves (500 IU, 1,000 IU, and 1,500 IU, respectively) resulted in edematization and a transient elevation of body temperature. Hale *et al.* (1995) concluded that vitamin E injected into neonatal piglets daily at 50 IU/kg/day for 13 days caused toxicity due to massive accumulation of vitamin E in mononuclear phagocyte system cells, liver, and spleen or muscles depending on the via of injection.

An adverse effect of excessive vitamin E intake is its interference with vitamin D utilization, particularly when the vitamin D level is marginal. Excess supplementation of α-tocopherol could be detrimental to the other vitamin E forms. In humans, extra supplementation of diets with α-tocopherol reduced serum concentrations of γ- and δ-tocopherols (Huang and Appel, 2003; Wolf, 2006). The effects of high supplemental α-tocopherol levels on other forms of vitamin E are unknown for livestock.

Vitamin K

Chemical structure and properties

The generic term vitamin K refers to different fat-soluble compounds of the quinone group that exhibit an antihemorrhagic effect. The primary molecule is a naphthoquinone (2-methyl-1.4-napthoquinone), and the various vitamers differ in the nature and length of the side chain (Figure 4.13).

- Vitamin K$_1$ or phylloquinone derived from plants.
- Vitamin K$_2$, or menaquinone (MK), is mainly the form produced by bacterial fermentation. Vitamin K$_2$ can be divided into subtypes indicated with MK-n, where n stands for the number of isoprenoid residues in the aliphatic side chain: for example, short-chain for menaquinone-4 or MK-4 or long-chain for menaquinone-7 or MK-7. MK-4 is synthesized in

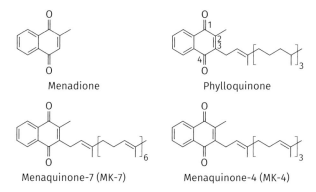

Menadione

Phylloquinone

Menaquinone-7 (MK-7)

Menaquinone-4 (MK-4)

Figure 4.13 Vitamin K structures

the liver from ingested menadione or changed to a biologically active menaquinone by intestinal microorganisms (Suttie, 2013).

- Vitamin K_3, or menadione, is produced by chemical synthesis. This form, partially water-soluble and highly stable, is typically used in compound feeds for animal nutrition.

Natural sources
Naturally occurring sources of vitamin K are fat-soluble, stable to heat, and destabilized by oxidation, alkali conditions, strong acids, light, and irradiation. Vitamin K_1 is a golden yellow, viscous oil. It is slowly degraded by atmospheric oxygen but fairly rapidly destroyed by sunlight or ultraviolet light. Vitamin K_1 is present in fresh dark-green plants, e.g., dried alfalfa contains 10 mg/kg vitamin K_1, cereals around 0.2–0.3 mg/kg (NRC, 1998), and it is abundant in pasture and green roughages, thus providing high quantities of vitamin K to grazing livestock. Light is essential for its formation, and parts of plants that do not usually form chlorophyll contain little vitamin K_1. However, the natural loss of chlorophyll as the yellowing of leaves does not bring about a corresponding change in vitamin K_1. Swine, poultry, and feedlot animals would receive little vitamin K_1 from diets based on grains and oilseed meals.

Vitamin K_2 produced by bacterial flora in animals can be found in all by-product feedstuffs of animal origin, including fish meal (2 mg/kg) and fish liver oils, especially after they have undergone extensive bacterial putrefaction. Vitamin K_2 is also produced by intestinal bacterial flora and is especially important in providing the vitamin K requirements of most mammals. However, pigs do not receive sufficient vitamin K_2 from intestinal microbial synthesis (Ullrey, 1991; Crenshaw, 2000; Monegue, 2013). In reality, the site of synthesis is the lower gut, an area of poor absorption. Thus, availability to the host is limited unless the animal practices coprophagy, in which case the synthesized vitamin K is highly available. The type of diet, independent of vitamin K concentration, will influence total K_2 synthesis.

Commercial sources
Vitamin K supplementation in animal diets is provided by the synthetic product, namely vitamin K_3, in the form of various bisulfite complexes or water-soluble salts, which are more stable and potent (Huyghebaert, 1991; Ullrey, 1991; Suttie, 2013). The feed industry does not utilize vitamin K_1 due to cost and lack of a stabilized form. The various products used by the feed industry and their respective content in menadione are listed in Table 4.1.

Menadione dimethylpyrimidinol bisulfite (MPB) was tested in 3 experiments for growing swine by Seerley et al. (1976), observing positive effects to overcome all effects of vitamin K deficiency. Encapsulation techniques have been gradually applied to feed additives, which may improve the stability of vitamins. Mujica-Álvarez et al. (2020) reported that microencapsulation could enhance the stability of vitamins. The EFSA (European Food Safety Authority) (2014) reported that pelleting reduced MSB (menadione sodium bisulfite) of crystal to about 53% of the initial content (pelleting at 90°C, 6 mg MSB/kg feed) and reduced MNB (menadione nicotinamide bisulfite) of crystal by about 52% of the initial content (pelleting at 70°C, 4.5 mg MNB/kg feed).

Recently, Wang et al. (2021) evaluated the effects of sources or formulations of vitamin K_3 on its stability during extrusion or pelleting in swine feed. Extrusion or pelleting significantly reduced the recovery of vitamin K_3. Those authors suggested that MNB (MSB) should be recommended as the vitamin K_3 source, the micro-capsule formulation should be advised during pelleting, and the crystal formulation should be recommended during extrusion. Furthermore, the temperature and length-to-diameter ratio should be reduced as much as possible during the thermal processing of feed to reduce the loss of vitamin K_3 potency. Development of

Table 4.1 Menadione salts used for diet supplementation

Vitamin K$_3$ salt	Menadione (K$_3$) concentration (%)	Amount of menadione salt to provide 1 g of menadione (K$_3$)
		(g)
Menadione sodium bisulfite (MSB)	50	2
Menadione dimethylpyrimidinol bisulfite (MPB)	45.4	2.2
Menadione nicotinamide bisulfite (MNB)	43	2.3
Menadione sodium bisulfite complex (MSBC)	33	3

micro-capsule and micro-sphere carriers and further technical updates are needed to improve vitamin stability.

Moisture, choline chloride, trace elements, and alkaline conditions impair the stability of these K$_3$ supplements in premixes and diets. Menadione sodium bisulfite complex (MSBC) or MPB may lose almost 80% of bioactivity if stored for 3 months in a vitamin–trace mineral premix containing choline. Still, losses were considered far less if stored in a similar premix containing no choline. Coated K$_3$ supplements are generally more stable than uncoated supplements.

Metabolism

Absorption and transport

Like all fat-soluble vitamins, vitamin K is absorbed in association with dietary fats and requires the presence of bile salts and pancreatic juice for adequate uptake from the alimentary tract. The absorption of vitamin K depends on its incorporation into mixed micelles, and the optimal formation of these micellar structures requires the presence of both bile and pancreatic juice. Thus, any malfunction of the fat absorption mechanism (e.g., biliary obstruction, malabsorption syndrome) reduces the availability of vitamin K (Ferland, 2006). Menaquinone is absorbed by a passive process in the small intestine and colon. The digestibility of menaquinone is much greater than that of phylloquinone. Griminger and Donis (1960) observed in rats that around 60% of the phylloquinone had been eliminated in feces 24 hours after ingestion, while in the case of menaquinone, elimination was only 11%. Unlike phylloquinone and menaquinones, menadione salts, relatively water-soluble, are absorbed satisfactorily from low-fat diets. Male animals are more susceptible to dietary vitamin K deprivation than females, apparently due to a stimulation of phylloquinone absorption by estrogens, and the administration of estrogens increases absorption in both male and female animals (Duello and Matschiner, 1971; Jolly et al., 1977; Suttie, 2013).

The absorption of various forms differs significantly. In pigs, the absorption takes place mainly in the small intestine, although it has been shown that it can also occur in the colon. The lymphatic system and portal circulation form the major transport route of absorbed phylloquinone from the intestine. An energy-dependent process absorbs ingested phylloquinone from the proximal portion of the small intestine (Hollander, 1973). Shearer et al. (1970) demonstrated the association of phylloquinone with serum lipoproteins, but little is known about the existence of specific carrier proteins. In contrast to the active transport of phylloquinone, menaquinone is absorbed from the small intestine by a passive noncarrier-mediated process. Menadione can be absorbed from both the small intestine and the colon by a passive approach and transformed into a biologically active form.

The measured efficiency of vitamin K absorption ranges from 10% to 70%, depending on the form of the vitamin administered. Some reports have indicated that menadione is completely absorbed, whereas phylloquinone is absorbed only at a rate of 50%. The complete absorption of menadione may be due to the aqueous solubility of the menadione salts (Crenshaw, 2000; Monegue, 2013).

Storage and excretion

Duello and Matschiner (1971) characterized the vitamin K forms stored in the liver of pigs. Their mass spectrometry results of purified samples from pig liver gave molecular ions for menaquinones (MK-7, MK-7 (H2), MK-8, MK-8 (H2), MK-8 (H4), MK-8 (H6), MK-9, MK-9 (H2), MK-9 (H4), MK-9 (H6), MK-10, and MK-10 (H2)). The maximum amount of these compounds that could have been present in pig liver but remain undetected was estimated to be 10–11% of the biological activity in the extracted lipid.

In other organs menaquinones also exceed phylloquinone. As such, phylloquinone had equally as good biological activity upon prothrombin synthesis as menaquinone found in the pig's liver following the feeding of menadione. Therefore, MK-4 (menaquinone-4) is most likely produced if menadione is fed or if the intestinal microorganisms degrade the dietary K_1 or K_2 to menadione. However, the formation of MK-4 is not required for the metabolic activity of vitamin K since phylloquinone is equally active in synthesizing the vitamin K-dependent, blood-clotting proteins.

Menadione is widely distributed in all tissues and is very rapidly excreted. Although phylloquinone is quickly concentrated in the liver, it does not have a long retention time in this organ (Thierry et al., 1970). The inability to rapidly develop a vitamin K deficiency in most species results from the difficulty in preventing the absorption of the vitamin from the diet or intestinal synthesis rather than from significant storage of the vitamin.

Rats were found to excrete about 60% of ingested phylloquinone in the feces within 24 hours of ingestion but only 11% of ingested menadione (Griminger, 1984). However, 38% of ingested menadione and only a small amount of phylloquinone were excreted via the kidneys during the same period. The conclusion was that although menadione is well absorbed, it is poorly retained in the liver, while the opposite is true for phylloquinone. The excretion in pigs could be similar (Crenshaw, 2000).

Normal human subjects were found to excrete less than 20% of a large (1 mg) dose of phylloquinone in feces. Still, as much as 70–80% of the ingested phylloquinone was excreted unaltered in the feces of patients with impaired fat absorption caused by pancreatic insufficiency or adult celiac disease (Suttie, 2013). Some breakdown products of vitamin K are excreted in the urine. One of the main excretory products is a chain-shortened and oxidized derivative of vitamin K, which forms γ-lactone and is probably excreted as a glucuronide (Suttie, 2013).

Biochemical functions
Blood clotting
The principal function of vitamin K is controlling the blood coagulation period since it activates plasmatic prothrombin (Ullrey, 1991). A complex series of reactions are involved in converting circulating fibrinogen into a fibrin clot. Many proteins with different metabolic functions participating in the "cascade" of blood coagulation require vitamin K for their biosynthesis (Figure 4.14).

Vitamin K is required for the synthesis of the active form of prothrombin (Factor II) and other plasma clotting factors, namely Factor VII (proconvertin), Factor IX (Christmas factor), and Factor X (Stuart-Prower factor). These factors are synthesized as inactive precursors

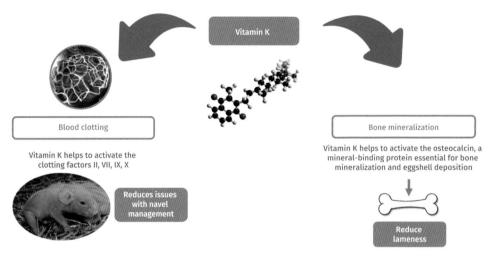

Figure 4.14 Vitamin K functions (source: Crenshaw, 2000; Monegue, 2013)

(zymogens), and vitamin K is necessary for their conversion into biologically active proteins (Suttie and Jackson, 1977). Thus, in the case of vitamin K deficiency, blood coagulation time increases because of the lack of conversion of these factors. In deficiency, vitamin K administration produces a prompt response in 4 to 6 hours; in the absence of the liver, this response does not occur (Suttie, 2013).

Vitamin K-dependent proteins can be identified by γ-carboxyglutamic acid residues (Gla), an amino acid common to all vitamin K proteins. The discovery of this new amino acid clarified the role of vitamin K in blood coagulation and led to the discovery of additional vitamin K-dependent proteins (e.g., bone proteins) (Ferland, 2006; Monegue, 2013; Suttie, 2013).

Bleeding disorders result from an inability of a liver microsomal enzyme, currently called the vitamin K-dependent carboxylase (Esmon *et al.*, 1975), to carry out the average post-translational conversion of specific glutamyl residues in the vitamin K-dependent plasma proteins to γ-carboxy glutamyl residues (Nelsestuen *et al.*, 1974). Therefore, the result of low vitamin K serving as a cofactor for this enzyme decreases thrombin generation.

Converting inactive precursor proteins to biologically active forms involve the carboxylation of glutamic acid residues in the inactive molecules. Carboxylation allows prothrombin and the other procoagulant proteins to participate in a specific protein-calcium phospholipid interaction necessary for their biological role (Suttie and Jackson, 1977; Monegue, 2013; Suttie, 2013). Four other vitamin K-dependent proteins have also been identified in plasma: proteins C, S, Z, and M. Protein C and protein S play an anticoagulant rather than a procoagulant role in normal hemostasis (Suttie and Olson, 1990). Protein C inhibits coagulation and, stimulated by protein S, promotes fibrinolysis. Also, a protein C–S complex can partially hydrolyze the activated factors V and VIII and thus inactivate them. Protein S can also regulate bone turnover (Binkley and Suttie, 1995). The function of proteins M and Z is unclear, and protein Z has been shown to have an anticoagulant role under some conditions (Suttie, 2013). When given to humans at pharmacological doses, menaquinone protects against fracture risk and bone loss in the spine (Shea and Booth, 2008).

The blood-clotting mechanism can be stimulated by either an intrinsic system, in which all the factors are in the plasma or an extrinsic system. In the extrinsic coagulation system, tissue thromboplastin converts prothrombin in the blood to thrombin in the presence of various elements and calcium. The enzyme thrombin facilitates the conversion of the soluble fibrinogen into insoluble fibrin. Fibrin polymerizes into strands and enmeshes the blood-formed elements, especially the red blood cells, to create the blood clot (Griminger, 1984). The final active component, in both the intrinsic and extrinsic systems, it appears to activate the Stuart factor, which leads to prothrombin activation (Monegue, 2013).

Continuing research has revealed that vitamin K-dependent reactions are present in most tissues, not just blood. A reasonably large number of proteins are subjected to this post-translational carboxylation of specific glutamate residues γ-carboxyglutamate residues (Vermeer, 1986). Atherocalcin is a vitamin K-dependent protein in atherosclerotic tissue. A vitamin K-dependent carboxylase system in the skin is related to calcium metabolism (de Boer-van den Berg *et al.*, 1986).

Bone mineralization

Two of the best-characterized vitamin K-dependent proteins not involved in hemostasis are osteocalcin or bone Gla protein (BGP), matrix Gla protein, which was initially discovered in bone, and protein S (Crenshaw, 2000; Monegue, 2013). Vitamin K is a cofactor for forming γ-carboxyglutamate (Gla) residues in proteins. Proteins that undergo carboxylation reactions all participate in reactions that require calcium. Osteocalcin contains 3 Gla residues that give this protein its mineral-binding properties. Osteocalcin appears in embryonic chick bone and rat bone matrix at the beginning of mineralization of the bone (Gallop *et al.*, 1980). It accounts for 15% to 20% of the non-collagen protein in the bone of most vertebrates and is one of the most abundant proteins in the body.

Osteocalcin is produced by osteoblasts, with synthesis controlled by 1,25-dihydroxy vitamin D. About 20% of the newly synthesized protein is released into circulation. It can be used to measure bone formation. As is true for other non-blood vitamin K-dependent proteins, the physiological role of osteocalcin remains largely unknown. However, reduced osteocalcin content of cortical bone (Vanderschueren *et al.*, 1990) and alteration of osteocalcin distribution within osteons (Ingram *et al.*, 1994) are associated with aging. It remains unknown whether any of these findings are related to the age-related increased risk of fracture. Osteocalcin may play a role in the control of bone remodeling because it has been reported to be a chemoattractant for monocytes, the precursors of osteoclasts. Serum osteocalcin is a good predictor of bone turnover in pigs (Hall *et al.*, 1986; Carter *et al.*, 1996; Crenshaw, 2000). This suggests a possible role for osteocalcin in bone resorption (Binkley and Suttie, 1995; Suttie, 2013).

Several cell types in the body secrete matrix Gla protein (matrix γ-carboxyglutamate-protein) and protein S. However, matrix Gla protein is highly accumulated in bone and cartilage and found in the calcification of blood vessels. It contains 5 vitamin-K-dependent γ-carboxyglutamic acid residues with high affinity to calcium and phosphate ions and can bind to hydroxyapatite crystals of mineralized tissue (Coen *et al.*, 2009). Matrix Gla protein-deficient mice have abnormal calcification leading to osteopenia, fractures, and premature death owing to arterial calcification (Booth, 1997; Crenshaw, 2000). Laenoi *et al.* (2010) reported that matrix Gla protein could be involved in osteochondrosis for young fast growing pigs, which is a significant welfare issue. Potentially vitamin K levels may play a role in regulating the gene expression of these proteins essential for ossification.

Several observations in humans indicate that vitamin K could be involved in the pathogenesis of bone mineral loss (Binkley and Suttie, 1995; Cashman and O'Connor, 2008):

1   low blood vitamin K in patients with bone fractures
2   concentration of circulating under γ-carboxylated osteocalcin associated with age, low bone mineral density, and hip fracture risk
3   anticoagulant therapy is associated with decreased bone density
4   decreased bone loss and calcium excretion with vitamin K supplementation
5   Crenshaw (2000) discussed the role of vitamin K in calcium and phosphorus metabolism and its interactions with vitamin D. Hall *et al.* (1985, 1991) reported a hemorrhagic syndrome induced by high dietary calcium levels in growing pigs that increased vitamin K requirements.

Nervous system
Another vitamin K-dependent protein is Gas 6; the function of this protein has a possible role in nervous system function, vascular cell function, and platelet activation (Suttie, 2007). To date, both *in vitro* and *in vivo* studies suggest a role of vitamin K in regulating multiple enzymes involved in sphingolipid metabolism within the myelin-rich regions in the brain (Denisova and Booth, 2005). The brain is enriched with sphingolipids, essential membrane constituents, and major lipid signaling molecules that have a role in motor and cognitive behavior.

Nutritional assessment
Traditional assessment of vitamin K status includes evaluation of blood-clotting time. As discussed above, the vitamin K family comprises K_1 (phylloquinone from plants) and K_2 (menaquinone from carnivorous and bacterial sources). Moreover, we must include the other vitamers indicated with MK-n, like MK-4 and MK-7. The various forms have very different pharmacokinetics, with a half-life of 1–2 hours for MK-4 and K_1, 3 days or more for MK-7, and longer chain MKs (Schurgers and Vermeer, 2002).

Vitamin K status may be assessed by measuring the circulating concentration of each relevant vitamers or by measuring the circulating concentration of uncarboxylated Gla-proteins. Direct measurement of circulating K-vitamers is generally accomplished by reversed-phase HPLC or ultra-performance liquid chromatography (UPLC) with fluorescence or mass spectrometric detection. However, many menaquinones are not available as reference compounds. The concentration in circulation reflects recent dietary exposure rather than true status concentrations (Höller *et al.*, 2018). ELISA-based methods for measuring uncarboxylated Gla-proteins are currently the most reliable for assessing vitamin K status. These tests can determine tissue-specific proteins like uncarboxylated osteocalcin (ucOC) for bone.

Deficiency signs
Vitamin K deficiency is produced by ingesting the antagonist, dicumarol, or by feeding sulfonamides (in monogastric species) at levels sufficient to inhibit the intestinal synthesis of vitamin K. Supplementation of vitamin K will overcome the anticoagulation effect of dicumarol. Vitamin K antagonists increase the need for this vitamin. Mycotoxins are also antagonists that may cause vitamin K deficiency (Ullrey, 1991).

The primary clinical sign of vitamin K deficiency in all species is impairment of blood coagulation. Other clinical symptoms include low prothrombin levels, increased clotting time, and hemorrhaging, as observed in baby pigs by Schendel and Johnson (1962). In its most severe form, a lack of vitamin K will cause subcutaneous and internal hemorrhages, which can be fatal or cause anemia, anorexia, and weakness. Schendel and Johnson (1962) reported that after 4 or 5 weeks of deficiency, piglets could die if they do not receive some source of this vitamin.

But piglets responded 2 to 4 hours after an oral dose or intramuscular injection of vitamin K (menadiol sodium diphosphate). The minimum dietary requirement estimated at that time was 5 µg per kg of body weight per day, and the minimal curative injected dose was less than 20 µg per kg of body weight.

Vitamin K deficiency can arise from dietary deficiency, lack of microbial synthesis within the gut, inadequate intestinal absorption, or inability of the liver to use the available vitamin K. In addition, a deficiency can be caused by the ingestion of vitamin K antagonists like dicumarol, present in some plants, or by feeding sulfonamides (in monogastric species) at levels sufficient to inhibit the intestinal synthesis of vitamin K. Supplementation with vitamin K will overcome the anticoagulation effect of dicumarol. A characteristic symptom is increased coagulation time of the umbilical cord in piglets after birth. Other symptoms are blood in the urine and subcutaneous hemorrhages (Hoppe, 1987).

Hall *et al.* (1991) accidentally produced vitamin K deficiency characterized by increased blood-clotting times and high death losses when feeding excess calcium (2.7%) without supplemental vitamin K. Either supplemental vitamin K or reduced dietary calcium prevented the disease. Pigs on a high-sugar diet suffered heart lesions and hemorrhagic syndrome, which could be controlled by providing vitamin K (Brooks *et al.*, 1973). Several field trials in the United States and other countries have reported a hemorrhagic syndrome for growing pigs (Newsholme *et al.*, 1985). In one study, hemorrhagic syndrome occurred 9 days after pigs were fed a standard diet, while those receiving either 2.5% dehydrated alfalfa meal or supplemental vitamin K remained in good health (Fritschen *et al.*, 1970). Gross visible signs of hemorrhagic syndrome include extensive subcutaneous hemorrhages, blood in the urine, and abnormal breathing. Additional clinical signs from field observations are that some pigs will develop enlarged blood-filled joints and become lame (Newsholme *et al.*, 1985).

In contrast, other animals may have swellings along the body wall filled with unclotted blood. Hematomas (or blood swellings) in the ears also occur (Cunha, 1977). Hemorrhagic conditions (Figure 4.15) in the growing pig have sometimes been associated with the ingestion of molds, such as *Aspergillus* or moldy materials, and have usually responded to vitamin K therapy.

Even though inadequate dietary vitamin K alters bone osteocalcin, signs associated with the skeletal system are not as apparent as blood-clotting problems. Although blood clotting was impaired and there was a reduction in bone γ-carboxyglutamic acid concentrations, vitamin K deficiency did not functionally impair skeletal metabolism. Vitamin K-dependent γ-carboxylated proteins have been identified as ligands for a unique family of receptor tyrosine kinases with transforming ability. The involvement of vitamin K metabolism and function in 2 well-characterized birth defects, warfarin embryopathy, and vitamin K epoxide reductase deficiency, suggests that developmental signals from vitamin K-dependent pathways may be required for normal embryogenesis (Park *et al.*, 2014).

Several considerations influence the likelihood of a vitamin K deficiency in swine, including dietary sources of the vitamin, level of vitamin K in the maternal diet, intestinal synthesis, coprophagy, presence of sulfa drugs, and other non-nutrients in the diet, and disease conditions. When sulfaquinoxaline or certain other drugs are present in the feed or the drinking water or when coccidiosis is being treated, supplementary vitamin K is needed at higher levels, up to 10 times the amount is required in the absence of these drugs (Joachim and Shrestha, 2019). Antimicrobial agents suppress intestinal bacteria that synthesize vitamin K (Crenshaw, 2000), and in their presence, the pig may be entirely dependent on dietary vitamin K (NRC, 1998).

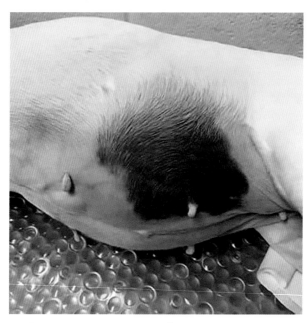

Figure 4.15 Vitamin K deficiency. Internal hemorrhaging (source: https://www.vet.cornell.edu/animal-health-diagnostic-center/testing/protocols/vitamin-k-deficiency)

Moreover, swine cannot utilize the vitamin K synthesized by intestinal flora because the synthesis is too close to the distal end of the intestinal tract to permit significant absorption unless the animal practices coprophagy. The rate of digesta passage through the digestive tract may influence vitamin K synthesis in swine, especially when there are enteric issues. Mycotoxins are also antagonists that may cause vitamin K deficiency: for example, its anticoagulant action is impaired by aflatoxins (Suttie, 2013).

Safety

The toxic effects of the vitamin K family are manifested mainly as hematologic and circulatory derangements. Not only is species variation encountered, but profound differences are observed in the ability of the various vitamin K compounds to evoke a toxic response (Barash, 1978).

Vitamin K_1 and vitamin K_2 are nontoxic at very high dosage levels. Synthetic menadione compounds have shown toxic effects when fed to humans, rabbits, dogs, and mice in excessive amounts. However, the toxic dietary level of menadione is at least 1,000 times the dietary requirement (NRC, 2012).

There is somewhat more information on the interaction of vitamin K with other fat-soluble vitamins. Vitamin K activity is impaired by excessive vitamins A (up to 100,000 IU/kg) and E (4,000 mg/kg) levels, with repercussions on coagulation time (3 times longer). Some water-soluble menadiol sodium diphosphate and water-miscible formulations of phylloquinone may react with free tissue sulfhydryl groups when administered intramuscularly to neonates (Ullrey, 1991). Menadione compounds can safely be used at low levels to prevent the development of a deficiency but should not be used as a pharmacologic treatment for a hemorrhagic condition. In studies with various monogastric species, the main effects of toxic levels of menadione were hemolytic anemia, hyperbilirubinemia, kernicterus, brain damage, and a high mortality rate (Crenshaw, 2000).

WATER-SOLUBLE VITAMINS

Among the water-soluble vitamins are the B complex vitamins plus vitamin C and choline. Most cannot be synthesized by pigs or not in sufficient quantities to cover their requirements in different physiological situations. Some can be supplied through the metabolism of the microbiota of the intestinal tract (Briggs and Beeson, 1951; Aufreiter *et al.*, 2011). Still, since absorption is limited to the posterior sections of the digestive tract, this process is inefficient and depends on subsequent coprophagy (De Passille *et al.*, 1989; Dove and Cook, 2000).

Generally, water-soluble vitamins are not stored in significant quantities in the body (except vitamin B_{12}), which prevents toxicity problems but requires regular supplementation in the ration (Matte and Lauridsen, 2022).

Vitamin B1 (thiamine)
Chemical structure and properties

Thiamine consists of a molecule of pyrimidine and a molecule of thiazole linked by a methylene bridge, and it contains both nitrogen and sulfur atoms (Figure 4.16). A hydroxyl (OH) group at one end allows it to form ester bonds with phosphoric acid, producing thiamine mono, di- or triphosphate. Most of the vitamin B_1 in animal tissues is in the form of thiamine diphosphate (TDP), also known as thiamine pyrophosphate (TPP) or cocarboxylase. Thiamine is isolated in pure form as white, crystalline thiamine hydrochloride. The vitamin has a characteristic sulfurous odor and a slightly bitter taste (Bettendorff, 2013).

Thiamine is mainly found in the form of chloride hydrochloride ($C_{12}H_{17}N_4OSCl.HCl$, molecular mass 337.27 g mol^{-1}) that decomposes at 198°C (Bettendorff, 2013). Thiamine hydrochloride is a hydrophilic molecule: it can form a hydrate even under normal atmospheric conditions by absorbing nearly 1 mole of water and has a solubility of ~1 g/ml of water at 25°C. Under ordinary conditions, thiamine hydrochloride is more hygroscopic than mononitrate salt. However, both products should be kept in sealed containers to avoid deterioration.

Thiamine is sparingly soluble in alcohol and insoluble in fat solvents. It is very sensitive to alkali, in which the thiazole ring opens at room temperature when the pH is above 7. In a dry state, thiamine is stable at 100°C for several hours, but moisture greatly accelerates

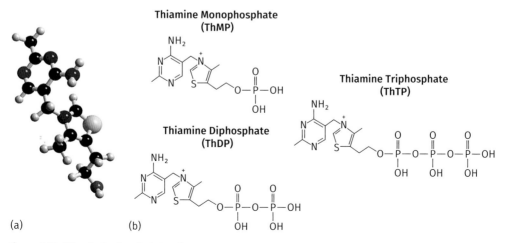

(a)   (b)

Figure 4.16 Vitamin B_1 chemical structures

destruction, and thus it is much less stable to heat in fresh than in dry foods. It is destroyed by ultraviolet light.

Natural sources

High amounts of thiamine are found in the main raw materials of plant origin, like cereals and soy used in the typical swine feed formulation. Cereal grains and their by-products, soybean meal, cottonseed meal, and peanut meal, are relatively rich sources of thiamine. However, brewer's yeast is the richest known natural source of thiamine (usually 3–6 mg/kg). Soy contains up to 7 mg/kg of whole soy, peas 2 mg/kg, and around 1.5 mg/kg of soy cake.

Since vitamin B_1 is present primarily in the germ and seed coats, by-products containing the latter are richer (7–20 mg/kg) than the whole kernel, while highly milled flour is very deficient. In humans, beriberi was prevalent in countries where polished rice is the dietary staple. Rice may have 5 mg/kg of thiamine, but the content is much lower for polished rice (0.3 mg/kg) and higher for rice bran (23 mg/kg) (Marks, 1975). Wheat germ ranks next to yeast in thiamine concentration. The level of thiamine in grain rises as the protein level rises: it depends on species, strain, and use of nitrogenous fertilizers (Bettendorff, 2013).

Using nongravid sows fed a low-thiamine compound feed supplemented with 0 g, 225 g, or 675 g wheat bran per day and 0 g, 575 g, or 1150 g alfalfa meal per day, the availability of wheat-bran thiamine was found to be better than that of alfalfa meal thiamine (Roth-Maier and Kirchgessner, 1994). The same authors also reported that "the bacterially fermentable substances from wheat bran and alfalfa meal included a higher bacterial thiamine synthesis than pectin". Roth-Maier and Kirchgessner (1993a) indicated that high pectin supplementation (400 g daily) did not affect thiamine bioavailability for sows.

Nevertheless, the frequent presence of mold or antagonists, such as mycotoxins, and high susceptibility of thiamine to inactivation by heat must be considered. Analyses of moldy feed showed a thiamine content of less than 0.1 ppm, whereas the same feed not contaminated had a thiamine content of 5.33 ppm. Reddy and Pushpamma (1986) studied the effects of 1 year of storage and insect infestation on the thiamine content of feeds. Thiamine losses were high in several sorghums and pigeon peas (40% to 70%) and lower in rice and chickpea (10% to 40%). Since thiamine is water-soluble and unstable to heat, significant losses may result during certain feed manufacturing processes (McDowell, 2000a; Bettendorff, 2013).

Recently, Witten and Aulrich (2018) found that in cereals and grain legumes thiamine (and riboflavin) content was influenced by variety, harvest year, and cultivation site. Hence, due to wide variations, it is difficult to estimate the amounts of both B vitamins in samples of cereals and grain legumes and the use of mean values can be deceptive. The authors recommended expressing table values as ranges and stating the number of underlying analyzed samples.

Commercial sources

Thiamine sources available for addition to feed are the thiamine chloride hydrochloride (337.28 g/mol; 98%) and thiamine mononitrate (327.36 g/mol; 98%) salts (Figure 4.17). Both are fine granular, white to pale yellow powders. Because of its lower solubility in water, the mononitrate salt has somewhat better stability characteristics in dry products than the hydrochloride (Bettendorff, 2013). Thiamine mononitrate is prepared from thiamine hydrochloride by dissolving the hydrochloride salt in a mildly alkaline solution, followed by precipitation of the nitrate half-salt with a stoichiometric amount of nitric acid. The concentration and requirements of vitamin B_1 are usually expressed in milligrams (mg).

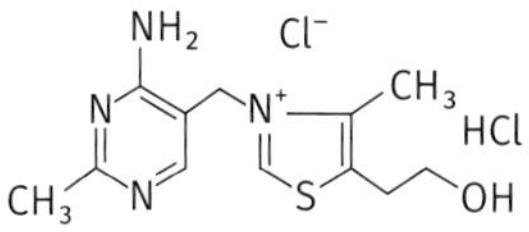

(a) Thiamine chloride hydrochloride 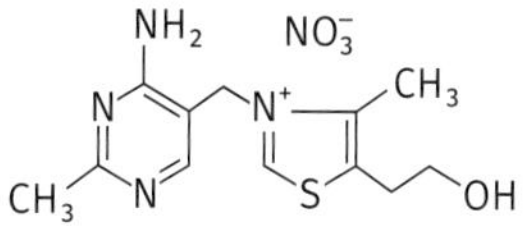   (b)   Thiamine mononitrate

Figure 4.17 Vitamin B$_1$ forms used in animal nutrition

Metabolism
Absorption and transport
Thiamine appears to be readily digested and released from naturally occurring sources. A precondition for normal thiamine absorption is sufficient stomach hydrochloric acid production. Phosphoric acid esters of thiamine are split in the intestine. The free thiamine formed is soluble in water and easily absorbed, especially in the jejunum.

The mechanism of thiamine absorption is not yet fully understood, but both active transport and simple passive diffusion are involved. There is active sodium-dependent transport of thiamine at low concentrations against the electrochemical potential, whereas, at high concentrations, it diffuses passively through the intestinal wall. Thiamine synthesized by the gut microflora in the cecum, or large intestine, is largely unavailable to animals except by coprophagy (De Passille et al., 1989).

Specific proteins (transporters and carriers) in the cell membrane have binding sites for thiamine, allowing it to be solubilized within the cell membrane. This permits the vitamin to pass through the membrane and ultimately reach the aqueous environment on the other side (Rose, 1990; Bates, 2006). Absorbed thiamine is transported via the portal vein to the liver with the carrier plasma protein. Thiamine is efficiently transferred to the embryo.

Thiamine phosphorylation can occur in most tissues, particularly in the liver. Almost 80% of thiamine in animals is phosphorylated in the liver under the action of ATP to form the metabolically active enzyme form TPP (diphosphate or cocarboxylase). Of total body thiamine, about 80% is TPP, about 10% is TTP, and the remainder is thiamine monophosphate (TMP) and free thiamine.

Storage and excretion
Although thiamine is readily absorbed and transported to cells throughout the body, it is one of the most poorly stored vitamins. Most mammals on a thiamine-deficient diet will exhaust their body stores within 1–2 weeks, so a continuous thiamine supply is required (Ensminger et al., 1983). The thiamine content in individual organs varies considerably, and the vitamin is preferentially retained in organs with high metabolic activity. Thiamine is contained in the greatest quantities in major organs such as the liver, heart, brain, and kidneys during deficiencies. Although liver and kidney tissues have the highest thiamine concentrations, approximately 50% of the total thiamine body stores are in muscle tissue (Polegato et al., 2019). For unknown reasons, however, tissue concentration in pigs is very high (Muroya et al., 2018). Studies carried out more than 5 decades ago showed that pigs receiving feed lacking in thiamine can live for at least 2 months without showing signs of deficiency.

Thiamine intakes above current needs are rapidly excreted. Absorbed thiamine is passed in urine and feces, with small quantities excreted in other secretions. Fecal thiamine may originate from feed, synthesis by microorganisms, or endogenous sources (i.e., via bile or excretion through the mucosa of the large intestine). When thiamine is administered in large doses, urinary excretion reaches saturation, and the fecal concentration increases considerably

(Bräunlich and Zintzen, 1976). Roth-Maier and Kirchgessner (1993a, 1994) determined in 2 separate investigations that more than 90 to 95% of excess thiamine is excreted via feces.

Biochemical functions

Thiamine is one of the enzymes critical in the metabolism of lysine, branched-chain amino acids, carbohydrates, and lipogenesis (Bettendorff, 2013). The main functions of thiamine are illustrated in Figure 4.18. Primarily, thiamine is important in carbohydrate and energy metabolism, especially in the heart and nervous system (Bâ, 2008; Muroya et al., 2018). For this reason, thiamine recommendations increase when the primary energy source supplied by the feed is carbohydrates.

The TPP (or TDP or cocarboxylase) is the active thiamine derivative involved in the tricarboxylic acid (TCA) cycle (citric acid, or Krebs cycle). Thiamine is the coenzyme for all enzymatic decarboxylations of α-keto acids. Thus, it functions in the oxidative decarboxylation of pyruvate to acetate, which in turn is combined with coenzyme A (CoA) for entrance into the TCA cycle. Thiamine is essential in 2 oxidative decarboxylation reactions in the TCA cycle that takes place in cell mitochondria and one reaction in the cytoplasm of the cells.

Decarboxylation in the TCA cycle removes carbon dioxide, and the substrate is converted into the compound having the next lower number of carbon atoms:

1   pyruvate –> acetyl-CoA + CO_2
2   α-ketoglutaric acid –> succinyl-CoA + CO_2.

These reactions are essential for the utilization of carbohydrates to provide energy. Vitamin B_2 (riboflavin), pantothenic acid, and niacin are also involved with thiamine in this biochemical process.

Thiamine plays a crucial role in glucose metabolism. TPP is a coenzyme in the transketolase reaction that is part of the direct oxidative pathway (pentose phosphate cycle) of glucose

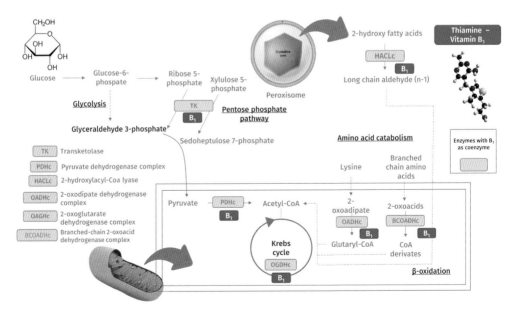

Figure 4.18 Vitamin B_1 roles in metabolism

metabolism in the liver, brain, adrenal cortex, and kidney cell cytoplasm, but not skeletal muscle. The pentose phosphate cycle is the only mechanism known for ribose synthesis needed for nucleotide formation. This cycle also reduces nicotinamide adenine dinucleotide phosphate (NADPH), essential for lowering carbohydrate metabolism intermediates during fatty acid synthesis (Bettendorff, 2013; Muroya et al., 2018).

Thiamine is, together with vitamin B_6 (pyridoxine) and B_{12} (cobalamin), one of the commonly called "neurotropic" B vitamins, playing particular and essential roles both in the central nervous system (CNS) and the peripheral nervous system (PNS) (Muralt, 1962; Cooper et al., 1963; Bâ, 2008; Calderón-Ospina and Nava-Mesa, 2020). The maintenance of nerve membrane function and the synthesis of myelin and several types of neurotransmitters (e.g., acetylcholine, serotonin, and amino acids) are essential in transmitting nervous impulses. Another thiamine function in the transmission of nervous impulses is due to its participation in the passive transport of sodium (Na^+) to excitable membranes, which is important for the transmission of impulses at the membrane of ganglionic cells. However, thiamine's above-described role in energy metabolism explains a significant part of its activity in the nervous system by providing energy to nerve cells (Bâ, 2008).

Nutritional assessment

Thiamine nutritional status is typically determined by measuring the thiamine-dependent erythrocyte transketolase activity (ETKA) or thiamine (free or phosphorylated) concentrations.

The ETKA assay is the most acceptable for a functional assessment of thiamine deficiencies by measuring the relative increase of erythrocyte transketolase activity in response to in vitro addition of TDP. However, analytical variability is reported due to standardization and sample stability issues (Sauberlich, 1999; Höller et al., 2018). HPLC-based methods to quantify free thiamine and the phosphorylated form require further improvements.

Deficiency signs

Cereals and soy have a high thiamine content but being present primarily in the germ and seed coats milled products contain much less thiamine. Thiamine is also highly susceptible to inactivation by heat. Moreover, in nature there are many anti-thiamine substances, causing its inactivation (more details at the end of the paragraph). Therefore, in theory, natural dietary content seems unlikely to lead to a deficiency but in practice supplementation is required. On occasion, deficiencies have been confirmed in the field, with symptoms such as anorexia, decreased body weight, vomiting, polyneuritis, and foot problems. The heart can be affected by bradycardia, arrhythmia, hypertrophy, myocardial degeneration, and sudden death associated with heart failure. Symptoms of thiamine deficiency are relatively unspecific (Barnhart et al., 1957). The loss of appetite can become extreme depending on the degree of deficiency involved. Vitamin B_1 requirements increase if the diet is high in carbohydrates, so the body's reserves are rapidly exhausted if there is a thiamine deficiency.

The detailed pathophysiology and biochemistry of thiamine deficiency-induced processes in the brain have been studied in human subjects, animal models, and cultured cells (Gibson and Zhang, 2002; Martin et al., 2003; Ke and Gibson, 2004; McCandless, 2010). Neurodegeneration becomes apparent as a reversible lesion and later irreversibly in specific areas of the brain, notably the sub-medial thalamic nucleus and parts of the cerebellum, especially the superior cerebellar vermis (Bates, 2006; McCandless, 2010; Bettendorff, 2013).

The classic pathological syndrome or disease caused by thiamine deficiency in humans is called beriberi (McCandless, 2010). It involves the nervous and circulatory systems, with symptoms also observed in various animal species. This is explained by the fact that the brain covers its energy requirement chiefly by the degradation of glucose and is therefore dependent on biochemical reactions in which thiamine plays a key role (Bâ, 2008; McCandless, 2010).

Of all nutrients, a thiamine deficiency has the most marked effect on appetite. Animals consuming a low-thiamine diet soon show severe anorexia, lose all interest in food, and will not resume eating unless given thiamine (Figures 4.19a and 4.19b). Thiamine must be force-fed or injected to induce animals to continue eating if the deficiency is severe.

The classic disease of polyneuritis in pigs represents a late stage of thiamine deficiency resulting from peripheral neuritis, perhaps caused by an accumulation of intermediates of carbohydrate metabolism. Low body temperature, muscular weakness, progressive dysfunction of the nervous system and occasionally vomiting, breathing disorders, and sudden death from heart failure. The inactivation of decarboxylase pyruvic acid leads to an accumulation of lactic acid and a drop in intracellular pH. As acetyl-coenzyme A is an important metabolite in fatty acid synthesis, deficiency reduces lipogenesis or fat synthesis (McCandless, 2010).

One case was reported by Hough *et al.* (2015), where they described a thiamine-responsive neurological disease and the methodology leading to its diagnosis. The initial case involved one nursery farm, approximately 5% of pigs 5 to 7 days after weaning exhibited CNS signs (Figure 4.19c). Over the next 3 weeks, 16 of the company's 41 nursery farms had pigs with similar clinical signs. One month later, several sow farms observed neurologic symptoms in unweaned piglets. Pigs were weaned at approximately 19 days and moved to off-site nurseries. Live pigs and fresh and formalin-fixed samples from acutely affected pigs were sent to diagnostic laboratories. Feed samples were submitted for mycotoxin and nutrient analyses. Initial reports revealed no precise cause of the neurological condition; however, polioencephalomalacia (PEM) was subsequently identified in affected pigs. A field trial determined the response to treatment with atropine, a vitamin A, D, and E preparation, or vitamin B_{12} plus thiamine. Pigs treated with injections of thiamine recovered from the neurological condition. Upon implementation of thiamine injections on a company-wide basis, neurological signs associated with

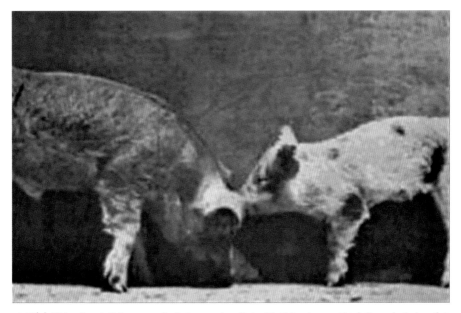

Figure 4.19(a) Thiamine deficiency: a pig fed a regular diet with thiamine on the left, a pig fed a diet lacking thiamine on the right

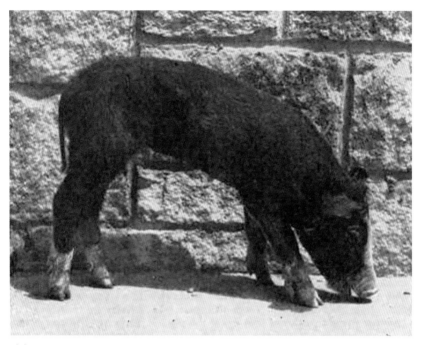

Figure 4.19(b) Thiamine deficiency: pig fed a diet lacking thiamine (source: Madsen, 1942)

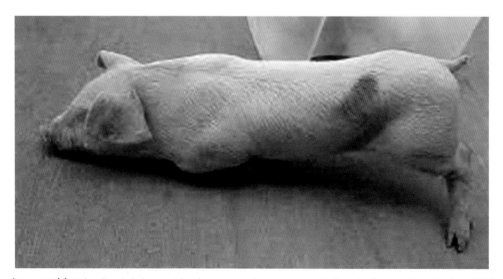

Figure 4.19(c) Thiamine deficiency: thiamine-responsive neurological disorder (source: Hough *et al.*, 2015)

PEM were no longer evident. The authors do not recommend routine thiamine injections under normal circumstances. In this case, compromised dietary thiamine levels during feed manufacturing possibly contributed to the PEM.

Substances with anti-thiamine activity, hence causing a deficiency, are relatively common in nature and include structurally similar antagonists and structure-altering antagonists. For example, fish meal contains thiaminases. The synthetic compounds pyrithiamine, oxythiamine, and amprolium (an anticoccidial) are structurally similar antagonists. Their mode of action is competitive inhibition, interfering with thiamine at different points in metabolism.

Pyrithiamine blocks the esterification of thiamine with phosphoric acid, inhibiting the thiamine coenzyme cocarboxylase. Oxythiamine competitively inhibits thiamine's binding to the carboxylase complex, blocking critical metabolic reactions. The coccidiostat amprolium inhibits the intestinal absorption of thiamine and blocks the phosphorylation of the vitamin (McDowell, 2000a). Thiaminase activity destroys thiamine by altering the structure of the vitamin (Bettendorff, 2013). Two types of thiaminase enzymes, I and II, have been described. Thiaminase I substitutes a new base for the thiazole ring. This leads to less thiamine, but it also results in thiamine analogs consisting of the pyrimidine ring of the original thiamine and another ring from the "cosubstrate." This thiamine-analog may be absorbed and inhibit thiamine-requiring reactions (McCandless, 2010). Thiaminase II cleaves the vitamin at the methylene bridge between the thiazole and the pyrimidine rings. Certain microorganisms (bacteria and molds) and plants (e.g., bracken fern) produce thiaminases.

Sulfur has been shown to be antagonistic to thiamine enzymes (Gibson et al., 1987). The sulfite ion has been shown to cleave thiamine from enzymes at the methylene bridge and, analytically, will imitate thiaminase. In premixes that include choline and trace minerals, thiamine stability is relatively low, and at ambient temperature, its content may be reduced by up to 50%. This occurs to a greater extent in feed contaminated by mycotoxin-producing fungi such as *Aspergillus* and *Fusarium*, where the B_1 concentration can drop by a factor of up to 10 (Nagaraj et al., 1994). Thiamine content was reduced from 43 to 50% for 2 cultivars of wheat infested with *Aspergillus flavus* compared to the uncontaminated sound wheat (Kao and Robinson, 1972).

Heinemann et al. (1946) reported that the pig could utilize stored thiamine over a long time, as 56 days was required for the pigs to lose their appetites after beginning a thiamine-deficient diet. Death has been reported 74 days after pigs began a thiamine-free but otherwise adequate diet (Loew, 1978). For young pigs, severe thiamine deficiency has resulted in death at 3 to 4 weeks. The first signs of thiamine deficiency in pigs are reduced feed consumption and vomiting, with a sharp reduction in weight gain (Van Etten et al., 1940; Miller et al., 1955; Barnhart et al., 1957; Peng and Heitman, 1973).

Functional and structural cardiac changes are the main findings in experimentally deficient swine; in contrast to clinical reports, nervous system lesions were not detected (Follis et al., 1943). Electrocardiographically demonstrable changes in heart tissue are also seen, with enlarged hearts obtained from pigs receiving thiamine-deficient diets (Figure 4.19d). Van Etten et al. (1940) reported that the heart could be flabby with myocardial degeneration. On microscopic examination, it is possible to recognize inflammations and necrotic changes in the myocardial fibers.

Thiamine-deficient animals have elevated plasma pyruvate concentrations (Miller et al., 1955; Barnhart et al., 1957) since, with this vitamin deficiency, there is an accumulation of intermediates of carbohydrate metabolism. The red blood cell enzyme transketolase is lowered in thiamine-deficient pigs. This enzyme is an indicator of thiamine status (McDowell, 2000a). Peng and Heitman (1973) determined that erythrocyte transketolase and TPP stimulation were very useful, sensitive, and specific methods for studying the thiamine status of growing-finishing pigs.

Safety

Thiamine ingested in large amounts orally is not toxic, and the same is true of parenteral doses. Dietary intake of thiamine up to 1,000 times the requirement is safe for most animal

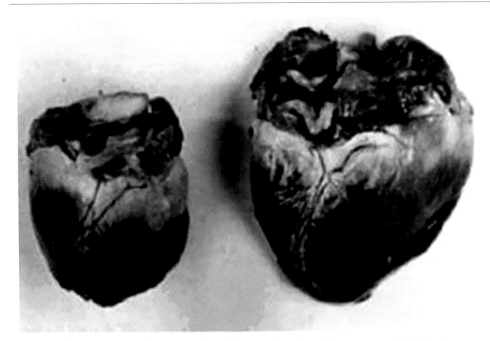

Figure 4.19(d) Thiamine deficiency: an enlarged heart. The enlarged heart on the right is due to a deficiency of thiamine. The heart on the left is from a similar pig fed the same diet plus thiamine (source: Courtesy of T.J. Cunha, Washington State University)

species (NRC, 1998). Levels as high as 100 mg/kg of body weight have been fed to young pigs with no ill effects (Crenshaw, 2000). Lethal doses with intravenous injections were 125, 250, 300, and 350 mg/kg of bodyweight for mice, rats, rabbits, and dogs, respectively (Bates, 2006). The effects of excessive intakes of thiamine have not been studied in swine (NRC, 1998).

Vitamin B$_2$ (riboflavin)
Chemical structure and properties
Riboflavin exists in 3 forms in nature: free dinucleotide riboflavin and the 2 coenzyme derivatives, flavin mononucleotide (FMN) and flavin adenine dinucleotide (FAD) (Pinto and Rivlin, 2013). It is composed of a dimethylisoalloxazine nucleus combined with ribitol. Riboflavin is a water-soluble, odorless, bitter, orange-yellow compound that melts at about 280°C. The molecular structure of riboflavin is shown in Figure 4.20.

Riboflavin is only slightly soluble in water but readily soluble in dilute basic or strongly acidic solutions. It is quite stable to heat in neutral and acid but not alkaline solutions, and very little (3–4%) is lost in feed processing (Lewis *et al.*, 2015; Yang *et al.*, 2020). Aqueous solutions are unstable to visible and UV light, and instability is increased by heat and alkalinity. Both light and oxygen have been found to induce riboflavin degradation (Becker *et al.*, 2003). When dry, riboflavin is appreciably less affected by light. An essential factor when pigs are given liquid feed.

Natural sources
Vitamin B$_2$ was first isolated from egg albumin in 1933 and subsequently detected in milk and liver. Overall, only a few feedstuffs fed to swine contain enough riboflavin to meet the

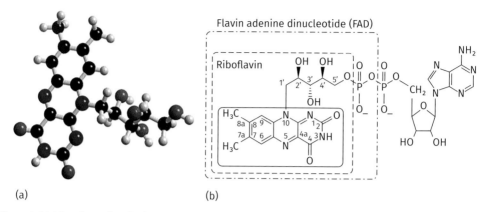

Figure 4.20 Vitamin B$_2$ chemical structure

requirements of young growing pigs (Chen, Huang, Lui *et al.*, 2019; Chen, Wang, Li *et al.* 2019; McDowell, 2000a). Riboflavin is found in appreciable quantities in green plants, in by-products of animal origin (buttermilk 28 mg/kg, fishmeal 5–10 mg/kg), and in dehydrated alfalfa (alfalfa 15 mg/kg). However, its content is limited to cereals and protein ingredients of plant origin, primarily used in swine diets. Riboflavin is also synthesized by yeast, fungi, and some bacteria except *Lactobacilli*, including intestinal bacteria such as *Faecalibacterium prausnitzii*.

Riboflavin is more bioavailable from animal products than from plant sources, as the flavin complexes in plants are more stable for digestion than in animal sources. Riboflavin is present at a low concentration in cereals (1.0–1.4 mg/kg, except for sorghum and rice, which contain up to 4 mg/kg). Cereal by-products contain slightly higher amounts (wheat bran contains approximately 3 mg/kg). Concentrates of vegetable protein generally contain appreciable amounts (whole soy 2.6 mg/kg, soy cake 3.0–4.0 mg/kg, sunflower meal 7 mg/kg, peanut 6 mg/kg). Corn-soy diets usually contain 2–2.6 mg/kg of riboflavin, 60% of which is bioavailable (Chung and Baker, 1990). The increase in pelleting temperatures and the use of expanders to control contamination by *Salmonella* has increased its degradation (Yang *et al.*, 2020). The bioavailability of riboflavin was less for chicks fed corn-soybeans than those fed purified amino acid diets. Riboflavin is one of the most stable vitamins, but, as said before, it is susceptible to light (especially ultraviolet light). For this reason, processing and storage conditions may represent significant losses if exposure to sunlight is not limited. Recently, Witten and Aulrich (2018) found that in cereals and grain legumes riboflavin (and thiamine) content was influenced by variety, harvest year, and cultivation site. Because of the wide variations, it is difficult to estimate the amounts of both B vitamins in samples of cereals and grain legumes and the use of mean values can be deceptive. The authors recommended to express table values as ranges under the mention of the number of underlying sample.

Commercial forms

Riboflavin is commercially available to the feed, food, and pharmaceutical industries as a feed-grade crystalline compound produced by chemical synthesis or fermentation, formulated in spray-dried powders containing 80% riboflavin. Riboflavin 5′-phosphate sodium salt (75–79% riboflavin) is available for applications requiring a water-dispersible source of riboflavin.

High-potency, USP, or feed-grade crystalline powders are electrostatic, hygroscopic, and dusty and, thus, do not flow freely and show the poor distribution in feeds. In contrast, 80% of commercial spray-dried powders show reduced electrostaticity and hygroscopicity for better feed flowability and distribution (Adams, 1978).

Metabolism
Absorption and transport
Riboflavin covalently bound to protein is released by proteolytic digestion. Phosphatases hydrolyze phosphorylated forms (FAD, FMN) of riboflavin in the upper gastrointestinal tract to free the vitamin for absorption. Cells from deficient animals have a greater maximal absorption uptake of riboflavin (Rose *et al.*, 1986). At low concentrations, riboflavin absorption is an active carrier-mediated process. At high concentrations, however, riboflavin is absorbed by passive diffusion, proportional to concentration. Mucosal cells absorb free riboflavin via a dynamic saturable transport system in all parts of the small intestine (Pinto and Rivlin, 2013). Free riboflavin is absorbed very efficiently throughout the small intestine of the pig. Riboflavin is phosphorylated to FMN in mucosal cells by the enzyme flavokinase (Rivlin, 2006). The FMN then enters the portal system, is bound to plasma albumin, transported to the liver, and converted to FAD, the form most present in plasma and tissues.

Transport of flavin by blood plasma involves loose associations with albumin and tight associations with some globulins (McCormick, 1990). A genetically controlled riboflavin-binding protein is present in serum. Thyroid hormones, particularly triiodothyronine (T_3), regulate the activities of the flavin biosynthetic enzymes, the synthesis of the apoflavoproteins, and the formation of covalently bound flavins (Pinto and Rivlin, 2013).

Storage and excretion
Hepatic cells from deficient animals have a relatively greater maximal absorption uptake of riboflavin (Rose *et al.*, 1986). Hepatic cell riboflavin absorption occurs via facilitated diffusion. The absorption of methionine also increased if the maximum concentration was used. Animals do not appear to be able to store appreciable amounts of riboflavin, with the liver, kidneys, and heart having the most significant concentrations.

The liver, the primary storage site, contains about one-third of the total body riboflavin. Intakes of riboflavin above current needs are rapidly excreted in the urine, primarily as free riboflavin. Minor quantities of absorbed riboflavin are excreted in feces and bile.

Biochemical functions
Riboflavin, in its phosphorylated form (FMN and FAD) or as a constituent of the flavoproteins, is a coenzyme and cofactor of more than 100 enzymes, namely flavoenzymes, involved in the transfer of electrons in redox reactions, in the metabolism of carbohydrates and amino acids and the synthesis and oxidation of fatty acids and transporting proteins (Pinto and Rivlin, 2013). Figure 4.21 shows the most important functions of riboflavin. Hence recommendations in swine rise when the quantity of fat or protein in the feed increases.

Interaction of flavin coenzymes with their respective apoflavoproteins involves both non-covalent and covalent associations, but only 25 coenzymes have been identified to be covalently linked. The conversion to FMN and FAD is regulated by nutritional status, particularly protein-calorie malnutrition, metabolic rate, hormones, and drugs. Flavoenzymes function within an eclectic array of cellular processes that involve (Pinto and Rivlin, 2013):

- electron transport, accepting and passing hydrogen in the cytochrome system in the generations of ATP
- metabolism of lipids, drugs, and xenobiotic substances

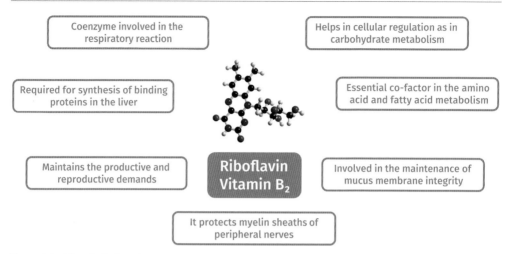

Coenzyme involved in the respiratory reaction

Helps in cellular regulation as in carbohydrate metabolism

Required for synthesis of binding proteins in the liver

Essential co-factor in the amino acid and fatty acid metabolism

Maintains the productive and reproductive demands

Riboflavin Vitamin B$_2$

Involved in the maintenance of mucus membrane integrity

It protects myelin sheaths of peripheral nerves

Figure 4.21 Vitamin B$_2$ functions

- cell signaling
- protein folding.

If riboflavin levels are low, the respiration process becomes less efficient, and 10 to 15% more feed is required to meet energy needs (Christensen, 1983). The enzymes that function aerobically are called oxidases, and those that function anaerobically are called dehydrogenases. The general function is in the oxidation of substrate and generation of energy (i.e., ATP). Collectively, the flavoproteins show great versatility in accepting and transferring 1 or 2 electrons with various potentials.

Many flavoproteins contain a metal (e.g., iron, molybdenum, copper, zinc). The combination of the flavin and metal ion is often involved in adjusting these enzymes in transfers between single- and double-electron donors. Xanthine oxidase contains the metals molybdenum and iron. It converts hypoxanthine to xanthine and the latter to uric acid. It also reacts with aldehydes to form acids, converting retinal (vitamin A aldehyde) to retinoic acid.

There is a close relationship between riboflavin and niacin because flavoproteins may accept a hydrogen ion (H$^+$) directly from the substrate, thus catalyzing the oxidation of the substrate, or it may catalyze the oxidation of some other enzyme by accepting a hydrogen ion from it. For example, from the niacin-containing coenzymes, nicotinamide adenine dinucleotide (NADH) and NADPH.

Flavoprotein enzymes may be arbitrarily classified into 3 groups:

1   NADH$_2$ dehydrogenases: reduced pyridine nucleotide is a substrate, and the electron acceptor is either a member of the cytochrome system or some other acceptor besides oxygen.
2   Dehydrogenases: accept electrons directly from the substrate and pass them to one of the cytochromes.
3   Oxidases (true): accept electrons from the substrate and pass them directly to oxygen (O$_2$ is reduced to H$_2$O$_2$); they cannot reduce cytochromes.

Riboflavin functions in flavoprotein-enzyme systems to help regulate cellular metabolism, although they are also specifically involved in the metabolism of carbohydrates. Riboflavin is also an essential factor in amino acid metabolism as part of amino acid oxidases. These enzymes oxidize amino acids, which results in the decomposition of the amino acids, yielding ammonia and a keto acid. Distinct oxidized D-amino acids (prosthetic group FAD) and L-amino acids (prosthetic group FMN) are produced. In the methionine and homocysteine metabolism, riboflavin plays a role as a coenzyme in the same way that cobalamin, folate, and pyridoxine do (Pinto and Rivlin, 2013).

Riboflavin not only is a critical link in the utilization of dietary folates and cobalamins but also controls homocysteine re-methylation and trans-sulfuration in association with methyl donor flavoenzymes within the one-carbon cycle as well as the FAD/FMN diflavin enzyme, methionine sulfoxide reductase (MSR), the FAD-dependent N5,N10-methylenetetrahydrofolate reductase (MTHFR) necessary for methionine formation. This function affects cardiovascular disease and osteoporosis (Pinto and Rivlin, 2013).

In addition, riboflavin plays a role in fat metabolism (Rivlin, 2006), and a FAD flavoprotein is an important link in fatty acid oxidation. This includes the acyl-coenzyme A dehydroge-nases, which are necessary for the stepwise degradation of fatty acids. An FMN flavoprotein is required for the synthesis of fatty acids from acetate. Thus, flavoproteins are needed to degrade and synthesize fatty acids.

Riboflavin and other vitamins play an important role in skin development, tensile strength, and healing rates (Lakshmi et al., 1989). A riboflavin deficiency can slow the epithelialization of wounds by 4–5 days (Lakshmi et al., 1989), reduce collagen content by 25%, and decrease the tensile strength of injuries by 45%. Riboflavin deficiency can increase skin homocysteine by 2- to 4-fold, ultimately impairing collagen's cross-link formation (Lakshmi et al., 1990). Marginal field deficiencies of riboflavin could increase skin tears, cause longer healing times, and ultimately increase costly downgrades.

Among the enzymes that require riboflavin is the FMN-dependent oxidase responsible for converting phosphorylated pyridoxine (vitamin B_6) to a functional coenzyme. Riboflavin deficiency also decreases the conversion of the vitamin B_6 coenzyme pyridoxal phosphate to the main vitamin B_6 urinary excretory product of 4-pyridoxic acid.

Riboflavin, coenzyme Q_{10} and niacin are associated with poly (ADP-ribose) polymer-ase (PARP), a family of proteins involved in several cellular processes, which function in post-translational modification of nuclear proteins. The poly ADP-ribosylated proteins func-tion in DNA repair, replication, and cell differentiation (Premkumar et al., 2008; Pinto and Rivlin, 2013).

It plays an important role in maintaining the integrity of mucous membranes and the ner-vous system (Pinto and Rivlin, 2013). It interacts with other vitamins: pyridoxine, niacin, and pantothenic acid.

It has been possible to observe that uterine flow during the first moments of gestation contains a high riboflavin concentration and that this concentration varies with the supply of this vitamin in the feed for sows (Moffatt et al., 1980; Murray et al., 1980; Frank et al., 1984; Bazer and Zavy, 1988). The specific reasons for this high concentration remain to be identified. Pettigrew et al. (1996) observed that riboflavin must perform an essential function in the initial moments of gestation, metabolically adapting the uterine tissue. The needs of riboflavin for sows during lactation were evaluated by Frank et al. (1984). These authors observed that gilts fed diets with 1.25 mg riboflavin/kg feed had higher piglet mortality, reduced feed intake, and lost more weight. The optimum levels were estimated at 16.2–16.3 mg/day. Miller et al. (1953) determined the riboflavin requirement of the baby pig for optimum growth and feed efficiency in 3.0 mg/kg of diet. However, currently, 4–7 mg/kg of feed are recommended for piglets (NRC, 2012; Rostagno et al., 2017).

Nutritional assessment

The assessment of the riboflavin nutritional status is not simple, and it seems that the sensitivity to changes in riboflavin intake is relatively low. The typical functional test used the erythrocyte glutathione reductase activity coefficient (EGRac) assay, which allows for determining the degree of tissue saturation with riboflavin (Sauberlich, 1999).

The riboflavin vitamers – free riboflavin and the coenzymes FMN and FAD – can be analyzed directly in serum (or homogenized erythrocytes) using liquid chromatography coupled to tandem mass spectrometry (LC-MS/MS), and data can be compared with EGRac. Correlations between plasma riboflavin and EGRac showed good, and all vitamers but not FAD seem suitable to assess riboflavin status (Höller et al., 2018).

Deficiency signs

Riboflavin is more likely than other vitamins to become deficient under practical conditions, especially under stressful conditions like cold stress (McMillen et al., 1949; Mitchell et al., 1950; Forbes and Haines, 1952; Terrill et al., 1955; Seymour et al., 1968; Christensen, 1973; Pinto and Rivlin, 2013; Pinto and Zempleni, 2016) and when aflatoxins are present, for which reason an ample safety margin should be applied in swine nutrition. Typical swine diets mainly based on grains would often be borderline to deficient in riboflavin levels. Only a few feedstuffs fed to swine contain enough riboflavin to meet their requirements (McDowell, 2000a).

Riboflavin deficiency affects iron metabolism, with less iron absorbed and an increased rate of iron loss due to an accelerated rate of small intestinal epithelial turnover (Christensen, 1973; Powers et al., 1991, 1993). A primary deficiency of dietary riboflavin has broad implications for other vitamins, as flavin coenzymes are involved in the metabolism of 5 vitamins: folic acid, vitamin B_6, vitamin K, niacin, and vitamin D (Pinto and Rivlin, 2013). Signs of lack of vitamin B_2 in pigs are quite unspecific. Usually, they involve the tissues and functions most dependent on energy from carbohydrates: epithelial and nervous tissue and reproduction functions. Signs typically include loss of appetite, growth retardation, poorer feed conversion, vomiting, dermatitis, alopecia, and inflammation of the anal mucosa. A decrease in consumption of up to 30% has been described in sows receiving feeds containing low levels of riboflavin (Frank et al., 1988).

Reduced feed intake was demonstrated in gilts given a lactation diet containing 1.3 mg/kg of riboflavin. These gilts consumed 30% less feed than those who received diets with 2.3–5.3 mg/kg of riboflavin (Frank et al., 1988). Typical clinical signs often involve the eye, skin, and nervous system. Symptoms of riboflavin deficiency in the young growing pig include anorexia, slow growth (Figure 4.22a), rough hair coat, dermatitis, alopecia, abnormal stiffness, unsteady gait, scours, ulcerative colitis, inflammation of anal mucosa, vomiting, cataracts, light sensitivity, and eye lens opacities (Hughes, 1940; Lehrer and Wiese, 1952; Terrill et al., 1955; Cunha, 1977; NRC, 1998).

In severe riboflavin deficiency in pigs, researchers have observed increased blood neutrophil granulocytes and neutrophilia (Mitchell et al., 1950), decreased immune response, discolored liver and kidney tissue, fatty liver, collapsed follicles, degenerating ova, and degenerating myelin of the sciatic and brachial nerves (Luce et al., 1990; NRC, 1998). Lehrer and Wiese (1952) indicated that the external deficiency symptoms observed in their study could be reversed by supplementation of 1–1.5 mg of riboflavin per day for 16 days. However, the internal tissue changes were not corrected during this supplementation interval. In 1954, Miller et al. observed gross and microscopic lesions in piglets receiving less than 2.0 mg of riboflavin per kilogram of solids.

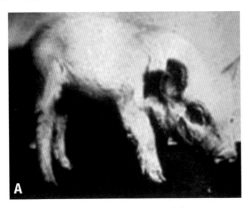
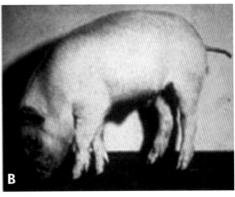

Figure 4.22(a) Vitamin B₂ deficiency: (A) pig that received no dietary riboflavin; (B) control pig (source: courtesy of the R.W. Luecke, Michigan Agricultural Experimentation Station, and J. Nutrition)

Riboflavin deficiency harms reproduction with anestrus, embryonic death, and reabsorption, the birth of weak piglets which die in the first 48 hours, edema in piglets, premature birth (up to 2 weeks), litters without hair, etc. (Esch *et al.*, 1981; Luce *et al.*, 1990; Pettigrew *et al.*, 1996). In the last few years, riboflavin deficiency has been observed to affect young sows' reproductive systems. Pigs fed a diet only marginally deficient in riboflavin often recover spontaneously. The condition is curable in the early stages, but in its chronic phase, it is irreversible (NRC, 2012).

Miller *et al.* (1953) reported that riboflavin deficiency seriously impaired reproduction in pigs. Sows receiving 0.55 mg riboflavin per kg of feed failed to reproduce or experienced death. Offspring from riboflavin-deficient sows are shown in Figure 4.22b. Cunha (1977) summarized the clinical signs for gilts fed a riboflavin-deficient diet during reproduction and lactation as follows:

1. erratic or, at times, complete loss of appetite
2. poor gains
3. parturition four to 16 days prematurely
4. one case of death of a fetus in an advanced stage with resorption in evidence
5. all pigs either were dead at birth or died within 48 hours thereafter
6. enlarged front legs in some pigs due to gelatinous edema in the connective tissue and generalized edema in many others
7. hairless litters.

The longer the period on riboflavin-deficient diets, the more severe the deficiency signs became. Christensen (1980) likewise reported the resorption of fetuses and premature farrowing for riboflavin-deficient sows.

Hepatic architecture is markedly disrupted in riboflavin deficiency with hepatic lipid peroxidation in experimental animals. Mitochondria in riboflavin-deficient mice progress through a series of morphological changes ranging from the elongation of cristae to the development of cristae clusters that result in cup-shaped mitochondria that tend to nest within each other. Although these cell structural abnormalities occur, changes in oxidative metabolism appear marginal, as minor losses are observed in the activity of the flavin-dependent components of the electron transport chain, namely, complexes I and II. Other critical organelles markedly

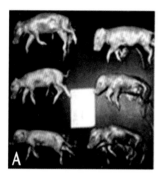
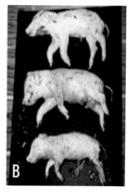
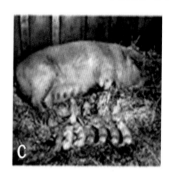

Figure 4.22(b) Vitamin B$_2$ deficiency. (A) All the pigs in this litter were born dead. Some were in the process of resorption. A few had edema and enlargement of the front legs due to gelatinous edema. (B) Pigs from a litter in which gelatinous edema was more pronounced. (C) Seven of the 10 pigs farrowed were born dead, and the other 3 were dead within 48 hours. The sow received a riboflavin-deficient diet for a shorter period than the sows farrowing the other 2 litters (source: courtesy of T.J. Cunha, Washington State University)

impaired during riboflavin deficiency are peroxisomes. These organelles contribute to several crucial metabolic processes such as β-oxidation of fatty acids, biosynthesis of ether phospholipids, and metabolism of ROS. Within erythrocytes, riboflavin deficiency causes a reduction in the activity of glucose-6-phosphate dehydrogenase (Pinto and Rivlin, 2013).

Riboflavin deficiency has led to anestrus (Esch *et al.*, 1981). Lack of riboflavin in post-pubertal gilts has reduced ovarian cyclicity without overt signs of deficiency. Gilts fed a riboflavin-deficient diet had a progressively longer average time interval between consecutive estrus periods until becoming anestrus 63 days after the beginning of the study. Teratogenic effects have been observed, including skeletal abnormalities, shortened bones, and fusions between ribs (Zintzen, 1975).

Safety
A large body of evidence has accumulated that supplementation with riboflavin over nutritional requirements has very little toxicity for animals and humans (Pinto and Rivlin, 2013). There are no reports of riboflavin toxicity studies in pigs. Most data from rats suggest that dietary levels between 10 and 20 times the requirement (possibly 100 times) can be tolerated safely (NRC, 1998). Campbell and Combs (1990a) fed diets containing up to 0.7% supplemental riboflavin to growing and finishing pigs and observed no effect on performance. When massive amounts of riboflavin are administered orally, only a small fraction of the dose is absorbed, the remainder being excreted in the feces.

Lack of toxicity is probably partly down to limitations in the transport system necessary for riboflavin absorption across the gastrointestinal mucosa, which becomes saturated limiting riboflavin absorption (Christensen, 1973). Also, the capacity of tissues to store riboflavin and its coenzyme derivatives appears to be limited when excessive amounts are administered.

Vitamin B$_6$ (pyridoxine)
Chemical structure and properties
The term vitamin B$_6$ refers to a group of 3 pyridine derivatives named according to the functional group in the position 4 (Dakshinamurti and Dakshinamurti, 2013):

- pyridoxol or pyridoxine (PN), the alcohol form
- pyridoxal (PL), the aldehyde form
- pyridoxamine (PM), the amine form.

These 3 compounds have a similar vitamin activity and are interconvertible in the animal's body. Pyridoxine is the predominant plant form, whereas pyridoxal and pyridoxamine are vitamin forms generally found in animal products.

Three additional vitamin B$_6$ forms are the phosphorylated forms pyridoxine 5′-phosphate (PNP), pyridoxal-5′-phosphate or codecarboxylase (PLP), and pyridoxamine 5′-phosphate (PMP). The natural, free forms of the vitamers could be converted to the key coenzymatic form, PLP, by the action of 2 enzymes, a kinase and an oxidase. Various forms of vitamin B$_6$ found in animal tissues are interconvertible, with vitamin B$_6$ metabolically active mainly as PLP and, to a lesser degree, as PMP (Figure 4.23).

Vitamin B$_6$ is stable to heat, acid, and alkali; however, exposure to light is highly destructive, especially in neutral or alkaline media. The free base and the commonly available hydrochloride salt are soluble in water and alcohol (Rosenberg, 2012)

Natural sources
Vitamin B$_6$ is widely distributed in feedstuffs. Most vitamin B$_6$ in animal products is in the form of pyridoxal and pyridoxamine phosphates, whereas in plants and seeds, the usual form is pyridoxine (McDowell, 2000a). The vitamin B$_6$ present in cereal grains (barley 3 mg/kg, corn 6 mg/kg, sorghum 3 mg/kg, oats 1 mg/kg) is concentrated mainly in the bran, with the rest of the grain containing only small amounts.

Most of the ingredients are good sources of this vitamin, but its bioavailability is relatively low (40–60%): 65% in soybean meal and 45 to 56% in corn (Chen, Huang, Liu *et al.*, 2019; Chen, Wang, Li *et al.* 2019;). The levels of vitamin B$_6$ contained in feedstuffs are also affected by processing and subsequent storage. Loss during processing, refining, and storage has been

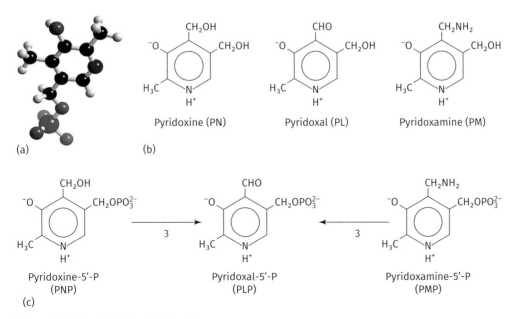

Figure 4.23 Vitamin B$_6$ chemical structure

reported to be as high as 70% (Shideler, 1983) or in the range of 0–40% (Birdsall, 1975). Of the forms, pyridoxine is far more stable than either pyridoxal or pyridoxamine. Therefore, the processing losses of vitamin B_6 tend to be highly variable (9–40%), with plant-derived foods (which mostly contain pyridoxine) losing little if any of the vitamin and animal products (mostly pyridoxal and pyridoxamine) losing large quantities (Lewis *et al.*, 2015; Yang *et al.*, 2020). The bioavailability of feedstuffs can be as low as 40–50% after heating. There was little difference in availability between corn samples not heated and those heated to 120°C. However, corn heated to 160°C contained significantly less available B_6.

Besides heat, losses may be caused by light and various agents promoting oxidation. Blanching of rehydrated lima beans resulted in a loss of 20% of the vitamin B_6, but, more significantly, the availability of the vitamin was reduced by almost 50% (Ekanayake and Nelson, 1990).

Coprophagy is a source of vitamin B_6 of microbial origin from microbial synthesis (De Passille *et al.*, 1989). However, it is not demonstrated that vitamin B_6 from posterior digestive tract sections is absorbed and used in significant quantities by monogastric animals.

Pyridoxine-5′-β-D-glucoside (PNG), a conjugated form of vitamin B_6, is abundant in various plant-derived foods (McCormick, 2006). This form of B_6 may account for up to 50% of the total vitamin B_6 content of oilseeds, such as soybeans and sunflower seeds. The utilization of dietary PNG relative to pyridoxine is 30% in rats and 50% in humans (Gregory *et al.*, 1991a). The glycosylated PNG can quantitatively alter the metabolism of pyridoxine *in vivo*. Hence, it partially impairs the metabolic utilization of co-ingested non-glycosylated forms of vitamin B_6 (Nakano and Gregory, 1995; Nakano *et al.*, 1997).

There are several vitamin B_6 antagonists, which either compete for reactive sites of apoenzymes or react with PLP to form inactive compounds. The presence of a vitamin B_6 antagonist in linseed meals is of particular interest to animal nutritionists. This substance was identified in 1967 as linatine, I-((N-γ-L-glutamyl) amino)-D-proline and was found to have antibiotic properties (Parsons and Klostermann, 1967). Pesticides (e.g., carbaryl, propoxur, or thiram) can be antagonistic to vitamin B_6. Feeding a diet enriched with vitamin B_6 prevented disturbances in the active transport of methionine in rats intoxicated with pesticides (Witkowska *et al.*, 1992; Dakshinamurti and Dakshinamurti, 2013).

Early studies conducted by Miller *et al.* (1957) indicated that the minimum requirement for growth and feed consumption was 0.5 mg/kg of solids. Still, blood hemoglobin, red blood cell, lymphocyte counts, and urinary xanthurenic acid indicated a minimum requirement between 0.75 mg and 1.0 mg of pyridoxine per kilogram of feed. Unfortunately, sow milk is a poor dietary source of vitamin B_6 (Benedikt *et al.*, 1996), with approximately 0.44 µg/ml. This is believed to cover less than half the amount required to sustain the piglet growth rate (Coburn, 1994). These authors concluded that vitamin B_6 concentration in blood and milk reflects dietary supply, whereby in lactation milk concentration is less influenced than in blood. The reduced quality and increased quantity of protein in the post-weaning feed, as opposed to dam's milk, would further increase the B_6 needs because of an increased interconversion and oxidation of amino acids. Those metabolic pathways are, in many cases, B_6-dependent (Matte *et al.*, 2005).

Commercial forms

Commercially, vitamin B_6 is available as fine crystalline powder of pyridoxine hydrochloride 99% and dilutions. Supplemental vitamin B_6 is reported to have higher bioavailability and stability than naturally occurring vitamins. Pyridoxine hydrochloride contains 82.3% vitamin B_6 activity. Dry premixes are used in feeds, and the crystalline product is used in parenteral and oral pharmaceuticals.

Metabolism

Absorption and transport

Digestion of vitamin B_6 would first involve splitting the vitamin, as it is bound to the protein portion of the feed. The 3 vitamin B_6 compounds are absorbed from the diet in dephosphorylated forms, carried to the liver by enterohepatic circulation, where they convert mainly to pyridoxal phosphate. Both niacin and vitamin B_2 participate in this conversion. The small intestine is rich in alkaline phosphatases for the dephosphorylation reaction. Sakurai *et al.* (1992) reported that a physiological dose of pyridoxamine was rapidly transformed into pyridoxal in the intestinal tissues and then released into the portal blood.

Vitamin B_6 is absorbed mainly in the jejunum and the ileum by passive diffusion. Absorption from the colon is insignificant, even though colon microflora synthesizes the vitamin. However, Durst *et al.* (1989) administered vitamin B_6 in the cecum of sows and concluded that the vitamin was absorbed in this location.

After absorption, B_6 compounds quickly appear in the liver, where they are mostly converted into PLP, considered the most active vitamin form in metabolism. Under normal conditions, most of the vitamin B_6 in the blood is present as PLP, which is linked to proteins, largely albumin in the plasma and hemoglobin in the red blood cells (McCormick, 2006). Both niacin (as NADPH-dependent enzyme) and riboflavin (as the flavoprotein pyridoxamine phosphate oxidase) are essential for the conversion of vitamin B_6 forms and phosphorylation reactions (Kodentsova *et al.*, 1993).

Although other tissues also contribute to vitamin B_6 metabolism, the liver is responsible for forming the PLP found in plasma. Pyridoxal and PLP found in circulation are associated primarily with plasma albumin and red blood cell hemoglobin (Mehansho and Henderson, 1980). Pyridoxal phosphate accounts for 60% of plasma vitamin B_6. Researchers disagree on whether pyridoxal or PLP is the transport form of B_6 (Coburn *et al.*, 1992).

Storage and excretion

Vitamin B_6 is widely distributed in various tissues, mainly as PLP or pyridoxamine phosphate, with the majority stored principally in muscular tissue. Only small quantities of vitamin B_6 are stored in the body. Russell *et al.* (1985) investigated B_6 metabolism in swine muscle: they indicated that under the conditions of their study, muscle tissue acts as an immobile reservoir of PLP, and 60–95% of muscle PLP was bound to muscle glycogen phosphorylase. Excess dietary vitamin B_6 increased whole-muscle total PLP.

Pyridoxic acid is the major excretory metabolite of the vitamin, eliminated via urine. Also, small quantities of pyridoxol, pyridoxal, pyridoxamine, and phosphorylated derivatives are excreted in urine (Henderson, 1984). However, Roth-Maier and Kirchgessner (1997) reported that 60–70% of vitamin B_6 was excreted via feces in a study evaluating its metabolism in sows fed suboptimal vitamin B_6 supply. Vitamin B_6 concentration in feces amounted to 10–12 µg/g dry matter.

Vitamin B_6 metabolism is altered in renal failure, as observed in rats exhibiting plasma pyridoxal phosphate 43% lower than controls (Wei and Young, 1994). On fecal excretion, Roth-Maier and Kirchgessner (1993b, 1997) concluded that vitamin B_6 was enlarged linearly by increasing fibrous supplementation to sows. Bacterially fermentable substrates from wheat bran induced a higher bacterial vitamin B_6 synthesis than cellulose.

Biochemical functions

Vitamin B_6, primarily as PLP, and, to a lesser extent, as PMP, plays an essential role in the amino acid, carbohydrate, and fatty acid metabolism and the energy-producing citric acid cycle, with over 60 enzymes known to depend on vitamin B_6 coenzymes. Pyridoxal phosphate functions in practically all reactions involved in amino acid metabolism, including transamination, decarboxylation, deamination, desulfhydration, and the cleavage or synthesis of amino acids. The largest group of vitamin B_6-dependent enzymes are transaminases. Aminotransferase is involved in the interconversion of a pair of amino acids into their corresponding keto acids, e.g., amino groups transferred from aspartate to α-ketoglutarate forming oxaloacetate and glutamate (McCormick, 2006; Dakshinamurti and Dakshinamurti, 2013).

The minimum requirements of vitamin B_6 have been proposed for rations with moderate protein levels and a balanced amino acid relationship (Russell *et al.*, 1985; Witkowska *et al.*, 1992; Matte *et al.*, 1997b, 2001, 2005). The recommended levels of vitamin B_6 supply increase with feeds with high protein levels or an amino acid profile distant from the ideal protein since more enzymes are needed to metabolize the excess amino acids, which depend on vitamin B_6.

Non-oxidative decarboxylations involve PLP as a coenzyme, e.g., converting amino acids into biogenic amines such as histamine, serotonin, γ-amino butyric acid (GABA), and taurine. Vitamin B_6 participates in functions that include (Marks, 1975; Driskell, 1984; McCormick, 2006; Dakshinamurti and Dakshinamurti, 2013):

1. deaminases: for serine, threonine, and cystathionine
2. desulfydrases and transulfurases: interconversion
3. synthesis of niacin from tryptophan: hydroxykynurenine is not converted to hydroxyanthranilic acid but rather to xanthurenic acid due to a lack of the B_6-dependent enzyme, kynureninase (Miller *et al.*, 1957; Harmon *et al.*, 1969)
4. formation of α-aminolevulinic acid from succinyl-CoA and glycine, the first step in porphyrin synthesis
5. conversion of linoleic to arachidonic acid in the metabolism of essential fatty acids (this function is controversial)
6. glycogen phosphorylase catalyzes glycogen breakdown to glucose-1-phosphate. Pyridoxal phosphate does not appear to be a coenzyme for the enzyme but rather affects the enzyme conformation
7. synthesis of epinephrine and norepinephrine from either phenylalanine or tyrosine–both norepinephrine and epinephrine are involved in carbohydrate metabolism and other body reactions
8. racemases – PLP-dependent racemases enable certain microorganisms to utilize D-amino acids. Racemases have not yet been detected in mammalian tissues
9. transmethylation involving methionine
10. incorporation of iron in hemoglobin synthesis
11. formation of antibodies–B_6 deficiency inhibits the synthesis of globulins that carry antibodies (Miller *et al.*, 1957)
12. inflammation-higher vitamin B_6 levels were linked to protection against inflammation (Morris *et al.*, 2010)
13. Decarboxylation of tryptophan to serotonin (McDowell, 2000a).

Matte *et al.* (1997a) investigated the relationship of B_6 in tryptophan metabolism in weanling piglets: they could not detect an effect on the oxidation of the tryptophan pathway but suggested that B_6 may stimulate another pathway in tryptophan metabolism. Matte *et al.* (1997b) investigated the importance of pyridoxine and tryptophan on glucose tolerance and insulin response to glucose in weanling piglets receiving a liquid diet through surgically inserted gastric tubes and detected an interaction between parenteral pyridoxine and duodenal infusion on changes in plasma insulin concentration. The most remarkable response was observed in the piglets that received 3 ml of pyridoxine HCl (5 g/l) intramuscularly and then an infusion of glucose. The insulin response was increased by approximately 55% in this group. They concluded that tryptophan and pyridoxine probably have different action modes on insulin sensitivity and release. These researchers suggested that the effect of vitamin B_6 on insulin response to a glucose load was perhaps linked to its role in the decarboxylation of tryptophan to serotonin. However, Matte *et al.* (1997b) indicated that results from his research have been inconsistent concerning the effect of pyridoxine supplementation on insulin metabolism and that further studies will be required.

Neurological functions

Pyridoxine is a coenzyme of several enzymes involved in the endogenous production of hydrogen sulfide, dopamine, norepinephrine, serotonin (5-HT), and GABA, as well as taurine, sphingolipids, and polyamines, which are molecules involved in cell signaling in the CNS (Dakshinamurti and Dakshinamurti, 2013).

Neurological disorders, including states of agitation and convulsions, result from reduced B_6 enzymes in the brain, including glutamate decarboxylase and γ-aminobutyric acid transaminase. Dopamine release is delayed with a vitamin B_6 deficiency, contributing to motor abnormalities (Tang and Wei, 2004). Maternal restriction of B_6 in rats adversely affected synaptogenesis, neurogenesis, neuron longevity, and progeny differentiation (Groziak and Kirksey, 1987, 1990).

Effects on immunity and as an antioxidant

Animal and human studies suggest that a vitamin B_6 deficiency affects both humoral and cell-mediated immune responses. In humans, vitamin B_6 depletion significantly decreased the percentage and the total number of lymphocytes, mitogenic responses of peripheral blood lymphocytes to T- and B-cell mitogens and interleukin 2 production (Miller *et al.*, 1957; Meydani *et al.*, 1991).

The role of PLP in affecting one-carbon metabolism is important in nucleic acid biosynthesis and immune system function. The PLP is also needed for gluconeogenesis by way of transaminases active on glucogenic amino acids and for lipid metabolism that involves several aspects of PLP function: for example, the production of carnitine needed to act as a vector for long-chain fatty acids for mitochondrial β-oxidation and of certain bases for phospholipid biosynthesis (McCormick, 2006).

Vitamin B_6 has antioxidant properties by inhibiting superoxide radicals, preventing lipid peroxidation, protein glycosylation, and Na^+, K^+-ATPase activity in high glucose–treated erythrocytes and hydrogen peroxide–treated monocytes and endothelial cells (Dakshinamurti and Dakshinamurti, 2013).

Metabolism of homocysteine and cardiovascular function

Vitamin B_6 has a central role in the metabolism of amino acids, which includes essential interactions with endogenous redox reactions through its effects on the glutathione peroxidase (GPX) system. In fact, B_6-dependent enzymes catalyze most reactions of the transsulfuration pathway, driving homocysteine to cysteine and further into GPX proteins. Homocysteine is a sulfur-containing amino acid formed during the metabolism of methionine. Pyridoxine is required as a coenzyme for the 2 key steps of the transsulfuration pathway catalyzed by

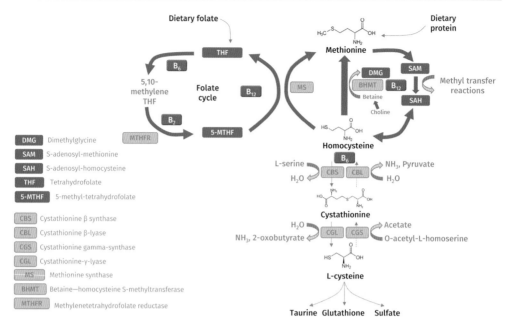

Figure 4.24 Pyridoxine, riboflavin, cyanocobalamin, choline and folate are involved in folate cycle, trans methylation and transsulfuration pathways

cystathionine synthetase and cystathionine γ-lyase. In this metabolic pathway, several B vitamins are involved (Figure 4.24).

Since mammals metabolize sulfur- and seleno-amino acids similarly, this vitamin plays a vital role in the fate of sulfur-homocysteine and its seleno counterpart between transsulfuration and one-carbon metabolism, especially under oxidative stress conditions. This is particularly important in reproduction because ovarian metabolism may produce excess ROS during the peri-estrus period, impairing ovulatory functions and early embryo development. Later in gestation, placentation raises embryo oxygen tension and may induce a higher expression of ROS markers and, eventually, embryo losses (Dalto and Matte, 2017).

Pyridoxine deficiency may increase blood pressure by stimulating smooth muscle in the blood vessels, creating endothelial dysfunction, generating ROS, and increasing susceptibility to oxidation. Homocysteine also enhances collagen synthesis, altering the elastin/collagen ratio, which contributes to the changes in the vessel wall that lead to systemic vascular resistance and hypertension (Dakshinamurti and Dakshinamurti, 2013).

As part of its role in amino acid metabolism, vitamin B_6 converts tryptophan to niacin, which again suggests the close relationship between different B complex vitamins and an association in the requirements of some of them (Kirchgessner and Kösters, 1977). Vitamin B_6 is also involved in the formation of adrenaline and noradrenaline from phenylalanine and tyrosine, in the transmethylation sulfuration of methionine, and in the incorporation of iron into the heme group of hemoglobin and myoglobin. On the other hand, there is evidence to suggest the role of vitamin B_6 in the conversion of linoleic acid to arachidonic acid and forming antibodies.

Nutritional assessment

The 6 interconvertible forms of vitamin B_6 can be measured in plasma to assess nutritional status. Nonetheless, PLP is the vitamer normally used, and its measurement in erythrocytes seems to provide a more appropriate evaluation (Sauberlich, 1999).

However, considering the complex metabolic pathways in which vitamin B_6 is involved, ratios between metabolites, or the possibility of quantifying numerous amino acids and metabolites related to PLP-dependent pathways, may provide a better insight into nutritional status (Höller *et al.*, 2018). Parameters to evaluate vitamin B_6 metabolism include fecal and urinary vitamin B_6 concentration and excretion, vitamin B_6 concentration in blood, hematological criteria, the activity of aspartate aminotransferase in erythrocytes (EAST), and xanthurenic acid excretion in the tryptophan load test (Roth-Maier and Kirchgessner, 1997).

Deficiency signs

Vitamin B_6 deficiency gives rise to several unspecific signs, including appetite loss, growth retardation, dermatitis, hair loss, epileptic-like convulsions, and anemia (Kirchgessner and Kösters, 1977; Rosenberg, 2012). Given its leading role in amino acid metabolism, deficiency in this vitamin is associated with a decreased capacity to utilize protein, with a marked drop in the nitrogen balance. In practice, problems of vitamin B_6 deficiency are uncommon due to its abundance in most ingredients used in swine nutrition.

Clinical signs of a vitamin B_6 deficiency in young growing animals appear within 2 to 3 weeks following the removal of the vitamin from the diet. An indication of a vitamin B_6 deficiency is elevated urinary levels of xanthurenic acid and kynurenic acid, indicating incomplete conversion of tryptophan (Dove and Cook, 2000). This evaluation is called the tryptophan-loading test. Vitamin B_6 facilitates the incorporation of iron into hemoglobin and the synthesis of immunoglobulins so that its deficiency will cause blood alterations. In order to evaluate status, Driskell (1984) concluded that the best assessment parameter for vitamin B_6 status in clinical cases is the measurement of either the coenzyme stimulation or erythrocyte alanine aminotransferase activity or PLP level. Marginal deficiencies provoke microcytic, normochromic polycythemia, and deficient pigs show a decreased IgM and IgG response to antibody challenge (Cartwright *et al.*, 1944; Dove and Cook, 2000). An extreme deficiency leads to microcytic, polychromatic, and hypochromic anemia (Cartwright *et al.*, 1948; Coburn, 1994).

In growing pigs, clinical signs of vitamin B_6 deficiency include a poor appetite, slow growth (Figure 4.25a), microcytic hypochromic anemia, epileptic-like fits or convulsions (Figure 4.25b), fatty infiltration of the liver, diarrhea, rough hair coat, scaly skin, a brown exudate around the eyes, demyelination of peripheral nerves and subcutaneous edema (Sewell *et al.*, 1964; Bauernfeind, 1974; Bräunlich, 1974; Cunha, 1977). Hughes and Squibb (1942) reported many of these deficiency symptoms and an unsteady gait in pyridoxine-deficient pigs. Almost identical symptoms of B_6 deficiency were reported in baby pigs (Lehrer *et al.*, 1951; Sewell *et al.*, 1964).

Follis and Wintrobe (1945) explicitly reported on the effects of pyridoxine deficiency on the tissues of the nervous system. Myelin degeneration of the peripheral portion of the sensory nerve was observed to be the initial neural change in pyridoxine-deficient animals. Based on morphologic data, the preliminary site of injury in pyridoxine-deficient animals is in the myelin sheath and axon. Like some other vitamins, vitamin B_6 deficiency reduces the immune responses of the pig (Harmon *et al.*, 1963). The first and most conspicuous sign in baby pigs is a loss of appetite. This may appear in less than 2 weeks if the deficiency is severe and may be accompanied by reduced growth, vomiting, diarrhea, and a peculiar compulsion to lick.

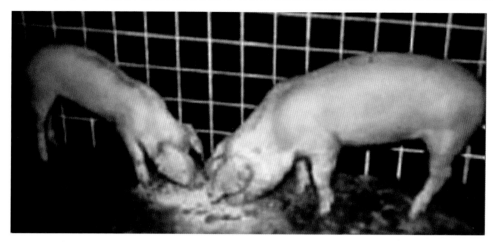

Figure 4.25(a) Vitamin B$_6$ deficiency in growing pigs: the pig on the left is vitamin B$_6$ deficient, the pig on the right received a vitamin B$_6$-fortified diet

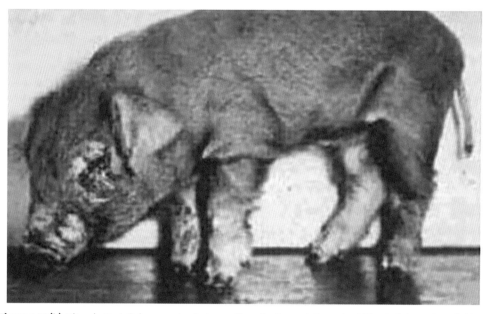

Figure 4.25(b) Vitamin B$_6$ deficiency: retarded growth and seizure. A 6-week-old B$_6$-deficient pig weighing only 3.6 kg (source: courtesy of E.H. Hughes and H. Heltman, California Agriculture Experimentation Station)

Kirchgessner and Kösters (1977) concluded that vitamin B$_6$ deficient piglets had 14.4% lower nitrogen retention than pair-fed controls fed diets with adequate pyridoxine after 5 weeks. Consequently, these deficient piglets also had lower metabolizable energy available.

When deficiency of vitamin B$_6$ reaches an advanced stage (probably due to degeneration of the peripheral nerves), disordered movement and ataxia appear. Finally, convulsions develop at irregular intervals but are apparently stimulated by excitement, as they are most often observed at feeding time. Between these convulsions, pigs lie down and are apathetic and unresponsive (Bräunlich, 1974). Bräunlich (1974) suggested that a vitamin B_6 deficiency may go unnoticed in swine because of a lack of visible signs explicitly associated with the deficiency.

In some experiments with vitamin B_6, protein retention by pigs deficient in the vitamin was reduced to less than half of that shown in animals receiving sufficient amounts of the vitamin. During reproduction and lactation, sows fed a corn-sorghum-soybean meal diet responded to a vitamin B_6 supplementation of 4.4 mg/kg feed (Adams et al., 1967). Vitamin B_6 supplementation of 11 mg/kg feed, produced a slightly superior daily weight gain, more piglets born alive, and a smaller number of resorbed fetuses compared with control sows that received only 1 mg/kg of vitamin B_6 (Ritchie et al., 1960). Knights et al. (1998) observed a tendency for reduced weaning-to-estrus intervals and increased nitrogen retention in Yorkshire and Hampshire sows. These researchers also observed an increased litter size in Yorkshire sows, the next feeding of 16 ppm pyridoxine daily to sows from weaning through the subsequent gestation. In rats, Roth-Maier et al. (1996) concluded that adequate levels of B_6 during lactation did not compensate for lack of B_6 during pregnancy and vice versa, as a high dose of B_6 during gestation was unable to alleviate all effects of a suboptimal supply of B_6 during lactation. These conclusions were based on data assessing rat liver B_6 status. Guilarte (1993) suggested that vitamin B_6 deficiency during gestation and lactation alters the function of N-methyl-D-aspartate receptors, a subtype of receptors of the glutamatergic neurotransmitter system thought to play an essential role in learning and memory.

There are vitamin B_6 antagonists that either compete for reactive sites of apoenzymes or react with PLP to form inactive compounds. The presence of a vitamin B_6 antagonist in linseed is of particular interest to animal nutritionists. In 1967 this substance was identified as hydrazic acid and was found to have antibiotic properties (Parsons and Klostermann, 1967).

Safety

Insufficient data are available to support estimates of the maximum dietary tolerable levels of vitamin B_6 for swine. It is suggested, primarily from dog and rat data, that nutritional levels at least 50 times the dietary requirements are safe for most species (NRC, 1987).

Signs of toxicity, which occur most obviously in the PNS, include changes in gait and peripheral sensation (Krinke and Fitzgerald, 1988; Xu et al., 1989), ataxia, muscle weakness, and incoordination at levels approaching 1,000 times the requirement (Dakshinamurti and Dakshinamurti, 2013).

Vitamin B_{12} (cyanocobalamin)
Chemical structure and properties
Nutritionists now consider vitamin B_{12} as the generic name for a group of compounds having vitamin B_{12} activity in which the cobalt atom is in the center of the corrin nucleus (cobalt-containing corrinoids), which contains 4 rings. When there is a cyanide group bound to cobalt, it is referred to as cyanocobalamin, which is the reference product. Cyanocobalamin has a molecular weight of 1,355 and is the most complex structure and heaviest compound of all vitamins (Figure 4.26). The empirical formula of vitamin B_{12} is $C_{63}H_{88}O_{14}N_{14}PCo$, and its unusual feature is the content of 4.5% cobalt. Vitamin B_{12} requirements and concentrations are expressed in mass units (usually µg per kg).

Vitamin B_{12} is a dark-red crystalline hygroscopic substance, freely soluble in water and alcohol but insoluble in acetone, chloroform, and ether. Oxidizing and reducing agents and exposure to sunlight tend to destroy its activity. Losses of vitamin B_{12} during feed processing are usually not excessive because vitamin B_{12} is stable at temperatures as high as 250°C,

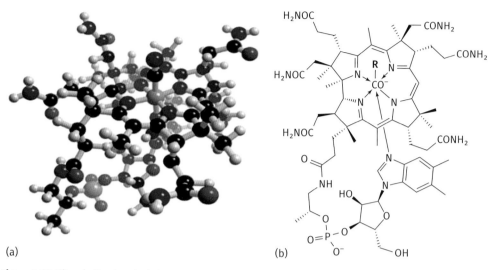

(a) (b)

Figure 4.26 Vitamin B$_{12}$ chemical structure

being the most stable vitamin during feed pelleting and storage processes (Lewis *et al.*, 2015; Yang *et al.*, 2020).

Adenosylcobalamin and methylcobalamin are naturally occurring forms of vitamin B$_{12}$ in feedstuffs and animal tissues. Cyanocobalamin is not a naturally occurring form of the vitamin but is the most widely used form of cobalamin in clinical practice because of its relative availability and stability (Green and Miller, 2013).

Natural sources

Feedstuffs of animal origin – meat, liver, kidney, milk, eggs, fish – or microorganisms, are reasonably good sources of vitamin B$_{12}$. The kidney and liver are excellent sources; these organs are richer in vitamin B$_{12}$ from ruminants than monogastrics. Vitamin B$_{12}$ presence in the tissues of animals is due to the ingestion of vitamin B$_{12}$ in animal feeds or from intestinal synthesis. The richest sources are fermentation residues, activated sewage sludge, and manure.

The concentration in fishmeal can reach more than 500 µg/kg, in meat meal is around 100 µg/kg, while in bloodmeal it exceeds 400 µg/kg. In the by-products of the dairy industry, it is much lower: for example, in whey, it rarely exceeds 10 µg/kg. It is important to point out the high variability in the concentration of this vitamin in the feedstuffs indicated.

Plant products are practically devoid of B$_{12}$. The vitamin B$_{12}$ reported in higher plants in small amounts may result from synthesis by soil microorganisms and excretion of the vitamin onto the soil, with subsequent absorption by the plant. The root nodules of certain legumes contain small quantities of vitamin B$_{12}$. Certain seaweed species (algae) have been reported to contain appreciable amounts of vitamin B$_{12}$ (up to 1 µg/g). Seaweed does not synthesize vitamin B$_{12}$: it is synthesized by the bacteria associated with seaweed and then concentrated by the seaweed (Bito and Watanabe, 2022). Dagnelie *et al.* (1991) reported that vitamin B$_{12}$ from algae is largely unavailable.

Bedding can be a source of vitamin B$_{12}$ for pigs housed on solid floors, although there are no data relating to its absorption level (Bilodeau *et al.*, 1989). Microorganisms synthesize vitamin B$_{12}$ in the intestinal tract (Firth *et al.*, 1953). However, cobalamin produced in the colon is represented by different corrinoids with lesser activity or not easily bioavailable because the receptors necessary for absorbing the vitamin are found primarily in the small intestine, upstream of the site of corrinoid production (Seetharam and Alpers, 1982; Bilodeau *et al.*, 1989). This cobalamin can be made available to the host via coprophagy (De Passille *et al.*, 1989).

Commercial forms
Commercial sources of vitamin B_{12} are produced from fermentation, available as cyanocobalamin, the most stable form of this vitamin. Little is known about the bioavailability of orally ingested B_{12} in feeds.

Metabolism
Absorption and transport
The dietary vitamin B_{12} binds to salivary protein. As the salivary protein is digested, the B_{12} is freed and bound to an unknown intrinsic factor secreted by the gastric parietal cells. The digestion of this vitamin first requires the release of the vitamin, which is frequently found in a protein matrix, by the action of digestive proteases, mainly trypsin. The absorptive site for vitamin B_{12} is the ileum, the lower portion of the small intestine. Substantial amounts of B_{12} are secreted into the duodenum and then reabsorbed in the ileum. Passage of vitamin B_{12} through the intestinal wall is a complex procedure and requires the intervention of particular carrier compounds able to bind the vitamin molecule (McDowell, 2000a). In most species, for the absorption of vitamin B_{12}, the following is required (Green and Miller, 2013):

1   adequate quantities of dietary vitamin B_{12}
2   production of the intrinsic factor for absorption of vitamin B_{12} through the ileum
3   normal stomach function for the breakdown of food proteins for the release of vitamin B_{12}
4   functional pancreas (trypsin secretion) required for the release of bound vitamin B_{12} before combining the vitamin with the intrinsic factor
5   functional ileum with receptor and absorption sites.

Gastric juice defects are responsible for most cases of food-vitamin B_{12} malabsorption in monogastrics (Carmel, 1994). Factors that diminish vitamin B_{12} absorption include protein, iron, and vitamin B_6 deficiencies, thyroid removal, and dietary tannic acid (Hoffmann-La Roche, 1984).

The absorption of vitamin B_{12} is limited by the number of intrinsic factor-vitamin B_{12} binding sites in the ileal mucosa so that not more than about 1 to 1.5 µg of a single oral dose of the vitamin in humans can be absorbed (Bender, 1992). The absorption is also slow: peak blood concentrations of the vitamin are not achieved for some 6 to 8 hours after an oral dose.

Intrinsic factors have been demonstrated in humans, monkeys, pigs, rats, cows, ferrets, rabbits, hamsters, foxes, lions, tigers, and leopards. It has not yet been detected in guinea pigs, horses, sheep, chickens, and other species. There are structural differences in the vitamin B_{12} intrinsic factors among species. Therefore, intrinsic factor concentrates prepared from the stomach of one animal species do not always increase B_{12} absorption in other animal species or humans. In pigs, Henderickx *et al.* (1964) demonstrated that 41.6–58% of the vitamin B_{12} labeled with cobalt 57 was absorbed in the colon of pigs and, consequently, vitamin B_{12} absorption could be not exclusive to the small intestine. Similarly, there are species differences in vitamin B$_{12}$ transport proteins (Polak *et al.*, 1979; Green and Miller, 2013). Vitamin B$_{12}$ is bound to transcobalamin (TC) and haptocorrin (HC) for transport in the blood, with about 20% being attached to TC and the rest to HC. The TC-bound cobalamin is the form most actively transported into tissues.

Storage and excretion

The storage of vitamin B$_{12}$ is found principally in the liver, and other storage sites include the kidney, heart, spleen, and brain (Green and Miller, 2013). Even though vitamin B$_{12}$ is water-soluble, Kominato (1971) reported a tissue half-life of 32 days, indicating considerable tissue storage.

The main excretion routes for absorbed vitamin B$_{12}$ are urinary, biliary, and fecal. Urinary excretion of the intact vitamin B$_{12}$ by kidney glomerular filtration is minimal. Biliary excretion via feces is the major excretory route. Most cobalamin excreted in bile is reabsorbed; at least 65–75% is reabsorbed in the ileum utilizing the intrinsic factor mechanism.

Biochemical functions

Although the most essential tasks of vitamin B$_{12}$ concern the metabolism of nucleic acids and proteins, it also functions in the metabolism of fats and carbohydrates. Overall, protein synthesis is impaired in vitamin B$_{12}$-deficient animals (Anderson and Hogan, 1950; Colby and Ensminger, 1950; Friesecke, 1980). Moreover, the promotion of red blood cell synthesis and the maintenance of nervous system integrity are functions attributed to vitamin B$_{12}$ (McDowell, 2000a; Green and Miller, 2013). Vitamin B$_{12}$ is metabolically related to other essential nutrients, such as choline, methionine, and folic acid. (Savage and Lindenbaum, 1995; Stabler, 2006).

A summary of vitamin B$_{12}$ functions includes (Figure 4.27):

- purine and pyrimidine synthesis
- transfer of methyl groups
- formation of proteins from amino acids
- carbohydrate and fat metabolism.

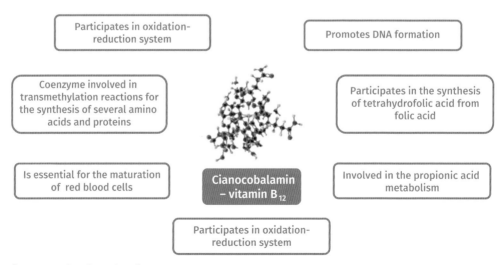

Figure 4.27 Vitamin B$_{12}$ functions

Vitamin B_{12} is an essential cofactor in the following functions:

- the maintenance of normal DNA synthesis: failure of this metabolic pathway can lead to megaloblastic anemia
- the regeneration of methionine for the dual purposes of maintaining protein synthesis and methylation capacity
- the avoidance of homocysteine accumulation, an amino acid metabolite implicated in vascular damage, thrombosis, and several associated degenerative diseases, including coronary artery disease, stroke, and osteoporosis (Green and Miller, 2013).

Erythrocyte synthesis and maintenance of the integrity of the nervous system stand out among the many functions that are affected by and regulate this vitamin since it is in these functions that deficiency symptoms first present themselves.

Gluconeogenesis and hemopoiesis are critically affected by cobalt deficiency, and carbohydrate, lipid, and nucleic acid metabolism depend on adequate B_{12} and folic acid metabolism. Cyanocobalamin is involved in the metabolism of fatty acids, the synthesis of proteins, and reactions involving the transfer of methyl and hydrogenated/hydrogen groups (Green and Miller, 2013). Vitamin B_{12} is a cofactor of 2 crucial metabolic reactions in the cells, one mitochondrial involving adenosylcobalamine and the other cytoplasmic, mostly related to methylcobalamine.

In the mitochondrial reaction, B_{12} in the form of 5'-deoxy-adenosylcobalamin is required for the enzyme methylmalonyl CoA mutase, a vitamin B_{12}-requiring enzyme (5'-deoxyadenosylcobalamin) that catalyzes the conversion of methylmalonyl-CoA to succinyl-CoA (Green and Miller, 2013). This is an intermediate step in transforming propionate to succinate during the oxidation of odd-chain fatty acids and the catabolism of ketogenic amino acids. In animal metabolism, propionate of dietary or metabolic origin is converted into succinate, entering the TCA (Krebs) cycle.

In the cytoplasmic reaction, B_{12} in the form of methylcobalamin is required in the folate-dependent methylation of the sulfur amino acid homocysteine to form methionine catalyzed by the enzyme methionine synthase. Apart from being necessary for adequate protein synthesis, methionine is also a key precursor for maintaining methylation capacity through synthesizing the universal methyl donor S-adenosylmethionine. Additionally, the methionine synthase reaction is finally necessary for normal DNA synthesis. The methyl group transferred to homocysteine during methionine synthesis is donated by the folate derivative methyltetrahydrofolate (methyl-THF), forming THF. THF is later transformed to 5,20-methylenetetrahydrofolate (methylene-THF) by a one-carbon transfer during serine conversion to glycine. Methylene-THF can be reduced again to form methyl-THF. Still, it also serves as the critical one-carbon source for the *de novo* synthesis of thymidylate from deoxyuridylate, which is required for DNA replication.

Various studies have also demonstrated the importance of vitamin B_{12} in reproduction (McDowell, 2000a). Its role as a limiting factor for the effect of folic acid in the prevention of malformations (Guay *et al.*, 2002) and the differences between gilts and sows with several litters, since sows with their first litters have lower levels of vitamin B_{12} in their tissues than other breeder sows (Matte *et al.*, 2006).

Deficiency of vitamin B_{12} induces a folic acid deficiency by blocking the utilization of folic acid derivatives as previously described. It has been suggested that vitamin B_{12} status may affect the systemic metabolism of folic acid during early pregnancy (Guay *et al.*, 2002).

Wagle *et al.* (1958) demonstrated that rats and baby pigs deprived of vitamin B$_{12}$ were less able to incorporate serine, methionine, phenylalanine, and glucose into liver proteins. There is good reason to believe that impairment of protein synthesis is the principal reason for the growth depression frequently observed in animals deficient in vitamin B$_{12}$ (Nesheim *et al.*, 1950; Friesecke, 1980).

Finally, an additional function of vitamin B$_{12}$ relates to immune function. In mice, vitamin B$_{12}$ deficiency affected Ig production and cytokine levels (Funada *et al.*, 2001).

Nutritional assessment

Historically, vitamin B$_{12}$ was measured using microbiological assays such as the *Lactobacillus delbrueckii* method, which was later adapted for high-throughput use (Sauberlich, 1999). Measuring the total vitamin B$_{12}$ concentration in serum is the first-line clinical test for determining vitamin B$_{12}$ deficiency. The current assays are primarily based on the competitive binding of the serum vitamin to intrinsic factor, followed by radiometric or fluorescence-based detection (Höller *et al.*, 2018).

TC-bound cobalamin, the form most actively transported into tissues, can be measured and considered a relevant marker of vitamin B$_{12}$ status. A newer method estimates holotranscobalamin (holoTC) as a fraction of vitamin B$_{12}$ carried by TC in serum and, therefore, available for tissue uptake (Höller *et al.*, 2018).

Deficiency signs

Problems of vitamin B$_{12}$ deficiency are much more frequent in young animals than in adults, whose intestinal flora can synthesize a part of the requirements. Nevertheless, the need for cobalt, which enables microorganisms to synthesize this vitamin, must be emphasized, as well as the possible effect of the design of the farm and the possibility of the pig having contact with feces (Anderson and Hogan, 1950; Neumann *et al.*, 1950b; Colby and Ensminger, 1950; Richardson *et al.*, 1951; Bauriedel *et al.*, 1954).

Vitamin B$_{12}$ deficiency has profound pathophysiological effects on the blood, nervous system, and possibly other organs. The most noticeable effect of vitamin B$_{12}$ deficiency is megaloblastic anemia, caused by the disruption of DNA synthesis. Vitamin B$_{12}$ deficiency reduces body weight gain, feed intake, and feed conversion in growing pigs (Nesheim *et al.*, 1950; Neumann *et al.*, 1950b; Catron *et al.*, 1952; Bauriedel *et al.*, 1954).

The most frequent signs include dermatitis, poor hair condition, anemia, and high mortality. Growth retardation is attributed essentially to difficulty in protein synthesis and not to a problem related to energy metabolism, as occurs with other B complex vitamins (Figure 4.28). Nervous signs are also frequently apparent, characterized by uncoordinated movement, mainly affecting the hind legs. Nervous disorders in the pig include increased excitability, unsteady gait, and posterior incoordination.

The most common cause of clinically evident B$_{12}$ deficiency is malabsorption due to gastric issues affecting intrinsic factors. These issues include pernicious anemia, an autoimmune loss of intrinsic factor responsible for the uptake of cobalamin that is fatal if untreated, or ileal mucosa issues. However, inadequate dietary intake cause or contributes to B$_{12}$ deficiency. Antibiotics can control gut health issues and improve vitamin B$_{12}$ absorption in pigs (Sewell *et al.*, 1952). Microcytic to normocytic anemia with high neutrophils with concomitantly low lymphocyte counts is typical, and many researchers, including Neumann *et al.* (1950a), have reported high neutrophil and low lymphocyte counts. However, observations on anemia are not unanimous and are sometimes contradictory. Even observations within one study show a wide variety of effects concerning hematologic manifestations of vitamin B$_{12}$ deficiency, as

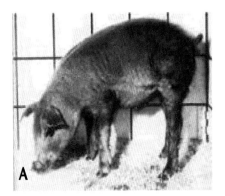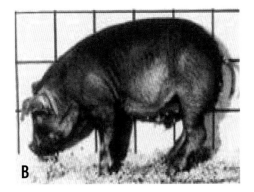

Figure 4.28 Vitamin B$_{12}$, growth retardation. (A) Pig deficient in vitamin B$_{12}$, rough hair coat, and dermatitis compared with the control pig. (B) Control pig, which had received adequate levels of vitamin B$_{12}$ (source: Catran D.V., Iowa State University)

sometimes anemia does not develop at all, and at other times moderately severe anemia occurs (Cartwright *et al.*, 1951; Catron *et al.*, 1952; Bauriedel *et al.*, 1954).

A deficiency of vitamin B$_{12}$ will induce folic acid deficiency by blocking the utilization of folic acid derivatives. The reduction of methylene-THF to methyl-THF is an irreversible reaction under physiological conditions. Consequently, when B$_{12}$ is deficient, and THF synthesis is impaired through interdiction of the methionine synthase reaction, methyl-THF has no metabolic outlet, forward to THF or backward to methylene-THF, and it becomes trapped (Green and Miller, 2013). This explains why the hematological damage of vitamin B$_{12}$ deficiency is indistinguishable from that of folacin deficiency, resulting in an inadequate quantity of methylene-THF to participate adequately in DNA synthesis. The thymus and spleen become atrophied, while the liver and tongue may be enlarged due to the proliferation of granulomatous tissue. Vitamin B$_{12}$ deficiency can be generated with the addition of high dietary levels of propionic acid.

In the breeder pigs, vitamin B$_{12}$ deficiency can cause reduced litter size and pig survival. Abortions, small litter, low birth weights, deformities, and inability to rear young occur in breeding sows (Teague and Grifo, 1966). Late estrus produces fewer *corpora lutea* and fewer embryos in vitamin B$_{12}$-deficient animals. During reproduction and lactation, vitamin B$_{12}$ supplementation has been shown to increase birth weights and the survival of young pigs. Heavier piglets at farrowing generally indicate better postnatal growth performance and carcass quality (Rehfeldt and Kuhn, 2006; Rehfeldt *et al.*, 2008). Frederick and Brisson (1961) found that sows deficient in vitamin B$_{12}$ had fewer pigs and had lower viability than those born from sows supplemented with vitamin B$_{12}$. Successive litters from deficient sows become progressively weaker. In a study of sows supplemented with vitamin B$_{12}$ at 80 to 100 μg daily during pregnancy, there were improved piglet and litter weights and a decreased percentage of stillbirths (Reinisch and Gebhardt, 1987). Under some conditions, the reproductive performance of sows has been improved by the inclusion of higher than recommended levels of dietary vitamin B$_{12}$ (Cunha, 1977). The response is evidenced by an increase in litter size and the birth weight of pigs.

Safety

Adding vitamin B$_{12}$ to feeds in amounts far above requirement or absorbability appears to be without hazard. Dietary levels of at least several hundred times the requirement are considered safe for most species (NRC, 1987). Vitamin B_{12} is reported to be toxic with around 5 mg/kg diet. No data are available about vitamin B_{12} safety in swine.

Niacin (vitamin B_3)
Chemical structure and properties
The 2 forms of niacin or vitamin B_3, nicotinic acid (pyridine-3-carboxylic acid) and nicotinamide (or niacinamide; pyridine-3-carboxylic acid amide), are functional parts of the coenzymes nicotinamide adenine dinucleotide (NAD) and NADPH, involved in the cellular respiration processes (Kirkland, 2013). As conversion takes place quickly and very efficiently, it is considered that both forms possess the same vitamin activity. Frequently, the term niacin is used for both the free acid form and the amide form.

The empirical formula is $C_6H_3O_2N$ (Figure 4.29). Both nicotinic acid and nicotinamide are white, odorless, crystalline solids soluble in water (nicotinic acid only sparingly, approx. 1.5 g/100 ml) and alcohol. They are resistant to heat, air, light, alkali, and oxidation and thus are stable in feeds. Niacin is also stable in the presence of the usual oxidizing agents: however, it will undergo decarboxylation at a high temperature in an alkaline medium.

An additional source of supplemental niacin would be the vitamin K supplement menadione nicotinamide bisulfite (MNB), with a content ≥31 % nicotinamide. Results with chicks suggest MNB is fully effective as a source of vitamin K and niacin activity (Oduho and Baker, 1993).

Natural sources
Niacin is widely distributed in feedstuffs of both plant and animal origin. Good sources are animal and fish by-products (50–150 mg/kg), distiller grains, yeast, peanut meal (150–200 mg/kg), various distillation and fermentation solubles, cereals, and certain oilseed meals. Sunflower meal (>200 mg/kg) and soy meal (20–60 mg/kg) content are good to moderate, although around 40% of the niacin in oilseeds is in a combined form that pigs cannot utilize. Cereals and their derivatives show an appreciable niacin content (for example, wheat or corn, around 60 mg/kg and 20 mg/kg, respectively, and wheat bran up to 300 mg/kg). Pigs usually obtain less than 30% of this niacin, so it is common practice to ignore its contribution.

Niacin in feedstuffs is reasonably stable under normal conditions, but its bioavailability is low, at least in monogastric animals, especially in wheat and sorghum (10–15%) and in corn (0–30%), as it is found in combination with a peptide or a carbohydrate (Luce et al., 1966, 1967). In oilseeds, bioavailability is 40%. Oilseeds contain about 40% of their total niacin in bound form, while only a small proportion of the niacin in pulses, yeast, crustacean, fish, animal tissue, or milk is bound.

Two types of bound niacin were initially described: (1) a peptide with a molecular weight of 12,000 to 13,000, the so-called niacinogens, and (2) a carbohydrate complex with a molecular weight of approximately 2,370 (Darby et al., 1975). The name niacytin has been used to

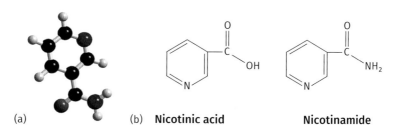

(a)   (b) **Nicotinic acid**   **Nicotinamide**

Figure 4.29 Niacin chemical structure

designate this latter material from wheat bran. Using a microbiological assay, Ghosh *et al.* (1963) reported that 85 to 90% of the total nicotinic acid in cereals is in a bound form. Using a rat assay procedure, for 8 samples of mature cooked cereals (corn, wheat, rice, and milo), only about 35% of the total niacin was available (Carter and Carpenter, 1982).

Therefore, in calculating the niacin content of formulated diets, probably all the niacin from cereal grain sources should be ignored or at least given a value no greater than one-third of the total niacin. In immature seeds, niacin is part of biologically available coenzymes necessary for seed metabolism. In rat growth assays for available niacin, corn harvested immaturely ("milk stage") gave values from 74 to 88 µg/g. In contrast, corn harvested at maturity gave assay values of 16 to 18 µg/g (Carpenter *et al.*, 1988). Niacin binding to carbohydrates by ester linkages may cause it to be retained in the mature seed until it is utilized. Hence, the vitamin availability for man and animals is thus impaired.

Because tryptophan can give rise to body niacin, both the niacin and tryptophan content should be considered together in expressing the niacin values of feeds. Most species can use the essential amino acid tryptophan, from which niacin can be synthesized. It has been demonstrated experimentally that the pig can convert tryptophan to nicotinic acid, albeit inefficiently (Luecke *et al.*, 1947, 1948; Powick *et al.*, 1948). The capacity to carry out this conversion depends mainly on the activity of a hepatic carboxyl, which acts specifically on picolinic acid, such that the greater the activity of this enzyme, the lower the capacity to obtain niacin from tryptophan. Its action in pigs is markedly greater than in rats, humans, or chickens, so the ability to produce niacin is proportionally small. According to studies by Firth and Johnson (1956), around 50 mg of tryptophan is needed to make 1 mg of niacin. However, tryptophan is preferably used for protein synthesis (Harmon *et al.*, 1969; Kodicek *et al.*, 1974; Kirkland, 2013). Consequently, it is unlikely that tryptophan conversion greatly contributes to the niacin supply since feedstuffs used in most diets tend to be low in tryptophan. As a result, adding niacin to feed pigs is usually considered necessary (Copelin *et al.*, 1980).

Commercial forms

Crystalline products are used in feeds and pharmaceuticals, and dry dilutions in feeds. Nicotinic acid and niacinamide are both available commercially as fine granular powder formulations containing 99% activity. However, niacinamide significantly increased ($p<0.05$) in milk, milk fat, and 4% fat-corrected milk over controls during lactation (Ivers *et al.*, 1993; Lauridsen and Matte, 2017). These production parameters were also higher than nicotinic acid-supplemented animals, but not significantly ($p<0.05$). As previously said, an additional supplemental niacin source is the vitamin K supplement menadione nicotinamide bisulfite (MNB).

Metabolism

Absorption and transport

Niacin in foods and feed occurs mainly in its coenzyme forms. Pyrophosphatase activity in the upper small intestine metabolizes NAD and NADP to yield nicotinamide, which is then hydrolyzed to form nicotinamide riboside and eventually free nicotinamide, which is hydrolyzed during digestion, yielding nicotinamide, which seems to be absorbed as such without further hydrolysis in the gastrointestinal tract (Kirkland, 2013). In the gut mucosa, nicotinic acid is converted to nicotinamide (Stein *et al.*, 1994). Nicotinic acid and nicotinamide are rapidly absorbed from the stomach and the intestine at either physiological or pharmacologic doses (Nabokina *et al.*, 2005; Jacob, 2006).

At low concentrations, absorption appears to be via sodium-dependent high-affinity transporters. Once absorbed from the lumen into the enterocyte, nicotinamide may be converted via the Preiss–Handler pathway to NAD or released into the portal circulation. Although some nicotinic acid moves into the blood in its native form, the enterocyte's bulk of nicotinic acid is converted to NAD. The intestinal mucosa contains niacin conversion enzymes such as NAD glycohydrolase (Henderson and Gross, 1979). As required, NAD glycohydrolases in the enterocytes release nicotinamide from NAD into the plasma, as the principal circulating form of niacin, for transport to tissues that synthesize NAD as needed.

Blood transport of niacin is associated mainly with red blood cells. Erythrocytes effectively take up nicotinic acid and nicotinamide by facilitating diffusion, converting them to nucleotides to maintain a concentration gradient. However, niacin rapidly leaves the bloodstream and enters the kidney, liver, and adipose tissues.

The amino acid tryptophan is a precursor for niacin synthesis in the body. There is considerable evidence that synthesis can occur in the intestine, and there is also evidence that synthesis can take place elsewhere within the body. The extent to which the metabolic requirement for niacin can be met from tryptophan will depend first on the amount of tryptophan in the diet and second on the efficiency of conversion of tryptophan to niacin (Matte et al., 2016). The kynurenine pathway of tryptophan conversion to nicotinic acid and, finally, NAD in the body is shown in Figure 4.30.

The conversion of tryptophan to nicotinic acid-NAD is irreversible (Kirkland, 2013). Protein, energy, vitamin B_6, and vitamin B_2 nutritional status and hormones affect one or more steps in the conversion sequence and hence can influence the yield of niacin from tryptophan. Two enzymes require iron to convert tryptophan to niacin, with a deficiency reducing tryptophan utilization. At low levels of tryptophan intake, the conversion efficiency is high, and it decreases when niacin and tryptophan levels in the diet are increased (Matte et al., 2016).

The variability in the efficient conversion of tryptophan to niacin among species is probably due to inherent differences in liver levels of picolinic acid carboxylase, the enzyme that diverts one of the intermediates (2-amino, 3-acroleylfumaric acid) to the picolinic acid pathway

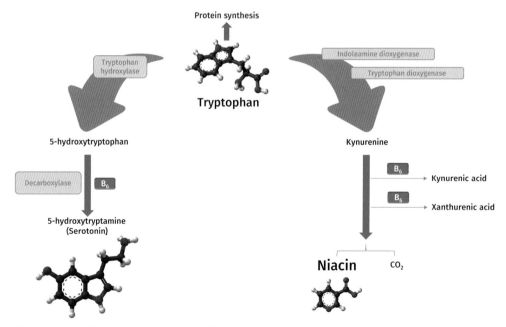

Figure 4.30 Overview of tryptophan metabolism to produce niacin

instead of allowing this compound to condense to quinolinic acid, the immediate precursor of nicotinic acid (Kirkland, 2013).

Picolinic acid carboxylase activity in livers of various species has a positive correlation to experimentally determined niacin requirements. The rat diverts very little of its dietary tryptophan to carbon dioxide and water and, thus, is relatively efficient in converting tryptophan to niacin. In practice, the production of niacin from tryptophan is minimal since this amino acid is not typically found in excess in diets. Moreover, high levels of fat in feed, especially saturated fat, will inhibit this reaction (Kirkland, 2013; Matte *et al.*, 2016). Finally, tryptophan is preferably used for protein synthesis (Harmon *et al.*, 1969; Kodicek *et al.*, 1974; Kirkland, 2013).

Consequently, it is unlikely that tryptophan conversion dramatically contributes to the niacin supply since feedstuffs used in most diets tend to be low in tryptophan. However, there are genetic differences in pigs. Le Floc'h *et al.* (2017) found that genetics contributes to the variability in the conversion of tryptophan to nicotinamide. They concluded that nicotinamide endogenous synthesis capacity from tryptophan is greater in Duroc than in Piétrain crossbred pigs, but this was apparent only at weaning.

Storage and excretion

Although niacin coenzymes are widely distributed in the body, no true storage occurs. The liver is the site of the greatest niacin concentration in the body, but the amount stored is minimal. The tissue content of niacin and its analogs, NAD and NADP, is a variable factor, dependent on the diet and several other factors, such as strain, sex, age, and treatment of animals (Hankes, 1984).

The liver is a central processing organ for niacin. Aside from its role in converting tryptophan to NAD, it receives nicotinamide and some nicotinic acid via the portal circulation, and nicotinamide is released from other extrahepatic tissues. In the liver, nicotinic acid and nicotinamide are metabolized to NAD or to yield compounds for urinary excretion, depending on the niacin status of the organism. Urine is the primary pathway of excretion of absorbed niacin and its metabolites, methylated or oxidized derivatives. The excretion of these metabolites is measured in studies of niacin requirements and niacin metabolism.

Biochemical functions

There are several metabolic reactions in which niacin participates, forming part of the NAD and NADP coenzymes. Therefore, it is essential in the metabolism of carbohydrates, amino acids, and fatty acids and for obtaining energy through the Krebs cycle. NAD and NADP coenzymes are essential in the metabolic reactions that furnish energy to the animal. Like the riboflavin coenzymes, the NAD- and NADP-containing enzyme systems play an important role in biological oxidation-reduction, including more than 200 reactions in the metabolism of carbohydrates, fatty acids, and amino acids, due to their capacity to serve as hydrogen-transfer agents. Hydrogen is effectively transferred from the oxidizable substrate to oxygen through a series of graded enzymatic hydrogen transfers. Nicotinamide-containing enzyme systems constitute one such group of hydrogen-transfer agents.

Important metabolic reactions catalyzed by NAD and NADP are summarized as follows (McDowell, 2000a; Kirkland, 2013):

1   carbohydrate metabolism:
    ○   clycolysis: anaerobic and aerobic oxidation of glucose
    ○   TCA or Krebs cycle

2   lipid metabolism:
    o   glycerol synthesis and breakdown
    o   fatty acid oxidation and synthesis
    o   steroid synthesis
3   protein metabolism:
    o   degradation and synthesis of amino acids
    o   oxidation of carbon chains via the TCA cycle
4   photosynthesis
5   rhodopsin synthesis.

Niacin, riboflavin, and coenzyme Q_{10} are associated with poly (ADP-ribose) synthesized in response to DNA strand breaks and are involved in the post-translational modification of nuclear proteins (Kirkland, 2013). The poly ADP-ribosylated proteins function in DNA repair, replication, and cell differentiation (Carson et al., 1987; Premkumar et al., 2008). These functions may be necessary for tissues with high turnover rates, like the skin, intestines, CNS (Kirkland, 2013; Gasperi et al., 2019), and the immunological system (Harmon et al., 1970). Rat data have shown that even a mild niacin deficiency decreases liver poly ADP-ribose concentrations, and those levels are also altered by feed restriction (Rawling et al., 1994). Zhang et al. (1993) suggested that a severe niacin deficiency may increase the susceptibility of DNA to oxidative damage, likely due to the lower availability of NAD.

Nutritional assessment
Niacin and its metabolites can be measured in plasma via gas chromatography (GC), HPLC, or simultaneously via LC-MS/MS. However, the central gap is the lack of reliable ranges, even in humans, making the assessment extremely complicated. Determination of the activity of erythrocyte nicotinic acid mononucleotide pyrophosribosyl transferase has been used as a possible method to assess the nutritional status of niacin in swine (Höller et al., 2018).

Deficiency signs
Severe metabolic disorders in the skin and digestive organs characterize niacin deficiency. The first signs are loss of appetite, retarded growth, weakness, digestive disorders, and diarrhea (Powick et al., 1947a; McMillen et al., 1949). Burroughs et al. (1950) observed these signs of niacin deficiency in rations that were calculated to contain less than 15 mg of niacin per kilogram of diet. However, the weanling pigs supplied with the same rations plus an additional 60 mg of niacin daily grew and developed normally. Cartwright and Wintrobe (1949) reported that pigs fed a low-protein diet without niacin developed moderately severe normocytic anemia that could be relieved by supplementation of niacin or protein. The pigs did not develop significant anemia when fed this low-protein diet but with supplemental niacin.

Niacin deficiency is found in human and animal populations that are overly dependent on foods, mainly corn, that are low in available niacin and its precursor, tryptophan (Powick et al., 1947a; Kodicek et al., 1956, 1959). Therefore, niacin is one of the B vitamins that would be expected to be deficient for typical swine diets, particularly when corn is fed (McMillen et al., 1949). Wide variation has been observed in the severity of clinical signs of niacin deficiency in pigs with similar breeding and environmental backgrounds. Occasionally, animals appear to thrive with no niacin, and other animals seem to vary in their requirement (Cunha, 1977).

It was impossible to produce niacin deficiency during gestation and lactation with sows fed a purified diet with either 18 or 26.1% casein (Ensminger et al., 1951). Evidently, the diet contained enough tryptophan to supply niacin needs, or the experiment's duration was insufficient for the animals to develop a niacin deficiency. Signs of niacin deficiency include poor appetite, decreased growth rate (Figure 4.31a), stomatitis, normocytic anemia (Cartwright *et al.*, 1948), and achlorhydria, followed by severe diarrhea, occasional vomiting, and an exfoliating type of dermatitis and hair loss (Cunha, 1977). Nervous system degenerative changes are reported in the ganglion cells in the posterior root, with extensive chromatolysis in the dorsal root (Wintrobe *et al.*, 1945). Powick *et al.* (1947b) and Braude *et al.* (1946) observed deficiency symptoms that were similar but not identical to those reported by Cunha (1977).

Niacin-deficient pigs have inflammatory lesions of the gastrointestinal tract. Ulcerative necrotic lesions of the large intestine swarm with fusiform bacteria and spirochetes (Figure 4.31b). Diarrhea with foul-smelling feces mainly involves the large intestine, which thickens, is very red, and appears weak and "rotten." Enteric conditions may be due to niacin deficiency, bacterial infection, or both. Deficient pigs respond readily to niacin therapy, but infectious enteritis is not benefited. However, adequate dietary niacin may aid the pig in maintaining its resistance to bacterial invasion (Luecke, 1955; Yen *et al.*, 1978).

Safety
Harmful effects of nicotinic acid occur at levels far above requirements. Limited research has indicated that nicotinic acid and nicotinamide are toxic at dietary intakes greater than 350 mg/kg of body weight per day (NRC, 1998, 2012). Nicotinic acid and niacinamide tolerance in swine have not been determined. Campbell and Combs (1990b, 1991) fed up to 68 g of niacin per kilogram feed to starting pigs. They reported a significant decrease in feed intake and average daily gain compared to pigs fed diets containing 34 g of niacin per kilogram feed.

Pantothenic acid (vitamin B₅)
Chemical structure and properties
In popular literature, pantothenic acid is often referred to as vitamin B_5, though the origin of this designation is obscure (Rucker and Bauerly, 2013). Pantothenic acid is an amide consisting of pantoic acid joined to β-alanine (3-[(2,4-dihydroxy-3, 3-dimethyl-1-oxobutyl) amino]propanoic acid) found forming part of the coenzymes, especially coenzyme A (CoA), containing the vitamin as an essential component, and the Acyl groups Carrier Protein (ACP). The structural formula and crystalline structure are shown in Figure 4.32.

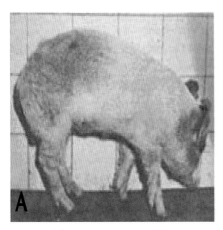
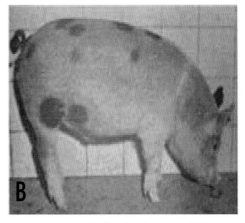

Figure 4.31(a) Niacin deficiency. (A) The pig has not received adequate niacin. The difference is less growth and a poorer condition than the previous pig. (B) Control pig (source: courtesy of D.E. Becker, Illinois Agriculture Experiment Station)

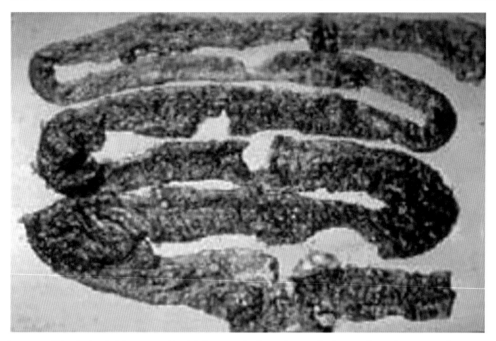

Figure 4.31(b) Niacin deficiency: gut health issues. The intestine of niacin-deficient pig shows thickened and hemorrhagic mucous membrane, also denuded areas (source: courtesy of R.W Luecke, Michigan State University)

The free acid of the vitamin is a viscous, pale yellow oil readily soluble in water and ethyl acetate. It crystallizes as white needles from ethanol and is reasonably stable to light and air. The oil is highly hygroscopic and easily destroyed by acids, bases, and heat. Maximum heat stability occurs at pH 5.5 to 7.0 (Rucker and Bauerly, 2013).

Pantothenic acid is optically active (characteristic of rotating a polarized light). It may be prepared either as the pure dextrorotatory (d) form or the racemic mixture (dl) form. The racemic form has approximately one-half the biological activity of d-calcium pantothenate, the commercial form used in animal nutrition. Only the dextrorotatory form, d-pantothenic acid, is effective as a vitamin.

Natural sources

Pantothenic acid is widely distributed in feedstuffs of animal and plant origin. Corn and soybean meal diets are likely to be low in pantothenic acid. Alfalfa hay, peanut meal, cane molasses, yeast, rice bran, green leafy plants, wheat bran, brewer's yeast, fish solubles, and rice polishings are good sources of vitamins for animals. Milling by-products, such as rice bran and wheat bran, are good sources, 2 to 3 times higher than the respective grains.

The concentration in cereals is around 10 mg/kg, ranging from 5–6 mg/kg in corn to 15 mg/kg in oats. According to Southern and Baker (1981), the availability of pantothenic acid in barley, wheat, and soy is high but much lower in sorghum. By-products of cereals generally have a much higher concentration (rice bran 22 mg/kg, wheat bran 18–30 mg/kg). Amounts in vegetable protein concentrate vary. While peanut meal contains 47 mg/kg, soy and linseed contain around 15 mg/kg, and sunflower only 10 mg/kg. Legumes have a lower concentration (peas 5 mg/kg). The concentration in milk by-products is between 20 and 45 mg/kg and in

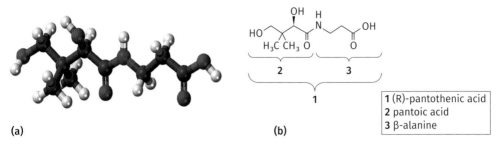

Figure 4.32 Structure of pantothenic acid

fishmeal is between 10 and 20 mg/kg. Finally, in fibrous foods, such as alfalfa, concentration is around 30 mg/kg.

Many swine diets are borderline sufficient in supplying pantothenic acid requirements, and many are deficient in this vitamin. The biological availability of pantothenic acid is high in corn and soybean meal but low in barley, wheat, and sorghum, approximately 60% (McMillen *et al.*, 1948; Bowland and Owen, 1952; Southern and Baker, 1981). Changing processing methods can significantly alter vitamin feed levels. For example, with changes in sugar technology, literature values for the pantothenic acid content of beet molasses have decreased from 50 to 100 mg/kg in the 1950s to about 1 to 4 mg/kg as recently assessed (Palagina *et al.*, 1990).

Pantothenic acid is relatively stable in feedstuffs during long storage periods (Chen, Huang, Liu *et al.*, 2019; Chen, Wang, Li *et al.* 2019). Heating during processing may cause considerable losses, especially if temperatures attain 100–150°C for long periods and pH values above 7 or below 5. Gadient (1986) considers pantothenic acid to be slightly sensitive to heat, oxygen, or light but very sensitive to moisture. As a general guideline, pantothenic acid activity in regular pelleted feed over 3 months at room temperature should be 80–100%. Although this vitamin is found in practically all feedstuffs, complementary supplementation is advisable in rations for swine to ensure a high production level.

Commercial forms

Pantothenic acid is available as a commercially synthesized product for feed use known as d- or dl-calcium pantothenate. Because livestock (and poultry) can biologically utilize only the d-isomer of pantothenic acid, nutrient requirements for the vitamin are routinely expressed in the d-form.

One gram of d-calcium pantothenate is equivalent to 0.92 g of d-pantothenic acid activity. Therefore 1.087 g of d-calcium pantothenate is required to get the activity of 1 g of d-pantothenic acid. Sometimes a racemic mixture (i.e., equal parts d- and dl-calcium pantothenate) is offered to the feed industry. The racemic mixture of 1 g of the dl-form has 0.46 g of d-pantothenic acid activity. Hence with this product, 2.174 g is needed to get the activity of 1 g of d-pantothenic acid. Products sold based on racemic mixture content can be misleading and confusing to a buyer not fully aware of the biological activity supplied by d-calcium pantothenate. To avoid confusion, the label should clearly state the grams of d-calcium pantothenate or its equivalent per unit weight and the grams of d-pantothenic acid. Moreover, the racemic mixture can create handling problems because of its hygroscopic and electrostatic properties.

Verbeeck (1975) reported calcium pantothenate to be stable in premixes with or without trace minerals, regardless of the mineral form. Losses of calcium pantothenate may occur in premixes that are highly acidic. Recently Lewis *et al.* (2015) and Yang *et al.* (2020) reported that pelleting causes only small losses of pantothenic acid.

Metabolism
Absorption and transport
Pantothenic acid is found in feeds in both bound (primarily as CoA) and free forms. It is necessary to liberate the pantothenic acid from the bound forms in the digestive process before absorption. Work with pigs and rats indicated that pantothenic acid, its salt, and the alcohol are absorbed primarily in the jejunum by a specific transport system that is saturable and sodium ion-dependent (Fenstermacher and Rose, 1986; Miller et al., 2006). The alcohol form, panthenol, oxidized to pantothenic acid in vivo, appears to be absorbed somewhat faster than the acid form.

After absorption, pantothenic acid is transported to various tissues in the plasma. Most cells take it up via another active-transport process involving the cotransport of pantothenate and sodium in a 1:1 ratio (Olson, 1990). Pantothenic acid is converted to CoA and other compounds within tissues, where a vitamin is a functional group (Sauberlich, 1985).

Storage and excretion
Livestock does not appear to have the ability to store appreciable amounts of pantothenic acid: organs such as the liver and kidneys have the highest concentrations. Most pantothenic acid in blood exists in red blood cells as CoA, but free pantothenic acid is also present. The serum does not contain CoA but does contain free pantothenic acid.

Urinary excretion is the major route of body loss of absorbed pantothenic acid, and excretion is prompt when the vitamin is consumed in excess. Most pantothenic acid is excreted as a free vitamin, but some species (e.g., dogs) pass it as b-glucuronide (Taylor et al., 1972). Smith and Song (1996) described that pantothenic acid's urinary and fecal excretion was 4 to 6 times the intake when semi-synthetic diets were fed. Pantothenic acid excretion increased as crude protein intake increased. An appreciable quantity of pantothenic acid (~15% of daily intake) is completely oxidized and excreted across the lungs as carbon dioxide.

Biochemical functions
Pantothenic acid is involved in several metabolic pathways critical in endogenous metabolism energy exchange in all tissues. Its main functions include (Rucker and Bauerly, 2013):

- utilization of nutrients
- synthesis of fatty acids, cholesterol, and steroid hormones
- synthesis of neurotransmitters, steroid hormones, porphyrins, and hemoglobin
- participation in the citric acid cycle or Krebs cycle, as a constituent of acetyl-coenzyme A (3-phospho-adenosine-5-diphospho-pantothene) and other enzymes and coenzymes
- energy-yielding oxidation of fats, carbohydrates, and amino acids (Pond et al., 1960; Sewell et al., 1962)
- participation in the production of antibodies, the adrenal glands' activity, and the acetylation of choline for nervous impulse transmission
- its relationship with vitamin B_{12}; if the latter is deficient, it accentuates the lack of pantothenic acid (Luecke et al., 1952)
- interactions with folic acid, biotin, and copper (Menten et al., 1987).

CoA's most critical function is acting as a carrier mechanism for carboxylic acids (Lehninger, 1982; Miller et al., 2006; Rucker and Bauerly, 2013). When bound to CoA, such acids have a high potential for transfer to other groups, and such carboxylic acids are normally referred to as "active." The most important of these reactions is the combination of CoA with acetate to form "active acetate" with a high-energy bond that renders acetate capable of further chemical interactions. Combining CoA with two-carbon fragments from fats, carbohydrates, and certain amino acids to form acetyl-CoA is essential in their complete metabolism because the coenzyme enables these fragments to enter the TCA cycle.

For example, acetyl-CoA is utilized directly by combining with oxaloacetic acid to form citric acid, entering the TCA cycle. Coenzyme A, along with ACP, functions as a carrier of acyl groups in enzymatic reactions involved in synthesizing fatty acids, cholesterol, sphingosine, porphyrins, and other sterols; oxidation of fatty acids, pyruvate, and α-ketoglutarate; and biological acetylations. Decarboxylation of α-ketoglutaric acid in the TCA cycle yields succinic acid, which is then converted to the "active" form by linkage with CoA. Active succinate and glycine are involved in the first step of heme biosynthesis.

In the form of acetyl-CoA, acetic acid can also combine with choline to form acetylcholine, a chemical transmitter at the nerve synapse, and can be used to detoxify various drugs, such as sulfonamides. Pantothenic acid also stimulates the synthesis of antibodies, increasing animal resistance to pathogens. It appears that when pantothenic acid is deficient, the incorporation of amino acids into the blood albumin fraction is inhibited, which would explain why there is a reduction in the titer of antibodies (Axelrod, 1971).

Nutritional assessment

Early assays used pantothenic acid-dependent microorganisms such as *Lactobacillus plantarum* for quantification (Sauberlich, 1999). This assay is prone to various interferences, and therefore more specific radioimmunoassay (RIA) or enzyme-linked immunosorbent assay (ELISA) tests have been developed (Sauberlich, 1999) and used to measure it in blood plasma to determine body status (Höller *et al.*, 2018).

Deficiency signs

Many swine diets are borderline sufficient in supplying pantothenic acid, and many are deficient in the vitamin (McMillen *et al.*, 1948; Neumann *et al.*, 1949; Pond *et al.*, 1960; Palm *et al.*, 1968; Cunha, 1977; Roth-Maier and Kirchgessner, 1977). Pantothenic acid deficiency is rare in practice, although pigs bred in intensive conditions may occasionally present some deficiency symptoms.

Early researchers documented various deficiency signs, including those reported by Luecke *et al.* (1950) and Wiese *et al.* (1951) in baby pigs. Owing to the relationship with multiple biochemical processes, inadequate intake of pantothenic acid causes a series of unspecific signs and symptoms, including growth retardation (Figure 4.33a), reduced appetite, bloody diarrhea, hair loss, dermatitis, and loss of immune response capacity.

As has been pointed out for other B group vitamins involved in the process of obtaining energy (mainly from glucose), deficiency also shows in nervous degeneration, the characteristic "goose stepping" (Figure 4.33b), and the effects on epithelial tissue and functions linked to reproduction.

Other changes caused by pantothenic acid deficiency included fatty liver degeneration, an enlarged heart with some related flaccidity of the myocardium, and intramuscular hemorrhages. Histopathologic studies showed degenerative changes and necroses of the tissue cells. Stothers *et al.* (1955) observed a decrease in the thickness of the glomerular layer of the adrenals in addition to the other symptoms of pantothenic acid deficiency reported by other researchers. Follis and Wintrobe (1945) compared the influence of pyridoxine or pantothenic acid deficiencies on the nervous tissues of young pigs. These authors reported that while the most prominent and initial feature in pyridoxine deficiency was degeneration of the peripheral

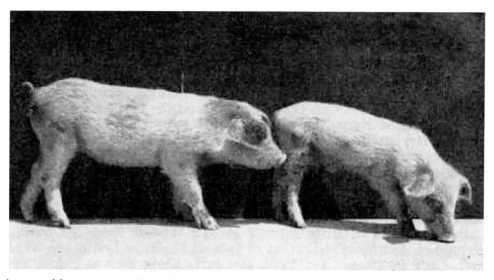

Figure 4.33(a) Pantothenic acid deficiency. Both these pigs were fed the same purified diet, except that the pig on the right did not get a supplement of pantothenic acid. This animal has a poor appetite, is weak and emaciated, and suffers from severe diarrhea (source: Madsen, 1942)

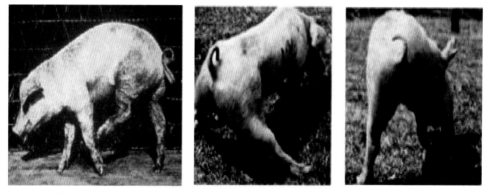

Figure 4.33(b) Pantothenic acid deficiency: goose stepping (source: courtesy R.W. Leucke, Michigan State Station)

process of the sensory neurons, chromatolysis was the first evidence of damage to the afferent neuron in animals subjected to pantothenic acid deficiency.

Pantothenic acid is particularly important in sow fertility, with insufficient quantities of the vitamin resulting in complete reproductive failure (Ullrey *et al.*, 1955). Estrus occurred, but the sows failed to retain the embryos following breeding. In gestating and lactating sows, fatty liver has been observed, as well as enlargement of the adrenal glands, hemorrhages, rectal congestion, atrophy of ovaries, and reduced estrogen and progesterone synthesis, leading to uterine atrophy (Ullrey *et al.*, 1955). Even with moderate deficiency, fertility decreases, and embryonic development is compromised.

Davey and Stevenson (1963) reported in their trials that litter weights at weaning were reduced with lower pantothenic acid levels and appeared to be due to a reduction in litter size. The incidence of stillbirths was inversely related to dietary pantothenic acid levels. The data from their experiments suggested that reproductive performance and growth could be improved if pantothenic acid was increased from 4.4 mg/kg to 11.9 mg/kg feed. These authors concluded that a minimum of 11.9 mg of pantothenic acid per kilogram diet is required in swine diets for maximum reproduction. Ensminger et al. (1951) reported that although gilts on a low-pantothenic acid diet became pregnant, they did not farrow or show any signs of pregnancy. Necropsy of gilts revealed macerating fetus in the uterine horns in all cases. Minimal pantothenic acid sufficient to result in normal farrowing may still result in abnormal locomotion in suckling pigs from sows that had received diets low in the vitamin (Teague et al., 1971). Sucking movements in deficient piglets are impaired, as is the use of the tongue (Christensen, 1983).

The pantothenic acid concentration in the liver is reduced during deficiency, and the liver is hypertrophied and varies in color from faint yellow to dirty yellow. Nerves and fibers of the spinal cord show myelin degeneration, and these degenerating fibers occur in all cord segments down to the lumbar region (Follis and Wintrobe, 1945; Goodwin, 1962; Fox, 1991).

Luecke et al. (1950) experimentally produced a pantothenic acid deficiency by feeding a low-protein ration containing corn and soybean oil meal supplemented with thiamine, riboflavin, nicotinic acid, and pyridoxine. Two pigs in the pantothenic acid-deficient lot were completely paralyzed in the hind quarters. Blood levels of pantothenic acid in pigs showing symptoms of deficiency were approximately two-fifths of those in the normal control group. These authors reported that the basal ration contained 9.3 mg of pantothenic acid per kilogram of ration. Adding supplemental pantothenic acid (22 mg calcium pantothenate per kilogram) without the other B vitamins resulted in significantly greater gains than that of pigs fed the unsupplemented basal ration. McKigney et al. (1957) reported that chlortetracycline at 22 mg/kg of feed could ameliorate some of the adverse effects of pantothenic acid deficiency.

A characteristic sign of a pantothenic acid deficiency in the pig is locomotor disorder (especially of the hindquarters), which was described by Goodwin (1962). In the early stages of such a deficiency, the movement of the back legs becomes stiff and jerky. Standing animals show a slight tremor of the hindquarters. When deficiency persists, this particular action of the rear legs grows more exaggerated and resembles the characteristic military gait, termed "goose stepping" (Figure 4.33b) (Luecke et al., 1953).

The condition may be so severe that, as the pig moves forward, the back legs will touch the belly. Finally, increasingly severe paralysis of the hindquarters develops. Affected pigs will frequently fall sideways or have their back legs spread apart in a posture resembling that of a sitting dog (Figure 4.33c and 4.33d). The chief microscopic lesion is chromatolysis of isolated cells of the dorsal root ganglia, followed by a demyelinating process in brachial and sciatic nerves. Recently, Lorenzett et al. (2023) reported a motor and somatosensory degenerative myelopathy responsive to pantothenic acid in piglets. All signs previously described were present. The ultrastructural study of the thoracic nucleus neurons and motor neurons showed the dissolution of Nissl granulation. The topographical distribution of the lesions indicated damage to the second-order neurons of the spinocerebellar tract, first-order axon cuneocerebellar tract, and dorsal column-medial lemniscus pathway as the cause of the conscious and unconscious proprioceptive deficit, and damage to the alpha motor neuron as the cause of the motor deficit. These authors indicated that clinical signs reversed and no new cases occurred after pantothenic acid levels were corrected in the ration, and piglets received parenteral administration of pantothenic acid.

Pigs suffering from pantothenic acid deficiency have scaly skin, thin hair, and a brownish secretion around the eyes. The dermatosis associated with deficiency appears principally on

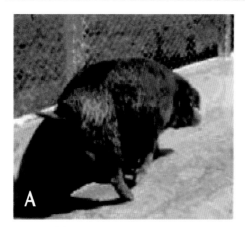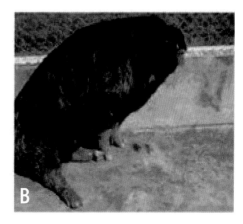

Figure 4.33(c) Pantothenic acid deficiency: abnormal postures. (A) Locomotor incoordination (goose stepping) with pantothenic acid deficiency. (B) Pig affected with the pantothenic acid deficiency will often fall sideways or, with its back legs spread apart, assume a posture resembling that of a sitting dog.

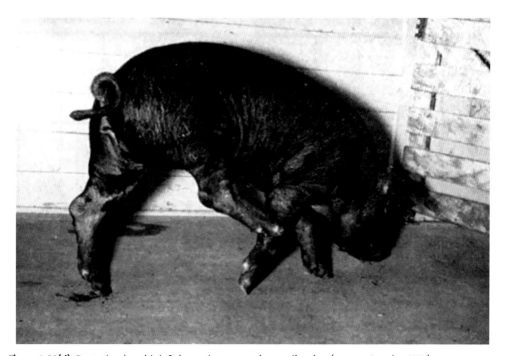

Figure 4.33(d) Pantothenic acid deficiency: locomotor incoordination (source: Luecke, 1955)

the shoulders and behind the ears; the skin appears dirty and scaly. Skin becomes reddened, and the bristles on the rump and along the spine loosen and fall (Figure 4.33e). The dermatosis extends to the intestinal mucosa, manifesting as necrotic enteritis, ulceration, and hemorrhages in the large intestine (Colby et al., 1948; Luecke, 1955; Ullrey et al., 1955). As a consequence the feces contain blood. Goodwin (1962) observed various degrees of gastritis and, occasionally, peritonitis and intestinal fissures.

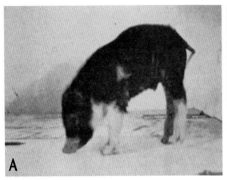 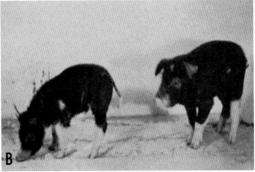

Figure 4.33(e) Pantothenic acid deficiency in baby pigs. (A) Pantothenic acid-deficient diet for 30 days. Note poor hair coat and dermatitis on legs. (B) Comparison of pantothenic acid-deficient pig and a fitter mate control animal on the right (source: Wiese *et al.*, 1951)

The most common antagonist of pantothenic acid is omega-methyl-pantothenic acid, which has been used to produce a vitamin deficiency in humans (Hodges *et al.*, 1958). Other antivitamins include pantoyltaurine, phenylpantothenate hydroxocobalamin (c-lactam), an analog of vitamin B$_{12}$, and anti-metabolites of the vitamin-containing alkyl or aryl ureido and carbamate components in the amide part of the molecule (Fox, 1991; Brass, 1993; Rucker and Bauerly, 2013).

Safety
Pantothenic acid is generally regarded as nontoxic. Excesses are primarily excreted in the urine. Pantothenic acid can become toxic at around 2,000 mg/kg. First, diarrhea and gastrointestinal disturbances can be observed, followed by a reduced growth rate associated with liver damage (Alhadeff *et al.*, 1984; Rucker and Bauerly, 2013). These levels are around 100 times the recommended supplementation for all species. Calcium pantothenate, sodium pantothenate, and panthenol are not mutagenic in bacterial tests.

Biotin (vitamin B$_7$)
Chemical structure and properties
The chemical structure of biotin includes a sulfur atom in its ring (like thiamine) and a transverse bond across the ring (Figure 4.34). Biotin is a bicyclic compound, a monocarboxylic acid with sulfur as a thioether linkage. One of the rings contains a ureido group (-N-CO-N-), and the other is a tetrahydrothiophene ring. The tetrahydrothiophene ring has a valeric acid side chain. With its rather unique structure, biotin contains 3 asymmetric carbon atoms; therefore, 8 different isomers are possible. Of these isomers, only d-biotin has vitamin activity (Mock, 2013).

Biotin crystallizes from water as long, white needles. Its melting point is 232–233°C. Free biotin is soluble in dilute alkaline solutions and hot water and practically insoluble in fats and organic solvents. Biotin is relatively stable under ordinary conditions. It is destroyed by nitric acid, other strong acids, strong bases, and formaldehyde and is inactivated by oxidative rancidity reactions. It is gradually destroyed by UV radiation (Camporeale and Zempleni, 2006; Said, 2012).

Structurally related biotin analogs can vary from no activity to partial replacement of biotin activity to anti-biotin action. Mild oxidation converts biotin to sulfoxide, and strong oxidation converts it to sulfone. Strong agents result in sulfur replacement by oxygen, resulting in oxybiotin and desthiobiotin. Previously biotin has been known as vitamin H or coenzyme

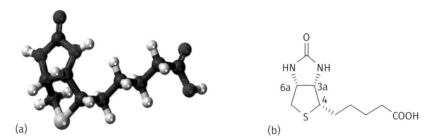

(a)   (b)

Figure 4.34 D-biotin chemical structure

R. Requirements, and concentrations are usually expressed in mass units (mg or µg/kg) (Camporeale and Zempleni, 2006; Said, 2012).

Natural sources

Biotin is present in common swine feedstuffs; however, corn, wheat, other cereals (0.1–0.2 mg/kg), meat, and fish are relatively poor sources of biotin (Table 4.2). Of all the vitamins present in feed ingredients of plant origin, biotin is the one that presents the most variable content, being affected by numerous environmental factors (Frigg, 1976, 1984, 1987; Misir and Blair, 1984; Kopinski et al., 1989a; Mock, 2013; Chen, Huang, Liu et al., 2019; Chen, Wang, Li et al. 2019). For example, 59 samples of corn analyzed for biotin varied between 56 and 115 µg/kg, and 62 samples of meat meal ranged from 17 to 323 µg/kg (Frigg, 1987). Compared to cereal grains, oilseed meals are better sources of total biotin. Soybean meal, for instance, contains a mean biotin content of 270 µg/kg with a range of 200 to 387 µg/kg (Frigg and Volker, 1994). Milling wheat or corn reduced biotin concentrations (Bonjour, 1991).

Biotin is present in feedstuffs and yeast in both bound and free forms: therefore, it is crucial

Table 4.2 Biotin content in feedstuffs (source: adapted from Frigg, 1987)

Feedstuffs	Mean bioavailable biotin content (ug/kg)	Feedstuffs	Mean bioavailable biotin content (ug/kg)
Barley	14	Safflower seed meal	305
Corn	79	Sunflower seed meal	346
Corn gluten meal	189	Fish meal	135
Oats	86	Meat meal > 50% CP	88
Rye	0	Meat and bone meal < 50% CP	76
Rice polishings	74	Skim milk powder	165
Sorghum	58	Whey powder	316
Wheat	0	Cassava meal	3
Wheat bran	72	Grass meal	238
Wheat middlings	17	Alfalfa	407
Wheat germ	150	Molasses, beet	331
Rapeseed meal	68	Molasses, cane	1080
Soybean meal	270	Brewer's yeast	634

to know the form of biotin, i.e., bound or unbound, and its overall content in the feed. Much of the bound biotin to protein or lysine is unavailable to animal species as covalent bonds hinder its digestion and availability for the animal. Less than one-half of the microbiologically determined biotin in a feedstuff is biologically available (Frigg, 1984, 1987; Kopinski *et al.*, 1989a). For alfalfa meal, corn, cottonseed meal, and soybean meal, the bioavailability of biotin is estimated at 100%. However, biotin availability is variable for other feedstuffs, for example, 11–50% in barley, 62% in corn gluten meal, 30% in fish meal, 10–60% in sorghum, 32% in oats, and 0–62% in wheat (Kopinski *et al.*, 1989a; McDowell, 2004; Chen, Huang, Liu *et al.*, 2019; Chen, Wang, Li *et al.* 2019). Diets based on these cereals without biotin supplementation led to higher mortality and slower growth rates.

Other factors influencing biotin availability (and requirement) are some nutrients, such as fiber, which interfere with its intestinal absorption (Tagwerker, 1974; Misir and Blair, 1984; Kopinski *et al.*, 1989a,b,c,d), protein level, with greater requirements at 18% than at 22% (Kopinski *et al.*, 1989d; Sauer *et al.*, 1988), the level of choline and the other water-soluble vitamins, which at high levels reduce the bioavailability of biotin (Kopinski *et al.*, 1989a,b,c,d); the proportion of added fat and even the composition of the fat.

The cecal microbiota of the pig can synthesize biotin, but the quantity is variable, and the importance of its utilization by the host does not seem to improve growth (Brooks, 1982; Bilodeau *et al.*, 1989; Bonomi *et al.*, 1996). Bilodeau *et al.* (1989) reported that biotin concentration in feces was 16-fold more remarkable than in the feed. As with most of the vitamins of the B group, there is a certain amount of recycling through coprophagy, but at 3 weeks, this is not very important, and at 7 weeks, it only amounts to 0.01 mg/kg (De Passille *et al.*, 1989). Scholtissek *et al.* (1990) quantified that under basal conditions 1.7–17% of the metabolic allowance of biotin can be covered by colonic biotin produced by microbes.

Biotin is unstable in oxidizing conditions and, therefore, is destroyed by heat, especially under conditions that support simultaneous lipid peroxidation by solvent extraction and improper storage conditions. At the same time, steam pelleting does not affect the stability of biotin (McGinnis, 1986b), and there has even been an increase of 10% measured in its bioavailability (McGinnis, 1986a,b).

Commercial forms
Biotin is commercially available normally as a 100% crystalline product or as various triturated dilutions premixed, and low-potency – 2% and 10% – spray-dried preparations, allowing a better distribution in premixes and feeds. The d-form of biotin is the biologically active form. It is the form that occurs in nature and is also the commercially available form.

Metabolism
Absorption and transport
After feed ingestion, biotinidase, present in pancreatic juice and intestinal mucosa, catalyzes the hydrolysis of biocytin, the biotin-bound form, to biotin and free lysine during the luminal phase of proteolysis. In most species that have been investigated, physiological concentrations of biotin are absorbed from the intestinal tract by a sodium-dependent active-transport process, which is inhibited by dethiobiotin and biocytin (Said and Derweesh, 1991).

Absorption of biotin by a sodium ion-dependent process was noted to be higher in the duodenum than in the jejunum, which was, in turn, more elevated than that in the ileum. It was concluded that the proximal part of the human small intestine was the site of maximum biotin transport (Said *et al.*, 1988, Said, 2011). Biotin is absorbed intact in the first third to half of the small intestine (Bonjour, 1991).

Biotin is also absorbed from the hindgut of the pig, with 50–61% of infused biotin disappearing between the cecum and feces. This is accompanied by a more than a 4-fold increase in plasma biotin concentration and more than a 6-fold increase in urinary biotin excretion (Barth et al., 1986).

Biotin exits the enterocyte across the basolateral membrane. This transport is also carrier-mediated. However, this carrier is sodium ion-independent, is electrogenic, and cannot accumulate biotin against a concentration gradient (Said et al., 1992; Said, 2011; Mock, 2013). Biotin transport is regulated by multiple factors, including biotin nutritional status, enterocyte maturity, anatomic location, and ontogeny (Said, 2011). Biotin transport is more active in the villus cells than in the crypt cells. Transport is most active in the upper small intestine and progressively less active aborally into the colon.

Biotin appears to circulate in the bloodstream free and bound to a serum glycoprotein, which also has biotinidase activity and catalyzes biocytin's hydrolysis. In humans, 81% of biotin in plasma was free, and the remainder was bound (Mock and Malik, 1992; Mock, 2013). In the plasma of chickens, 2 biotin-binding proteins have been detected, which appear to be functionally different. Information on biotin transport, tissue deposition, and storage in animals and humans is minimal. Mock (1990) reported that biotin is transported as a free water-soluble component of plasma, is taken up by cells via active transport, and is attached to its apoenzymes (Cooper et al., 1997).

Storage and excretion

All cells contain some biotin, with larger quantities in the liver and kidney. The intracellular distribution of biotin corresponds to known locations of biotin-dependent carboxylase enzymes, especially the mitochondria (Cooper et al., 1997; Mock, 2013). Investigations of biotin metabolism in animals are difficult to interpret, as biotin-producing microorganisms are present in the intestinal tract distal to the cecum.

The amount of biotin excreted in urine and feces often exceeds the total dietary intake, whereas urinary biotin excretion is usually less than the intake (Scholtissek et al., 1990). The efficient conservation of biotin and the recycling of biocytin released from the catabolism of biotin-containing enzymes may be as crucial as the intestinal bacterial synthesis of the vitamin in meeting biotin requirements (Bender, 1992). 14C-labeled biotin showed the major portion of intraperitoneally injected radioactivity to be excreted in the urine and none in the feces or as expired CO_2 (Lee et al., 1973). Biliary excretion of biotin and metabolites in rats and pigs is negligible (Zempleni et al., 1997).

Biochemical functions

Biotin is a coenzyme essential for gluconeogenesis, lipogenesis, and the elongation of essential fatty acids. It converts carbohydrates to protein and vice versa, transforming protein and carbohydrates into fat. Biotin is a cofactor of various enzymes that allow carbon dioxide to be fixed or eliminated in organic molecules (pyruvate carboxylase, propionyl coenzyme A carboxylase, acetyl-coenzyme A carboxylase, among others). All the enzymes involved in biotin require ATP and magnesium for activation. Biotin is vital for the normal functioning of the reproductive and nervous systems and the thyroid and adrenal glands.

Biotin also plays an important role in maintaining normal blood glucose levels from the metabolism of protein and fat when the dietary intake of carbohydrates is low. As a component of 5 carboxylating enzymes, it can transport carboxyl units and fix carbon dioxide (bicarbonate) in tissue (Camporeale and Zempleni, 2006; Mock, 2013).

The 5 biotin-dependent carboxylases are:

1   propionyl-CoA carboxylase (PCC)
2   methylcrotonyl-CoA carboxylase (MCC)
3   pyruvate carboxylase (PC)
4   acetyl-CoA carboxylase 1 (ACC1)
5   acetyl-CoA carboxylase 2 (ACC2).

All except ACC2 are mitochondrial enzymes. In carbohydrate metabolism, biotin functions in both carbon dioxide fixation and decarboxylation, with the energy-producing citric acid cycle dependent upon the presence of this vitamin. The hydrolysis of ATP drives the reaction to ADP and inorganic phosphate. Specific biotin-dependent reactions in carbohydrate metabolism are:

- carboxylation of pyruvic acid to oxaloacetic acid
- conversion of malic acid to pyruvic acid
- interconversion of succinic acid and propionic acid
- conversion of oxalosuccinic acid to α-ketoglutaric acid. In protein metabolism, biotin enzymes are important in protein synthesis, amino acid deamination, purine synthesis, and nucleic acid metabolism.

Biotin is required for transcarboxylation in the degradation of various amino acids. Vitamin deficiency in mammals hinders the standard conversion of the deaminated chain of leucine to acetyl-CoA. Depleting hepatic biotin reduces the hepatic activity of methylcrotonyl-CoA carboxylase, which is needed for leucine degradation (Mock and Mock, 1992; Mock, 2013). Likewise, the ability to synthesize citrulline from ornithine is reduced in liver homogenates from biotin-deficient rats. The urea cycle enzyme ornithine transcarbamylase was significantly lower in the livers of biotin-deficient rats (Maeda et al., 1996).

Acetyl-coenzyme A (CoA)-carboxylase catalyzes the addition of carbon dioxide to acetyl-CoA to form malonyl CoA, the first reaction in the synthesis of fatty acids. Biotin is required for normal long-chain unsaturated fatty acid synthesis and is vital for essential fatty acid metabolism. Deficiency in rats and chicks inhibited arachidonic acid (20:4) synthesis from linoleic acid (18:2) while increasing linolenic acid (18:3) and its metabolite (22:6) (Watkins and Kratzer, 1987a). The reduced synthesis of arachidonic acid (20:4) in chicks reduces plasma prostaglandin E_2 (PGE$_2$) since arachidonic acid is a precursor of prostaglandin (20:4) (Watkins and Kratzer, 1987b,c; Watkins, 1989a,b). Biotin supplementation in pigs has been shown to alter fatty acid metabolism and carcass composition (Kopinsky et al., 1989; Partridge and McDonald, 1990).

Evidence has emerged that biotin plays unique roles in cell signaling, epigenetic control of gene expression, and chromatin structure (Rodríguez-Meléndez and Zempleni, 2003; Riveron-Negrete and Fernandez-Mejia, 2017). In rats, biotin regulates the genetic expression of holo-carboxylase synthetase and mitochondrial carboxylases (Rodríquez-Meléndez et al., 2001). Manthey et al. (2002) report that biotin affects the expression of biotin transporters, biotiny-lations of carboxylases, and the metabolism of interleukin-2 in Jurat cells. These cells are an immortalized line of human T-lymphocyte cells used to study acute T-cell-related diseases like leukemia, T-cell signaling, and the expression of various chemokine receptors susceptible to viral entry, particularly HIV.

Nutritional assessment

Biotin status analysis can be measured in plasma using different methods, including microbiological, GC, avidin binding, colorimetric, polarographic, and isotope dilution assays (Sauberlich, 1999). Research is ongoing in humans on several markers of biotin status, but more clinical validation is needed. One of these tests is determining blood pyruvate carboxylase activity as an indicator of biotin status in pigs (Höller *et al.*, 2018).

Deficiency signs

Biotin is essential for the normal function of the thyroid and adrenal glands, reproductive tract (Tagwerker, 1974; Halama, 1979), and nervous system. Its effect on the cutaneous system is most dramatic since severe dermatitis is the significant obvious clinical sign of biotin deficiency in livestock. Biotin deficiency was produced in 1946 in swine by feeding a purified diet containing sulfathalidine or raw egg white (Lindley and Cunha, 1946; Cunha *et al.*, 1946).

For many years, biotin supplementation was considered unnecessary since it is synthesized by intestinal microorganisms and is widely distributed in feed. Nevertheless, feed company personnel and scientists observed clinical signs of deficiency under field conditions. Not until the 1970s did a greater awareness of biotin field deficiencies arise (Cunha, 1984). Biotin deficiency results in reduced growth rate and impaired feed conversion and produces various clinical signs (Hamilton *et al.*, 1983).

Lehrer *et al.* (1952) observed many symptoms of biotin deficiency in suckling pigs. Clinical signs associated with biotin deficiency include alopecia, dermatitis characterized by dryness, roughness, and a brownish exudate; ulceration of the skin; inflammation of the oral mucosa; hindleg spasticity; and transverse cracking of the soles and tops of hooves (Tagwerker, 1974; Cunha, 1977; Grandhi and Strain, 1980). Figure 4.35a and Figure 4.35b show clinical signs of biotin deficiency in swine.

The hoof horn becomes soft, rubbery, and poorly resistant to abrasions in a biotin deficiency. The slow growth and repair process in the hoof tissue and the weight on the feet add to the problem. Depending on the type of flooring on which the animal is kept, this may have little effect or may lead to the development of cracks and necrotic lesions, resulting in extreme lameness (Glättli *et al.*, 1975; Grandhi and Strain, 1980; Pluym *et al.*, 2011).

Secondary infections may gain entry through hoof cracks and infect the joints, leading to premature removal from the herd (Figure 4.35c). Feeding and breeding are also adversely affected. With hoof defects, the sow cannot support the boar's weight (Smith and Robertson, 1971). Also, because the hog's eating ability may be impaired, these problems lead to economic losses (Kilbride *et al.*, 2009, 2010; Lisgara *et al.*, 2015).

Supplementing the diet of breeding sows with biotin from an early stage of development significantly contributed to the maintenance of hoof horn integrity (Halama, 1979; Grandhi and Strain, 1980; Penny *et al.*, 1980; Simmins, 1985; Simmins and Brooks, 1985, 1988; Bryant *et al.*, 1985a,c; Luce *et al.*, 1995). Tagwerker (1983) noted that foot lesions accounted for 4–8% of all sows culled in Europe. Also, he commented on a Denmark study that reported 8.5% of biotin-supplemented sows having hoof lesions, compared with 25% for controls (Pedersen and Udesen, 1980). After biotin supplementation in Holland, the culling rate due to lameness decreased from 25 to 14% (de Jong and Sytsema, 1983). Webb *et al.* (1984) observed improvements in the compressive strength of the mid-abaxial sidewall region of the pig's hoof when they were supplemented with 1 mg d-biotin/kg feed. However, the hardness of the heel bulb was decreased.

Cunha (1984) noted that in most of the 40 countries he had visited during the past 30 years, biotin deficiency signs were observed in swine operations. Deficiency signs observed under

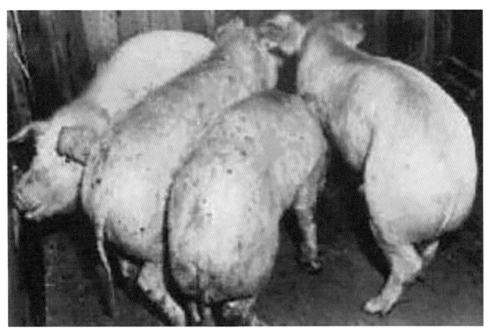

Figure 4.35(a) Biotin deficiency: poor growth and dermatitis. The 2 pigs in the middle are biotin deficient. Note the hair loss and dermatitis (source: Courtesy of T.J. Cunha, Washington State University)

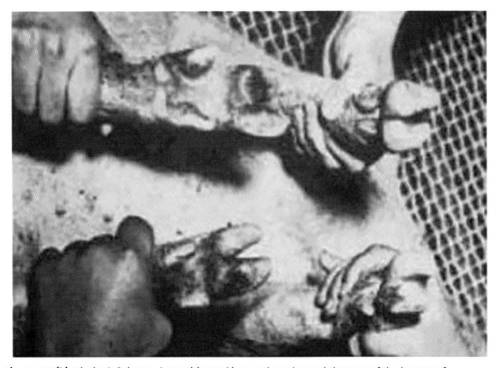

Figure 4.35(b) Biotin deficiency: dermatitis cracking on the soles and the tops of the hooves of biotin-deficient pigs (source: Courtesy of T.J. Cunha, Washington State University)

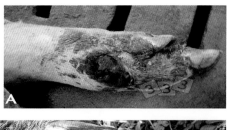
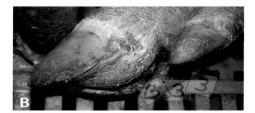
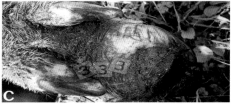

Figure 4.35(c) Biotin deficiency. (A) Septic laminitis. (B) Hoof lesions. (C) Lameness (source: https://www.pig333.com/pig-diseases/biotin-deficiency_13; A and B S. McOrist; C J. Borobia)

field conditions occurred in only 10–20% of sows or fewer. Baby pigs nursing these sows usually showed no biotin deficiency signs but responded to biotin supplementation. Piglets fed milk substitutes with low levels of biotin may have more deficiency signs, and a minimum of 10 µg biotin/kg feed in dry matter is needed for piglets up to 28 days of age (Newport, 1981). Unfortunately, many swine producers believe it is natural for a swine herd to have a few animals with hair loss, dermatitis, and cracked feet. Therefore, they are not overly concerned when a small percentage of sows exhibit these clinical signs (Cunha, 1984). Biotin supplementation in sow diets has significantly improved reproductive performance, including the number of pigs farrowed and weaned, litter weaning weight, and the number of days from weaning to estrus (Brooks *et al.*, 1977; Simmins and Brooks, 1983; Hamilton and Veum, 1984; Misir and Blair, 1984; Bryant *et al.*, 1985c; Kornegay, 1986).

In an earlier study (Brooks *et al.*, 1977), sows fed supplemental biotin had more pigs born alive (9.8 *vs.* 8.1), more pigs weaned (7.8 *vs.* 6.8), increased litter weight at weaning (71.0 *vs.* 64.5 kg) and reduced time interval from weaning to first estrus after weaning (6.2 *vs.* 15.3 days), compared with unsupplemented controls.

In a field study, sows had severe lameness and impaired reproduction (Fonge, 1977; Halama, 1979; Penny *et al.*, 1981). After these sows received supplemental biotin, normal foot health, and reproductive performance were restored. Researchers found that sows housed in total confinement showed a positive response in conception rate and interval from weaning to first estrus and a trend to larger litters when supplemented with biotin (Bryant *et al.*, 1985b).

Biotin deficiency adversely affects cellular and humoral immune function (Camporeale and Zempleni, 2006). The synthesis of antibodies is reduced in biotin-deficient rats. Biotin deficiency in mice decreases the number of spleen cells and the percentage of B lymphocytes in the spleen.

Safety
Studies with swine indicate that these species can safely tolerate dietary biotin levels 4 to 10 times their nutritional requirements (NRC, 1987). Pigs are very tolerant of high levels of biotin, and toxicity is rare because the vitamin is excreted intact (Alhadeff *et al.*, 1984; Mock, 2013; Riveron-Negrete and Fernandez-Mejia, 2017).

Folic acid (vitamin B₉)
Chemical structure and properties
Folacin is the generic descriptor for the original vitamin folic acid and related compounds that qualitatively show folic acid activity. The terms folacin, folate, and folic acid can be used interchangeably and refer to many compounds that possess folic acid's biological activity. Folic acid is structurally one of the most complex vitamins.

The pure substance is designated pterylomonoglutamic acid. The basic folate molecule is 5,6,7,8-tetrahydropteroylglutamate, also referred to as tetrahydrofolate (THF) monoglutamate, which consists of a 2-amino-4-hydroxy-pteridine (pterin) moiety linked via a covalent bond, methylene group at the C-6 position to a p-aminobenzoyl-glutamic acid. Its chemical structure contains 3 distinct parts: glutamic acid, a para-aminobenzoic acid (PABA) residue, and a pteridine nucleus (Figure 4.36).

In most naturally occurring folates, the number of glutamate units in the side chain varies from 5 to 8. The PABA portion of the vitamin structure was once considered a vitamin. Research has shown that if the folic acid requirement of the organism is met, there is no need to add PABA to the diet. Folic acid is a synthetic, fully oxidized monoglutamate form of the vitamin used commercially in supplements, fortified/enriched foods, and feeds (Bailey et al., 2013).

Folic acid is a yellowish-orange crystalline powder that is tasteless, odorless, and insoluble in alcohol, ether, and other organic solvents. It is slightly soluble in hot water in the acid form and more so in the salt form. It is fairly stable exposed to air and heat in neutral and alkaline solutions but unstable in acid solutions. From 70–100% of the folic acid activity is destroyed on autoclaving at pH 1.0 (O'Dell and Hogan, 1943). It is readily degraded by light and UV radiation, and heating can considerably reduce folic acid activity, particularly under oxidative conditions (Gregory, 1989).

Many microorganisms in the large intestine of humans and piglets (Kim et al., 2004) can synthesize folate. In piglets, the folate content of feces was 301.3±145.7 nmol/d, representing 36% of their dietary folate intake. Piglet fecal folate was predominantly present as short-chain folate (68.1±12.6%), with the predominant species being 5-methyl-THF, 29.3±33.2% of which was monoglutamylated. The hindgut microbial production of folate can potentially affect folate status in pigs. However, feed additives can reduce this source. Sulfonamides are the folic acid biosynthetic intermediate PABA analogs widely used as antibacterial agents (Brown, 1962). By competing with PABA, sulfonamides prevent folic acid synthesis so that microorganisms cannot multiply, reducing or eliminating an important source of folic acid to the animal. The stimulation of symbiotic bacterial load in the piglet colon with dietary inulin

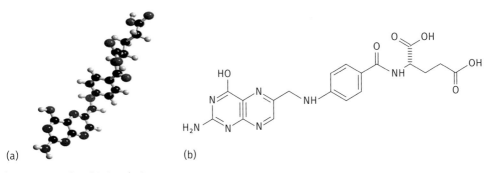

(a) (b)

Figure 4.36 Folic acid chemical structure

and galacto-oligosaccharides was insufficient to modify indices of whole-body folate status (Aufreiter *et al.*, 2011). Consequently, supplementation has been recommended for several years (Lindemann and Kornegay, 1986).

Natural sources
Much of the naturally occurring folic acid in feedstuffs is conjugated with varying numbers of different glutamic acid molecules, reducing its absorption efficiency. Folic acid is present in most of the ingredients of swine diets, almost exclusively THF acid derivatives, especially in those of animal origin, but in insufficient quantity (Lindemann, 1988; Chen, Huang, Lui *et al.*, 2019; Chen, Wang, Li *et al.* 2019). Good sources are soybeans, other beans, nuts, and cereal grains (1.8 mg/kg). It is also found in oilseeds (2.5 mg/kg), especially in whole seeds (soybean 3.5 mg/kg compared with 0.5 mg/kg in soy meal). Products of animal origin also have moderate concentrations (blood meal 0.8 mg/kg, fishmeal between 0.2 and 1.0 mg/kg, whey 0.9 mg/kg, etc.). The stable THF acid derivatives have a methyl or formyl group in the 5-position and generally possess 3 or more glutamic acid residues in glutamyl linkages. Only limited amounts of free folic acid occur in natural products, and most feed sources contain predominantly polyglutamyl folic acid.

The mean availability of folic acid in 7 separate food items was found to be close to 50%, ranging from 37% to 72% in the monoglutamate form (Babu and Skikantia, 1976). The bioavailability of orally administered 5-methyl folic and 5-formyl folic acid was equal to folic acid for rats (Bhandari and Gregory, 1992). Folic acid bioavailability in various foods generally exceeded 70% (Clifford *et al.*, 1990). The bioavailability of monoglutamate folic acid is substantially greater than polyglutamyl forms (Gregory *et al.*, 1991b; Clifford *et al.*, 1990).

A considerable loss of folic acid (50–90%) occurs during feed manufacturing. Folic acid is sensitive to light and heating, particularly in acid solutions. Under aerobic conditions, the destruction of most folic acid forms is significant with heating.

Commercial forms
Spray-dried folic acid and dilutions of crystalline folic acid are the most widely used product forms in animal feeds. Several lines of evidence indicate higher bioavailability of added folic acid than naturally occurring folates in many foods, with approximately 50% lower availability (Gregory, 2001). Synthesized folic acid is the monoglutamate (MG) form.

Supplementation with synthetic pteroylmonoglutamate form, N5-formyl-5,6,7,8,-tetrahydrofolic acid (THFA), or commercial bacterial cell powder sources rich in reduced folates had similar biopotency (Harper *et al.*, 2003). Although folacin is only sparingly soluble in water, sodium salt is quite soluble and is used in injections and feed supplements (McGinnis, 1986).

Metabolism
Absorption and transport
Polyglutamate forms of folic acid are digested via hydrolysis to pteroylmonoglutamate before transport across the intestinal mucosa. The enzyme responsible for the hydrolysis of pteroylpolyglutamate is a carboxy-peptidase known as folate conjugase (Baugh and Krumdieck, 1971). Most likely, several conjugase enzymes are responsible for the hydrolysis of the long-chain folate polyglutamates to the monoglutamates, which then enter the mucosal cell (Rosenberg and Newmann, 1974).

Pteroylmonoglutamate is absorbed predominantly in the duodenum and jejunum, apparently by an active process involving sodium. Folates are also absorbed by a simple diffusion mechanism when concentrations are at pharmacological levels or when the intestinal pH is above 6.0. The uptake of folic acid in the cecum raises the likelihood of absorption of bacterial-derived folic acid.

Most folacin is reduced to tetrahydrofolic acid (FH4) and can also be methylated. Kesavan and Noronha (1983) suggested from rat results that luminal conjugase is a secretion of pancreatic origin. The hydrolysis of folic acid polyglutamate forms occurs in the lumen rather than at the mucosal surface or within the mucosal cell. Studies showed that about 79–88% of labeled folic acid is absorbed, and absorption is rapid since serum concentrations usually peak about 2 hours after ingestion (Harper *et al.*, 1991).

After hydrolysis and absorption from the intestine, dietary folates are transported in plasma as monoglutamate derivatives, predominantly as 5-methyl-tetrahydrofolate. The monoglutamate derivatives then enter cells by specific transport systems. The pteroylpolyglutamates, the primary folic acid form in cells, are built up stepwise by an enzyme, folate polyglutamate synthetase. Polyglutamates keep folic acid within the cells since only the monoglutamate forms are transported across membranes, and only monoglutamates are found in plasma and urine (Wagner, 2001).

Storage and excretion

Folic acid is widely distributed in tissues, mainly in the conjugated polyglutamate forms of folic acid, usually containing 3–7 glutamyl residues linked by peptide bonds. The natural coenzymes are abundant in every tissue examined (Wagner *et al.*, 1984). Specific folate-binding proteins (FBPs) that bind folic acid mono- and polyglutamate are known to exist in many tissues and body fluids, including the liver, kidney, small intestinal brush border membranes, leukemic granulocytes, blood serum, and milk (Tani and Iwai, 1984). Giguère *et al.* (1998) reported a high-affinity FBP in cow, pig, and sheep serum. The physiological roles of these FBPs are unknown. However, they have been suggested to play a role in folic acid transport analogous to the intrinsic factor in the absorption of vitamin B_{12}.

The amount of folate-binding protein secreted by the endometrium during pregnancy was not affected by giving sows daily intravenous infusions of iron and tetrahydrofolate (Vallet *et al.*, 1999). In swine, sequence variation in the secreted iron-binding protein (FBPin) gene is associated with different factors affecting litter size, including ovulation rate, fertilization rate or embryonic survival, and uterine capacity (Thaler *et al.*, 1989; Vallet *et al.*, 1999, 2005). The dietary iron level also may alter folate utilization in sows and piglets (O'Connor *et al.*, 1989). Iron at 125 mg/kg of sow diet was associated with higher folate levels in sow serum and milk and concentrations in piglet livers.

Serum folate levels for gilts fed a single meal containing varying amounts of supplemental folic acid confirm that maximal levels are obtained within 2 hours post-feeding (Harper *et al.*, 1991). Kokue *et al.* (1998) reported that additional synthetic folic acid competes with the reduced folates in the intestinal mucosa for the absorption pathway.

Urinary excretion of folic acid represents a small fraction of total excretion. Fecal folic acid concentrations are quite high, often higher than intake, meaning not only undigested folic acid but, more importantly, the many bacterial syntheses of the vitamin in the intestine. Bile contains high levels of folic acid due to enterohepatic circulation, with most biliary folic acid reabsorbed in the intestine (Bailey *et al.*, 2013).

Biochemical functions

The principal functions of folic acid are related to:

- the synthesis of protein and purines, and pyrimidines, which make up the nucleic acids needed for cell division (Bailey *et al.*, 2013)

- the interconversions of various amino acids
- the maturation process of red corpuscles and the functioning of the immune system.

This means that there are multiple coenzyme forms in transferring one-carbon activity (Bailey *et al.*, 2013). In THF form folic acid is indispensable in transferring single carbon units in various reactions, a role analogous to that of pantothenic acid in the transfer of two-carbon units (Bailey and Gregory, 2006; Bailey *et al.*, 2013). The one-carbon teams can be formyl, methylene, or methyl groups. Some biosynthetic relationships of one-carbon units are shown in Figure 4.37.

The major *in vivo* pathway providing methyl groups involves the transfer of a one-carbon unit from serine to tetrahydrofolate to form 5,10-methylenetetrahydrofolate, which is subsequently reduced to 5-methyltetrahydrofolate. Methyltetrahydrofolate then supplies methyl groups to remethylate homocysteine in the activated methyl cycle, providing methionine for synthesizing the critical methyl donor agent S-adenosylmethionine (Krumdieck, 1990; Jacob *et al.*, 1994; Bailey *et al.*, 2013).

The critical physiological function of THF consists of binding the one-carbon units to the vitamin molecule, thus transforming them to "active formic acid" or "active formaldehyde." These are interconvertible by reduction or oxidation and transferable to appropriate acceptors. Folic acid polyglutamates work at least as well as or better than the corresponding monoglutamate forms in every enzyme system examined (Wagner, 2001). It is now accepted that the pteroylpolyglutamates are the acceptors and donors of one-carbon units in amino acid and nucleotide metabolism, while the monoglutamate is merely a transport form.

Specific reactions involving single carbon transfer by folic acid compounds are:

- purine and pyrimidine synthesis for nuclei acids
- interconversion of serine and glycine

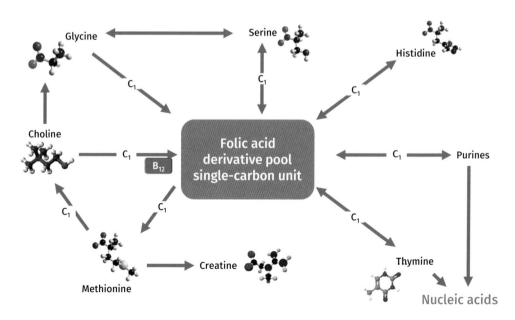

Figure 4.37 Folic acid metabolism requires single carbon units

- glycine–carbon as a source of C_1 units for many syntheses
- histidine degradation
- synthesis of methyl groups for such compounds as methionine, choline, and thymine (a pyrimidine base).

As folacin is involved in the interconversion of serine and glycine, in the degradation of histidine, and in the addition of methyl groups to compounds such as methionine, choline, and thiamine, inadequate levels of other methyl group donors – such as vitamin B_{12}, serine, methionine, betaine, and choline – increase folic acid requirements (Bailey et al., 2013). Logically, high protein levels in the diet raise the dietary recommendations for folate.

Folic acid may play a role in the expression of the hormone leptin and its receptor in early gestation maternal-fetal cross-talk (Pharazyn and Aherne, 1987; Guay et al., 2001). Sows supplemented with 15 ppm folic acid, and 0.6% glycine had lower expression levels of leptin and its receptor in both endometrial and embryonic tissues. This research group discussed this mechanism as a possible explanation of folic acid effects in decreasing embryonic mortality and improving litter size by 10% (Matte et al., 1984b; Tremblay et al., 1986, 1989; Pharazyn and Aherne, 1987; Harper et al., 1989, 1996). Habibzadeh et al. (1986) had reported that supplementation of folic acid and vitamin C during early gestation reduced embryo mortality in guinea pigs.

Folic acid is also essentially involved in all the reactions of labile methyl groups. The metabolism of labile methyl groups plays an essential role in methionine biosynthesis from homocysteine and choline from ethanolamine. Folic acid has a sparing effect on the requirements of choline. The choline chapter discusses the critical role of both folic acid and vitamin B_{12} in synthesizing choline.

Folic acid is needed to maintain the immune system. The blastogenic response of T-lymphocytes to certain mitogens is decreased in folic acid-deficient humans and animals, and the thymus is preferentially altered (Dhur et al., 1991). Its function in metabolism is closely linked to that of vitamin B_{12}, choline, and vitamin C, but also to vitamin B_6 because of its role in reassembling the profile of amino acids circulating in plasma on explicit demand by ribosomes which regulate the process of protein synthesis. Plasma folates change during the life cycle in pigs (Natsuhori et al., 1994).

Several studies have recently been carried out to determine the metabolic functions of folic acid, using piglets as a model because of the similarity between their digestive and circulatory systems and those of humans (Nijhout et al., 2008; Asrar and O'Connor, 2005). These authors emphasize the importance of consuming folic acid in humans to prevent diseases such as megaloblastic anemia, Down's syndrome, and various types of cancer, especially those related to the gastrointestinal tract and leukemia (Shulpekova et al., 2021). These effects are also valid for swine production (Ambrosi et al., 1999; Douglass et al., 2021).

Nutritional assessment

Serum/plasma folate is a good indicator of current folate status and is used as a first-line clinical indicator of folate deficiency. (Sauberlich, 1999). Folates can be measured using HPLC-MS/MS, electrochemical or fluorescence-based techniques, radio- and immuno-based assays, and the traditional *Lactobacillus casei* growth assay. This microbiological approach measures all biologically active folate species, including di- and tri-glutamates of the species, but cannot differentiate between the species (Höller et al., 2018).

As folate and cobalamin (B$_{12}$) jointly participate in one-carbon metabolism and thus have close biological links, both are usually measured concurrently since the deficiency will interact with the blood status markers of the other (Höller *et al.*, 2018).

Deficiency signs

Folacin deficiency produces unspecific symptoms, such as megaloblastic anemia, leucopenia, and growth retardation. Deficiency symptoms are uncommon as microorganisms can synthesize this vitamin in the digestive tract of pigs. However, special attention must be paid to young animals, where intestinal flora is still insignificant, and when substances with antimicrobial action are administered in the feed. Vitamin degradation during storage can also reduce its bioavailability (Yang *et al.*, 2021b) and consequently cause a reduction in plasma levels.

Tissues that have a rapid rate of cell growth or tissue regeneration, such as the epithelial lining of the gastrointestinal tract, epidermis, and bone marrow, are most affected (Hoffbrand, 1978). Until recently, folic acid deficiency in swine had only been produced by the simultaneous feeding of sulfa drugs. Deficiencies were not observed when young pigs were fed only purified diets or natural diets low in folic acid alone (Johnson *et al.*, 1950), indicating that intestinal synthesis was adequate to meet the animal's needs. Feeding a purified diet containing 2% sulfasuxidine to weanling pigs reduced gains and alopecia (Cartwright and Wintrobe, 1949).

The pigs also developed mild normochromic, normocytic anemia. In the bone marrow, there was a decrease in the ratio of leukocytes to erythrocytes and an increase in the number of immature nucleated red blood cells. A positive response was obtained after supplementation with folic acid. Cunha *et al.* (1948) found that folic acid was needed for normal hematopoiesis with 8-week-old pigs fed a purified diet for 21 weeks with sulfasuxidine. Folic acid prevented normocytic anemia, whereas more severe anemia was produced by using a crude folic acid antagonist. A combination of folic acid and biotin was more effective than folic acid in counteracting anemia.

Lindemann and Kornegay (1986) reported that a combination of the antibiotic mixture ASP 250 (includes chlortetracycline, sulfamethazine, and penicillin) and folic acid in a corn-soybean meal diet increased gains and feed consumption with no effect on either fed alone. More severe deficiency signs that responded to folic acid supplementation were induced by feeding diets containing a sulfonamide and a folic acid antagonist (Welch *et al.*, 1947). Under such circumstances, pigs became listless, had a reduced growth rate, and developed diarrhea. Hematologic manifestations were severe macrocytic anemia, leukopenia with a more marked reduction in the number of polymorphonucleocytes, and mild thrombocytopenia (Cartwright *et al.*, 1950). Cartwright *et al.* (1952) reported a combined folic acid and vitamin B$_{12}$ deficiency in pigs receiving a purified soybean protein diet with a folic acid antagonist. The growth rate was reduced, and macrocytic anemia, leukopenia, and neutropenia developed with erythroid hyperplasia of the bone marrow. Folic acid supplementation immediately resulted in a normal blood and bone marrow profile, but growth was decreased, and blood parameters subsequently relapsed.

In addition to sulfa drugs and other folic acid antagonists, moldy feeds can increase the need for the vitamin. In 7 swine feeding trials involving more than 1,000 pigs fed corn with a mold infestation, additional folic acid increased the growth rate to 15% and improved feed efficiency by up to 9% (Purser, 1981). Folic acid supplementation was of no value when regular corn was fed.

Inadequate folic acid has been associated with the suboptimal reproductive performance of sows. A dramatic decrease in serum folic acid concentrations was observed during early and mid-gestation, which may, in part, be associated with embryonic mortality

(Matte *et al.*, 1984a; Pharazyn and Aherne, 1987; Vallet *et al.*, 2005). In another trial, when folic acid was administered intramuscularly according to a schedule that maintained serum folic acid concentrations at approximately the same level between weaning and 60 days of gestation (Matte *et al.*, 1984b; Vallet *et al.*, 1999), the average live litter size was 12 piglets per litter for sows receiving folic acid and flushing treatments compared with 10.5 piglets for sows receiving no treatment.

Lindemann and Kornegay (1989) found the number of matings required per female farrowing was less with folic acid supplements (1.07 *vs.* 1.16 for controls). The effect of folic acid and glycine (to provide a methyl group to folic acid) supplementation was studied on embryo development in early pregnancy (Guay *et al.*, 2002). Folic acid was found to be adequate during the first 25 days of gestation, but in multiparous Yorkshire-Landrace sows, the folic acid + glycine supplement appeared to optimize embryo development. However, Giguère *et al.* (2000) did not observe the effect of folate on uterine prostaglandin. Additional research is required to determine if supplemental dietary folic acid will reduce embryonic death loss under differing management systems to improve the overall efficiency of production (i.e., to optimize pig survival and litter size).

With a folic acid deficiency, there is a reduction in the biosynthesis of nucleic acids essential for cell formation and function. Hence, folic acid deficiency leads to impaired cell division and alterations in protein synthesis. These effects are most noticeable in rapidly growing tissues such as red blood cells, leukocytes, intestinal mucosa, embryos, and fetuses. In the absence of adequate nucleoproteins, normal maturation of primordial red blood cells does not occur, and hematopoiesis is inhibited at the megaloblast stage. As a result of this megaloblastic arrest for normal red blood cell maturation in bone marrow, the first sign of folic acid deficiency is represented by characteristic macrocytic anemia. White blood cell formation is also affected, resulting in thrombopenia, leukopenia, and multi-lobed neutrophils. Vitamin B_{12} is necessary to reduce one-carbon compounds in the oxidation stage of formate and formaldehyde. In this way, it participates with folic acid in the biosynthesis of labile methyl groups (Savage and Lindenbaum, 1995).

The effects of folic acid deficiency on humoral immunity have been more thoroughly investigated in animals than in humans. The antibody responses to several antigens have been shown to decrease. As *de novo* synthesis of methyl groups requires the participation of folic acid coenzymes, the effect of folic acid deficiency on pancreatic exocrine function was examined in rats (Balaghi and Wagner, 1992; Balaghi *et al.*, 1993). Pancreatic secretion was significantly reduced in the deficient group compared with the pair-fed control groups after 5 weeks.

Safety
Folic acid is generally considered a nontoxic vitamin (NRC, 1998). No adverse responses to the ingestion of folic acid have been documented in swine. Fuchs *et al.* (1995) reported that supplying a shock dose of 30 mg/kg every 7 days, which provides much greater levels than the requirement for folic acid, had no adverse effect on changes in selected biochemical and hematologic indices in pregnant sows.

Vitamin C
Chemical structure and properties
Vitamin C is named ascorbic acid (2-oxo-L-threo-hexono-1,4-lactone-2,3-enediol), and there are 4 stereoisomers: D- and L-ascorbic acid and D- and L-isoascorbic acid (with the D-form also named erythorbic acid). However, the term vitamin C refers only to the compounds with L-ascorbic acid activity, which are biologically active, and it includes 2 forms (Figure 4.38):

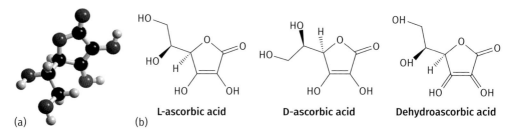

(a)
(b)

L-ascorbic acid   D-ascorbic acid   Dehydroascorbic acid

Figure 4.38 Vitamin C chemical structure

- L-ascorbic acid: reduced form
- dehydro-L-ascorbic acid: oxidized form.

Although in nature, the vitamin is primarily present as ascorbic acid, and both forms are biologically active, but not the D-isomers. In nature, the reduced form of ascorbic acid may reversibly oxidize to the dehydroxidized form, i.e., dehydroascorbic acid (Johnston et al., 2013), and dehydroascorbic acid is irreversibly oxidized to the inactive diketogulonic acid. The latter can be further oxidized to oxalic acid and L-threonic acid. Since this change takes place readily, vitamin C is susceptible to destruction through oxidation, accelerated by heat and light. Reversible oxidation-reduction of ascorbic acid with dehydroascorbic acid is vitamin C's most important chemical property and the basis for its known physiological activities and stabilities (Moser and Bendich, 1991).

Vitamin C is a white to yellow-tinged crystalline powder. It crystallizes, out of water, in square or oblong crystals. It is slightly soluble in acetone and has lower alcohol. A 0.5% solution of ascorbic acid in water is strongly acid with a pH of 3. The vitamin is more stable in acid than in an alkaline medium. Crystalline ascorbic acid is relatively stable in the air without moisture. However, vitamin C is the least stable and, therefore, most easily destroyed of all the vitamins. Several chemical substances, such as air pollutants, industrial toxins, heavy metals, and some pharmacologically active compounds, are antagonistic to vitamin C and can lead to increased vitamin requirements (Johnston et al., 2013).

Natural sources

The main sources of vitamin C are fruits and green plants. Vitamin C occurs in significant quantities in animal organs, such as the liver and kidney, but in only small amounts in meat. However, vitamin C is very low in cereals and oil seeds used in swine nutrition. Post-harvest storage values vary with time, temperature, damage, and enzyme content (Zee et al., 1991; Johnston et al., 2013).

Commercial forms

Ascorbic acid is commercially available as:

- 100% crystalline L-ascorbic acid
- sodium ascorbate
- 97.5% L-ascorbic acid – ethyl cellulose-coated (EC)
- 35% phosphorylated Na/Ca salt of L-ascorbic acid (Ca or Na ascorbyl-2-phosphate; $C_6H_9O_9P$ molecular mass 256.11 g/mol)
- 50% phosphorylated Na salt of L-ascorbic acid (Ca or Na ascorbyl-2-phosphate; $C_6H_6O_9Na_3P \cdot H_2O$ molecular mass 358.08 g/mol).

When providing supplemental ascorbic acid in heat-treated feeds, it is strongly advisable to use a stabilized form like EC-coated or phosphorylated forms. In storage experiments, ascorbic acid protected in this manner was 4 times more stable than untreated ascorbic acid crystals (Kolb, 1984). Adams (1978) reported that EC-coated ascorbic acid showed higher retention after processing than the crystalline form, 84 versus 48%. Retention of ascorbic acid in mash feed was reasonably good, but stability was poor in crumbled meals with elevated storage time and temperature.

Crystalline L-ascorbic acid and L-ascorbyl-2-polyphosphate forms had similar bioavailability (Mahan, 1993). However, a wide variation has been observed in the level of these responses and, therefore, in the zootechnical results obtained, which may be due to diverse factors, including the:

- low stability of vitamin C in feed, which improves significantly in phosphorylated forms and also in drinking water, especially if alkaline and/or unchlorinated (Brown, 1984)
- dietary energy level (Brown *et al.*, 1970, 1971)
- level and duration of dosage (Brown *et al.*, 1975)
- the age of the pigs (Chavez, 1983; Ching and Mahan, 1998)
- intensity and combination of stress factors (Riker *et al.*, 1967; Ivos *et al.*, 1971; Warriss, 1979, 1984; Dvorak, 1984), disease (Strittmatter, 1977), immunological challenge (Schwager and Schulze, 1997, 1998), or injury (Rajkhowa *et al.*, 1996).

Through modern technological advances a form of ascorbic acid is currently being marketed as a phosphate ester, which is stable to heat processing and storage conditions. The product L-ascorbyl-2-monophosphate (Rovimix Stay-C 35®) contains 35% ascorbic acid (Cafantaris, 1996; Schultze and Willy, 1997). The phosphate ester allows the ascorbic acid to withstand heat processing. When entering the digestive tract of swine, the phosphate ester is cleaved off, and the ascorbic acid is available for adsorption. Magnesium-L-ascorbyl-2-phosphate is a stable form of vitamin C that was shown to be available in swine diets (Mahan *et al.*, 1994).

Metabolism
Synthesis
Pigs can synthesize ascorbic acid. L-Gulono-γ-lactone oxidase [EC 1.1.3.8] (GLO) is present in the microsomes of liver cells and is responsible for ascorbic acid biosynthesis. The enzyme converts L-gulono-γ-lactone to L-keto-gulono-γ-lactone, after which L-ascorbic acid is produced through isomerization.

Brown *et al.* (1970, 1971) evaluated the influence of the level of energy and ascorbate supplementation on hydroxyproline excretion in swine. Their data suggested that when energy is limited, the capacity of swine to synthesize ascorbic acid is limited and supplementary ascorbate might increase the polymerization of precursor collagen into stable forms.

GLO activity in fetal pigs at mid-gestation (60 days) is relatively high but declined by ~70% to birth (Ching *et al.*, 2001a). In contrast, fetal liver ascorbic acid concentration increased by 12-fold during this period, suggesting that an increasing amount of ascorbic acid was transferred from the dam as gestation progressed. Consequently, fetal ascorbic acid synthesis appears to be the primary source of the vitamin during early development. During the latter gestation period, however, the maternal source becomes the primary vitamin supplier to the fetus. Sow colostrum and later milk supply a large quantity of ascorbic acid to nursing pigs (Matte and Audet, 2020). These large amounts of ascorbic acid in milk suppress the liver GLO activity of nursing pigs, but upon weaning, the liver GLO activity of pigs increased in a linear manner (Ching *et al.*, 2001b).

Absorption and transport

Vitamin C is absorbed like carbohydrates (monosaccharides) in the small intestine with an availability of 80%. Intestinal absorption in vitamin C-dependent animals requires sodium-dependent vitamin C transporters (SVCT1 and 2) (Johnston, 2006; Johnston *et al.*, 2013). It is assumed that those not-scurvy-prone species like swine have an absorption mechanism through diffusion, mainly in the duodenum and jejunum (Spencer *et al.*, 1963).

Ascorbic acid is readily absorbed when the quantities ingested are small, but limited intestinal absorption occurs when excess ascorbic acid is ingested. The bioavailability of vitamin C in feeds is limited, but 80–90% appears to be absorbed (Kallner *et al.*, 1977). In experimental animals, the absorption site in guinea pigs is in the duodenal and proximal small intestine, whereas in rats the highest absorption takes place in the ileum (Hornig *et al.*, 1984).

In its metabolism, ascorbic acid is first converted to dehydroascorbate by several enzymes or non-enzymatic processes and can then be reduced back to ascorbic acid in cells (Johnston *et al.*, 2013). Absorbed vitamin C readily equilibrates with the body pool of the vitamin. No specific binding proteins for ascorbic acid have been reported, and it is suggested that the vitamin is retained by binding to subcellular structures.

Storage and excretion

Ascorbic acid is widely distributed throughout the tissues in animals capable of synthesizing vitamin C and in those dependent on an adequate dietary amount of the vitamin. In experimental animals, the highest concentrations of vitamin C are found in the pituitary and adrenal glands, and high levels are also found in the liver, spleen, brain, and pancreas. Tissue levels are decreased by virtually all forms of stress, which also stimulates the biosynthesis of the vitamin in those animals capable of synthesis.

Ascorbic acid is excreted mainly in urine, with small amounts in sweat and feces. In guinea pigs, rats, and rabbits, oxidation to carbon dioxide is the major excretory mechanism for vitamin C. Primates generally do not utilize the carbon dioxide catabolic pathway, with the major loss occurring in the urine. Urinary excretion of vitamin C depends on body stores, intake, and renal function.

Biochemical functions

Unlike other species, pigs can synthesize ascorbic acid from glucose in the liver (Brown and King, 1977) depending on the animal's live weight (Ching and Mahan, 1998; Johnston, 2006). Evidence suggests that in some circumstances, this endogenous synthesis may be insufficient (Riker *et al.*, 1967; McCampbell *et al.*, 1974; Chiang *et al.*, 1985). The capacity for vitamin C synthesis varies with age and hereditary predisposition. Palludan and Wegger (1984) studied plasma concentration at 11–14 weeks of life in pigs from different litters, which were handled identically and observed a considerable degree of homogeneity in the values among pigs of the same litter but marked differences between litters, with average values between 1.8 and 5.6 mg/l. Ascorbic acid is involved in fundamental biological and metabolic processes, and its function is related to its reversible oxidation and reduction characteristics. Its action is essential in the following:

- calcification processes
- immune response

- adaptation to stress
- maintenance of electrolytic balance.

Vitamin C's biochemical and physiological functions have been reviewed (Moser and Bendich, 1991; Padh, 1991; Gershoff, 1993; Johnston, 2006; Johnston *et al.*, 2013). However, the exact role of this vitamin in the living system is not entirely understood since a coenzyme form has not yet been reported.

In more detail, the main biochemical functions of vitamin C are (Figure 4.39):

- antioxidant and immune role (stimulation of phagocytic activity)
- biosynthesis of collagen
- control of glucocorticoid synthesis
- conversion of vitamin D_3 to its active form
- absorption of minerals (iron).

Antioxidant and immune role (stimulation of phagocytic activity)

One of the most interesting properties of vitamin C is its ability to act as a reducing agent or electron donor. Ascorbic acid converts to dehydroascorbic acid and is subsequently reduced in the cell cytoplasm, playing an essential part in electron transfer (oxidation-reduction). It reacts rapidly with free radicals and acts synergistically with vitamin E, facilitating the regeneration of the reduced form of α-tocopherol in biological systems (Kornegay *et al.*, 1986; Eichenberger *et al.*, 2004), hence accounting for the observed sparing effect on this vitamin (Jacob, 1995). In the process of sparing fatty acid oxidation, tocopherol is oxidized to the tocopheryl free radical. Ascorbic acid can donate an electron to the tocopheryl free radical, regenerating the reduced antioxidant form of tocopherol (Hoppe *et al.*, 1989).

Tissue defense mechanisms against free-radical damage generally include vitamin C, vitamin E, and β-carotene as the major vitamin antioxidant sources. In addition, several metalloenzymes that include glutathione peroxidase (selenium), catalase (iron), and superoxide

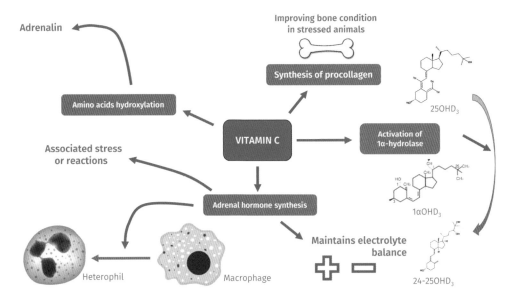

Figure 4.39 Some vitamin C biochemical functions

dismutase (copper, zinc, and manganese) are also critical in protecting the internal cellular constituents from oxidative damage (Yen *et al.*, 1985).

The dietary and tissue balance of all these nutrients is vital in protecting tissue against free-radical damage (Benito and Bosch, 1997; Cadenas *et al.*, 1998). Both *in vitro* and *in vivo* studies showed that antioxidant vitamins generally enhance cellular and noncellular immunity (Mahan, 1994b). The antioxidant function of these vitamins could, at least in part, enhance immunity by maintaining the functional and structural integrity of critical immune cells. A compromised immune system will reduce animal production efficiency through increased susceptibility to diseases, thereby leading to increased animal morbidity and mortality (Williams *et al.*, 1997; Lauridsen and Jensen, 2005).

Ascorbic acid is reported to have a stimulating effect on the phagocytic activity of leukocytes, the function of the reticuloendothelial system, and the formation of antibodies. Ascorbic acid levels are very high in phagocytic cells, with these cells using free radicals and other highly reactive oxygen-containing molecules to help kill pathogens that invade the body. Ascorbic acid, as an effective scavenger of ROS, minimizes the oxidative stress associated with the respiratory burst of activated phagocytic leukocytes, thereby functioning to control the inflammation and tissue damage associated with immune responses (Rojas *et al.*, 1996; Chien *et al.*, 2004; Bacou *et al.*, 2021).

Biosynthesis of collagen
The beneficial effects of ascorbic acid in collagen biosynthesis are extensively documented and represent the most clearly established role for vitamin C. Collagens are the tough, fibrous, intercellular materials (proteins) that are the principal components of skin and connective tissue, the organic matrix of bones and teeth and the ground substance between cells (Moser and Bendich, 1991; Padh, 1991; Gershoff, 1993; Tsuchiya and Bates, 1997; Johnston, 2006; Johnston *et al.*, 2013).

In the case of vitamin C deficiency, the impairment of collagen synthesis appears to be due to lowered ability to hydroxylate lysine and proline, which constitutes the basis for the crossover of tropocollagen molecules, giving rise to structures of great size and consistency. Also, its hydroxylation capacity is essential in carnitine synthesis and may be indirectly involved in fatty acid and cholesterol metabolism (Hutagalung *et al.*, 1969). In addition to the relationship of ascorbic acid to hydroxylase enzymes, Franceschi (1992) suggests that vitamin C is required for the differentiation of connective tissue such as muscle, cartilage, and bone derived from mesenchyme (embryonic cells capable of developing into connective tissue). Beneficial effects result from ascorbic acid synthesizing "repair" collagen. Alteration of basement membrane collagen synthesis and its integrity in the mucosal epithelium during vitamin C restriction might explain the mechanism by which the capillary fragility is induced in scurvy and the increased incidences of periodontal disease under vitamin C deprivation. Failure of wounds to heal and gum and bone changes resulting from vitamin C undernutrition are direct consequences of reducing insoluble collagen fibers. Ascorbic acid is a cofactor in extracellular matrix metabolism because it affects collagen, laminin, various cell-surface integrins, and elastin. Vitamin C is a cofactor for enzymes key to the post-translational modification of matrix proteins (Johnston *et al.*, 2013).

Ascorbic acid is thought to contribute to the prevention of muscle degeneration causing pale, soft, and exudative pork (Rajic, 1971; Sevkovic *et al.*, 1976), and affecting meat color (Rajic *et al.*, 1977). It is proposed that the collagen matrix produced by ascorbic acid-treated cells provides a permissive environment for tissue-specific gene expression. A common finding in all studies is that vitamin C can alter the expression of multiple genes as cells progress through specific differentiation programs (Ikeda et al., 1997).

Control of glucocorticoid synthesis
Vitamin C controls the synthesis of glucocorticoid norepinephrine in the adrenal gland. The protective effects of vitamin C (also vitamin E) on health may partially result from reducing glucocorticoid circulating levels (Nockels, 1990). During stress conditions (e.g., heat stress, weaning), glucocorticoids, which suppress the immune response, are elevated (Yen et al., 1985). Vitamin C reduces adrenal glucocorticoid synthesis, helping to maintain immunocompetence.

Conversion of vitamin D_3 to its active form
Because of its relationship to hydroxylation enzymes, vitamin C directly affects the C-1 hydroxylation of $25OHD_3$ to the active form $1,25(OH)_2D_3$ (Suter, 1990; Cantatore et al., 1991).

Absorption of minerals (iron)
Ascorbic acid has a role in metal ion metabolism due to its reducing and chelating properties. This results in enhanced absorption of minerals from the diet and their mobilization and distribution throughout the body. Ascorbic acid promotes non-heme iron absorption from food (Olivares et al., 1997). It reduces the ferric iron at the acid pH in the stomach and forms complexes with iron ions that stay in solution at alkaline conditions in the duodenum (Volker et al., 1984).

Some other functions of ascorbic acid are the following.

1   Owing to the ease with which ascorbic acid can be oxidized and reversibly reduced, it probably plays an essential role in reactions involving electron transfer in the cell. Almost all terminal oxidases in plant and animal tissues can directly or indirectly catalyze the oxidation of L-ascorbic acid. Such enzymes include ascorbic acid oxidase, cytochrome oxidase, phenolase, and peroxidase. In addition, its oxidation is readily induced under aerobic conditions by many metal ions and quinones.

2   Ascorbic acid has a role in the metabolic oxidation of specific amino acids, including tyrosine.

3   Carnitine is synthesized from lysine and methionine and depends on 2 hydroxylases containing ferrous iron and L-ascorbic acid. Vitamin C deficiency can reduce the formation of carnitine, resulting in the accumulation of triglycerides in the blood and the physical fatigue and lassitude associated with scurvy (Ha et al., 1994). About 98% of total body carnitine is in muscle; skeletal and heart muscle carnitine concentrations are reduced by 50% in vitamin C-deficient guinea pigs compared with controls (Johnston et al., 2013).

4   Interrelationships between vitamin C and the B vitamins are known: tissue levels and urinary excretion of vitamin C are affected in animals in case of deficiencies of thiamine, riboflavin, pantothenic acid, folic acid, and biotin.

5   Vitamin C has been demonstrated to inhibit nitrosamines, which are potent carcinogens (Mirvish, 1986).

6   Ascorbic acid is found in up to a 10-fold concentration in seminal fluid compared to serum levels and decreasing levels have caused nonspecific sperm agglutination (Dvorak and Podany, 1966, 1971; Cleveland et al., 1983; Lin et al., 1985; Palludan and Wegger, 1988). In a review of ascorbic acid and fertility, Luck et al. (1995) suggested 3 of ascorbic acid's principal functions: its promotion of collagen synthesis, its role in hormone production, and its ability to protect cells from free radicals, which may explain its reproductive actions.

7   Vitamin C has a biological role in keratinocytes. Because the skin must provide the first line of defense against environmental free-radical attack (e.g., sunburn, skin aging, and skin cancer), it has developed a complex antioxidant network that includes enzymatic and non-enzymatic components (Duarte and Almeida, 2012). The epidermis is composed of several layers of keratinocytes supplied with enzymes (superoxide dismutase, catalase, thioredoxin reductase, and glutathione reductase) and low-molecular-weight antioxidant molecules (tocopherol, glutathione, and ascorbic acid) (Podda and Grundmann-Kollmann, 2001). Furthermore, since ascorbic acid is essential in collagen formation, its presence increases the capacity to heal skin wounds, as observed in chickens (Rajkhowa *et al.*, 1996) and humans (Vaxman *et al.*, 1995; Duarte and Almeida, 2012). In pigs, Darr *et al.* (1992) reported that topical application of vitamin C elevates its levels, which correlates with skin protection from UVB damage measured by erythema and sunburn cell formation. This protection is related to the reducing properties of the molecule. In addition, vitamin C protects porcine skin from UV light-mediated phototoxic reactions. In keratinocytes, vitamin C counteracts oxidative stress via transcriptional and post-translational mechanisms. Vitamin C can: (a) act directly by scavenging ROS generated by stressors; (b) prevent ROS-mediated cell damage by modulating gene expression; (c) regulate keratinocyte differentiation by maintaining a balanced redox state; and (d) promote cell cycle arrest and apoptosis in response to DNA damage (Catani *et al.*, 2005). Pullar *et al.* (2017) reviewed the roles of vitamin C in skin health.
8   Vitamin C is also involved in many hormone activation processes. Hormones like melanotropins, calcitonin, growth hormone-releasing factors, corticotrophin and thyrotropin, vasopressin, oxytocin, cholecystokinin, and gastrin undergo amidations where ascorbic acid serves as a reductant to maintain copper in a reduced state at the active site of the enzyme (Johnston *et al.*, 2013).
9   The high concentration of vitamin C in the testicle (Lin *et al.*, 1985; Lechowski, 2009; Horký *et al.*, 2016; Lechowski *et al.*, 2018) and ovarian corpus luteum (Petroff *et al.*, 1996) suggests a physiological role linked to reproduction (Yen and Pond, 1983; Palludan and Wegger, 1988; Carmona-Garcia, 1984; Audet *et al.*, 2004).

Nutritional assessment

Several biological compartments, such as whole blood, erythrocytes, leucocytes, and plasma or serum, can be used to assess vitamin C status. However, serum or plasma ascorbate concentration is the most reliable marker (Rojas *et al.*, 1996). Analysis of ascorbic acid in biological samples is complicated by the high susceptibility of this compound to oxidation which requires the use, for example, of EDTA (Höller *et al.*, 2018).

Several approaches have been developed to measure vitamin C in biological materials: HPLC provides an efficient means to quantify vitamin C with good selectivity and sensitivity (Höller *et al.*, 2018).

Deficiency signs

According to Zintzen (1975), the signs of vitamin C deficiency in swine include weakness, fatigue, dyspnea, bone pain, skin hemorrhages, musculature, adipose tissue, and specific organs (e.g., liver, spleen, and brain). Schwager and Schulze (1998) suggested that ascorbic acid is involved in pigs' osteoblast formation, matrix mineralization, and bone resorption. In research with a relatively small number of pigs conducted by Grøndalen and Hansen (1981), there was a tendency for less severity of lesions in the elbow joint, distal epiphysial ulna plate, or medial femur condyle in pigs that received vitamin C supplementation versus control pigs.

Ascorbic acid appears to play a prominent role in collagen synthesis related to the hydroxylation of proline and lysine intracellularly during the formation of tropocollagen. Therefore, some of the effects of vitamin C deficiency are due to collagen failing to cross-link correctly and the lack of hydroxyproline and hydroxylysine. A specific clinical leg-weakness syndrome in growing pigs manifests as crooked and (or) deviated forelegs. These signs are indicated by contracted flexor tendons and weak joint ligaments, which become apparent in pigs weighing 30–45 kg and seem to indicate an impaired development in growing loaded connective tissues (Nielsen and Vinther, 1984).

Ascorbic acid deficiency and reproduction

According to Chatterjee (1967), degeneration of the ovaries and testes occurs in guinea pigs on an ascorbic acid-free diet, but the effects are associated with general inanition. There is evidence for reduced testosterone synthesis by Leydig cells in the testes of vitamin C-deficient male guinea pigs. The precise role of ascorbic acid in sex steroid biosynthesis has not been established.

In females, there are considerable demands for collagen synthesis and degradation during pregnancy as uterine growth, placental development, and fetal development depend on rapid increases in connective tissue components, of which ascorbic acid plays a critical role.

In a study of pregnant sows, Wegger (1994) reported that maternal ascorbic acid deficiency impairs mineralization in fetal bone and normal osteoid formation. Defective collagen synthesis and decreased proteoglycan synthesis were suggested to be involved. Wegger and Palludan (1994) described the skeletal abnormalities during fetal development in swine resulting from maternal vitamin C deficiency (Figure 4.40).

Ascorbic acid is also known to enhance iron absorption from the intestine (Volker *et al.*, 1984). In hematopoiesis, ascorbic acid facilitates the transfer of iron from transferrin (a plasma protein) to ferritin (an organ protein), which stores iron in the bone marrow, spleen, and liver. Ascorbic acid deficiency disrupts this iron transport between blood plasma and storage organs.

In the reproductive tissues of the sow, the transfer of iron from uteroferrin to transferrin (Buhi, 1981) is likewise facilitated by ascorbic acid. Gipp *et al.* (1974) reported dietary ascorbic acid supplementation increased the plasma iron level, the degree of saturation of plasma transferrin, and the rate of removal from plasma and uptake by red blood cells of iron-59. They suggested that ascorbic acid may help overcome iron deficiency induced by high dietary copper either by interfering with copper absorption or increasing iron absorption and utilization.

Voelker and Carlton (1969) had reported previously that excess dietary ascorbic acid had adverse effects on the absorption, transport, and excretion of copper in miniature swine. These interactions between ascorbic acid and copper were also discussed by Tsuchiya and Bates (1997), who concluded that copper intake significantly affected blood and tissue copper concentrations and superoxide dismutase activity, and ascorbic acid intake significantly affected adrenal ascorbate levels and the deoxypyridinoline:pyridinoline cross-links ratio, especially in bone. Perks and Miller (1996) added ascorbic acid to iron-fortified cow's milk. They could not detect a long-term effect of ascorbic acid on iron absorption when fortified milk was supplied to piglets.

Uteroferrin is a purple, progesterone-induced glycoprotein secreted by the sow and mare's uterine endometrial epithelium. It transports iron to the developing conceptus (Roberts and Bazer, 1980). Presumably, this is achieved by the ascorbic acid acting as a chelator to transfer iron from uteroferrin to transferrin. Transferrin would then transfer iron to cells of the hematopoietic system of the liver, spleen, and bone marrow to meet the need for hemoglobin

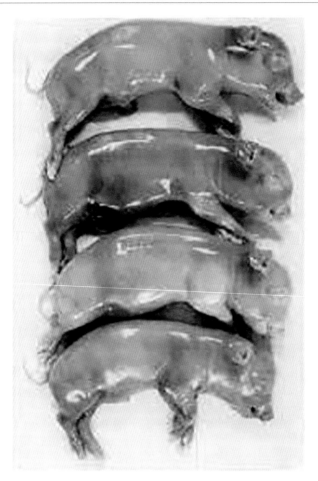

Figure 4.40 Vitamin C deficiency: hematological and skeletal abnormalities during fetal development in swine (source: Wegger and Palludan, 1994)

synthesis and erythrocyte development. This process begins around day 14 of pregnancy as blood islets form in the yolk sac endoderm and continue until the end of pregnancy when the hematopoietic centers reside principally in the bone marrow.

The ascorbic acid content in the sow's uterus increases during early pregnancy with a doubling in uterine length and a significant increase in uterine collagen content (Renegar *et al.*, 1981). The placental membranes and fetuses are also rich in collagen, the synthesis of which is dependent upon vitamin C.

The possible role of ascorbic acid in steroid metabolism within the pregnant uterus is unknown. However, the decreased cholesterol content of the adrenal gland is characteristic of ascorbic acid-deficient guinea pigs and would reduce substrate availability for the synthesis of sex steroids (Chatterjee, 1967). The interconversion of $NADPH_2$ and NADPH can be influenced by the electron transfer from ascorbic acid to dehydroascorbic acid. The production of reducing equivalents ($NADPH_2$) is required for numerous hydroxylation reactions in sex steroid biosynthesis.

The establishment and maintenance of pregnancy in all farm animals depend upon the maintenance of a corpus luteum that produces progesterone and, in some species, estrogen production by the placenta. Since adequate ascorbic acid concentrations in tissue may be essential for normal sex steroid metabolism by ovarian and fetal-placental tissue, vitamin C would appear crucial to the reproductive process. Petroff *et al.* (1996) measured total ascorbate and oxidized ascorbate levels in the ovarian stroma, follicles, and corpora lutea throughout the estrus cycle and during pregnancy. They reported that maximal luteal and follicular function periods are associated with elevated concentrations of total ascorbate within these tissues. In addition, aging of the corpora lutea was associated with a high partitioning of reduced ascorbate. Petroff *et al.* (1996) demonstrated that prostaglandin (PGF_2) depletes the porcine corpus luteum of vitamin C by inducing the secretion of the vitamin into the bloodstream. Thus, these findings support the hypothesis that vitamin C depletion contributes to the demise of the porcine corpus luteum.

Ivos *et al.* (1971) reported an inverse relationship between ambient temperature and conception rate in sows. Additionally, these authors reported that the average conception rate in sows increased when boars were supplemented with either 1 or 2 g of ascorbic acid daily compared to controls. Lin *et al.* (1985) observed increased sperm concentration per ejaculate in heat-stressed working boars that received 300 mg of ascorbic acid daily compared to unsupplemented boars. Boars that received the supplemental ascorbic acid also had fewer abnormal sperm cells per ejaculation. Using a Danish mutant strain of pigs unable to synthesize ascorbic acid – osteogenic disorder (OD) pigs – Palludan and Wegger (1988) investigated the influence of ascorbic acid status on boar performance. Boars from the OD line had histologic anomalies in the spermatogenic epithelium.

Dvorak and Podany (1971) indicated that the high ascorbic acid content of boar testes is related to the optimum development of the gonad. Healthy, fertile boar testis averaged 0.4 mg ascorbic acid per gram, greater than the liver's ascorbic acid concentration. Testis' total ascorbic acid content decreases to about 250 mg in adult life (Dvorak and Podany, 1966). Dvorak (1984) reported that the ascorbic acid concentration in boar semen was higher than in blood serum. However, the concentration of ascorbic acid is affected by accessory gland secretion. He also indicated that the high ascorbic acid level of the male gonadal glands is related to reproductive function. This also applies to accessory glands, as evidenced by the ascorbic acid concentration of these tissues, and their secretions were reduced by half one month after castration (Dvorak and Podany, 1971). The role of ascorbic acid in these processes is likely associated with producing male reproductive cells.

Ascorbic acid's high concentration in semen is a physiological manifestation of the sexual activity of the boar and, therefore, a desirable characteristic. Disease conditions have been found to affect vitamin C metabolism. Vitamin C can protect tissues by enhancing humoral and cellular immune responses to disease (Nockels, 1988). With a vitamin C deficiency, impaired chemotaxis in macrophages and depressed T-lymphocyte response have been reported (Beisel, 1982). Mozalene *et al.* (1991) reported that dietary vitamin C had a normalizing effect in pigs on the pathologic reaction induced by infection with *Trichuris suis*. Their conclusion was based on ceruloplasmin levels, indicative of the degree of inflammatory response and changed immunological reactivity of the host.

Vitamin C deficiency in young and growing pigs.
Swine nutritionists have generally formulated diets without vitamin C because the young pig can synthesize ascorbic acid within 1 week of birth, as demonstrated by Braude *et al.* (1950), and both sow colostrum and milk are a source of the vitamin to the nursing pig (Wegger and Palludan, 1984). Hidiroglou and Batra (1995) indicated that the ascorbic acid content of colostrum is more than twice that of the subsequently produced milk when measured

at 7 days of age. In addition, the concentration of ascorbic acid in the plasma of piglets at birth (13.1 mg/ml) following colostrum uptake slowly declined during the first 28 days of age to 3.2 mg/ml. Birke *et al.* (1993), in a study with a minimal number of sows, indicated that restriction of milk intake in piglets, by allowing only 12 hours of suckling per day, did not influence plasma or tissue ascorbic acid content. The NRC (1998 and 2012) suggested that including vitamin C in swine diets is unnecessary.

However, the modern pig may not be able to synthesize adequate amounts of ascorbic acid to meet its need during periods of adverse environmental conditions, disease, or exposure to other stressors (Wariss, 1984). Some swine researchers have indicated that under certain situations, pigs may need supplemental vitamin C for maximum weight gain and feed use (Mahan *et al.*, 1966; Yen and Pond, 1981; Mahan and Saif, 1983; Mahan *et al.*, 1994; de Rodas *et al.*, 1998). However, nearly an equal number of reports did not show enhanced performance (Brown *et al.*, 1970; Partridge and Brown, 1971; Leibbrandt, 1977; Yen and Pond, 1983, 1984, 1987; NRC, 1998, 2012). This inconsistency may be because unpredictable environmental and psycho-logical stresses imposed on swine may increase requirements for ascorbic acid. In explaining the lack of vitamin C effect on weight gain in their study, Yen and Pond (1988) suggested that the weight gain of the control pigs was so high that further improvement by dietary manipu-lation may have been unachievable. The age of the pigs studied can influence the response to vitamin C (Mahan *et al.*, 1994). Likewise, Cromwell *et al.* (1969, 1970) reported no benefit in adding vitamin C to the diets of growing pigs.

The level of available dietary energy is a significant factor in determining the amount of ascorbic acid available to the pig (Brown *et al.*, 1970, 1975; Brown, 1984). Serum ascorbic acid concentrations and urinary output are directly related to the level of energy in the diet. It was also found that minor stress, such as individual penning, will evoke a positive growth response from supplementary ascorbic acid, especially in animals fed a "low-energy" diet. Dietary energy can cause a shift in ascorbic acid synthesis because of restrictions on the amount of free glucose available for this synthesis. Brown and King (1977) suggested that glucose levels may control the production of ascorbic acid. Dvorak (1974b) also concluded that glucose con-centration is an important and positive factor influencing the amount of endogenous synthesis of ascorbic acid.

When there is a need for dietary vitamin C, the newly weaned pig is the class of swine most likely to be deficient. Sow's milk contains a high concentration of vitamin C at parturition, but the level drops dramatically toward weaning. For the baby pig, the general consensus is that ascorbic acid blood level increases with colostrum intake, drops at weaning and slowly increases after 7 weeks to the mature level (Wegger and Palludan, 1984).

Handling practices at weaning (especially early weaning), which are generally considered stressful, including transport and mixing with unfamiliar pigs, have been shown to deplete ascorbate from the body in the same way that endotoxins do (Rojas *et al.*, 1996). Wariss (1979) investigated the concentration of ascorbic acid in the adrenal glands of pigs subjected to var-ious pre-slaughter treatments. Wariss (1979) concluded that depletion of ascorbic acid from the adrenal glands could be utilized as a measure of the stress experienced by animals during the pre-slaughter period. Wariss (1981) also investigated the effect of body size on ascorbic acid content and the weight of adrenal glands. He concluded that in pigs, the concentration of ascorbic acid remained relatively constant as body size increased while the relative adrenal gland weight decreased. However, Kornegay *et al.* (1986) did not find a significant effect of nursery temperature on the response of weanling pigs to supplemental vitamin C.

The humoral immune response and corticoid levels were not yet influenced by supplemen-tal vitamin C, in view of decreased plasma vitamin C concentration and dramatic nutritional and social changes. Other environmental factors associated with weaning suggested that the beneficial response from supplemental vitamin C with weanling pigs might be related to the suppression of post-weaning subclinical disease (Yen and Pond, 1981). In a study with growing pigs between the age of 4 and 7 weeks, Park and Harrison (1990) reported an improvement in nursing pig performance (6% improvement in daily gain; 5% improvement in gain:feed) resulting from vitamin C supplementation in tap drinking water.

Spontaneous scurvy due to a genetic defect was observed in a swine production herd among 2–3-week-old piglets (Jensen et al., 1983; Jensen and Basse, 1984). Closer observation revealed that all pigs were from the same boar. Analysis of their blood and tissues revealed only a minimal concentration of vitamin C. The 3 : 1 ratio between normal and affected pigs was characteristic of simple autosomal recessive inheritance in matings between nonaffected carriers. Liver microsomes were shown incapable of synthesizing ascorbic acid *in vitro*, even with L-gulonolactone as substrate (Jensen and Basse, 1984). Schwager and Schulze (1997, 1998) utilized vitamin E-deficient pigs as animal models to investigate the effect of ascorbic acid on lymphocytes and leukocytes. They reported that ascorbic acid selectively influences the proliferation of B-lymphocytes and negatively acts on interleukin-2 production by T-lymphocytes when a threshold of saturation is exceeded. Furthermore, ascorbic acid influences leukocyte function as the production of reactive oxygen intermediates by polymorphonuclear leukocytes decreased in pigs supplemented with ascorbic acid. In agreement with other evidence that vitamin C has a stimulatory effect on the immune responsiveness of swine, Kristensen et al. (1986) indicated that vitamin C-deficient pigs' lymphocytes had a reduced response to the mitogens concanavalin A and phytohemagglutinin.

Safety
Several studies with poultry, swine, and laboratory animals had shown no deleterious effect when the animals were fed high levels of vitamin C (NRC, 1998). Research with swine (Brown *et al.*, 1975; Chavez, 1983) has indicated that the dietary vitamin C intake of as much as 1% of the diet did not adversely affect the animals. These studies, however, were less than 60 days in duration. In guinea pigs, extremely high levels (8.7%) fed for 6 weeks caused decreased bone density and decreased urinary hydroxyproline compared to control animals fed 0.2% ascorbic acid (Bray and Briggs, 1984). However, no significant bone changes were observed.

Choline
Chemical structure and properties
Choline is considered a vitamin, although it does not fulfill some of the prerequisites of this definition. For example, pigs require high quantities of choline (less than 1%), similar to amino and essential fatty acids. It can be synthesized in the liver of pigs from serine and methyl groups, requiring 3 moles of methionine for each mole of choline synthesized. However, for most metabolic processes, the quantity and rate of synthesis are insufficient to cover requirements, especially when the supply of precursors such as methionine, vitamin B_{12}, or folacin is limited.

Choline is a β-hydroxyethyl-trimethyl-ammonium hydroxide (Figure 4.41). Pure choline is a colorless, viscous, strongly alkaline liquid that is notably hygroscopic. Choline is soluble in water, formaldehyde, and alcohol and has no definite melting or boiling point. The chloride salt of this compound, choline chloride, is produced by chemical synthesis for use in the feed industry, although there are other forms. Choline chloride consists of deliquescent white crystals, which are very soluble in water and alcohol. Aqueous solutions are almost pH neutral (Jiang *et al.*, 2013).

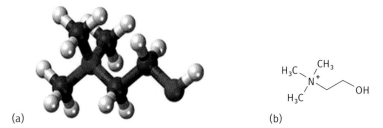

(a)   (b)

Figure 4.41 Choline structure

Natural sources

All naturally occurring fats contain some choline, and thus, it is supplied by all feeds that contain fat. Egg yolk, glandular meats, and the brain are the richest animal sources, whereas the
germ of cereals, legumes, and oilseed meals are the best plant sources (DuCoa, 1994). Corn is
low in choline, with wheat, barley, and oats containing approximately twice as much choline
as corn.

Choline in all plant and animal cells is mainly in the form of the phospholipids phosphatidylcholine (lecithin), lysophosphatidylcholine, choline plasmalogens, and, to a lesser
extent, in free form or as sphingomyelin – essential components of all membranes (Zeisel,
1990).

Since betaine can spare the choline requirements, it would be helpful to know its concentration in feeds. Unfortunately, most feedstuffs contain only small amounts of betaine.
However, wheat and wheat by-products contain over twice as much betaine as choline. Thus,
the choline needs of swine fed with wheat-based diets would be much lower than those provided based on other grains. Sugar beets are also high in betaine.

Little is known about the biological availability of choline in natural feedstuffs. Using a
chick assay method it has been assessed that in soybean, canola, and peanut meals a substantial proportion of choline is unavailable (Emmert and Baker, 1997). However, according to
Chen, Huang, Liu et al. (2019) and Chen, Wang, Li et al. (2019) in dehulled regular soybean meal
and whole soybeans, availability ranges from 75 to 100%. The availability of choline is 100% in
corn. Soybean lecithin products are equivalent to choline chloride in bioavailability (Emmert
and Baker, 1997). Although 3 times as rich in total choline as soybean meal, canola meal has
less bioavailable choline (Emmert and Baker, 1997). In their work with chicks, the production of
trimethylamine (resulting from bacterial degradation of choline) in the intestine was greater
in chicks fed canola meal than in those fed soybean meals.

Commercial forms

Commercially, choline is produced by chemical synthesis, and choline salts are used in dietary
supplementation (Hongtrakul et al., 1997). The available forms are:

• choline chloride 75% solution in water
• choline chloride on a carrier (50–70 wt. %)
• choline chloride crystals (>95%).

The 75% liquid is very corrosive and requires special storage and handling equipment. It
is not suitable for inclusion in concentrated vitamin premixes but is most economical to add
directly to concentrate swine feed mixtures. The physical properties of choline chloride should

be considered for mixing and storing vitamins and vitamin–trace mineral premixes, especially if they will be stored for several months. Choline chloride is highly hygroscopic and can attract moisture to vitamin and vitamin–trace mineral premixes.

Coelho (2002) concluded that after 6 months of storage, the loss of vitamin in a vitamin premix without choline chloride was 1–5%. But, with choline chloride in the premix, the vitamin losses were up to 32% of its activity. In a vitamin–trace mineral premix, the impacts were even more harmful. Without the choline in the vitamin–trace mineral premix, after 6 months of storage, the loss of vitamins was 12–30%, but with the choline chloride, vitamins lost was 23–52%. Yang et al. (2021d) reported that choline (40,000 mg/kg) and high concentrations of copper (500 mg/kg) and zinc (8,000 mg/kg) significantly increased vitamin A, K_3, B_1, and B_2 loss during storage ($p<0.05$). These values are lower than previously reported in the literature about vitamin stability in the presence of chloride, copper, and zinc. The reason is that most vitamin products have improved stability in the past years (Yang et al., 2021d).

Metabolism
Synthesis
Most animals can significantly synthesize choline (Chan, 1991; Garrow, 2007). Therefore, absorption from the intestine may not be critical under normal conditions. The biosynthesis of choline results from the decarboxylation of the amino acid serine to ethanolamine in a pyridoxal dependent reaction. Ethanolamine is then progressively methylated to form choline. Excess dietary methionine is one of the primary sources of the methyl groups used in the biosynthesis of choline (Jiang et al., 2013; Côté-Robitaille et al., 2015).

Absorption and transport
Choline is present in the unsupplemented diet mainly in phosphatidylcholine or lecithin, with less than 10% present either as the free base or as sphingomyelin. Choline is released from lecithin and sphingomyelin by hydrolysis by digestive enzymes of the gastrointestinal tract, although 50% of ingested lecithin enters the thoracic duct intact (Chan, 1991). Pancreatic secretions and intestinal mucosal cells contain enzymes capable of hydrolyzing lecithin in the diet. Phospholipase A_2 cleaves the α-fatty acid within the gut mucosal cell, and phospholipase B cleaves both fatty acids. Quantitatively, digestion by pancreatic lipase is the most crucial process (Zeisel, 1990). The net result is that most ingested lecithin is absorbed as lysophosphatidylcholine.

These lipid components are incorporated into mixed micelles and enter the enterocytes, mainly within the duodenum and jejunum, by passive diffusion. Choline is also absorbed primarily in the jejunum and ileum by the energy and sodium-dependent carrier mechanism. Only one-third of ingested choline in monogastric diets appears to be absorbed intact (Hegazy and Schwenk, 1984). Choline seems to be absorbed through a transport system in the small intestine that is not dependent on cellular energy (Jiang et al., 2013).

The extent to which choline is absorbed from raw materials is unknown (Workel et al., 2002). Absorbed choline is transported into the lymphatic circulation primarily in lecithin bound to chylomicron and is transported to the tissues predominantly as phospholipids associated with the plasma lipoproteins (De La Huerga and Popper, 1952). Phospholipase C cleaves lecithin yielding a diglyceride and phosphorylcholine. Free choline can be oxidized in the mitochondria to yield betaine aldehyde, further converted into betaine, which is the actual source of methyl groups. The small fraction of choline acetylated provides the important neurotransmitter acetylcholine.

Storage and excretion

Most of the choline deposited in tissues exists in esterified forms, particularly phosphatidyl-choline, and phospholipids, accounting for 90% of all choline in the liver. Free choline accounts for only 0.5%–1% of the total choline deposited. Glycerophosphocholine and betaine are over-represented in the kidney, whereas acetylcholine is found in relatively high amounts in the brain (Jiang *et al.*, 2013).

Dietary choline is the main factor governing excretion. Two-thirds of ingested choline is metabolized by microbiota to trimethylamine and excreted in urine within 6 to 12 hours after ingestion (De La Huerga and Popper, 1952). When an equivalent amount of choline is ingested as lecithin, trimethylamine excretion is lesser and appears within 12 to 24 hours after intake.

Biochemical functions

Lecithin contains the predominant phospholipid (>50%), phosphatidylcholine, in most mammalian membranes. In the lung, desaturated lecithin is the primary active component of surfactant (Brown, 1964), a lack of which results in respiratory distress syndrome in pre-mature infants. Endotoxic shock with *E. coli* LPS, simulating an infection, induces impaired pulmonary phosphatidylcholine biosynthesis and associated respiratory illness (Benito and Bosch, 1997). These effects are reduced by the antioxidant protective effects of ascorbic acid. The various metabolic functions and synthesis of choline are depicted in Figure 4.42. The main functions of choline can be grouped into 8 categories (Zeisel, 2006; Garrow, 2007; Jiang *et al.*, 2013).

It is a metabolic essential for building and maintaining cell structure

As a phospholipid component, choline is a structural part of lecithin, certain plasmalogens, and sphingomyelins. Lecithin is a part of animal cell membranes and lipid transport moieties in cell plasma membranes. Both phosphatidylcholine and sphingomyelin are preferentially localized to the outer leaflet of the lipid bilayer, thereby contributing to the lipid asymmetry

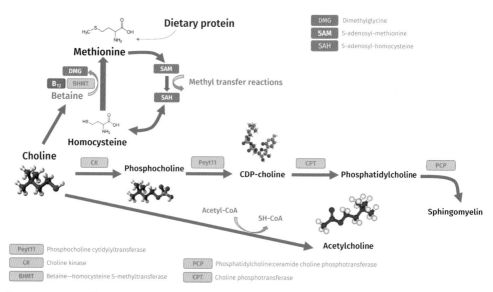

Figure 4.42 Metabolic pathway for the synthesis of choline and related compounds

of cellular membranes. These choline-containing phospholipids undergo dynamic *trans-* and *inter-* membrane movements, facilitating membrane trafficking (Jiang *et al.*, 2013). Choline is required as a constituent of the phospholipids needed for the normal maturation of the cartilage matrix of the bone, which facilitates its growth.

Choline plays an essential role in fat metabolism in the liver

Choline prevents abnormal accumulation of fat (fatty livers) by promoting its transport as lecithin or increasing the utilization of fatty acids in the liver itself (Kroening and Pond, 1967; Boyd *et al.*, 1982; Xu *et al.*, 2010). Phosphatidylcholine is the major phospholipid on the surface of VLDLs: it is packaged with triglyceride droplets in the Golgi cisternae, producing VLDLs that are exported out of the liver. Choline is thus referred to as a "lipotropic" factor due to its acting on fat metabolism by hastening removal or decreasing fat deposition in the liver. Phosphatidylcholine is also the major phospholipid (>95%) in bile and is derived primarily from HDL-phosphatidylcholine (Kroening and Pond, 1967; Jiang *et al.*, 2013).

Forming acetylcholine

Choline is essential for forming acetylcholine, a substance that allows the transmission of nerve impulses: it is the agent released at the termination of the parasympathetic nerves. With acetylcholine, nerve impulses are transmitted from presynaptic to postsynaptic fibers of the sympathetic and parasympathetic nervous systems.

Metabolites as second messengers

Phosphatidylcholine and sphingomyelin contained in cellular membranes are sources of choline-derived second messengers, including lysophosphatidylcholine, lysosphingomyelin, arachidonic acid, diacylglycerol (DAG), phosphatidic acid, ceramide, and sphingosine. These second messengers influence signaling pathways involved in inflammation, growth, differentiation, eicosanoid generation, cell cycle arrest, and apoptosis.

Platelet-activating factor.

The platelet-activating factor (PAF) is produced from phosphatidylcholine. PAF is involved in processes such as platelet activation, blood pressure regulation, and inflammation. PAF releases arachidonic acid to form eicosanoids (Jiang *et al.*, 2013).

Methyl groups

Choline is a source of labile methyl groups or methyl group donors for transmethylation reactions important in forming many substances. Choline furnishes labile methyl groups to form methionine from homocysteine and creatine from guanidino acetic acid (Nesheim and Johnson, 1950). This is a role it shares with methionine and betaine, which means that all these substances can partially substitute for each other. However, their interrelations, reviewed by Simon (1999), are complex (Lovett *et al.*, 1986; Pillai *et al.*, 2006a,b).

  Folic acid and Vitamin B_{12} also take part in these reactions. Thus, their requirements increase with insufficient choline supply (Ryu *et al.*, 1995). Methyl groups function in synthesizing purine and pyrimidine, which are used to produce DNA. Methionine is converted to S-adenosylmethionine in a reaction catalyzed by methionine adenosyl transferase. S-adenosylmethionine is the active methylating agent for many enzymatic methylations. A disturbance in folic acid or methionine metabolism changes choline metabolism and vice versa (Zeisel, 1990). The involvement of folic acid, vitamin B_{12}, and methionine in methyl group metabolism and *de novo* choline synthesis may allow these substances to substitute partly for choline. A severe folic acid deficiency has been shown to cause secondary liver choline deficiency in rats (Kim *et al.*, 1994).

The demand for choline as a methyl donor is probably the primary factor determining how rapidly a diet deficient in choline will induce pathology. The pathways of choline and 1-carbon metabolism intersect at the formation of methionine from homocysteine. Methionine is regenerated from homocysteine in a reaction catalyzed by betaine homocysteine methyltransferase (BHMT), in which betaine, a metabolite of choline, serves as the methyl donor (Finkelstein *et al.*, 1982). Pigs show low choline oxidase activity, as in humans, and deficiencies in methionine do not affect hepatic BHMT but increase its activity in the kidney. Emmert *et al.* (1998) detected elevations in liver activity by adding choline and betaine, whereas choline does not affect the renal enzyme. Although statistically significant changes in hepatic and renal BHMT activity occurred in both experiments conducted by Emmert *et al.* (1998), the magnitude of the responses was probably not physiologically important. Therefore, in contrast to previous findings with rats and chicks, it does not seem that hepatic and renal BHMT activity in pigs is influenced substantially by methionine deficiency or by surfeit levels of choline or betaine (Kroening and Pond, 1967; Emmert *et al.*, 1998).

To be a source of methyl groups, choline must be converted to betaine, which has been shown to perform methylation functions in some cases. Since choline contains biologically active methyl groups, methionine can partly be spared by choline and homocysteine (Russett *et al.*, 1979a,b; Simon, 1999; Jiang *et al.*, 2013). Maxwell *et al.* (1987) observed that choline supplementation had a more significant effect on litter size and pig and litter weight when the gestation diet contained 12% crude protein compared to 16% crude protein.

Influence on brain structure
Choline has been shown to influence brain structure and function. For rodents, choline was critical during fetal development, affecting stem cell proliferation and apoptosis, thereby altering brain structure and function. Memory is permanently enhanced in rodents exposed to choline during the latter part of gestation (Zeisel and Niculescu, 2006), and brain development is affected in piglets from sows with choline deficiency (Seerley *et al.*, 1981; Jiang *et al.*, 2013; Mudd *et al.*, 2016a,b; 2018). Choline supplementation may affect gut inflammation by altering the gut microbiota and lipid metabolism in weaned piglets (Qiu *et al.*, 2021).

Carnitine homeostasis
Choline supplementation alters carnitine homeostasis (Daily and Sachan, 1995). Lower urinary excretion of carnitine has been observed in humans, and guinea pigs supplemented with choline.

Nutritional assessment
Plasma choline (and betaine) concentrations are strongly correlated with choline intake amounts, but in severe deficiency, choline concentrations do not fall according to the low nutritional intake (Hongtrakul *et al.*, 1997).

Deficiency signs
In the baby pig, choline deficiency resulted in slower weight gain and fatty infiltration of the liver (Johnson and James, 1948; Hongtrakul *et al.*, 1997). Choline deficiency in the young pig results in failure to grow, poor conformation (short-legged and pot-bellied), lack of coordination in movements, a characteristic lack of proper rigidity in joints (particularly

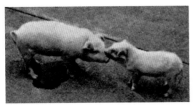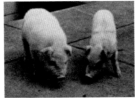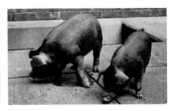

Figure 4.43(a) Pigs on the complete diet (left) and pigs on the choline-low diet (right) (source: Connor and Marian, 1948)

the shoulders), fatty infiltration of the liver (Figure 4.43a), characteristic renal glomerular occlusion and some tubular epithelial necrosis (Cunha, 1977). These clinical signs resulted from low-methionine diets (0.8%) and were prevented with 1.6% dietary methionine inclusion.

Recently, Mudd *et al.* (2016a,b) demonstrated that prenatal choline deficiency delays neurodevelopment by structural and metabolic magnetic resonance imaging (MRI) assessments. These authors used a factorial arrangement of 4 treatments with choline-deficient (CD) or choline-sufficient (CS) sows as prenatal factor levels. Piglets from these sows were stratified in CD and CS milk replacer groups for postnatal factor levels and fed up to 30 days of age when MRI procedures. The single-voxel spectroscopy (SVS) analysis revealed postnatally CS piglets had higher ($p<0.001$) concentrations of glycerophosphocholine–phosphocholine than postnatally CD piglets. Volumetric analysis indicated smaller ($p<0.006$) total brain volumes in prenatally CD piglets compared with prenatally CS piglets. Differences ($p<0.05$) in the corpus callosum, pons, midbrain, thalamus, and right hippocampus, were observed as larger region-specific volumes proportional to total brain size in prenatally CD piglets compared with CS piglets. Diffusion tensor imaging (DTI) suggested interactions ($p<0.05$) between prenatal and postnatal choline status in fractional anisotropy values of the thalamus and right hippocampus. Prenatally, CS piglets had lower cerebellar radial diffusivity ($p = 0.045$) than prenatally CD piglets. All these observations clearly explain the reasons for signs previously observed by previous researchers.

"Spraddled hindleg" is a problem occasionally seen in newborn pigs, and some evidence suggests that the incidence has a vital genetic component. This condition, which is often attributed to choline deficiency, is sometimes prevented by supplementation of the vitamin. However, some reports fail to relate a choline deficiency to the incidence of spraddle-legged pigs (Luce *et al.*, 1985). Similarly, Stockland and Blaylock (1974) found no consistent relationship between the number of sows farrowing pigs with spraddled legs and the level of dietary choline. Whether folic acid and vitamin B_{12} are involved in the condition is unknown, but choline requirements are increased under deficiencies of these vitamins. Spraddled legs can be described as a congenital disorder in which the newborn pig cannot stand or walk because of the leg condition (Figure 4.43b). The problem seems to be worst on slippery floors. Nursing is also hindered, which affects weaning weights.

Spraddled legs started to appear as swine producers began to decrease feed allowances given to sows during gestation from 2.7–3.2 kg daily to 1.4–2.0 kg (Cunha, 1977), which resulted in reduced intakes of both choline and methionine. Studies from Colombia, South America revealed death losses due to spraddled legs. Some of these pigs recuperated by the tenth day after birth, indicating that the sow's milk could correct the condition.

Other reports have indicated that a high proportion of baby pigs affected by spraddled legs were able to recover after a few days, especially if the hindlegs are bound temporarily

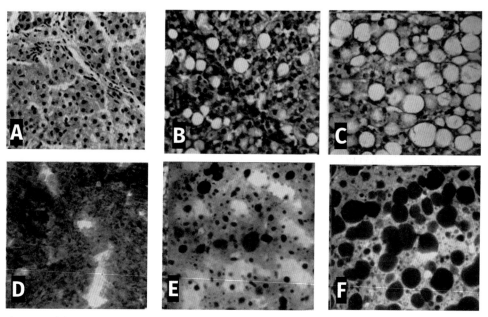

Figure 4.43(b) Photomicrographs of liver sections of pigs. Magnification 225× (original 300× reduced). (A) and (D) Liver showing the typical appearance and normal distribution of fat. (B) and (E) Liver from choline omitted and show some fat infiltrations. (C) and (F) Liver choline, inositol, and p-aminobenzoic acid omitted with a large amount of fat infiltration (source: Connor and Marian, 1948)

to allow them to move and suckle. Research reports have shown that sows without choline had a significantly lower conception rate and farrowing rate and farrowed significantly fewer total pigs and fewer live pigs per litter. No difference was found in the average birth weight. Still, sows with choline supplementation weaned significantly more pigs per litter, and sows without choline farrowed a slightly higher percentage of pigs with spraddled legs. Pigs from CD sows were unthrifty in appearance and became increasingly so with age (Ensminger *et al.*, 1947). Stockland and Blaylock (1974) reported that sows fed a diet without choline had significantly lower conception rates (57% *vs.* 73%), lower farrowing rates (62% *vs.* 78% bred sows), fewer total pigs per litter farrowed (9.3 *vs.* 10.1) and fewer live pigs per litter at farrowing (8.0 *vs.* 9.1) than sows that received diets containing 412 mg or 824 mg choline per kilogram ration.

The North Central Region (NCR-42) Committee on Swine Nutrition (1976) evaluated the effects of supplemental choline at 770 mg/kg diet during gestation and lactation on litter size at birth and weaning. Nine stations participated in 22 trials on 551 sows. The diet was a 15% protein corn-soybean meal type during gestation, and 7.5% beet pulp was substituted for an equal amount of corn during lactation. Results indicated that sows fed supplemental choline farrowed more total pigs per litter (10.54 *vs.* 9.89), live pigs per litter (9.33 *vs.* 8.64), and weaned more pigs per litter (7.72 *vs.* 7.29). Kornegay and Meacham (1973) evaluated the effect of adding choline to a fortified corn-soybean meal gestation-lactation diet for sows. Sows fed 880 mg of supplemental choline per kg diet during breeding and gestation farrowed more live pigs than the sows without supplemental choline. The most prominent response to choline supplementation occurred during the fifth and sixth parities. Kornegay and Meacham (1973) saw no benefit of choline supplementation on several pigs weaned.

Safety

Limited data with pigs indicated a high tolerance for choline (NRC, 1998). However, a more extensive study showed that pig diets should avoid excess choline if the maximum gain is achieved (Southern et al., 1986). Excess supplemental choline (2,000 mg/kg) given throughout the weanling, growing, and finishing phases of growth (121 to 126 days) reduced daily gain but had no effect on feed utilization.

Choline at 2,000 mg/kg did not affect pig gain when given only during the growing and finishing stages (68 to 86 days). Bryant et al. (1977) also found no detrimental effects of choline on the performance of young or grow-finish pigs fed diets containing 2,000 mg choline per kilogram of complete feed. Very high levels of choline (>5 g per day) in humans have been associated with a fishy body odor, excessive sweating and salivation, vomiting, and gastrointestinal distress (Garrow, 2007).

Chapter 5

Optimum vitamin nutrition for swine

INTRODUCTION

Vitamins are organic compounds necessary in small quantities to maintain physiological functions for optimum growth, reproduction, and health. As vitamins act primarilily as regulators of metabolism, and have several interactions among them, establishing the requirements and recommendations for each single vitamin under diverse conditions and age phases has been challenging, much more so than for similar work on amino acids which are the building block of proteins, i.e., structural components of the body. This chapter will discuss the scientific evidence available related to the effects of dietary vitamin levels on multiple parameters of swine live performance, health, welfare, reproduction, and pork quality. Additionally, the trends of recommendations from multiple sources and the current utilization of vitamins in the swine industry will be discussed.

There are several factors behind the difficulties in establishing the effects of vitamins. First, the variability in results observed in research publications across time. Micronutrients may provoke multiple simultaneous variations in metabolism that are not easily quantifiable and may have long-term effects. Not all the potential effects of vitamin levels can be detected during the experimental period. Second, the variation in published results can also be related to the analytical methodologies used to assess each vitamin from laboratory to laboratory and over time. More precise instruments have been developed to analyse vitamins in recent years, but methods are not entirely standardized across labs.

Third, in most cases, the ingredients used in feed formulation contain vitamins in variable concentrations and bioavailability, differing depending on storage conditions, time, and feed processing treatments applied. When the level of one vitamin is tested, the level of other vitamins, certain amino acids, fatty acids, minerals, and other nutrients and antinutrients can affect the responses (Miller and Kornegay, 1983; Gebert *et al.*, 1999a; McDowell, 2006; Yang *et al.*, 2021a,d). Nutrient levels fed to pigs have changed over time, and feedstuffs used may have variable nutrient composition, digestibility, or bioavailability.

All these factors increase the difficulty of precisely establishing the quantity and the forms of vitamins ingested by animals. All this means that, in practice, it is impossible to invoke the factorial methodology to calculate vitamin requirements. Therefore, it is necessary to adopt empirical tests where different levels of vitamins are added to a basal diet, and the response is measured.

Usually, these tests are done by including vitamins in conventional feeds. But this basal diet may contain a more or less constant concentration of naturally occurring vitamins and obtaining a dose–response curve that shows the optimum vitamin concentration should be included to supplement that provided by the ingredients. The dose–response curve obtained in this type of trial is similar to those obtained for any other nutrients (Figure 5.1). However, it is not common today to evaluate the lack of an essential nutrient, such as vitamins, for

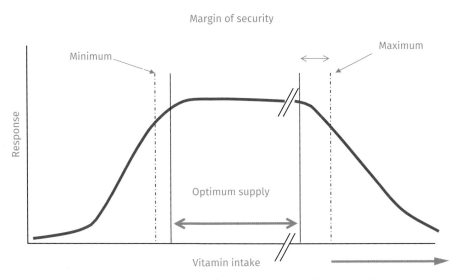

Figure 5.1 Relation between the quantity of vitamin intake and theoretical productive response

a sufficiently prolonged period because these deficiencies are incompatible with current production levels and health.

Thus, any increment in supply allows a substantial improvement in effective response, which may be adjusted according to an exponential equation following the law of diminishing returns from a certain point. That is to say that the benefit obtained by increasing the concentration of the nutrient-like vitamins in feed is proportionally smaller every time until what may be called a plateau phase is reached where the maximum productive response is located. This curve enables the need for a particular nutrient to be determined, that is, the minimum quantity a healthy animal should receive daily to meet the requirements for maintenance and a given production level. As these are "minimum" quantities, the values are usually increased within so-called "safety margins," whose objective is to correct deviations resulting from the biological variability of both animals and feed. The values obtained are considered optimum nutrient provision and have a relatively wide range (Figure 5.1).

This optimum supply may sometimes be exceeded, leading to a surplus and even toxicity. In the case of vitamins, toxic effects have only been observed with vitamins A and D and only when administering quantities far greater than the ones used in practice. Since supplying a given nutrient in high concentrations increases the ration cost, a quantity is chosen, representing the minimum supply that provides the maximum productive response within a safety margin (Figure 5.1).

The introduction of the economic factor, essential in ration formulation and establishing nutrient restrictions, represents an additional difficulty. As the maximum productive response approaches, returns become smaller, and therefore increments in the concentration of nutrients may become economically unviable. For this reason, ultimately, the establishment of each recommendation has an economic base, hence the concept of "economic optimum," which may be the minimum concentration of a nutrient that produces the maximum response or even a slightly lower concentration that does not produce the maximum response but does produce the most significant economic benefit of the process. The need to introduce the economic factor in animal nutrition is linked to the fact that each productive situation is unique.

Therefore, the production strategy is also unique, and the definition of formulation need and criteria should also be specific to each case.

Calculating the most appropriate level of supplementation in conventional feed may be confusing because feeds considered normal in some geographical areas or production conditions may not be used in other parts of the world. For example, a good deal of North American production is obtained using feeds based on corn and soy. The content and availability of vitamins differ significantly from that in cassava, barley, wheat, or sunflower.

IS IT NECESSARY TO REVISE VITAMIN RECOMMENDATIONS FOR SWINE NUTRITION?

Most recommendations for vitamins in swine nutrition are based on studies carried out several decades ago. The question of revising these values is often discussed. However, this topic raises some controversy because, in some cases, the information is unclear, and commercial interests may sometimes make the need to update recommendations less desirable. Nevertheless, from our point of view, several reasons suggest the need to periodically review recommendations for vitamins (and other nutrients) for swine. These include the following.

- Most vitamin recommendations derived from different trials are expressed in concentration per kilogram feed. In pigs, genetic selection, nutrition, and technological developments to improve the FCR has indirectly reduced voluntary ingestion over the recent decades (Culbertson et al., 2017; Soleimani and Gilbert, 2020). Pig voluntary feed intake (VFI) decreased by 30 g/day annually during the early 1980s. However, time trends show that VFI stabilized around 1990, while the lean tissue growth rate grew 4 g/day annually (Knap, 2009). Then, nutrient metabolic efficiency plays a more significant role in improving FCR. These changes in FCR and feed intake do not affect pigs during all productive phases with the same intensity, nor is the effect on both sexes the same. Consequently, susceptibility to potential subclinical vitamin deficiencies is more considerable.
- There has been a marked increase in the productive capacity of the animals, ever approaching the physiological limit. As the productive limit is approached, more attention should be paid to the supply of the different nutrients to avoid imbalances. However, genetics continue to evolve (Culbertson et al., 2017; Lozada-Soto et al., 2022). We are probably on the threshold of a revolution thanks to the massive application of techniques based on molecular biology. It will therefore be necessary to optimize feed formulation to maintain that rate of improvement in production. In only 5 years, from 2016 to 2021, the USA swine herd has observed (Table 5.1) improvements in the average pigs per litter, piglets born alive or live-born per female per year, and the number of piglets weaned. However, sow and gilt mortality and culling rates are still growing issues that must be addressed. The forecast of swine genetic productivity for the next 10 years is very promising (Table 5.2). This higher genetic potential implies that nutrition precision should be enhanced to optimize final results.
- With increases in knowledge of the phenomena that regulate animal physiology and productive processes, studies must consider other factors besides those strictly related to a lack of deficiency or the mere optimization of response. Aspects like immune response capacity, breeder longevity, the viability of neonatal pigs, adaptation to environmental and immunological stress, response to vaccinations, susceptibility to pathological problems, and the capacity to overcome disease or develop resilience will require more consideration.

Table 5.1 Swine breeder and piglet performance summary (USA), 2016–2021 (https://www.pigchamp.com/news/benchmark-magazine)

	2016 (416 farms)	2017 (340 farms)	2018 (375 farms)	2019 (365 farms)	2020 (305 farms)	2021 (292 farms)	% change 2021/ 2016	% change/year 2021/2016
Average pigs/litter (n)	13.95	14.22	14.43	14.71	14.99	15.2	8.96	1.8
Average born alive/litter (n)	12.58	12.71	12.9	13.2	13.46	13.54	7.63	1.5
Liveborn female/year (n)	27.74	28.53	28.62	29.74	29.38	29.54	6.49	1.3
Pre-weaning mortality (%)	15.37	14.69	14.85	14.55	15.42	15.7	2.14	0.4
Average age at weaning (day)	20.54	20.71	20.74	20.82	20.66	20.84	1.46	0.3
Average litter weaning weight (kg)	148.32	141	132.95	130.33	131.86	124.54	−16.03	−3.2
Pigs weaned per litter weaned (n)	11.03	11.16	11.23	11.48	11.77	11.85	7.43	1.5
Pigs weaned per female/year (n)	23.06	23.82	24.11	24.86	24.84	24.83	7.67	1.5
Sows and gilts death rate (%)	10	10.73	11.68	12.31	13.91	14.86	48.6	9.7
Culling rate (%)	44.51	42.31	45.06	45.69	48.79	46.29	3.99	0.8

Table 5.2 Swine productivity commercial performance 2022 and forecast for 2032 (PIC data, adapted from Saskia Bloemhof-Abma, AMVEC 2022, unpublished)

	2022	Annual change (unit)	Annual change (%)	2032
Pigs/sow/year (n)	33.5	1.2	3.5	45.5
Weaned/litter (n)	13.4	0.49	3.6	18.3
Weaned weight/sow year (kg)	201	8.5	4.2	286
Pigs weaned sow/lifetime (n)	60.9	2.2	3.6	82.9
Weight sold sow/year (kg)	4,058	198	4.9	6,039
% sold	93.2	0.38	0.4	97
Average market weight (kg)	130	1.1	0.9	141.4
Whole-system feed efficiency	2.5	0.036	1.4	2.14

- Today, the variability among pig individuals in a herd, and not only the average values in any production parameter, deserves ever-increasing attention in modern swine production to achieve precision livestock nutrition. The effects of vitamin levels on achieving precision nutrition have not been evaluated in sufficient depth. Different response curves for the same vitamin can be expected according to the parameter measured, either growth, resistance to disease, meat quality, reproductive ability, or immune response (Lauridsen et al., 2021a,b; Matte and Lauridsen, 2022).
- Recently and increasingly, pork consumers play a more active role in shaping production and are becoming far more selective in their choices. For this reason, attention must be paid to their opinions and specific demands. Thus, aspects like diversification of production, animal well-being, the content of potentially toxic compounds or residues, fortification of food with natural compounds, etc., acquire ever increasing relevance. Optimum vitamin nutrition in swine offers attractive alternatives that must be studied and applied appropriately (Boler et al., 2009; Duffy et al., 2018a; Johnson et al., 2019).
- During the past few years, conditions in production have been modernized significantly, with improved genetics, facilities, etc. The technical revolution's consequences call for nutrition optimization (Matte and Lauridsen, 2022). The improvements in FCR, pig growth, number of piglets per litter, and livability vary depending on the technological production level. The potentially different trajectories that the swine sector could follow in the coming decades can significantly affect sustainability, FCR, feed composition, and even vitamin needs. These effects were studied by Lassaletta et al. (2019) using a methodology of modeling 5 potentially different shared socioeconomic pathways (SSP). The improvements in FCR are expected to continue if the scenario with rapid technological improvements (SSP5) increases in the coming years (Figure 5.2). Under these prevalent conditions worldwide, optimum vitamin nutrition can become more relevant.
- The costs of the different ingredients (including vitamins) used in pig feed are variable. Therefore, the vitamin levels permit the optimum economic return in each case. Scientific and technical processes and large-scale industrial production mean synthetic vitamins are more efficient. So, the cost of vitamin supply is becoming proportionally lower than of the other ingredients used in ration formulation. Therefore, the feed's vitamin concentration corresponding to the economic optimum tends to increase, ever approaching the recommended concentration for optimum production. This fact demands special attention

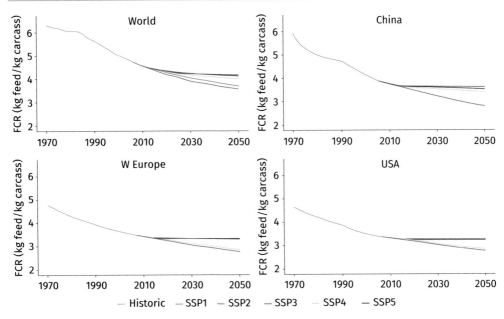

Figure 5.2 Trajectories of FCR aggregated for all production system levels at the global scale and for intensive systems in China, Western Europe, and the USA for 1970–2050 for the 5 socioeconomic pathway scenarios evaluated (feed is expressed as a kg DM) (Lassaletta *et al.*, 2019)

  since not all commercial vitamin preparations are of the same quality, nor are they equally beneficial to the animals.
- Changes to feed guidelines, e.g., the bans on ingredients of animal origin and antibiotics, and other changes that will undoubtedly occur, mean that the entire production strategy should be reviewed. This includes rethinking housing, vaccination plans, handling, and intestinal health in critical periods like weaning. This process entails re-evaluation in economic terms of the supply of different micronutrients in different phases of the productive cycle (Lauridsen and Matte, 2017; Lauridsen *et al.*, 2021a,b; Matte and Lauridsen, 2022).

Taking all these considerations into account, this review considers the study of vitamin requirements in swine nutrition and feed in light of the latest scientific research.

CURRENT VITAMIN RECOMMENDATIONS FOR SWINE

Despite the lack of conclusive research results to determine optimum vitamin levels, there are sources of information to consult when deciding the levels to use. Research and academic organizations like the National Research Council (NRC, 2012) in the USA, the Brazilian Tables (Rostagno *et al.*, 2017), and FEFANA (2015) in Europe have put together vitamin recommendations for piglets, growing pigs, gilts, and sows during gestation and lactation (Tables 5.3, 5.4 and 5.5). The leading genetic companies in the world also have their recommendations (Tables 5.6, 5.7, and 5.8), and recently several swine industry surveys (Tables 5.9, 5.10, and 5.11) have summarized the current use of vitamins in Brazil (Dalto and da Silva, 2020), the USA (Flohr *et al.*, 2016, Faccin *et al.*, 2022) and China (Yang *et al.*, 2021b). Based on all this information and recent research reports, DSM Nutritional Products (2022b) proposed the OVN™ levels (Tables 5.3, 5.4, and 5.5).

Table 5.3 Vitamin inclusion levels (mg/kg feed) for piglets according to research committees and academic or feed industry organizations

	Unit	Prestarter (3–20 days) 5–7 kg				Nursery I (21–35 days) 7–11 kg			
		NRC, 2012	FEFANA, 2015	Rostagno et al., 2017	OVN™ (DSM Nutritional Products, 2022b)	NRC, 2012	FEFANA, 2015	Rostagno et al., 2017	OVN™ (DSM Nutritional Products, 2022b)
Vitamin A	IU	2,200	15,000–25,000	12,304	10,500–22,500	2,200	15,000–25,000	12,304	10,500–16,000
Vitamin D$_3$	IU	220	1,800–2,000	2,707	1,890–2,100	220	1,800–2,000	2,707	1,890–2,100
25OHD$_3$ (HyD)®	mg	–	–	–	0.05	–	–	–	0.05
Vitamin E	mg	16	80–150	73.8	105–160	16	80–150	73.8	105–160
Vitamin K	mg	0.5	8–10	5.33	8.5–11	0.5	8–10	5.33	5.2–6.4
Vitamin B$_1$	mg	1.5	3.5–5.5	1.81	3.8–5.8	1	3.5–5.5	1.81	3.2–5.2
Vitamin B$_2$	mg	4	10–15	6.73	10.5–16	3.5	10–15	6.73	10.5–16
Vitamin B$_6$	mg	7	6–8	3.61	6.4–8.4	7	6–8	3.61	6.4–8.4
Vitamin B$_{12}$	mg	0.02	0.050–0.070	0.037	0.052–0.072	0.0175	0.050–0.070	0.037	0.042–0.062
Niacin	mg	30	60–80	53.3	63–84	30	60–80	53.3	38–58
D-Panthothenic acid	mg	12	30–50	27.1	32–52	10	30–50	27.1	26–46
Folic acid	mg	0.3	1.5–3.0	0.574	1.6–3.3	0.3	1.5–3.0	0.574	1.6–2.6
Biotin	mg	0.08	0.2–0.4	0.18	0.32–0.52	0.05	0.2–0.4	0.18	0.32–0.52
Vitamin C	mg	–	100–200	–	210–260	–	100–200	–	105–210
Choline	mg	600	500–800	360.9	525–840	500	500–800	360.9	260–420

Vitamin	Unit	Nursery II (36–49 days) 11–25 kg				Nursery III (50–70 days) 25–50 kg			
		NRC, 2012	FEFANA, 2015	Rostagno et al., 2017	OVN™ (DSM Nutritional Products, 2022b)	NRC, 2012	FEFANA, 2015	Rostagno et al., 2017	OVN™ (DSM Nutritional Products, 2022b)
Vitamin A	IU	1,750	15,000–25,000	10,931	10,500–16,000	1,300	10,000–20,000	10,931	10,500–16,000
Vitamin D_3	IU	200	1,800–2,000	2,405	1,890–2,100	150	1,800–2,000	2,405	1,890–2,100
25OHD$_3$ (HyD)®	mg	–	–	–	0.05	–	–	–	0.05
Vitamin E	mg	11	80–150	65.6	105–160	11	70–100	65.6	105–160
Vitamin K	mg	0.5	8–10	4.74	5.2–6.4	0.5	5–6	4.74	5.2–6.4
Vitamin B_1	mg	1	3.5–5.5	1.60	3.2–5.2	1	3–5	1.60	3.2–5.2
Vitamin B_2	mg	3	10–15	5.98	10.5–16	2.5	10–15	5.98	10.5–16
Vitamin B_6	mg	3	6–8	3.21	6.4–8.4	1	6–8	3.21	6.4–8.4
Vitamin B_{12}	mg	0.015	0.050–0.070	0.033	0.042–0.062	0.01	0.040–0.060	0.033	0.042–0.062
Niacin	mg	30	60–80	47.4	38–58	30	40–60	47.4	38–58
D-Panthothenic acid	mg	9	30–50	24.0	26–46	8	25–45	24.0	26–46
Folic acid	mg	0.3	1.5–3.0	0.510	1.6–2.6	0.3	1.5–2.5	0.51	1.6–2.6
Biotin	mg	0.05	0.2–0.4	0.16	0.32–0.52	0.05	0.2–0.4	0.16	0.32–0.52
Vitamin C	mg	–	100–200	–	105–210	–	100–200	–	105–210
Choline	mg	400	500–800	320.6	260–420	300	250–400	320.6	260–420

Note: OVN™ levels are ranges for consideration, depending on several factors, such as husbandry conditions and health status. https://www.dsm.com/anh/products-and-services/tools/ovn/ovn-calculator.html.

Table 5.4 Vitamin inclusion levels (mg/kg feed) for growing and finishing pigs according to research committees and academic or feed industry organizations

	Unit	Growing I (71–90 days) 50–75 kg				Growing II (92–112 days) 75–100 kg				Finisher 100 kg to market			
		NRC, 2012	FEFANA, 2015	Rostagno et al., 2017	OVN™ (DSM Nutritional Products, 2022b)	NRC, 2012	FEFANA, 2015	Rostagno et al., 2017	OVN™ (DSM Nutritional Products, 2022b)	NRC, 2012	FEFANA, 2015	Rostagno et al., 2017	OVN™ (DSM Nutritional Products, 2022b)
Vitamin A	IU	1,300	8,000–12,000	7,270	7,350–10,500	1,300	6,000–8,000	6,018	7,350–10,500	1,300	6,000–8,000	5,005	5,250–8,400
Vitamin D$_3$	IU	150	1,500–2,000	1,599	1,570–2,100	150	1,000–1,500	1,324	1,570–2,100	150	1,000–1,500	1,101	1,050–1,570
25OHD$_3$ (HyD®)	mg	-	-	-	0.05	-	-	-	0.05	-	-	-	0.05
Vitamin E	mg	11	60–80	43.6	64–105	11	40–60	36.1	64–105	11	40–60	30	64–105
Vitamin K	mg	0.5	2–4	3.15	2.1–4.2	0.5	2–4	2.61	2.1–4.2	0.5	2–4	2.17	2.1–4.2
Vitamin B$_1$	mg	1	2–3	1.07	2.1–3.1	1	1–2	0.88	2.1–3.1	1	1–2	0.73	1.1–2.1
Vitamin B$_2$	mg	2.5	7–10	3.97	7.3–10.5	2	6–10	3.29	7.3–10.5	2	6–10	2.74	6.3–10.5
Vitamin B$_6$	mg	1	2.5–4.5	3.13	2.6–4.7	1	2.0–3.5	1.77	2.6–4.7	1	2.0–3.5	1.47	2.1–3.7
Vitamin B$_{12}$	mg	0.005	0.030–0.050	0.022	0.032–0.052	0.005	0.030–0.050	0.018	0.032–0.052	0.005	0.030–0.050	0.015	0.032–0.052
Niacin	mg	30	30–40	31.5	21–50	30	20–40	26.1	21–50	30	20–40	21.7	21–42
D-Panthothenic acid	mg	7	25–45	16.0	26–47	7	25–45	13.2	26–47	7	25–45	11	26–47
Folic acid	mg	0.3	1.0–1.5	0.339	1.1–1.6	0.3	0.5–1.0	0.281	1.1–1.6	0.3	0.5–1.0	0.234	0.52–1.05
Biotin	mg	0.05	0.15–0.30	0.107	0.2–0.4	0.05	0.10–0.20	0.088	0.2–0.4	0.05	0.10–0.20	0.073	0.105–0.21
Choline	mg	300	150–300	213.3	157–315	300	100–200	176.5	157–315	300	100–200	146.8	105–210

Note: OVN™ levels are ranges for consideration, depending on several factors, such as husbandry conditions and health status. https://www.dsm.com/anh/products-and-services/tools/ovn/ovn-calculator.html

Table 5.5 Vitamin inclusion levels (mg/kg feed) for breeder pigs according to research committees and academic or feed industry organizations

	Unit	Gilts				Gestation			
		NRC, 2012	FEFANA, 2015	Rostagno et al., 2017	OVN™ (DSM Nutritional Products, 2022b)	NRC, 2012	FEFANA, 2015	Rostagno et al., 2017	OVN™ (DSM Nutritional Products, 2022b)
Vitamin A	IU		8,000–12,000	10,400	10,500–13,100	4,000	10,000–15,000	10,400	10,500–15,700
Vitamin D_3	IU		1,800–2,000	1,560	1,900–2,100	800	1,500–2,000	1,560	1,570–2,100
25OHD$_3$ (HyD®)	mg		–	–	0.05	–	–	–	0.05
Vitamin E	mg		–	58.5	84–105	44	60–80	58.5	105–160
Vitamin K	mg		1.5–3.0	2.6	2.5–4.4	0.5	4.5–5.0	2.6	4.7–5.2
Vitamin B_1	mg		1–2	1.3	1.05–2.2	1	2.0–2.5	1.3	2.1–2.6
Vitamin B_2	mg		6–10	5.2	6.3–10.5	3.75	6–10	5.2	6.3–10.5
Vitamin B_6	mg		3.5–5.5	1.95	5.3–8.4	1	3.5–5.5	1.95	3.7–5.7
Vitamin B_{12}	mg		0.030–0.050	0.026	0.032–0.052	0.015	0.030–0.050	0.026	0.032–0.052
Niacin	mg		30–40	32.5	30–50	10	30–40	32.5	32–47
D-Panthothenic acid	mg		15–30	20.8	16–33	12	30–35	20.8	37–42
Folic acid	mg		3.5–5.5	1.3	3.7–5.7	1.3	3.5–5.5	1.3	3.7–5.7
Biotin	mg		0.3–0.5	0.325	0.32–0.52	0.2	0.5–0.8	0.325	0.52–0.84
Vitamin C	mg		200–300	–	210–315	–	200–300	–	210–315
Choline	mg		250–500	780	270–525	1,250	500–800	780	525–840
β-carotene	mg		–	–	–	–	–	–	–

Table 5.5 (continued)

	Unit	Lactation				Boars			
		NRC, 2012	FEFANA, 2015	Rostagno et al., 2017	OVN™ (DSM Nutritional Products, 2022b)	NRC, 2012	FEFANA, 2015	Rostagno et al., 2017	OVN™ (DSM Nutritional Products, 2022b)
Vitamin A	IU	2,000	10,000–15,000	10,400	10,500–15,700	4,000	10,000–15,000	10,400	10,500–15,700
Vitamin D$_3$	IU	800	1,500–2,000	1,560	1,570–2,100	200	1,500–2,000	1,560	1,570–2,100
25OHD$_3$ (HyD®)	mg	–	–	–	0.05	–	–	–	0.05
Vitamin E	mg	44	40–53	58.5	105–190	44	–	58.5	105–160
Vitamin K	mg	0.5	4.5–5.0	2.6	4.7–5.2	0.5	4.5–5.0	2.6	4.7–5.2
Vitamin B$_1$	mg	1	2.0–2.5	1.3	2.1–3	1	1–2	1.3	1.05–2.2
Vitamin B$_2$	mg	3.75	6–10	5.2	6.3–10.5	3.75	6–10	5.2	6.3–10.5
Vitamin B$_6$	mg	1	3.5–5.5	1.95	3.7–5.7	1	3.5–5.5	1.95	3.7–5.7
Vitamin B$_{12}$	mg	0.015	0.030–0.050	0.026	0.032–0.052	0.015	0.030–0.050	0.026	0.032–0.052
Niacin	mg	10	30–40	32.5	40–100	10	30–40	32.5	32–47
D-Panthothenic acid	mg	12	30–35	20.8	37–42	12	20–30	20.8	21–33
Folic acid	mg	1.3	3.5–5.5	1.3	3.7–5.7	1.3	3.5–5.5	1.3	3.7–5.7
Biotin	mg	0.2	0.5–0.8	0.325	0.52–0.84	0.2	0.5–0.8	0.325	0.52–0.84
Vitamin C	mg	–	200–300	–	210–315	–	200–500	–	210–525
Choline	mg	1,000	500–800	780	525–840	1,250	500–800	780	525–840
β-carotene	mg	–	–	–	300*	–	–	–	–

Note: * For improved sow fertility the suggested level must be fed per animal per day immediately after weaning until confirmed conception. OVN™ levels are ranges for consideration, depending on several factors, such as husbandry conditions and health status. https://www.dsm.com/anh/products-and-services/tools/ovn/ovn-calculator.html

Table 5.6 Vitamin inclusion levels (mg/kg feed) for piglets according to 4 swine genetic companies

	Unit	Prestarter (3–20 days) 5–7 kg					Nursery I (21–35 days) 7–11 kg					Piglet references
		Topigs Norsvin, 2016	Hypor, 2017	PIC, 2021	Danbred, 2021	OVN™ (DSM Nutritional Products, 2022b)	Topigs Norsvin, 2016	Hypor, 2017	PIC, 2021	Danbred, 2021	OVN™ (DSM Nutritional Products, 2022b)	
Vitamin A	IU	16,000	12,000	5,000	9,600	10,500–22,500	16,000	12,000	5,000	9,600	10,500–16,000	Wang et al. (2020): 26,000–53,000 IU better ADG and Gain:Feed
Vitamin D₃	IU	1,800–2,000	1,500	1,600	960	1,890–2,100	1,800–2,000	1,500	1,600	960	1,890–2,100	–
25OHD₃ (HyD®)	mg	–	–	–	–	0.05	–	–	–	–	0.05	Upadhaya et al. (2022) 0.05 mg improved piglet performance; Konowalchuk et al. (2013) 0.05 mg/kg immunomodulaotory action; Yang et al. (2018) up to 0.155 mg/kg reduced inflammatory response and increased antioxidant response
Vitamin E	mg	100–150	85	51	168	105–160	100–150	85	51	168	105–160	Lopez-Bote et al. (2001): 200 mg improved intestinal mucous membrane integrity
Vitamin K	mg	3–6	3	3	2	8.5–11	3–6	3	3	2	5.2–6.4	–
Vitamin B₁	mg	4–5	2.5	–	2	3.8–5.8	4–5	2.5	–	2	3.2–5.2	–
Vitamin B₂	mg	7.5–15	7.5	8.00	5	10.5–16	7.5–15	7.5	8	5	10.5–16	–
Vitamin B₆	mg	4–8	4	–	4	6.4–8.4	4–8	4	–	4	6.4–8.4	Li et al. (2019): 7 mg better BW, ADG; Gain:Feed; Woodworth et al. (2000): 7.7 mg; Yin et al. (2020): 7 mg modulation of immune system
Vitamin B₁₂	mg	0.05–0.06	0.04	0.04	0.024	0.052–0.072	0.05–0.06	0.04	0.04	0.024	0.042–0.062	–
Niacin	mg	50–55	40	51	24	63–84	50–55	40	51	24	38–58	Real et al. (2002): 55 mg optimize gain:feed rate
D-Panthothenic acid	mg	17.5–45	25	29	12	32–52	17.5–45	25	29	12	26–46	–
Folic acid	mg	1.25–2.5	1.25	–	–	1.6–3.3	1.25–2.5	1.25	–	–	1.6–2.6	Wang et al. (2021): 9 mg better BW, ADG; DFI, health
Biotin	mg	0.1–0.4	0.2	–	0.24	0.32–0.52	0.1–0.4	0.2	–	0.24	0.32–0.52	–
Vitamin C	mg	200	–	–	–	210–260	200	–	–	–	105–210	Lauridsen and Jensen (2005): 500 mg better immunity
Choline	mg	250–300	200	–	–	525–840	250–300	200	–	–	260–420	–

Table 5.6 (continued)

	Unit	Nursery II (36–49 days) 11–25 kg					Nursery III (50–70 days) 25–50 kg					Piglet references
		Topigs Norsvin, 2016	Hypor, 2017	PIC, 2021	Danbred, 2021	OVN™ (DSM Nutritional Products, 2022b)	Topigs Norsvin, 2016	Hypor, 2017	PIC, 2021	Danbred, 2021	OVN™ (DSM Nutritional Products, 2022b)	
Vitamin A	IU	16,000	12,000	5,000	5,800	10,500–16,000	7,000–10,000	10,000	5,000	5,660	10,500–16,000	Wang et al. (2020): 26,000–53,000 IU better ADG and Gain:Feed
Vitamin D$_3$	IU	1,800–2,000	1,500	1,600	580	1,890–2,100	1,500–2,000	1,500	1,600	565	1,890–2,100	–
25OHD$_3$ (HyD®)	mg	–	–	–	–	0.05	–	–	–	–	0.05	Upadhaya et al. (2022) 0.05 mg improved piglet performance; Konowalchuk et al. (2013) 0.05 mg/kg immunomodulaotory action; Yang et al. (2018) up to 0.155 mg/kg reduced inflammatory response and increased antioxidant response
Vitamin E	mg	100–150	85	51	162	105–160	40–100	70	51	68	105–160	Lopez-Bote et al. (2001): 200 mg improved intestinal mucous membrane integrity
Vitamin K	mg	3–6	3	3	2	5.2–6.4	2–3	1.5	3	2	5.2–6.4	–
Vitamin B$_1$	mg	4–5	2.5	–	2	3.2–5.2	2–3	2	–	2	3.2–5.2	–
Vitamin B$_2$	mg	7.5–15	7.5	8	5	10.5–16	7–10	4.0	8	5	10.5–16	–
Vitamin B$_6$	mg	4–8	4	–	3	6.4–8.4	2–4	2	–	3	6.4–8.4	Li et al. (2019): 7 mg better BW, ADG; Gain:Feed; Woodworth et al. (2000): 7.7 mg; Yin et al. (2020): 7 mg modulation of immune system
Vitamin B$_{12}$	mg	0.05–0.06	0.04	0.04	0.023	0.042–0.062	0.03–0.05	0.035	0.04	0.023	0.042–0.062	–
Niacin	mg	50–55	40	51	23	38–58	20–40	35	51	23	38–58	Real et al. (2002): 55 mg optimize gain:feed rate
D-Panthothenic acid	mg	17.5–45	25	29	12	26–46	10–45	15	29	11	26–46	–
Folic acid	mg	1.25–2.5	1.25	–	–	1.6–2.6	0.4–1.5	0.5	–	–	1.6–2.6	Wang et al. (2021): 9 mg better BW, ADG; DFI, health
Biotin	mg	0.1–0.4	0.2	–	0.23	0.32–0.52	0.4	0.4	–	0.23	0.32–0.52	–
Vitamin C	mg	200	–	–	–	105–210	150–300	–	–	–	105–210	Lauridsen and Jensen (2005): 500 mg better immunity
Choline	mg	250–300	200	–	–	260–420	250–300	150	–	–	260–420	–

Table 5.7 Vitamin inclusion levels (mg/kg feed) for growing and finishing pigs according to 4 swine genetic companies

	Unit	Growing I (71–90 days) 50–75 kg					Growing II (91–112 days) 75–100 kg					Growing – finishing pigs references
		Topigs Norsvin, 2016	Hypor, 2017	PIC, 2021	Danbred, 2021	OVN™ (DSM Nutritional Products, 2022b)	Topigs Norsvin, 2016	Hypor, 2017	PIC, 2021	Danbred, 2021	OVN™ (DSM Nutritional Products, 2022b)	
Vitamin A	IU	7,000–10,000	10,000	5,000	4,880	7,350–10,500	7,000–10,000	7,500	3,750	4,880	7,350–10,500	–
Vitamin D$_3$	IU	1,500–2,000	1,500	1,600	440	1,570–2,100	1,500–2,000	1,500	1,200	440	1,570–2,100	–
25OHD$_3$ (HyD®)	mg	–	–	–	–	0.05	–	–	–	–	0.05	Upadhaya et al. (2022): 0.05 mg improved performance and meat quality (reduced drip loss)
Vitamin E	mg	40–100	70	51	43	64–105	40–100	50	37	43	64–105	Wang et al. (2017): 250 mg better milk and sow colostrum, immune and antioxidant response, weaning weight, ADG; Jin et al. (2018): 400 mg better meat quality, less meat waste
Vitamin K	mg	2–3	1.5	3	2	2.1–4.2	2–3	1	2.4	2	2.1–4.2	–
Vitamin B$_1$	mg	2–3	2	–	2	2.1–3.1	2–3	1.5	–	2	2.1–3.1	–
Vitamin B$_2$	mg	7–10	4	8	2	7.3–10.5	7–10	3.5	6.6	2	7.3–10.5	–
Vitamin B$_6$	mg	2–4	2	–	3	2.6–4.7	2–4	1.5	–	3	2.6–4.7	–
Vitamin B$_{12}$	mg	0.03–0.05	0.035	0.04	0.021	0.032–0.052	0.03–0.05	0.02	0.029	0.021	0.032–0.052	–
Niacin	mg	20–40	35	51	21	21–50	20–40	20	31	21	21–50	Real et al. (2002): 55 mg optimize gain:feed rate
D-Panthothenic acid	mg	10–45	15	28	11	26–47	10–45	12.5	18	11	26–47	Minelli et al. (2016): 100 mg better carcass yield, lean meat
Folic acid	mg	0.4–1.5	0.5	–	–	1.1–1.6	0.4–1.5	–	–	–	1.1–1.6	–
Biotin	mg	0.4	0.4	–	0.1	0.2–0.4	–	–	–	0.1	0.2–0.4	Wilt and Carlson, 2009 0.44 mg improved ADG
Choline	mg	150–300	150	–	–	157–315	150–300	100	–	–	157–315	–

Table 5.7 (continued)

	Unit	Finisher 100 kg to market					Growing – finishing pigs references
		Topigs Norsvin, 2016	Hypor, 2017	PIC, 2021	Danbred, 2021	OVN™ (DSM Nutritional Products, 2022b)	
Vitamin A	IU	5,000–7,500	7,500	2,500	4,880	5,250–8,400	–
Vitamin D₃	IU	1,000–1,500	1,500	800	440	1,050–1,570	–
25OHD₃ (HyD®)	mg	–	–	–	–	0.05	Upadhaya et al. (2022): 0.05 mg improved performance and meat quality (reduced drip loss)
Vitamin E	mg	30–75	50	25	43	64–105	Wang et al. (2017): 250 mg better milk and sow colostrum, immune and antioxidant response, weaning weight, ADG; Jin et al. (2018): 400 mg better meat quality, less meat waste
Vitamin K	mg	1.5–2	1	1.5	2	2.1–4.2	–
Vitamin B₁	mg	1–2	1.5	–	2	1.1–2.1	–
Vitamin B₂	mg	5–8	3.5	4.4	2	6.3–10.5	–
Vitamin B₆	mg	1.5–3	1.5	–	3	2.1–3.7	–
Vitamin B₁₂	mg	0.02–0.04	0.02	0.019	0.021	0.032–0.052	–
Niacin	mg	15–30	20	26	21	21–42	Real et al. (2002): 55 mg optimize gain:feed rate
D-Panthothenic acid	mg	7–35	12.5	14	11	26–47	Minelli et al. (2016): 100 mg better carcass yield, lean meat
Folic acid	mg	0.25–1	–	–	–	0.52–1.05	–
Biotin	mg	–	–	–	0.1	0.105–0.21	Wilt and Carlson, 2009 0.44 mg improved ADG
Choline	mg	100–200	100	–	–	105–210	

Table 5.8 Vitamin inclusion levels (mg/kg feed) for breeder pigs according to 4 swine genetic companies

	Unit	Gilts					Gestation					Breeders references
		Topigs Norsvin, 2016	Hypor, 2017	PIC, 2021	Danbred, 2021	OVN™ (DSM Nutritional Products, 2022b)	Topigs Norsvin, 2016	Hypor, 2017	PIC, 2021	Danbred, 2021	OVN™ (DSM Nutritional Products, 2022b)	
Vitamin A	IU	10,000	12,000	9,920	10,000	10,500–13,100	10,000	12,000	9,920	10,000	10,500–15,700	Lindeman et al. (2008): IM injections 250,000–500,000 IU gilts/sows, more born and weaned piglets
Vitamin D₃	IU	2,000	1,500	1,985	1,000	1,900–2,100	2,000	1,500	1,985	1,000	1,570–2,100	Lin et al. (2017): 2,000 IU increased the sperm motility and effective sperm number
25OHD₃ (HyD®)	mg	–	–	–	–	0.05	–	–	–	–	0.05	Coffey et al. (2012): 0.05 mg improved reproductive performance; Zhang et al. (2020): 0.05 mg improved immune and antioxidant response, bone strength, litter weight, piglet muscle development; Upadhaya et al. (2022): 0.05 mg improved piglet performance; Lin et al. (2017): 2,000 IU increased the sperm motility and effective sperm number
Vitamin E	mg	40	70	66	43	84–105	40	70	66	41	105–160	Wang et al. (2017): 250 mg better milk and sow colostrum, immune and antioxidant response, weaning weight, ADG
Vitamin K	mg	1	2	4.4	4	2.5–4.4	1	2	4.4	4.2	4.7–5.2	–
Vitamin B₁	mg	1–2	2	2.2	2.1	1.05–2.2	1–2	2	2.2	2.1	2.1–2.6	Audet et al. (2004): 20 mg improved sperm production and motility

Table 5.8 (continued)

	Unit	Gilts					Gestation					Breeders references
		Topigs Norsvin, 2016	Hypor, 2017	PIC, 2021	Danbred, 2021	OVN™ (DSM Nutritional Products, 2022b)	Topigs Norsvin, 2016	Hypor, 2017	PIC, 2021	Danbred, 2021	OVN™ (DSM Nutritional Products, 2022b)	
Vitamin B$_2$	mg	4–5	5	10	2.1–5.2	6.3–10.5	4–5	5	10	5.2	6.3–10.5	–
Vitamin B$_6$	mg	1–3	3	3.3	3.2	5.3–8.4	1–3	3	3.3	3.2	3.7–5.7	–
Vitamin B$_{12}$	mg	0.030–0.050	0.05	0.037	0.03	0.032–0.052	0.030–0.050	0.05	0.037	0.03	0.032–0.052	–
Niacin	mg	15–50	50	44	21.4	30–50	15–50	50	44	21.4	32–47	–
D-panthothenic acid	mg	15–30	15	33	11–15.3	16–33	15–30	15	33	15.3	37–42	Wang et al. (2017): 100 mg milk production and quality, litter weight, ADG
Folic acid	mg	3–4	4	1.3	1.6	3.7–5.7	3–4	4	1.3	2.0	3.7–5.7	Wang et al. (2011): up to 100 mg/kg improved milk yield and quality, milk production efficiency and weaning performance; Matte and Girard (1999): 10 mg improved metabolism
Biotin	mg	0.3–0.5	0.2	0.22	0.22	0.32–0.52	0.3–0.5	0.2	0.22	0.5	0.52–0.84	–
Vitamin C	mg	–	–	–	200	210–315	–	–	–	Recommended	210–315	Lin et al. (1985): 30 mg improved sperm production and motility; Lauridsen and Jensen (2005): 250 mg better immunity
Choline	mg	500–750	750	660	–	270–525	500–750	750	660	–	525–840	–
β-carotene	mg	–	–	–	–	–	–	–	–	–	–	–

	Unit	Lactation					Boars		Breeders references
		Topigs Norsvin, 2016	Hypor, 2017	PIC, 2021	Danbred, 2021	OVN™ (DSM Nutritional Products, 2022b)	PIC, 2021	OVN™ (DSM Nutritional Products, 2022b)	
Vitamin A	IU	12,000	14,000	9,920	10,000	10,500–15,700	9,920	10,500–15,700	Lindeman et al. (2008): IM injections 250,000–500,000 IU gilts/sows, more born and weaned piglets
Vitamin D$_3$	IU	2,000	1,000	1,985	1,000	1,570–2,100	1,985	1,570–2,100	Lin et al. (2017): 2,000 IU increased the sperm motility and effective sperm number
25OHD$_3$ (HyD®)	mg	–	–	–	–	0.05	–	0.05	Coffey et al. (2012): 0.05 mg improved reproductive performance; Zhang et al. (2020): 0.05 mg improved immune and antioxidant response, bone strength, litter weight, piglet muscle development; Upadhaya et al. (2022): 0.05 mg improved piglet performance; Lin et al. (2017): 2,000 IU increased the sperm motility and effective sperm number
Vitamin E	mg	60	100	66	186.5	105–190	66	105–160	Wang et al. (2017): 250 mg better milk and sow colostrum, immune and antioxidant response, weaning weight, ADG
Vitamin K	mg	1	3	4.4	4.5	4.7–5.2	4.4	4.7–5.2	–
Vitamin B$_1$	mg	1–3	3	2.2	2.3	2.1–3	2.2	1.05–2.2	Audet et al. (2004): 20 mg improved sperm production and motility

Table 5.8 (continued)

	Unit	Lactation					Boars		Breeders references
		Topigs Norsvin, 2016	Hypor, 2017	PIC, 2021	Danbred, 2021	OVN™ (DSM Nutritional Products, 2022b)	PIC, 2021	OVN™ (DSM Nutritional Products, 2022b)	
Vitamin B$_2$	mg	5–7.5	7.5	10	5.7	6.3–10.5	10	6.3–10.5	–
Vitamin B$_6$	mg	2–4	4	3.3	3.4	3.7–5.7	3.3	3.7–5.7	–
Vitamin B$_{12}$	mg	0.030–0.1	0.01	0.037	0.03	0.032–0.052	0.037	0.032–0.052	–
Niacin	mg	15–100	100	44	23	40–100	44	32–47	–
D-panthothenic acid	mg	15–30	17.5	33	17	37–42	33	21–33	Wang et al. (2017): 100 mg milk production and quality, litter weight, ADG
Folic acid	mg	3–5	3	1.3	2	3.7–5.7	1.3	3.7–5.7	Wang et al. (2011): up to 100 mg/kg improved milk yield and quality, milk production efficiency and weaning performance; Matte and Girard (1999): 10 mg improved metabolism
Biotin	mg	0.3–0.5	0.5	0.22	0.5	0.52–0.84	0.22	0.52–0.84	–
Vitamin C	mg	–	–	–	Recommended	210–315	–	210–525	Lin et al. (1985): 30 mg improved sperm production and motility; Lauridsen and Jensen (2005): 250 mg better immunity
Choline	mg	500–1,000	250	660	–	525–840	660	525–840	–
β-carotene	mg	–	–	–	–	300*	–	–	–

Note: * For improved sow fertility the suggested level must be fed per animal per day immediately after weaning until confirmed conception

Table 5.9 Vitamin inclusion levels (mg/kg feed) for piglets in Brazil, China, and the United States swine industries. Means or average weighted mean and in brackets standard deviation

	Unit	Prestarter (3–20 days) 3–5 kg				Nursery I (21–35 days) 5–10 kg			
		Brazil[1]	USA[2] 2016	USA[3] 2022	China[4]	Brazil[1]	USA[2] 2016	USA[3] 2022	China[4]
Vitamin A	IU	11,368 (6,319)	10,600 (832)	10,878 (2,975)	10,280 (3,848)	11,037 (2,918)	10,274 (3,373)	10,878 (2,975)	10,280 (3,848)
Vitamin D$_3$	IU	2,350 (1,404)	2,554 (2,303)	2,397 (1,605)	3,540 (1,726)	2,247 (715)	1,773 (528)	2,397 (1,605)	3,540 (1726)
Vitamin E	mg	106.2 (87.3)	73.9 (27.7)	93.4 (37.5)	29.4 (28.5)	77.9 (48)	63.4 (25.1)	93.4 (37.5)	29.4 (28.5)
Vitamin K	mg	10.8 (23)	4.0 (0.53)	3.74 (2.16)	4.47 (9.63)	4.1 (2.1)	4.0 (1.5)	3.74 (2.16)	4.47 (9.63)
Vitamin B$_1$	mg	3.1 (1.1)	2.9 (1.9)	8.25 (10.5)	2.77 (4.99)	2.4 (1.0)	2.9 (0.42)	8.25 (10.5)	2.77 (4.99)
Vitamin B$_2$	mg	8.3 (4.1)	9.0 (2.3)	12.5 (6.01)	5.95 (3.59)	6.5 (2.8)	8.6 (2.0)	12.5 (6.01)	5.95 (3.59)
Vitamin B$_6$	mg	4.8 (3.0)	3.7 (0.6)	7.38 (5.27)	3.31 (2.60)	3.6 (1.8)	4.0 (0.81)	7.38 (5.27)	3.31 (2.60)
Vitamin B$_{12}$	mg	0.032 (0.019)	0.0389 (0.024)	0.0408 (0.007)	0.185 (0.0884)	0.0319 (0.0126)	0.0385 (0.0119)	0.0408 (0.007)	0.185 (0.0884)
Niacin	mg	44.3 (23.4)	49.1 (11.4)	50.7 (13.2)	27.1 (14.3)	39.3 (14.0)	47.7 (15.2)	50.7 (13.2)	27.1 (14.3)
D-panthothenic acid	mg	25.1 (14.8)	30.1 (3.6)	36.6 (11.4)	21.3 (14.3)	23.7 (9.3)	29.7 (8.6)	36.6 (11.4)	21.3 (14.3)
Folic acid	mg	2.2 (1.6)	1.6 (4.8)	5.32 (6.01)	2.31 (5.87)	1.7 (1.3)	1.8 (0.9)	5.32 (6.01)	2.31 (5.87)
Biotin	mg	0.64 (1.45)	0.33 (0.90)	0.31 (0.12)	0.20 (0.12)	0.24 (0.21)	0.35 (0.22)	0.31 (0.12)	0.20 (0.12)
Vitamin C	mg	192.3 (151.2)	250	209.5	–	93.9 (8.7)	–	209.5	–
Choline	mg	711.2 (430.9)	245.5 (167)	372.3 (217.5)	448 (379)	521.1 (381.7)	209 (97)	372.3 (217.5)	448 (379)

Table 5.9 (continued)

	Unit	Nursery II (36–49 days) 10–20 kg				Nursery III (50–70 days) 20–29 kg			
		Brazil[1]	USA[2] 2016	USA[3] 2022	China[4]	Brazil[1]	USA[2] 2016	USA[3] 2022	China[4]
Vitamin A	IU	10,966 (3,441)	8,868 (3,676)	10,305 (3,234)	10,186 (3,124)	10,014 (3,308)	5,643 (1,057)	6,903 (2,645)	9,690 (3,103)
Vitamin D_3	IU	2,238 (821)	1,537 (552)	2,273 (1,664)	2,828 (1,239)	2,026 (690.9)	999 (166.5)	1,608 (644.3)	2,565 (1,227)
Vitamin E	mg	69.7 (49.8)	46.9 (20.5)	85.8 (34.3)	33.9 (31.9)	61.2 (43.2)	27.1 (7.7)	57.6 (25.9)	26.2 (22.29)
Vitamin K	mg	3.8 (2.0)	3.5 (1.6)	3.55 (2.2)	3.46 (6.40)	2.8 (1.10)	2.4 (0.57)	3.07 (1.42)	3.33 (5.09)
Vitamin B_1	mg	2.4 (1.0)	3.1 (0.16)	3.76 (2.2)	2.67 (4.80)	2.1 (0.9)	–	2.87 (1.63)	2.02 (2.98)
Vitamin B_2	mg	6.2 (2.6)	7.5 (2.4)	8.65 (1.69)	5.8 (3.78)	5.3 (2.2)	4.8 (1.3)	6.78 (1.89)	5.01 (3.24)
Vitamin B_6	mg	3.4 (1.9)	3.5 (1.9)	5.55 (2.17)	2.91 (2.32)	2.9 (1.6)	–	4.82 (2.24)	2.47 (2.33)
Vitamin B_{12}	mg	0.0311 (0.0129)	0.0332 (0.0136)	0.0381 (0.008)	0.106 (0.006)	0.0279 (0.0123)	0.022 (0.0031)	0.0296 (0.009)	0.069 (0.005)
Niacin	mg	34.8 (14.9)	41.6 (17.6)	47.5 (11.9)	26.4 (14.77)	30.6 (15.6)	27.5 (6.9)	36.4 (10.7)	23.2 (13.83)
D-panthothenic acid	mg	21.1 (9.7)	25.7 (9.7)	34.2 (10.4)	19.3 (11.84)	18.1 (9.4)	16.9 (2.9)	24.8 (7.03)	16.3 (10.4)
Folic acid	mg	1.6 (1.4)	1.9 (1.1)	2.11 (1.59)	2.38 (6.10)	1.3 (1.3)	–	2.53 (1.23)	1.33 (3.64)
Biotin	mg	0.25 (0.25)	0.26 (0.07)	0.32 (0.12)	0.19 (0.11)	0.23 (0.23)	0.07	0.40 (0.15)	0.38 (0.328)
Vitamin C	mg	93.9 (8.7)	–	–	–	45.9	–	–	–
Choline	mg	410.2 (383)	–	329.4 (207.0)	343 (244)	300.4 (371.5)	–	240.5 (170.4)	289 (204)

Note: [1]Dalto and Silva (2020); [2]Flohr et al. (2016); [3]Faccin et al. (2022); [4]Yang et al. (2021c).

Table 5.10 Vitamin inclusion levels (mg/kg feed) for growing and finishing pigs in Brazil, China, and the United States swine industries. Means or average weighted mean and in brackets standard deviation

	Unit	Growing I (71–90 days) 29–50 kg				Growing II (91–112 days) 50–75 kg			
		Brazil[1]	USA[2] 2016	USA[3] 2022	China[4]	Brazil[1]	USA[2] 2016	USA[3] 2022	China[4]
Vitamin A	IU	6,185.6 (2207.3)	5,643 (1057)	4,280 (1,536)	4,946 (2295)	6,185.6 (2207.3)	5,192 (955.2)	3,870 (1,399)	4,656 (1775)
Vitamin D$_3$	IU	1,392.5 (605.5)	998.8 (166.5)	1,167 (462.5)	2,145 (1071)	1,392.5 (605.5)	874.9 (150.7)	1,061 (448.6)	2,058 (963)
Vitamin E	mg	34.5 (25.4)	27.1 (7.7)	35.5 (11.8)	20.1 (24)	34.5 (25.4)	23.3 (7.9)	33.3 (11.7)	23 (30)
Vitamin K	mg	2.0 (0.9)	2.4 (0.57)	1.97 (1.34)	2.55 (1.83)	2.0 (0.9)	2.0 (0.46)	1.79 (1.34)	4.94 (29.97)
Vitamin B$_1$	mg	1.1 (0.6)	–	1.3 (1.65)	1.2 (0.68)	1.1 (0.6)	–	1.20 (1.13)	1.17 (1.70)
Vitamin B$_2$	mg	3.9 (2.0)	4.8 (1.3)	5.03 (0.98)	3.42 (1.65)	3.9 (2.0)	4.2 (1.4)	4.60 (0.99)	3.16 (1.41)
Vitamin B$_6$	mg	1.8 (0.9)	–	1.99 (0.05)	1.55 (1.54)	1.8 (0.9)	–	1.98 (0.16)	1.54 (1.99)
Vitamin B$_{12}$	mg	0.022 (0.00154)	0.022 (0.0031)	0.0023 (0.0042)	0.0148 (0.0084)	0.022 (0.0015)	0.0189 (0.0031)	0.0209 (0.0045)	0.047 (0.0032)
Niacin	mg	21.3 (8.9)	27.5 (6.9)	30.1 (7.08)	16.7 (12.69)	21.3 (8.9)	23.5 (5.1)	27.7 (6.61)	15 (7.45)
D-panthothenic acid	mg	13.9 (7.9)	16.9 (2.9)	18.9 (3.60)	12.4 (8.11)	13.9 (7.9)	14.5 (2.4)	16.6 (3.67)	10.7 (5.97)
Folic acid	mg	0.50 (0.36)	–	0.46 (0.24)	0.74 (1.86)	0.50 (0.36)	–		0.95 (2.93)
Biotin	mg	0.14 (0.17)	0.07	0.1	0.12 (0.07)	0.14 (0.17)	0.07	0.1	0.29 (1.08)
Vitamin C	mg	140.5 (84.2)	–		–	140.5 (84.2)	–		–
Choline	mg	270.6 (377)	–		263 (235)	270.6 (377)	–		188 (100)

Table 5.10 (continued)

	Unit	Finisher 75 kg to market			
		Brazil[1]	USA[2] 2016	USA[3] 2022	China[4]
Vitamin A	IU	5,091.2 (1818)	4,616 (999.2)	3,378 (1,314)	4,826 (1772)
Vitamin D$_3$	IU	1,149 (642.2)	781.7 (209)	932.1 (442.9)	2,005 (914)
Vitamin E	mg	26.9 (17.1)	20 (6.6)	29.9 (11.22)	23.9 (31.28)
Vitamin K	mg	1.7 (0.9)	1.8 (0.53)	1.60 (1.37)	6.79 (41.16)
Vitamin B$_1$	mg	0.94 (0.51)	–	1.15 (0.94)	1.19 (0.67)
Vitamin B$_2$	mg	3.3 (1.7)	3.5 (0.95)	4.06 (1.10)	3.22 (1.35)
Vitamin B$_6$	mg	1.5 (0.7)	–	1.97 (0.25)	1.54 (1.72)
Vitamin B$_{12}$	mg	0.0178 (0.0014)	0.0165 (0.0035)	0.0186 (0.005)	0.029 (0.00214)
Niacin	mg	17.1 (7.3)	20.2 (4.8)	24.6 (6.99)	15.3 (7.3)
D-panthothenic acid	mg	11.6 (6.6)	12.5 (3.1)	14.7 (3.75)	10.8 (5.93)
Folic acid	mg	0.43 (0.29)	–	0.46 (0.24)	0.77 (2.13)
Biotin	mg	0.10 (0.15)	0.04	0.1	0.18 (0.51)
Vitamin C	mg	122.9 (73.7)	–		–
Choline	mg	205.9 (297.3)	–		197 (0.109)

Note: [1]Dalto and Silva (2020); [2]Flohr *et al.* (2016); [3]Faccin *et al.* (2022); [4]Yang *et al.* (2021c).

Table 5.11 Vitamin inclusion levels (mg/kg feed) in Brazil, China, and the United States swine industries breeder pigs. Means or average weighted mean and in brackets standard deviation

	Unit	Gilts				Gestation			
		Brazil[1]	USA[2] 2016	USA[3] 2022	China[4]	Brazil[1]	USA[2] 2016	USA[3] 2022	China[4]
Vitamin A	IU	10,272.6 (3,731.9)	9,405 (2,444)	9,481 (2,243)	6,640 (2952)	10,486.8 (3020.4)	10,362 (1026)	10,511 (1,549)	7,721 (2119)
Vitamin D_3	IU	1,914.8 (549.6)	1,621 (497.2)	2,102 (965.1)	2,512 (1494)	2,154 (1814)	1,783 (360.4)	2,276 (805.9)	2,445 (918)
Vitamin E	mg	71.3 (30.5)	62.5 (29.7)	88.7 (26.9)	45.5 (38.03)	60.7 (42.5)	70 (25.1)	95.5 (22.9)	45.7 (31.5)
Vitamin K	mg	2.6 (0.9)	3.3 (1.1)	3.54 (1.75)	3.01 (1.79)	2.5 (1.5)	3.7 (0.99)	3.9 (2.10)	4.43 (2.11)
Vitamin B_1	mg	1.8 (0.7)	2.2 (0.77)	2.30 (1.11)	1.31 (0.616)	1.7 (0.8)	2.2 (0.77)	2.6 (1.94)	1.49 (0.66)
Vitamin B_2	mg	6.5 (2.0)	7.5 (2.0)	8.27 (1.88)	4.55 (1.95)	5.5 (2.4)	8.1 (1.4)	9.0 (1.26)	4.68 (1.66)
Vitamin B_6	mg	2.9 (1.0)	3.3 (1.1)	3.68 (1.4)	2.57 (2.27)	2.83 (1.27)	3.5 (1.1)	4.1 (1.65)	2.44 (1.52)
Vitamin B_{12}	mg	0.0277 (0.006)	0.0321 (0.0008)	0.0347 (0.007)	0.147 (0.007)	0.0178 (0.009)	0.0352 (0.0048)	0.0379 (0.0057)	0.053 (0.0031)
Niacin	mg	32.6 (7.4)	40.3 (10.8)	41.6 (9.6)	22.6 (10.95)	28.3 (12.7)	45.5 (11.7)	44.9 (9.3)	23 (9.76)
D-panthothenic acid	mg	20.0 (5.9)	25.1 (5.9)	28.9 (6.65)	16.1 (2.01)	17.8 (9.4)	27.3 (4.0)	31.8 (5.5)	17.2 (7.75)
Folic acid	mg	2.0 (1.3)	1.7 (0.73)	2.39 (1.48)	2.34 (4.11)	2.2 (1.5)	1.7 (0.59)	2.65 (1.32)	2.37 (2.45)
Biotin	mg	0.53 (0.42)	0.29 (0.09)	0.35 (0.12)	0.58 (1.63)	0.38 (0.32)	0.29 (0.07)	0.37 (0.10)	0.43 (0.79)
Vitamin C	mg	–	250	209.5	–	132.3 (95.8)	250	209.5	–
Choline	mg	242.7 (128.1)	541.2 (132)	431.6 (258.8)	349 (175)	359.9 (339.6)	610.7 (114.4)	533.3 (115.3)	394 (342)

Table 5.11 (continued)

	Unit	Lactation				Boars			
		Brazil[1]	USA[2] 2016	USA[3] 2022	China[4]	Brazil[1]	USA[2] 2016	USA[3] 2022	China[4]
Vitamin A	IU	10,930.4 (3247.8)	10,404 (918.5)	10,511 (1,549)	5,457 (1693)	11,255.9 (3208.7)	11,249 (1898)	11,193 (1,644)	7,071 (2570)
Vitamin D_3	IU	1,947.8 (704.9)	1,789 (348.7)	2,276 (805.9)	2,437 (904)	2,042.1 (849.8)	847 (442.9)	2,398 (885.9)	2,500 (841)
Vitamin E	mg	59.5 (34.7)	70.2 (24.9)	95.5 (22.9)	46.3 (32.5)	90.5 (73.8)	77.4 (31)	118.4 (34.6)	49.9 (36.3)
Vitamin K	mg	2.4 (1.2)	3.7 (0.99)	3.9 (2.10)	4.47 (14.92)	2.8 (1.7)	3.5 (1.0)	3.93 (1.32)	3.08 (1.8)
Vitamin B_1	mg	1.8 (1.0)	2.2 (0.77)	2.6 (1.94)	1.48 (0.74)	1.8 (1.0)	2.0 (1.2)	2.58 (1.50)	1.45 (0.62)
Vitamin B_2	mg	5.5 (2.0)	8.1 (1.4)	9.0 (1.26)	4.7 (1.66)	6.1 (2.7)	8.1 (1.5)	9.25 (1.36)	4.66 (1.69)
Vitamin B_6	mg	2.5 (1.3)	3.5 (1.1)	4.1 (1.65)	2.4 (1.65)	2.9 (1.6)	3.3 (1.6)	4.78 (2.00)	2.25 (1.18)
Vitamin B_{12}	mg	0.0263 (0.009)	0.0354 (0.005)	0.0379 (0.0057)	0.079 (0.004)	0.0304 (0.012)	0.0464 (0.0035)	0.0405 (0.011)	0.017 (0.006)
Niacin	mg	29.2 (12.0)	45.8 (11.7)	44.9 (9.3)	24.6 (11.69)	32.0 (14.0)	44.9 (6.6)	46.1 (6.52)	21.4 (7.57)
D-panthothenic acid	mg	17.6 (7.5)	27.3 (3.7)	31.8 (5.5)	17 (7.36)	20.1 (10.0)	27.7 (4.2)	32.9 (6.18)	19 (8.46)
Folic acid	mg	2.2 (1.4)	1.7 (0.59)	2.65 (1.32)	2.45 (2.98)	2.7 (1.6)	1.8 (0.7)	3.04 (1.59)	2.94 (4.67)
Biotin	mg	0.36 (0.31)	0.29 (0.07)	0.37 (0.10)	0.36 (0.54)	0.42 (0.31)	0.33 (0.15)	0.47 (0.14)	0.30 (0.18)
Vitamin C	mg	–	250	209.5	–	183.4 (125.5)	250	342.3	–
Choline	mg	408.9 (394.8)	533.9 (108.5)	523.2 (115.1)	350 (164)	433.3 (255.9)	715.7 (507.8)	455.7 (155.8)	401 (130)

Note: [1]Dalto and Silva (2020); [2]Flohr et al. (2016); [3]Faccin et al. (2022); [4]Yang et al. (2021c).

FAT-SOLUBLE VITAMINS

Vitamin A

As discussed in Chapter 4, vitamin A and carotenoids are very susceptible to oxidation reactions, so significant losses may result from feed being stored, ground, exposed to air, or heated. Therefore, it is difficult to determine the actual supply of vitamins from the ingredients used in pig feed. Stable vitamin A is often added in sufficient quantities to meet all the requirements, regardless of the contribution from other ingredients.

Vitamin A facilitates various vital processes and depends on many factors that are difficult to control. These include genetics, productive status, level of reserves in the liver, vitamin or provitamin content of ingredients, storage and technological treatments of feed, capacity for absorption of retinol or of different provitamin forms, capacity for conversion from provitamins to vitamin A, the oxidative status of the animals, consumption, etc. For these reasons, establishing precise recommendations is complicated.

The NRC (2012) recommends 2,200 IU/kg feed for piglets up to 11 kg and 1,750 for piglets up to 25 kg (Table 5.3). Above 25 kg the recommendation is 1,300 IU/kg (Table 5.4). In feeds for gestation, the recommendation increases to 4,000 IU/kg and in lactation, it reduces to 2,000 IU/kg (Table 5.5). These recommendations should be understood to be minimum values. A more realistic view could probably be obtained from research studies, recommendations from other research and academic groups, genetic companies, and surveys that picture the actual utilization in the swine industry.

The Brazilian Tables (2017) recommended supplementation of between 5.6 and 8.5 times more vitamin A, and FEFANA (2015) up to 15.38 times more for piglets (Table 5.3). For growing pigs, the Brazilian Tables suggested levels between 3.85 and 5.59 higher than NRC (2012), while FEFANA recommends between 4.62 and 9.23 times more (Table 5.4). In breeder pigs, the supplementation recommended by the Brazilian Tables is 2.6 to 5.2 times higher than NRC, and FEFANA indicates levels 3.75 to 7.5 times more than NRC (Table 5.5). The DSM Nutritional Products (2022b) OVN™ recommendations are between the Brazilian Tables and the maximum of FEFANA. In some cases, somewhat higher since the recent research discussed herein indicated the benefits of using even higher levels.

The current recommendations from genetic companies are between 5,000 and 22,500 IU/kg for piglets (Table 5.6), 3,750–10,000 for growing, and 2,500–7,500 IU/kg for finisher pigs (Table 5.7). These levels rise to 10,000–12,000 IU/kg for gilts and 10,000–14,000 IU/kg for gestation and lactation (Table 5.8). The variations in recommendations among the 4 swine genetic companies consulted are very high. The genetic companies generally have similar levels to FEFANA, except for PIC, which in 2021 reduced the levels to 5,000 IU/kg for piglets (Table 5.6). In any case, the high variability described indicates the lack of definitive information available and the prevailing confusion. However, compared to previous recommendations of genetic companies (Barroeta *et al.*, 2012), they have been increased.

In a past review (Barroeta *et al.*, 2012) of the vitamin content of feeds used in Spain, Fraga and Villamide (2000) found an average value of 13,800 IU/kg of feed for piglets, 7,800 IU/kg for fatteners and 11,765 IU/kg for breeders. In a similar study in the USA, Coelho (2000) obtained similar values, supporting the opinion that NRC's suggested levels are widely exceeded in practice.

The actual use in the swine industry has increased in the recent years (Tables 5.9, 5.10, and 5.11). Flohr *et al.* (2016) in the USA identified a wide variation in supplementation rates across populations, including higher vitamin A rates than recommended. In nursery diets, the rates were 3.2 times the recommended levels, while on gestation and boar diets (Table 5.11), the supplementations were 2.6 and 2.8 times higher, respectively. In Brazil, Dalto and da Silva (2020) reported levels higher than those observed in the USA and China, with more considerable variability. In the Chinese market survey by Yang *et al.* (2021c), a similar inclusion rate and variations were observed as in the American swine industry study published by Flohr *et al.* (2016). There was an exception in finishing pigs, where the inclusion levels were half of those observed in the USA (Table 5.10). However, Faccin *et al.* (2022) recently reported an increase of up to 2% in the supplementation of vitamin A for sows during gestation and lactation.

Not only have the levels been increasing, but there is also a common trend seeking higher quality in the commercial sources of the vitamins. Microencapsulation is one tendency. Yang *et al.* (2020) proved that microencapsulation of vitamins could improve piglets' bioavailability and growth performance when there was a supplementation of 13,500 IU of vitamin A.

A dosage of 13,500 IU of retinyl acetate was used in a later study by Yang *et al.* (2021a). They determined the relative bioavailability of microencapsulated vitamin supplements compared to the normal form. They proved that while there's no significant difference in the bioavailability measured as the area under the curve (AUC) of vitamin A of the 2 forms of supplements, there is a tendency to increase when vitamin A was formulated with lipid matrix microencapsulation; therefore, indicating that microencapsulation for vitamin A has the potential to improve its bioavailability.

Piglets

Animals in the early phases of growth may receive more benefits from vitamin A supplementation due to the fast growth rates at these stages. Lima *et al.* (2012) reported that administering an injectable ADE vitamin combination (135,000 IU vitamin A, 40,000 IU vitamin D, and 40 mg vitamin E/animal) via deep intramuscular injection at 20 and 40 days of age can increase weight gain. Their data also showed reduced oxidative stress and malondialdehyde production in treated animals at 60 days of age.

Jang *et al.* (2015) concluded that the plasma status of $25OHD_3$, α-tocopherol, and retinyl palmitate are differentially altered between types of vitamins administered and between administration routes. The injection route had a more significant increase and slower disappearance of plasma vitamin levels than the oral route during the suckling period of pigs. The relative bioavailability of oral administration compared with injection administration was 55.26%.

Gannon *et al.* (2017) confirmed that a single high-dose vitamin A supplementation to neonatal piglets increased liver storage of retinol. However, the distribution of injected vitamins varies depending on the vitamin. Jang *et al.* (2020) reported that fat-soluble vitamin injection increased the plasma status of α-tocopherol, retinol, retinyl palmitate, and $25OHD_3$. As plasma levels decreased post-injection, vitamin A levels in the liver and vitamin E levels in the muscle, heart, and liver increased. The α-tocopherol found in plasma after injection was distributed to various tissues but retinyl palmitate only to the liver.

Recently, Hu *et al.* (2020) demonstrated that a dietary supplementation of vitamin A (13,500 IU/kg) could improve serum retinol concentration (Figure 5.3) and immune function and antioxidant capacity (Figure 5.4) in 30-day-old weaned piglets with an initial average body weight of 9.11±0.03 kg. They compared the efficacy of gelatin or starch-encapsulated vitamin A on growth performance, immune status, and antioxidant capacity. The authors found that starch vitamin A is better than gelatin vitamin A, especially in promoting the growth performance of piglets, during an experimental period of 42 days.

Vitamin A interacts with other nutrients in metabolism. Zhou, Qin, Xiong *et al.* (2021) investigated the interactive effects of iron and vitamin A (2,500 IU) on intestinal development and

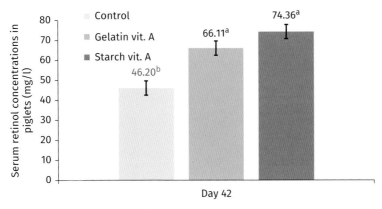

Figure 5.3 Effects of vitamin A (13,500 IU/kg) on serum retinol concentrations in piglets depending on the form of gelatin or starch (Hu *et al.*, 2020). Bars with a different superscript letter (a, b) are significantly different ($p<0.05$)

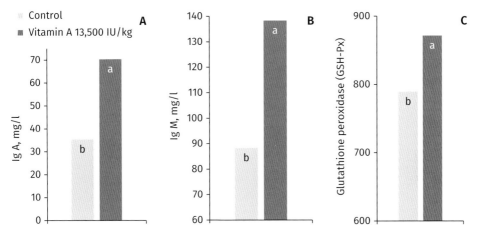

Figure 5.4 Effects of vitamin A (13,500 IU/kg) on immunoglobulin A and M concentrations and glutathione peroxidase in piglets (Hu *et al.*, 2020). Bars with a different superscript letter (a, b) are significantly different ($p<0.05$)

cell differentiation in suckling piglets. These piglets received oral doses of saline solution, 100 mg of ferrous sulfate, 2,500 IU of vitamin A, or 100 mg of ferrous sulfate combined with 2,500 IU of vitamin A on days 2, 7, 12, and 17. The results of this experiment indicated that iron could affect cell proliferation and promote intestinal maturation by improving the morphology of the intestine. Vitamin A stimulates intestinal development by promoting cell differentiation, regulating the expression of stem cell genes, and modulating the related signaling pathways.

Wang *et al.* (2020) indicated that 16 mg/kg of vitamin A (53,333 IU/kg) could improve piglet growth by regulating intestinal stem cells in the jejunum, thereby relieving the weaning stress of piglets. This study lasted 14 days and used 32 21-day-old weaned [(Yorkshire × Landrace) × Duroc] piglets with an average weight of 8.34±0.13 kg that were randomly divided into 4 treatment groups with (1) 2 mg/kg (6,667 IU/kg; control), (2) 4 mg/kg (13,333 IU/kg), (3) 8 mg/kg (26,667 IU/kg), and (4) 16 mg/kg (53,333 IU/kg) doses of vitamin A. The average daily gain

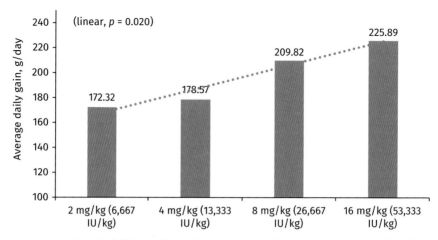

Figure 5.5 Average daily gain (g/dday) affected by vitamin A levels fed to weaned piglets (21 d) for 2 weeks (Wang *et al.*, 2020). The linear effect of vitamin A levels on average daily gain (*p* = 0.020)

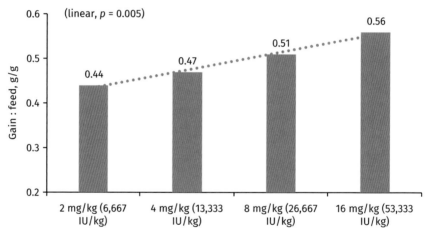

Figure 5.6 Gain-to-feed ratio (g : g) is affected by vitamin A levels fed to weaned piglets (21 d) for 2 weeks (Wang *et al.*, 2020). The linear effect of vitamin A levels on gain: feed ratio (*p* = 0.005)

(Figure 5.5) and feed conversion (Figure 5.6) improved linearly from days 8 to 14. The Lgr5[+] gene expression increased in the jejunum mucosa of piglets fed the 16 mg/kg of vitamin A. This gene is an important marker of intestinal stem cells. The morphology of the jejunum mucosa, including villus height, villi surface area, and crypt depth, were significantly increased in the piglets fed 4 and 8 mg/kg vitamin A, and the ratios of villus height to crypt depth significantly increased in the 16 mg/kg group. The activity of the enzymes maltase, sucrose, and alkaline phosphatase were significantly increased when supplemented with 4 mg/kg vitamin A. Moreover, the budding rates, budding number per organoid, and cell differentiation markers chromogranin A and Muc2 expression of piglet intestinal organoids were significantly reduced by vitamin A and its metabolite retinoic acid.

The effects observed with vitamin A dietary supplementation can be affected by factors like vitamin damage or interactions with other nutrients. Vitamin A is easily oxidized when exposed to heat, light, or humidity (Courraud *et al.*, 2013; Yang *et al.*, 2021a). Vitamin E can enhance vitamin A intestinal absorption and medium concentrations, increasing antioxidant capacity. However, high levels of vitamin A – between 20,000 and 40,000 IU/kg according to Hoppe *et al.* (1992) – can decrease serum levels of vitamin E, inhibit gut bacteria for vitamin K_2 synthesis, and interfere with the liver activity of vitamin K (Gonçalves *et al.*, 2015; Stacchiotti *et al.*, 2021). Vitamin A and C (ascorbic acid) can also interact with antioxidant activities. Zhou, Huang, Bi *et al.* (2021) tested the antioxidant activities of vitamin A 12,000 IU/kg with vitamin C. The combination of vitamins A and C improved immune parameters and antioxidant capacity.

Minerals such as iodine, iron, and zinc also affect vitamin A responses. Zinc is required for vitamin transport. Retinoic acid is involved in iodine uptake, and low vitamin A levels can decrease iodine and impact thyroid metabolism. Iron is necessary for converting β-carotene into retinol, and vitamin A increases iron absorption. These relationships are essential for piglets. Zhou, Qin, Xiong *et al.* (2021) evaluated the interaction effects caused by ferrous sulfate (100 mg) and vitamin A (2,500 IU as retinol acetate) using solutions fed every 5 days to weaned piglets. Researchers concluded that vitamin A could significantly promote intestinal development by enhancing intestinal enzyme activity (Figure 5.7), promoting cell differentiation, regulating the expression of stem cell genes, and modulating the related signaling pathways.

β-carotene can prevent weaning-induced intestinal inflammation by modulating gut microbiota in piglets. Li *et al.* (2021) used piglets weaned on day 21 and supplemented them with oral solutions of either 40 or 80 mg/kg body weight of β-carotene from day 12 to day 26. The results showed that β-carotene improved the growth performance, intestinal morphology and relieved inflammation. Furthermore, β-carotene significantly decreased the species from phyla *Bacteroidetes* and the genuses *Prevotella*, and *Blautia*, and increased the species from the phyla *Firmicutes*. These findings indicate that β-carotene could alleviate weaning-induced intestinal inflammation by modulating gut microbiota

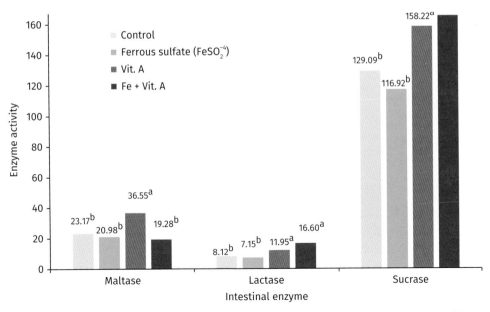

Figure 5.7 Effects of vitamin A and iron (ferrous sulfate) on intestinal enzyme activity in weaned piglets (Zhou, Qin, Xiong *et al.*, 2021). Bars with a different superscript letter (a, b) are significantly different ($p<0.05$)

in piglets. *Prevotella* bacteria may be a potential target of β-carotene in alleviating the weaning-induced intestinal inflammation in piglets.

Gestation and lactation

The risk of subclinical and clinical vitamin A deficiency increases with gestational age, accelerated fetus growth, and the physiological increase of blood volume in swine (Radhika *et al.*, 2002; Vlasova *et al.*, 2013). Vitamin A-deficient women with serum retinol levels at 0.70 µmol/l or below were more susceptible to some enteric and respiratory diseases, with young children at the highest risk (Glasziou *et al.*, 1993; Darlow and Graham, 2016).

Heat stress can play a role in the unavailability of essential micronutrients in the piglet. Amavizca-Nazar *et al.* (2019) reported that sows exposed to a hot environment post-partum have reductions in vitamin A levels in serum (0.21 µg/ml) compared to sows during the winter period (0.29 µg/ml). Consequently, dietary vitamin E and A supplementation could be potentially positive for sows and piglets during heat stress.

Vitamin A appears to improve the reproductive performance of gilts by decreasing embryonic mortality, resulting in more pigs per litter (Brief and Chew, 1985; Lindemann *et al.*, 2008). Weekly injections supplying 12,800 IU vitamin A and 32.6 mg β-carotene per gilt daily resulted in elevated levels of plasma vitamin A and β-carotene, reduced embryonic mortality, and produced more and heavier pigs alive at birth and weaning (Brief and Chew, 1985). Heavier piglets could be associated with better postnatal growth performance and carcass quality in pigs related to myogenesis (Rehfeldt and Kuhn, 2006; Rehfeldt *et al.*, 2008).

A regional study in the USA involving 182 sows was conducted in 5 cooperating experimental stations to determine the effects of intramuscular (IM) injection of high levels of vitamin A (control, 250,000 and 500,000 IU) at weaning and breeding on subsequent litter size of sows (Lindemann *et al.*, 2008). The results of this project demonstrated that injection of high doses of vitamin A in young sows at weaning and breeding improves the subsequent number of pigs born and weaned per litter. This indicates that vitamin A requirements for maximal performance may vary with age. Only sows in parity 1 and 2 were affected, compared to parity sows 3 to 6.

Using the same high-energy-feed gilt model, Whaley *et al.* (2000) reported that a treatment with vitamin A (100,000 IU) stimulated an earlier resumption of meiosis and altered the development of oocytes before ovulation, resulting in more uniform and advanced oocytes and early embryos. Previous reports have also shown improvements in the number of pigs born alive with injectable vitamin A (Coffey and Britt, 1991, 1993; Whaley *et al.*, 2000). Coffey *et al.* (1989) indicated that injecting multiparous sows with β-carotene at weaning increased litter size at the subsequent farrowing.

The liver, serum, and milk levels of vitamin A are affected by dietary supply. The vitamin A and fat concentrations of colostrum and milk were reported by Bowland *et al.* (1949a,b) and a more recent and comprehensive analysis has been published by Csapó *et al.* (1996). Vitamin A content of the milk fat increased at the end of lactation in sows under pasture but decreased in sows fed in intensive systems. Heying *et al.* (2013) demonstrated that high provitamin A carotenoids from orange maize fed during gestation and lactation could improve vitamin A liver levels more in the weanling piglets than a single oral dose of vitamin A (1.05 mmol retinyl palmitate in 5 ml soybean oil) provided to the sows post-conception. Orange maize is a biofortified variety of corn to contain more β-carotene and β-cryptoxanthin. The orange maize provitamin A concentrations before and after mixing with the diet were 14 and 12 µg/g, respectively. Sows fed the orange maize received ~40% more than the sows from the white maize and retinyl ester dose control treatment. Sows fed orange maize had a higher milk reti-nol concentration (1.36±1.30 µmol/l) than those fed white maize (0.93±1.03 µmol/l). Sow livers were collected at the end of the study (n = 3/group) and had identical retinol concentrations (0.22±0.05 µmol/g).

Vitamin A supplementation during lactation may improve the resistance of piglets to diseases. Langel *et al.* (2019) worked with gilts that received 30,000 IU daily oral retinyl acetate starting at gestation day 76 throughout lactation. At 3 and 4 weeks prepartum, vitamin A supplemented and non-supplemented gilts were inoculated with the porcine epidemic diarrhea virus (PEDV) or mock-inoculated. All piglets were PEDV-challenged at 3–5 days postpartum to determine if lactogenic immunity correlated with protection. The survival rate of PEDV + vitamin A litters was 74.2% compared with 55.9% in PEDV litters. Mock and mock + vitamin A litter survival rates were 5.7% and 8.3%, respectively. PEDV + vitamin A gilts had increased PEDV IgA antibody-secreting cells in the ileum and PEDV IgA antibodies in serum prepartum and IgA+β7+ (gut homing) cells in milk post piglet challenge compared with PEDV gilts. These findings suggested that dietary vitamin A supplementation of sows at 30,000 IU improved immunity. Meanwhile, vitamin A can improve the resistance of newborn weaned pigs to infection by PEDV and enhance the pro-tective effect of lactogenic immunity. Previous studies had demonstrated that the resistance of pigs to rotavirus and rotavirus vaccines was decreased when they were diets deficient in vitamin A (Chattha *et al.*, 2013; Kandasamy *et al.*, 2014).

Earlier studies involved treatments using both injections and enhanced dietary levels. In a study involving over 600 sows, Coffey *et al.* (1989) found that injecting β-carotene (0, 50, 100, or 200 mg) at the time of weaning linearly increased by approximately 14% the number of live-born pigs at the subsequent farrowing. Coffey *et al.* (1990) determined that injec-tion of β-carotene is much more effective than oral supplementation concerning the influ-ence on plasma and tissue concentrations. Coffey and Britt (1991) reported improvements in the number of pigs born alive when equivalent doses of vitamin A were utilized, confirming the positive effects of vitamin A on reproductive performance. Treatments consisted of 200 mg β-carotene injections, 50,000 IU vitamin A (palmitate), or vehicle (control) at weaning, breed-ing, and day 7 after breeding. In a subsequent report, Coffey and Britt (1993) provided addi-tional evidence that litter size could be enhanced by injecting either β-carotene or vitamin A into sows receiving sufficient quantities of dietary vitamin A.

These studies indicated that vitamins might impact reproductive efficiency post-weaning. This was confirmed in a study by Lindemann *et al.* (2008). The IM injection of high vitamin A concentrations (250,000 IU and 500,000 IU) to sows at different ages from weaning to breeding demonstrated positive effects in the number of piglets born and weaned from younger sows (1st and 2nd litters). In comparison, the effects were not as significant in older sows (3rd to 6th litters). Again, this study demonstrated that vitamin A requirements for maximum reproductive yield might vary according to age, raising the need to revise the current recommended. In 2013, Lindemann *et al.* concluded that fat supplementation to gestating sows could improve the vitamin status of newborn and nursing pigs.

Growing pigs

Another aspect of interest that should be considered when establishing dosage in the for-mulation of compound feeds is the possible interaction with other nutrients with similar characteristics, such as vitamin E. Evidence shows that high doses of vitamin A in feed cause vitamin E depletion in young pigs' tissue. However, the available data for fattening pigs is scarce and sometimes inconclusive. For example, while Hoppe *et al.* (1992) found interaction in the hepatic tissue when using doses of 20,000–40,000 IU of vitamin A upwards, no effects were found with lower concentrations (10,000 IU). In this study α-tocopherol plasma level after 150 days exceeded those at 42 days in treatments 1 to 3 (5,000, 10,000, and 20,000 IU/kg feed), but not in treatment 4 (40,000 IU/kg): hence the vitamin A dose having an impact on α-tocopherol in this trial was set between 20,000 and 40,000 IU/kg. Anderson et al. (1995a) found no interference in growing-fattening pigs when using concentrations of 20,000 IU of vitamin A. Olivares et al. (2009a) observed in 3 experiments that very high levels of vitamin A (100,000 IU) produced lower fat and liver α-tocopherol concentrations and increased susceptibility of muscle tissue to oxidation, even after 2 weeks of feeding these diets. These authors also did not observe the effects of vitamin A in the 1,300–13,000 IU/kg range on muscle, fat, and liver α-tocopherol concentrations. Still, liver α-tocopherol was higher when vitamin A was removed from the diet 5 weeks before slaughter. This research group also reported (Olivares et al., 2011) that vitamin A supplementation levels (0, 1,300, or 13,000 IU/kg) did not affect growth performance and carcass traits. Pigs fed 1,300 IU/kg had higher intramuscular fat in the longissimus dorsi compared to pigs fed 13,000 IU/Kg. Low vitamin A pigs had saturated fatty acid and decreased monounsaturated fatty acid/saturated fatty acids ratio (MUFA/SFA) in the subcutaneous backfat outer layers, but no muscle fatty acid composition changes were observed. The suppression of vitamin A in the diet fed 5 weeks before slaughter did not affect the intramuscular fat and fatty acid composition of the outer layer of the subcutaneous backfat. At the same time, the saturated fatty acids in the liver decreased, and the PUFA increased.

The effects of removing vitamin A on reducing adipocyte differentiation and fatty acid composition of intramuscular fat (higher MUFA and lower SFA content) were confirmed studied by Ayuso et al. (2015b) when feeding pigs from 35.8 kg live weight to slaughter (158 kg). Removing vitamin A early in life (16.3 kg) or during the growing period (35.8 kg) worsens growth and feed conversion efficiency (Ayuso et al., 2015a). These authors compared diets containing 10,000 IU vitamin A/kg diet with no supplementation (0 IU vitamin A/kg). Vitamin A restriction in young pigs increases lipogenesis without affecting other carcass traits. However, α-tocopherol increases in liver and fat when vitamin A is at low levels or removed.

Vitamin D

Under outdoor production systems, vitamin D may be obtained partially by endogenous synthesis. In practice, it is necessary to include a sufficient quantity of feed to meet the requirements for proper growth. The NRC (2012) recommends 220 IU/kg feed for piglets from 5 to 11 kg, 200 IU/kg for pigs between 11 and 25 kg, and 150 IU/kg during the remainder of the growing and fattening period (Tables 5.3 and 5.4). The quantity for breeders in gestation and lactation is 800 IU/kg (Table 5.5). These recommendations are to avoid deficiency symptoms.

In contrast, the Brazilian Tables (Rostagno et al., 2017), FEFANA (2015), DSM Nutritional Products (2022b) OVN™ and genetic companies recommend optimizing live performance. The Brazilian Tables (Rostagno et al., 2017), FEFANA (2015), and DSM Nutritional Products (2022b) OVN™ for piglets growing and finishing pigs (Tables 5.3 and 5.4) are around 10 times higher than the levels recommended by NRC (2012). For breeder pigs, the suggestions are 2 to 10 times higher than NRC (2012) (Table 5.5). Recommendations from the genetic companies range between 960 and 2,000 IU/kg for piglets (Table 5.6), 440 and 2,000 IU/kg for growing pigs, and 440 and 1,500 IU/kg for finishing pigs (Table 5.7). The genetic companies recommend between 1,000 and 2,000 IU/kg for gilts, sows in gestation, and lactation (Table 5.8).

However, the surveys from the industry indicated that producers have relied on higher levels of vitamin D for a long time. The previous surveys (Barroeta et al., 2012) indicated that the vitamin content in commercial feeds in Spain (Fraga and Villamide, 2000) were, on average, 2,120, 1,112, and 1,720 IU/kg feed for piglets, growing pigs, and breeders, respectively. In the USA, Coelho (2000) reported slightly smaller values with 1,528, 1,418, and 1,602 IU/kg for piglets, growing pigs, and gestating sows, respectively. Recent surveys in Brazil (Dalto and da Silva, 2020), the USA (Flohr et al., 2016; Faccin et al., 2022), and China (Yang et al., 2021b) indicated that vitamin D supplementation increased in the recent years in piglets, e.g., in USA from 999 IU/kg to 1,608 IU/kg for nursery pigs 20–29 kg (Table 5.9), 782–2,145 IU/kg in growing pigs (Table 5.10), 1,621–2,512 IU/kg in gilts, and 1,783–2,445 IU/kg in gestating and lactating sows (Table 5.11).

All these values from commercial recommendations and utilization practice are approximately 10 times more than the figures indicated by the NRC (2012). The coefficients of variation in utilization are still significant but smaller than those with vitamin A. Chinese producers tend to use higher vitamin supplementation levels than Brazilian, with the lowest being in the USA according to a survey conducted in 2016 (Flohr et al., 2016). The recent publication by Faccin et al. (2022), surveying 72% of US sow diets, indicated that there was a 27% increase from the values reported by Flohr et al. (2016). Thirteen of the 36 producers supplied vitamin D through 25OHD$_3$ as a single source or as a percentage of the supplied vitamin D$_3$.

Reproduction, lactation, and piglet performance

Several studies of vitamin D have been conducted in the reproductive and lactation phase. The NRC (1998) indicated that at that time no studies had been reported on the vitamin D requirement in sows during gestation or lactation. Consequently, the vitamin D recommendation for sows during gestation and lactation of 200 IU/kg feed (NRC, 1998) was not based on scientific reports. However, research published in subsequent years has contributed to the knowledge that has formed the basis of the recommendation for increased vitamin D supplementations in gestating and lactating sows to 800 IU/kg feed (NRC, 2012). But recent reports have evaluated even higher levels of supplementation or the use of vitamin D metabolites.

Lauridsen (2014) reviewed and compiled the most essential results from previous studies at the time, which indicated that the dietary vitamin D ranges ran from 200 to 2,500 IU/kg feed, as well as addressing the effects on vitamin D status, performance, reproduction, transfer of vitamin D to the neonate, and bone status markers of gilts and sows (Mahan and Vallet, 1997; Matte and Audet, 2020). Dietary treatments with ≥800 IU/kg feed have shown beneficial effects in bone mineral content and ultimate strength, decreased number of still born piglets, and greater vitamin D status compared with the dietary treatment of 200 IU/kg feed.

More recently, further observation of additional maternal vitamin D supplementation effects on the progeny have been undertaken. Zhao et al. (2022) evaluated the long-term effect of sow vitamin D$_3$ supplementation during gestation on the intestinal health of piglets. Two diets were tested with 800 IU D$_3$/kg or 2,000 IU D$_3$/kg during the gestation of gilts and a standard diet containing 3,000 IU vitamin D$_3$ during lactation. The results indicated that the 2,000 IU D$_3$/kg tended ($p = 0.08$) to reduce the sow body weight loss during lactation. The 2,000 IU D$_3$/kg supplementation improved piglet intestinal health by increasing the relative length and weight of the small intestine and villus height of the duodenum and ileum. Additionally, upregulation of multiple genes markers of gut development and mucosal tight junction integrity (IGF-1, IGF-2R, VDR, GLUT-2, Occludin, ZO-1, MUC2, PEPT1, and CAT1), higher concentrations of secretory immunoglobulin A (IgA) in the jejunum, and increased content of short-chain fatty acids and relative abundance of *Lactobacillus* and *Faecalibacterium* in the feces were observed.

Vitamin D metabolites have also been reported to improve piglet numbers. Coffey et al. (2012) observed that gilts fed diets containing 25OHD$_3$ had an increased number of fetuses on day 90 of gestation compared to vitamin D$_3$-fed gilts. Dietary 25OHD$_3$ may influence implantation through its immunomodulatory effect or its regulation of specific genes associated with implantation (Viganó et al., 2003), leading to a larger litter size. Supplementation of 25OHD$_3$ to sow feed can also affect progeny muscle development. Zhou et al. (2016) reported the benefits of maternal 25OHD$_3$ (50 µg/kg) on prenatal and postnatal skeletal muscle development of pig offspring by modulating the expressions of muscle transcription factors.

Zhou et al. (2017) also observed that sows fed diets supplemented with 25OHD$_3$ (50 µg/kg) during gestation and lactation had one more piglet at farrowing and 1.17 more piglets at weaning than sows fed basal diets with 50 µg/kg vitamin D$_3$. Body weight at weaning is considered a key indicator of the maternal ability of sows and is vital in controlling economic efficiency. Moreover, milk quality is essential for achieving optimum litter performance. Zhou et al. (2017) showed that the content of solids-not-fat, protein, fat, or lactose were improved in the 25OHD$_3$-supplemented sows. Additionally, the serum bone status markers of sows and the bone strength, density, and ash content of piglets were also improved by maternal 25OHD$_3$. Previous observations can explain these effects on milk quality. Zinser and Welsh (2004) reported that vitamin D might contribute to mammary cell turnover during the reproductive cycle via endocrine and autocrine signaling pathways.

These effects of 25OHD$_3$ on sow and piglet bones were confirmed by Zhang et al. (2019a). They used sows with an average body weight of 262.30±3.61 kg and average parity of 3.81±0.26 assigned randomly to 1 of 2 diets supplemented with 2,000 IU/kg vitamin D$_3$ or 50 µg/kg 25OHD$_3$. They concluded that maternal 25OHD$_3$ supplementation improved maternal and neonatal bone properties via modulating milk fatty acid composition and up-regulating mRNA expression levels of calciotropic genes. Bone development is improved by sow supplementation of 50 µg/kg 25OHD$_3$. Thayer et al. (2019) observed more muscle primary fibers (66,139 vs. 37,501) and secondary to primary muscle fibers at birth in piglets from sows supplemented when the basal diet contained 1,500 IU vitamin D$_3$. This indicates a potential for better muscle development with better initial hyperplasia, as demonstrated by Rehfeldt and Kuhn (2006), Rehfeldt et al. (2008) and Hines et al. (2013).

In a later study, Zhang et al. (2019b) determined the effects of maternal 25OHD$_3$ on nutrient digestibility, milk composition, and the fatty acid profile of lactating sows and gut bacterial metabolites in the hindgut of suckling piglets. Sows were assigned randomly to 1 of 2 dietary treatments: 2,000 IU vitamin D$_3$/kg feed or 50 µg 25OHD$_3$/kg feed. The experiment began on day 107 of gestation and continued until weaning on day 21 of lactation. The authors concluded that supplementing diets with 25OHD$_3$ during lactation improved total litter weight gain, calcium digestibility, fat milk content, milk IgG concentration, and milk 25OHD$_3$ content in lactating sows. Moreover, supplementing the lactation diet with 25OHD$_3$ changed gut bacterial fermentation profiles in the hindgut of suckling piglets. In particular, maternal 25OHD$_3$ supplementation enriched butyrate concentration in the cecal digesta of piglets. These results indicated the functional roles of maternal 25OHD$_3$ supplementation on the reproductive performance of lactating sows and gut bacterial metabolites in the hindgut of suckling piglets.

In the study conducted by Zhang et al. (2020), the effects of maternal vitamin D$_3$ (2,000 IU/kg) in the basal diet or the addition of 25OHD$_3$ during the last week of gestation and lactation was studied on serum parameters, intestinal morphology, and microbiota in suckling piglets. Higher litter weight at weaning were observed after maternal 25OHD$_3$ (50 µg/kg) supplementation, coupled with an increased total litter weight gain, which indicated that maternal 25OHD$_3$ supplementation improved the growth rate of piglets (Figure 5.8). This result could be partially explained by higher growth hormone and insulin-growth factor (IGF-I) in the serum of piglets.

The antioxidant capacity of colostrum and milk was also improved. Sows fed the diet with 25OHD$_3$ had higher antioxidant activities, better glutathione peroxidase (GSH-Px) activity in

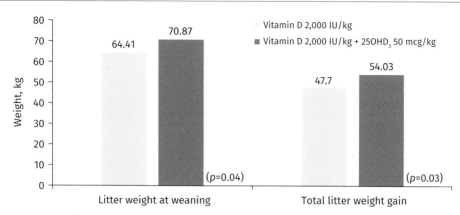

Figure 5.8 Effect of maternal sources of vitamin D (2,000 vitamin D_3 or 2,000 vitamin D_3 + 50 µg/kg 25OHD$_3$) on litter weight (Zhang *et al.*, 2020)

colostrum, and superoxide dismutase (SOD) and GSH-Px activities in milk than in sows fed the basal diet. Feeding 25OHD$_3$ to sows tended to increase ($p<0.10$) the species richness in the colonic digesta of suckling piglets and the relative abundance of colonic *Alloprevotella* and caecal *Lactobacillus*. In contrast, the population of the caecal *Eubacterium coprostanoligenes group* was lower. In conclusion, adding 50 µg/kg 25OHD$_3$ to maternal diets during lactation improved antioxidant capacity, enhanced growth performance and intestinal health, and regulated gut microbiota in suckling piglets.

In a more recent literature review, Zhang and Piao (2021) indicated that new research results suggested that dietary 25OHD$_3$ supplementation may improve milk quality via its effect on mammary glands thereby increasing milk fat, protein, and lactose content. Sow 25OHD$_3$ supplementation could improve the mRNA expressions of insulin-induced gene 1 (INSIG1) and sterol regulatory element-binding protein 1 (SREBP1) in the mammary gland cells from milk and increase the mRNA expressions of acetyl-CoA carboxylase α (ACCα) and fatty acid synthase (FAS) in the mammary gland tissue. Maternal 25OHD$_3$ supplementation improved growth performance and skeletal muscle development in piglets before and after parturition, while sows had a similar feed intake.

Several authors (Coffey *et al.*, 2012; Zhou *et al.*, 2017; Zhang *et al.*, 2019a,b) concluded that feeding 50 µg/kg 25OHD$_3$ to sows during gestation and lactation improved sow and newborn piglet serum 25OHD$_3$ concentrations, which resulted in improvements in reproductive performance, milk quality, sow and piglet bone metabolism, bone density, and breaking force. Finally, these authors discussed the effects of supplementing 25OHD$_3$ in sow diets on the gut microbiota metabolites of suckling piglets and proposed an indirect role of butyrate production on bone health.

Maternal supplementation with other vitamin D metabolites have shown similar effects in the progeny. Wang *et al.* (2022b) evaluated the supplementation of 1α,25(OH)$_2$D$_3$ in 140 crossbred gilts (Landrace × Yorkshire). Levels of 0, 1, 2, and 4 µg/kg of 1α,25(OH)$_2$D$_3$-glycosides were used. The results indicated that 4 µg/kg 1α,25(OH)$_2$D$_3$-glycosides significantly promoted the piglet birth weight, weaning weight, colostrum quality, and lactation ability of primiparous sows. This metabolite also may regulate mammary gland development and lactation by multiple signaling pathways. Proteomic analysis identified 48,868 unique peptides and 4,292 differentially abundant proteins in the mammary tissues for the 1α,25(OH)$_2$D$_3$-glycosides supplemented treatment. These peptides and proteins are involved in multiple potential signaling pathways, mainly including fatty acid metabolism, fatty acid biosynthesis, regulating lipolysis in fat cells, peroxisomes, and peroxisome proliferators-activated receptor (PPAR) signaling pathways.

Recently Hasan *et al.* (2023) published a review based on a data search on Web of Science and PubMed databases concerning the efficacy of vitamin D$_3$ in comparison with 25OHD$_3$ on pig physiology, i.e., reproductive capacities, growth performance, immunity, and bone development. Dietary intake of vitamin D$_3$ or 25OHD$_3$ did not influence the reproductive capacity of sows. Unlike Vitamin D$_3$, the maternal intake of 25OHD$_3$ significantly improved the growth performance of piglets, which might be attributed to maternally induced micronutrient efficiency. Consequently, even in the absence of maternal vitamin D$_3$ supplementation, 25OHD$_3$-fed offspring also demonstrated better growth than the offspring receiving vitamin D$_3$. Moreover, a similar superior 25OHD$_3$ impact was seen with respect to serum markers of innate and humoral immunity. Last but not least, supplements containing 25OHD$_3$ were found to be more effective than vitamin D$_3$ to improve bone mineralization and formation, especially in pigs receiving basal diets low in calcium and phosphorus. The insights are of particular value in determining the principal dietary source of vitamin D$_3$ to achieve its optimum utilization efficiency, nutritional benefits, and therapeutic potency and to further improve animal welfare across different management types.

Boars

Vitamin D can play a role in male reproductive ability. Lin *et al.* (2017) evaluated the effects of the different levels of dietary vitamin D on boar performance and semen quality. The author concluded that supplementing boar diets with 2,000 IU/kg vitamin D$_3$ increased sperm motility and sperm number and reduced sperm deformities (Figure 5.9). Additionally, these results aligned with the elevated concentrations of vitamin D in the seminal plasma, hormone secretion (testosterone and aromatase), and gene expression in sperm. Testosterone concentrations were 4.49, 6.21, and 5.88 ng/ml for boars fed 200, 2,000, and 4,000 IU of vitamin D$_3$, respectively. These higher levels of supplementation for boars have been adopted in China and Brazil but not in the USA yet (Table 5.9).

Piglets

The level and source of vitamin D can play an essential role in piglet growth and health. Vitamin D can impact the antioxidant systems, immunity, mineral utilization, and gut microbiota.

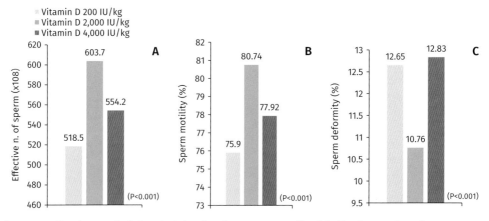

Figure 5.9 Effect (*p*<0.001) of vitamin D$_3$ level on boar sperm quality: (A) effective number of sperm (1×108); (B) sperm motility (%); (C) sperm deformity (%) (Lin *et al.*, 2017)

Environmental factors, weaning, and infection can induce oxidative stress, which leads to severe economic losses (Williams *et al.*, 1997). Vitamin D_3 adminstered as single injections or daily supplementation via drinking water are adequate to increase blood serum $25OHD_3$ in nursery pigs (Dal Jang *et al.*, 2018).

Mukhopadhyay *et al.* (2000) showed that vitamin D_3 acted as an antioxidant on rapidly proliferating neoplasms in mice. However, little work has been done on the antioxidative properties of vitamin D that can help with immunity in pigs. Konowalchuk *et al.* (2013) observed positive immunomodulatory effects of $25OHD_3$, increasing leukocyte cell numbers and phagocytic capacity across blood and bronchoalveolar compartments that may increase systemic and mucosal antimicrobial responses.

Zhao *et al.* (2014) demonstrated the effects of 5,000 IU/kg of vitamin D_3 (VD 5000 IU) compared to 200 IU/kg (VD 200 IU) in piglets challenged with porcine rotavirus (PRV). In this experiment, piglets recovered average daily feed intake (ADFI), average daily gain (ADG), and feed conversion (feed : gain ratio) post-challenge with rotavirus (Table 5.12). The same authors also observed that 5,000 IU/kg of vitamin D_3 improved the villi height and crypt depth, the immune response, and the consistency of feces post-challenge with PRV (Figure 5.10). Yang *et al.* (2019b) observed similar effects of $25OHD_3$ alleviating the PEDV by improving the intestinal structure and immune response in weaned pigs.

The effect of dietary $25OHD_3$ supplementation on growth performance, immune function, and antioxidant capacity in weaned piglets was studied by Yang *et al.* (2019a). Piglets were divided into 5 groups and fed diets supplemented with 5.5, 43.0, 80.5, 118.0, and 155.5 µg $25OHD_3$/kg, respectively. The treatment with 5.5 µg $25OHD_3$/kg (equivalent to 220 IU vitamin D/kg) was used as a control. Adding 80.5 and 118.0 µg $25OHD_3$/kg diet enhanced serum GSH-Px activity and malondialdehyde (Figure 5.11). GSH-Px is an antioxidative enzyme that helps control lipid and hydrogen peroxide levels (Rotruck *et al.*, 1973). Those results indicated that feeding high doses of $25OHD_3$ partly improved immune functions and the antioxidative capacity in weaned pigs.

Table 5.12 Effect of vitamin D_3 level on live performance response of piglets challenged with porcine rotavirus (PRV) (Zhao *et al.*, 2014)

Items	PRV (−)		PRV (+)	
	VD 200 IU/kg	VD 5,000 IU/kg	VD 200 IU/kg	VD 5,000 IU/kg
ADFI (g)				
Pre-challenge (0–7 days)	1,365.00	1364.5	–	–
Post-challenge (8–14 days)	1,350.1[a]	1398.5[a]	1067.5[c]	1251.5[b]
ADG (g)				
Pre-challenge (0–7 days)	669.6	658.8	–	–
Post-challenge (8–14 days)	669.4[a]	679.2[a]	430.6[c]	540.3[b]
Feed: gain ratio				
Pre-challenge (0–7 days)	2.04	2.07	–	–
Post-challenge (8–14 days)	2.02[c]	2.06[c]	2.49[a]	2.32[b]

Note: ADFI = average daily feed intake; ADG = average daily gain. a-c Means within a row with unlike superscript letters were significantly different ($p<0.05$).

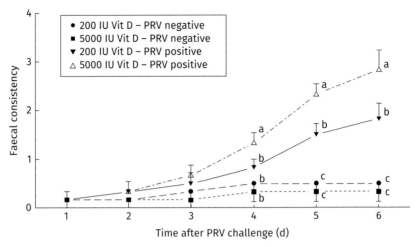

Figure 5.10 Fecal scoring of piglets fed with diets containing either 200 or 5,000 IU/kg of vitamin D$_3$ and challenged with porcine rotavirus (PRV). Fecal consistency scores: 0, solid; 1, semi-solid; 2, semi-liquid; 3, liquid (Zhao *et al.*, 2014)

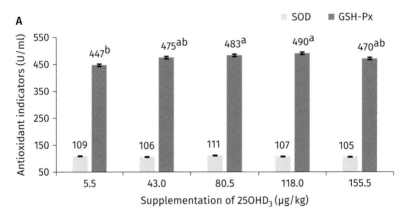

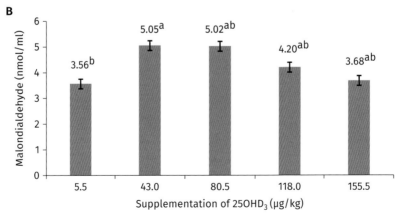

Figure 5.11 Effect of dietary levels of 25OHD$_3$ on (A) antioxidant indicators (U/ml) and (B) malondialdehyde in the serum of weaned piglets (Yang *et al.*, 2019a). Bars with different letters (a, b) indicate significant differences (*p*<0.05)

In a recent study, Zhou *et al.* (2022) observed that vitamin D_3 could not promote optimal antioxidant capacity when feeding diets containing a regular dose of 2,000 IU/kg of vitamin D_3 to weaned piglets. In contrast, piglets fed diets containing $25OHD_3$ at the same dosage (50 µg/kg) had better growth performance, an improved antioxidant capacity with better intestinal integrity and IgA content than those supplemented with vitamin D_3. In agreement with several studies showing that vitamin D_3 is critical in modulating immune function, also in this trial, the supplementation of $25OHD_3$ decreased the frequency of CD_3+CD_4+ and CD_3+CD_8+ T-cells linearly. The results indicated that feeding high doses of $25OHD_3$ (43.0, 80.5, 118.0, and 155.5 ug $25OHD_3$/kg) improved immune functions and the antioxidative capacity in weaned pigs and that a "regular" dosage of 2,000 IU/kg vitamin D_3 in the weaned piglets' diet did not achieve optimal antioxidant capacity and immune function.

Previous studies have shown that the proliferation of cytotoxic T-lymphocytes and T-helper cells was suppressed by regulatory cells (T_{reg}) (Käser *et al.*, 2011), which could be induced by $1,25(OH)_2D_3$ (Lucas *et al.*, 2014). The data collected by Zhao *et al.* (2022) referenced supplementation with 1,500 IU/kg of feed of phytase and 50 µg/kg of $25OHD_3$ for weaned piglets (21 days of age) could enhance dietary calcium and phosphorus utilization and promote bone development in low calcium diets.

Recently, Zhang *et al.* (2022) found that supplementing 50 µg/kg of $25OHD_3$ in a low calcium–phosphorus diet improved serum immunity, bone biochemical parameters, and fecal microbiota (such as decreased *Streptococcaceae* abundance and increased *Lachnospiraceae* abundance), which could subsequently promote the growth of piglets. The effects were similar to that of a regular calcium–phosphorus diet. These results indicate that although no differences in performance are observed in the first pig life stage, the physiological results may yield better performance results later.

Immediately post-weaning, piglets are prone to gastrointestinal infectious diseases. The active metabolite of vitamin D $1,25(OH)_2D_3$ has direct impact on immune cell function and responses. Thus, a low vitamin D status may compromise the immune responses during infectious diseases. Madsen *et al.* (2023) investigated the effect of supplementation of either vitamin D_3 or $25OHD_3$ on suckling piglets' vitamin D status at weaning and whether the vitamin D status could affect their immune development and robustness against *E. coli* challenge. Genetically *E. coli* F4 susceptible litters of piglets were divided into 2 treatment groups: group 1 (n = 16) provided milk formula supplemented with vitamin D_3 (Control: CON), and group 2 (n = 16) provided milk formula supplemented with $25OHD_3$ (Treated: TREAT). Piglets were offered the experimental milk formulas from day 3 after farrowing until weaning (at day 28 of age). Vitamin D status in piglets was investigated by collection of plasma samples on days 3, 15, 28 and 35 of age. In general, the vitamin D status of the piglets was low. However, piglets provided TREAT during the suckling period had increased vitamin D status at weaning compared to piglets provided CON. Vitamin D was used during activation of the immune system as pigs inoculated with *E. coli* had lower plasma concentrations of $25OHD_3$ than non-inoculated pigs possibly due to mobilizing of vitamin D in the liver. Hence, increased vitamin D status at weaning might improve piglets' resistance to *E. coli* infection.

Growing and finishing pigs, and pork quality

Very high vitamin D_3 has been fed to pigs for short periods before slaughter to increase meat quality (Wilborn *et al.*, 2004). Enright *et al.* (1998) fed swine diets containing 3 levels of vitamin D_3 (331, 55,031, or 176,000 IU/kg) to finishing pigs for the last 10 days before slaughter. They reported that feeding the higher levels of vitamin D_3 reduced feed intake and average daily gains while increasing serum calcium concentration. Reduced drip loss and color values (Hunter L* measurement) and improved subjective color and firmness scores were exhibited in the carcass due to increased dietary vitamin D_3. Tenderness was not evaluated in this study.

Sparks et al. (1998) determined that the optimal vitamin D_3 was 500,000 IU daily for 3 days before slaughter based on blood calcium concentration. The researchers stated that the results of feeding high vitamin D_3 in this initial study did not improve pork tenderness and other measures of pork quality.

Wiegand et al. (2002) fed finishing pigs 500,000 IU per day of vitamin D_3 3 days before slaughter. Vitamin D supplementation did not affect quality characteristics (measured by subjective scores) or tenderness (Warner-Bratzler shear force). However, the treatment improved Hunter's color values at 14 days of storage. Other researchers (Wilborn et al., 2004) observed that supra nutritional levels of vitamin D_3 (40,000, or 80,000 IU vitamin D_3/kg) improved pork color and increased pH in Duroc-cross pigs. Still, it took at least 44 days to observe significant effects and retarded growth if fed at 80,000 IU/kg.

Vitamin D metabolites supplementation has been used for several years with positive effects. Regassa et al. (2015) evaluated the effects of $25OHD_3$ at 50 and 100 µg/kg on top of a wheat-corn-soybean diet containing 150 IU/kg of vitamin D_3 in growing female pigs with an initial weight of 23.13±1.49 kg. At the end of the 42-day experimental period, these researchers evaluated bone density, calcium and phosphorus gut transporters gene expression, calcium and phosphorus fecal digestibility. Diets with $25OHD_3$ did not significantly improve bone mineralization or gene expression but reduced calcium and phosphorus excretion.

In contrast, Duffy et al. (2018a,b) observed positive results when investigating the effects of supplementing both $25OHD_3$ (50 µ/kg) and phytase (500 units/kg) on pig performance, nutrient digestibility, carcass characteristics, bone parameters, and pork quality in finisher pigs. A factorial design was used in a low-phosphorus diet. Pigs supplemented with $25OHD_3$ had higher phosphorus and nitrogen digestibility coefficients (Figure 5.12). In contrast, the phytase group had better apparent total tract digestibility of ash, phosphorus, and calcium than pigs that offered nonphytase-supplemented diets. The supplementation with $25OHD_3$ also improved meat color, increasing redness ($p = 0.009$), yellowness ($p = 0.009$), and saturation

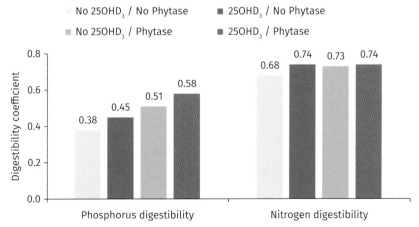

Figure 5.12 Effect of $25OHD_3$ and phytase on phosphorus and nitrogen digestibility after 45 days of feeding experimental diets to finishing pigs (Duffy et al., 2018a)

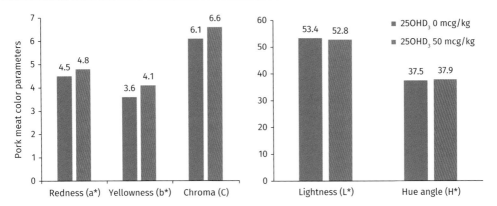

Figure 5.13 Effect of 25OHD$_3$ and phytase pork meat color after 55 days of feeding experimental diets to finishing pigs with 108±0.56 kg final live weight (Duffy *et al.*, 2018a)

values (*p* = 0.001) (Figure 5.13), mainly by increasing antioxidative capacity and decreasing the rate and extent of pH decline.

The enrichment of pork with vitamin D has been evaluated in several studies. Many factors can affect vitamin D uptake into the muscles. Rosbotham *et al.* (2021) used machine learning techniques to identify factors influencing the vitamin D bio-enrichment of pork. Their target variable was vitamin D activity calculated as vitamin D$_3$ + (25(OH)D$_3$ × 5) in bio-enriched pork, categorized as "high" (>19 µg/kg) or "low" (≤19 µg/kg). The models obtained F1 scores ranging from 57.1% to 77.1%. The K-nearest neighbor algorithm (KNN) and the C4.5 algorithm performed best (77.1% and 75%) in determining the best variables. Serum 25OHD$_3$ levels at the midpoint and endpoint of the study, body weight gain, and body weight at slaughter were commonly identified by Naïve Bayes, decision trees (C4.5 and classification and regression trees), and KNN as the 4 most important factors influencing vitamin D activity in bio-enriched pork. Results from all 5 classification models determined sex to be the least important feature influencing the bio-enrichment process.

Gestation, lactation, and growing-finishing pig performance

The effects of 25OHD$_3$ supplementation on gestating and lactating sows and their progeny during the growing and finishing period were evaluated by Flohr *et al.* (2014) and recently by Upadhaya *et al.* (2022). Forty-eight multiparous sows were fed either a basal diet containing 2,000 IU/kg vitamin D$_3$ and supplemented without (Control: CON) or with (Treated: TRT) 50 µg/kg 25 OHD$_3$. At weaning, 80 pigs each from CON and TRT sows were allocated to weaning. Growing-finishing basal diets were fortified with 2,500 and 1,750 IU/kg vitamin D$_3$ and supplemented without or with 50 µg/kg 25OHD$_3$. Sows fed 25OHD$_3$-supplemented diets improved the pre-weaning growth rate of nursing piglets, as previously reported in several studies.

At 42 days post-weaning, a significant effect of the sow and pig weaning diet was observed on the growth rate. Later, pigs consuming 25OHD$_3$-supplemented diets gained weight faster, ate more, and tended (*p* = 0.088) to convert feed to gain more efficiently than those fed a CON diet between days 98 and 140 post-weaning (Figure 5.14). The pork meat quality evaluation showed better water holding capacity and reduced drip loss for pork meat of 25OHD$_3$-supplemented pigs. On physiological parameters, supplemental 25OHD$_3$ produced higher interleukin-1 and lower interleukin-6 concentrations in blood circulation, downregulated myostatin, and up-regulated myogenic differentiation and myogenic factor 5 gene expressions. These data

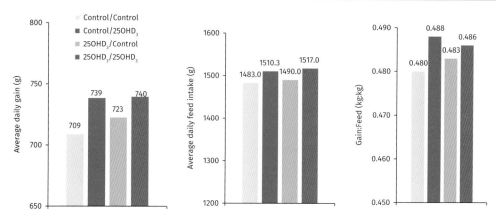

Figure 5.14 Effect of 25OHD$_3$ supplementation in the piglet diets on the live performance of piglets from sows fed diets with or without 25OHD$_3$ supplementation (Upadhaya *et al.*, 2022)

collectively indicated that growing pigs may benefit from 25OHD$_3$ supplementation improving the growth rate, feed conversion, meat quality, and immunity.

Vitamin E

With consideration of the multiple effects of the many processes in which vitamin E is involved and the possibility of using larger quantities to boost some aspects of health or the quality of products vitamin E recommendations can and have been established to achieve different end points. Consequently, the figures recommended for pigs in the bibliography also vary considerably. This review will first study the established recommendations to obtain optimum productive efficiency, pointing out, when necessary, the existence of data to indicate the possible usefulness of modifying the supply according to the situation or production objectives desired in certain circumstances. The second part will examine the possible usefulness of providing higher quantities to improve meat characteristics.

The vitamin E requirements needed to avoid classical deficiencies have been estimated by the NRC (2012) to be 16 IU/kg feed for piglets up to 11 kg live weight and 11 IU/kg feed for growing pigs up to 120 kg live weight (Tables 5.3 and 5.4). The recommendation for gestating and lactating sows and boars rises to 44 IU/kg (Table 5.5). These were the same values recommended by NRC (1998), while the productivity of pigs has improved in the past decades (Culbertson *et al.*, 2017). In contrast, recommendations from FEFANA (2015) and the Brazilian Tables (Rostagno *et al.*, 2017) are 4.6 to 9.4 times higher for piglets (Table 5.3), 2.72 to 9.1 times higher for growing pigs (Table 5.4), and 1.3 to 1.8 more prominent for sows in gestation and lactation (Table 5.5). Also the DSM Nutritional Products (2022b) OVN™ recommendations are overall in the same range of multiples compared to NRC (2012) with some higher levels in critical phases targeting specific responses (e.g. immune modulation).

The genetic companies recommend between 3.2 and 10.1 times more vitamin E for piglets (Table 5.6) than the NRC (2012), 2.3–9 times more for growing pigs (Table 5.7) and 1.5–2.3 times more for sows in gestation and lactation (Table 5.8). These practical recommendations differ considerably due to the variability of swine production systems and the broad range of vitamin E functions and expected results.

The inclusion levels in the swine industry have increased. Two decades ago, Fraga and Villamide (2000) reported levels of vitamin E for piglets of 31.4 IU/kg (with a range 3.3–100 IU/kg), 9.5 IU/kg for growing pigs (range 0–20 IU/kg) and breeders 23.6 IU/kg (range

5.4–53.6 IU/kg) in the Spanish swine industry. In the USA, Coelho (2000) found much higher concentrations, with average values for piglets, growers, fatteners, and breeders of 52, 28, 20, and 54 IU/kg, respectively. The recent surveys in Brazil (Dalto and da Silva, 2020), the USA (Flohr et al., 2016; Faccin et al., 2022), and China (Yang et al., 2021b) indicated levels 2–6.6 times higher than NRC (2012) in piglets (Table 5.9), 2 to 3 times in growing pigs (Table 5.10), and double in breeders (Table 5.11).

Sows and piglets

Several studies on breeder sows have demonstrated a positive relationship between vitamin E administration and the number of piglets born (Carrion et al., 1994). Mahan (1991) included 4 vitamin E concentrations (0, 16, 33, and 66 mg/kg) in feed for breeder sows during 3 consecutive reproductive cycles and observed a characteristic exponential response. However, some information indicates that the use of vitamin E in the breeder sow goes beyond improving the number of piglets born or survival to 7 days (Cargill et al., 1994). For example, some reproductive failures could be associated with the deficient production of prostaglandins close to farrowing, the concentration of which depends to quite an extent on the oxidative status of animals. Still, an increase in the duration of parturition has been shown when vitamin E intake is reduced, which could be due to inadequate contraction of the smooth musculature (on muscle contraction, being related with calcium availability, also vitamin D has an important influence). A relationship between vitamin E intake and the incidence of MMA has also been shown (Mahan, 1991, 1994a; Cargill et al., 1994; Carrion et al., 1994). It is worth pointing out that vitamin E transfer through the placenta is minimal, so piglets are born with deficient levels of α-tocopherol (Mahan and Vallet, 1997; Matte and Audet, 2020).

This is supremely important because it has been demonstrated experimentally that vitamin E increases immune response capacity (Wuryastuti et al., 1993). Iron administration in the neonatal period also overloads the piglet's limited antioxidant capacity (Hill et al., 1999). Thus, it has been recognized as necessary to establish strategies that increase the concentration of α-tocopherol in the piglet, foremost among them the dam's diet during the final stages of gestation and the lactation period (Mahan et al., 2000). Given good physiological conditions in sows fed with conventional feed, colostrum provides a very high concentration of α-tocopherol (more than 20 µg/ml), which permits a considerable increase of α-tocopherol in tissue concentration in piglets during the first few days of their life.

This is achieved by the sow drawing on her physical reserves of α-tocopherol, which in the days following parturition causes a sharp drop in the concentration of α-tocopherol in her serum which goes from a value close to 2–3 µg/ml (5–7 µmol/l) to a value less than 1 µg/ml (2.5 µmol/l). The concentration of α-tocopherol in the milk falls during lactation until it reaches a figure close to 2 µg/ml (5 µmol/l). Consequently, the concentration in the piglet serum also falls until it reaches a figure close to 3–4 µg/ml (7–9 µmol/l). This behavior seems to indicate that it might be helpful to increase the supply of vitamin E to the breeder sow in gestation and/or lactation so that there is a greater possibility of transfer to the piglet (Mahan and Vallet, 1997). Hidiroglou et al. (1993) observed a linear response in the α-tocopherol content of milk when between 22 and 88 mg of vitamin E/kg was included in feed. Babinszky et al. (1992) observed that increasing vitamin E supplementation up to 136 mg/kg in feed for sows during the pre-weaning period improved immune response in weaned piglets. When evaluating lower levels it has not been possible to observe these effects.

Vitamin E supplementation generally has synergic effects with selenium supplementation. Hayek et al. (1989) concluded that supplementation with vitamin E (1,000 IU) and/or selenium

(5 mg) as a single injection administered on day 100 of gestation augmented the transfer of immunity to pigs from sows fed levels of vitamin E and selenium that approximated the sow's requirement (NRC, 1998). Colostral immunoglobulin transfer is essential to the pig's immunity and survival. The newborn pig lacks circulating antibodies (Bourne et al., 1978; Hakkarainen et al., 1978b) and must draw on maternal immunoglobulins via colostrum during the first few hours postpartum (Butler, 1984).

Okere and Hacker (1997) evaluated whether prepartum injections of vitamin E and/or selenium to sows effectively enhanced reproductive performance and augmented the colostral transfer of immunoglobulins to piglets. Piglet serum IgG was significantly higher in the treatment groups at 24 hours postpartum, 7 days of age, and at weaning. These authors hypothesized that immune-deficient porcine neonates could benefit from the improved IgG transfer attributed to vitamin E and/or selenium supplementation of the sows (Matte and Audet, 2020).

This hypothesis was also explored by Hayek et al. (1987) with some positive results. In their study, Nemec et al. (1994) could not consistently confirm the positive effects of vitamin E supplementation on immunoglobulin transfer. Vitamin E-supplemented sows did have a significant dose-dependent increase in milk IgG levels but only on day 14 after parturition. However, for gilts that received 110 or 220 IU of vitamin E per kg of diet during lactation, offspring required less time to acquire phytohemagglutinin response and displayed a greater concanavalin A reply than did piglets from sows supplemented with 55 IU of vitamin E per kg. Thus, maternal vitamin E supplementation improved the ability of newborn pigs to acquire cellular immunity as measured by these responses.

In another study, Lauridsen and Jensen (2005) observed that the content in the sow's plasma and the milk rises linearly when the concentration of vitamin E in the feed is increased from 70 to 250 IU/kg and this response is maintained throughout lactation. Figure 5.15 shows the concentration of α-tocopherol in the hepatic tissue of piglets according to the concentration of vitamin E in the dam's feed during the lactation period. At the time of weaning (at 28 days), the concentration of α-tocopherol in the liver of piglets whose mothers received 250 IU is more than double that of piglets whose mothers received 70 IU.

In a field study evaluating the nutritional status of pig breeding herds in Norway, Sivertsen et al. (2007) observed that supplementation with 0.3 and 0.4 mg selenium per kg feed in the form of sodium selenite and 110 to 161 mg vitamin E per kg feed, as α-tocopheryl acetate, were probably suboptimal but the levels of these 2 nutrients partially compensate for each other

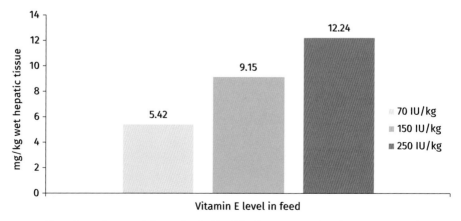

Figure 5.15 Effect of supplemental dietary (as-fed basis) all-*rac*-α-tocopheryl acetate to sow feed on the concentration of α-tocopherol in wet hepatic tissue piglets on day 28 (Lauridsen and Jensen, 2005)

in the weaning period. Mean plasma vitamin E was 4.0 µg/ml in the sows and 2.6 µg/ml in the piglets the day before farrowing, fell to 1.6 µg/ml in the weanling pigs at day 4, and remained low. Mean plasma selenium was 0.22 µg/g in the sows and 0.08 µg/g in the piglets before farrowing, rose to 0.10 µg/g in the weanlings at day 4, and continued rising. Consequently, these authors recommended higher levels of vitamin E supplementation for sows.

Combining vitamin E with other antioxidant vitamins like ascorbic acid or, as already observed, minerals like selenium has shown more efficacy (Yen et al., 1985). Sosnowska et al. (2011) reported that the addition of vitamin E (200 mg/kg) together with vitamin C (500 mg/kg) significantly reduced the body temperature of sows after farrowing and considerably reduced the number of sows culled after rearing. The concentrations of both vitamins in the blood serum of piglets increased, but no significant effects on piglet or litter performance were detected. Chen et al. (2016) evaluated the effects of selenium and vitamin E in sow diets on antioxidant status and reproductive performance. They fed multiparous sows with diets supplemented with 30 or 90 IU/kg of vitamin E. No interaction effects were detected with Se, and the higher vitamin E level (90 IU/kg) did not improve the main sow reproductive parameters.

In a recent study Wang et al. (2017) showed, in contrast, that high concentrations of vitamin E supplementation (250 IU/kg) in sow diet during the last week of gestation (107 days) and the lactation phase until weaning (day 21) significantly improved the immunological variables and antioxidative parameters in piglets. In this study, vitamin E improved colostrum and milk's composition and immunoglobulin levels (Table 5.13), the piglet weights at weaning, and enhanced humoral immune function and antioxidant activity in sows and piglets (Table 5.14). Amavizca-Nazar et al. (2019) reported that sows exposed to a hot environment have reductions in vitamin E levels in serum (0.90 µg/ml) and milk (1.81 µg/ml) compared to sows during the winter period (2.00 and 2.23 µg/ml, respectively). Similar effect was measured on retinol. Consequently, dietary vitamin E and A supplementation could be potentially positive for sows and piglets during heat stress.

Boars

For boars, little information is available on how supplementing feed with vitamin E influences sperm quality (Ribas-Maynou et al., 2021). Cerolini et al. (2000) observed that when including α-tocopherol in the diluting medium of semen, this vitamin is incorporated in spermatozoid membranes, increasing the spermatozoa's resistance to oxidative deterioration, maintaining a higher concentration of some PUFAs in phospholipids and significantly reducing the loss of viability of the ejaculate during storage.

Liu, Cottrell, Collins et al. (2017) provided a study that evidenced that boar supplementation with a diet that contained an n-6 : n-3 fatty acid ratio of 6 : 1 and 400 mg/kg of vitamin E improved boar sperm morphology by promoting the antioxidant capacity of serum, spermatozoa, and seminal plasma and preventing oxidative damage to spermatozoa. In a subsequent study, these researchers (Liu, Zhou, Duan et al., 2017b) evaluating 2 n-6 : n-3 ratios (14.4 and 6.6) and 2 vitamin E levels (200 and 400 mg/kg) concluded that a 6 : 6 ratio and 400 mg/kg vitamin E enhanced sperm motility by improving membrane integrity and membrane fluidity of the spermatozoa.

Piglets

Another critical moment in the pig's life is its weaning. Vitamin E plays a significant role as the pig's limited digestive capacity at this stage diminishes tissue concentration. In the case of blood serum, the concentration can fall to less than half in just 1 week after weaning. This

Table 5.13 Effect of sow supplementation (250 IU/kg feed) on colostrum and milk composition (Wang *et al.*, 2017)

	Vitamin E (mg/kg)		
	44	250	*p-value*
Colostrum			
α-tocopherol (mg/l)	18.51	26.97	*<0.01*
Fat (g/kg)	44.35	53.8	*<0.001*
Protein (g/kg)	196.83	198.6	*n.s.*
Lactose (g/kg)	24.5	23.27	*n.s.*
Total milk solids (g/kg)	265.93	255.13	*n.s.*
IgG (g/l)	52.78	63.45	*<0.001*
IgA (g/l)	8.02	9.01	*<0.01*
Milk			
α-tocopherol (mg/l)	4.16	7.97	*<0.01*
Fat (g/kg)	67.01	79.13	*<0.01*
Protein (g/kg)	50.4	50.63	*n.s.*
Lactose (g/kg)	50.61	50.11	*n.s.*
Total milk solids (g/kg)	197.37	200.57	*n.s.*
IgG (g/l)	0.89	0.96	*<0.05*
IgA (g/l)	3.81	4.11	*<0.05*

Table 5.14 Effect of vitamin E supplementation (250 IU/kg feed) to sows on piglet plasma (Wang *et al.*, 2017)

Piglet plasma	Vitamin E 44 mg/kg	Vitamin E 250 mg/kg	*p*
α-tocopherol (mg/l)	3.88	5.29	<0.01
IgG (g/l)	0.44	0.49	<0.05
IgA (g/l)	0.33	0.36	<0.05
T-AOC (IU/ml)	6.82	7.65	<0.05
GSH-Px (mmol/l)	621.69	651.34	n.s.
CAT (U/ml)	7.38	8.78	<0.05

implies a high susceptibility to suffering oxidation processes during this critical moment in the piglet's life (Amazan *et al.*, 2014). Teige *et al.* (1982) found an inverse relationship between the presentation of clinical symptoms after experimental infections and the intake of vitamin E and have consequently found an improvement in productive indices when the sanitary situation was poor. Since feed intake could be variable in weaned piglets, vitamin E–selenium injection has received positive evaluations (Mahan and Moxon, 1980).

Short-term inoculation of pigs with *E. coli* led to a decreased liver α-tocopherol status (Lauridsen *et al.*, 2011). Vitamin E and selenium supplementation in young pigs increased whole-cell agglutination against *E. coli* (Ellis and Vorhies, 1976). In this 56-day study, 6- to 8-week-old pigs were supplemented with a diet of 0, 22, or 110 IU of vitamin E per kg. Each pig was injected with *E. coli* bacteria intramuscularly on days 0 and 35. Supplementation with vitamin E increased antibody titers of pigs to *E. coli* bacteria 1.5 and 2.7 times for the 22 and 110 IU per kg treatments, respectively, compared to unsupplemented controls. Teige *et al.* (1977) also found that the response to *E. coli* endotoxin was affected by the vitamin E supply available to pigs. Hidiroglou *et al.* (1995) reported that when piglets were injected IM with 500 IU of α-tocopherol at birth and 1,000 IU of α-tocopherol at 7 and 14 days of age their antibody titers to Keyhole limpet hemocyanin were significantly higher than those of the control piglets.

Vitamin E is also used to counteract the adverse effects of peroxidized soybean oil on animal performance in weaned nursery pigs. In a study conducted by Silva-Guillen *et al.* (2020) with vitamin E (100 IU/l of RRR-α-tocopherol) and phytogenics added via drinking water observed that supplementation of vitamin E, but not phytogenics, increased the vitamin E body status. However, no effects of vitamin E or phytogenics were observed on growth performance, oxidative stress, or cytokine concentrations.

Related to stress post-weaning, Chen, Wang, Li *et al.* (2019) evaluated the dietary supplementation of vitamin E at 0, 16, 32, 80, and 160 IU/kg in weaned piglets [(Yorkshire × Landrace) × Duroc]. These researchers only observed a slight increase in growth performance indicators, such as average daily gain, feed intake, and gain-to-feed ratio in piglets fed at 80 IU/kg. However, they observed that the intestinal morphology (Figure 5.16) and functions were affected by inhibiting jejunal epithelial cell proliferation at this level. These findings suggest that 80 IU/kg of vitamin E may lessen weaning stress for post-weaned piglets.

Different strategies have been established to minimize the dramatic fall in the serum levels of α-tocopherol during weaning. Moreira and Mahan (2002) have demonstrated

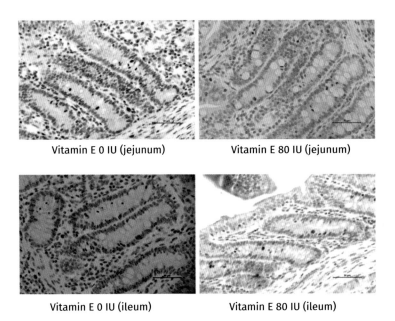

| Vitamin E 0 IU (jejunum) | Vitamin E 80 IU (jejunum) |
| Vitamin E 0 IU (ileum) | Vitamin E 80 IU (ileum) |

Figure 5.16 Intestinal epithelial cell proliferation within weaning piglets jejunal and ileal crypts fed 0 or 80 IU/kg feed of vitamin E (Chen, Wang, Li *et al.*, 2019)

that including vitamin E up to 200 IU/kg of feed increases the serum concentration of α-tocopherol. Nevertheless, effectiveness is limited due to digestive inefficiency and antagonism with other liposoluble compounds, such as vitamin A (Ching *et al.*, 2002). It is, therefore, necessary to supply a concentration in the feed of 100 IU/kg or more. The same authors demonstrated that the inclusion of fat in the feed (around 5%) effectively prevents a sharp fall in the concentration of α-tocopherol in recently weaned piglets, especially during the first few days after weaning, so that an intake of around 60 IU/kg feed might be sufficient.

A combination of antioxidant vitamins has been demonstrated to be effective. Szczubiał (2015) demonstrated that the supplementation of vitamin E (in combination with vitamin C and β-carotene) in sows, in a concentration of 200 mg (twice a week, intramuscularly), during the second half of pregnancy has beneficial effects on the antioxidative/oxidative balance in the postpartum period, by reducing lipid and protein peroxidation and increasing the antioxidant potential.

Conversely, Lauridsen and Jensen (2005) demonstrated the benefits of supplementing weaned piglet feed with vitamin C (500 mg/kg feed), especially if the piglets are starting with a low/moderate level of α-tocopherol in the liver, while this is less effective if the hepatic concentration of α-tocopherol is already high at the time of weaning. The supplementation of vitamins C and E (100 or 200 mg/kg) to piglets (9–10 kg) fed diets contaminated with crude oil (15 g/kg) were recently evaluated by Mbachiantim *et al.* (2022). This research group demonstrated that these vitamins (100 mg/kg each) reduced the negative toxic impacts of crude oil on the red and white blood parameters of growing pigs.

Growing pigs

Regarding growing pigs, the results of vitamin E supplementation are variable. Although some authors have found an improvement in zootechnical parameters when fortifying feeds with vitamin E (Wastell *et al.*, 1972; Asghar *et al.*, 1991), most of the available literature indicates no effect.

Vitamin E supplementation has been proven to affect the intestinal health of growing pigs, especially under stress. For example, López-Bote *et al.* (2001) found lesser epithelial desquamation of the small intestine's mucous membrane in pigs receiving 200 mg α-tocopherol acetate per kilogram of feed compared with those receiving 20 mg/kg feed. Considering the quantitative importance of the desquamation of intestinal cells in pigs, saving energy and amino acid could explain the possible zootechnical benefit in some cases. The relationship between vitamin E intake and the phenomenon of apoptosis (cell death) could be the basis to explain this phenomenon, and possibly the phenomena related to the decrease in the number of somatic cells in milk opening an exciting field of research. Liu *et al.* (2016) reported improved intestinal barrier function and reduced oxidative stress when heat-stressed growing pigs were supplemented with 1 mg/kg of selenium and 200 IU/kg of vitamin E.

Upadhaya *et al.* (2015) demonstrated that supplementation of 300 IU vitamin E and omega-3 fatty acids (obtained with 25% replacement of tallow to linseed oil as a source of n-3 fatty acids) significantly reduced the production of pro-inflammatory cytokine and prostaglandin E_2 (PGE_2), improved muscle growth, and average daily gain of growing-finishing pigs. These effects were observed after a challenge with intramuscular injection of *E. coli* lipopolysaccharide twice weekly over the 6-week experiment. However, no effects were observed in the inflammatory response of pigs on the supplementation, proving that immune system markers and production parameters are independent and not additive.

Effects of vitamin E on meat quality

Many studies have demonstrated a positive relationship between the administration of levels of vitamin E (between 200 and 400 IU/kg) in pig feed and meat quality attributes (Gray, 1990; Jensen *et al.*, 1998; Hoz *et al.*, 2003; Guo *et al.*, 2006a,b; Trefan *et al.*, 2011; Matte and Lauridsen, 2013). Therefore, it is essential first to find the possible positive effects and establish quantity and guidelines for appropriate administration in each case.

Genetics and nutrition can affect the responses to vitamin E supplementation. Kerth *et al.* (2001) have demonstrated that the effect of vitamin E on the quality of meat depends on whether the genotype carries the halothane gene, meaning that vitamin E supplementation to non-carrier pigs is more effective. The interaction of genotype with the action of vitamins (for both vitamin E and other vitamins) promises to be an exciting line of investigation in the coming years.

Genetic differences can be observed between pure and hybrid breeds. Szterk *et al.* (2016) demonstrated how the meat of Pure Polish Landrace and hybrid Polish Landrace 3 Duroc pig breeds was enriched with vitamin E when feed was supplemented with 100 and 200 mg/kg of vitamin E. Depending on feed enrichment, swine breed and the tested muscles, vitamin E levels increased from 1.7 to 4.9 mg/kg. However, the response varied between the 2 genetic groups confirming the hypothesis that meat from hybrid maternal breeds contains higher vitamin E meat levels than the meat of purebreds.

Regarding nutrition, the dietary lipid levels and fatty acid profile influence the impact of vitamin E supplementation. Huang *et al.* (2019) evaluated the inclusion of flaxseed oil (0%, 1%) plus poultry fat (1%, 3%, or 5%) and vitamin E (11 or 220 IU/kg) in a 4 × 2 factorial arrangement of treatments. Pigs were processed when they reached 110.0±3.0 kg. No interaction effects of growth performance were detected. As dietary lipid increased, feed intake decreased linearly, and the gain-to-feed ratio improved linearly. Similarly, dietary supplementation with 1% flaxseed oil + 1%, 3% or 5% poultry fat did not affect the subjective marbling score or ether extract content of loin muscle. Supplementation with 220 IU vitamin E increased carcass leanness with 6% dietary lipids but increased carcass backfat with 0–4% dietary lipids. Vitamin E supplementation increased subjective marbling score but did not affect loin muscle color, ham and loin muscle pH, loin muscle characteristics, or pork belly firmness.

Vitamin E and oxidative stability

Once an animal has been slaughtered, most of the mechanisms which control oxidative processes become inactive and oxidative reactions occur. These cause marked alterations in meat properties within a few days. Oxidative deterioration is regarded as the main reason for these alterations in the meat after microbial activity, although this can be controlled with appropriate storage temperatures. Numerous experiments have shown that supplementation of 300 to 600 mg/kg with α-tocopherol acetate produces a high tissue content of α-tocopherol, leading to an improvement in the oxidative stability of muscle in pigs (Monahan *et al.*, 1990; Asghar *et al.*, 1991; Buckley *et al.*, 1995; Morrissey *et al.*, 1996; Jensen *et al.*, 1998; Morrissey *et al.*, 2000), and backfat quality (Flachowsky *et al.*, 1997).

The effectiveness of vitamin E has also been observed in cooked muscle (Monahan *et al.*, 1990) and the presence of salt (Buckley and Connolly, 1980). Different studies have also been conducted to investigate the antioxidant effect of vitamin E concerning the fat composition of the ration. Monahan *et al.* (1992) observed a positive antioxidant effect of vitamin E when supplemented at 200 mg/kg to pig rations fortified with 3% soy oil and tallow.

Leskanich *et al.* (1997) observed similar effects. They also suggested that the greater the addition of unsaturated fatty acids, the greater the amount of vitamin E to be administered, since when adding the same quantity of vitamin E to diets containing 2% rapeseed oil and 1% fish oil and to control rations containing tallow and soy oil, the levels were lower in the former. Flachowsky *et al.* (1997) also observed positive antioxidative effects of 1 g of α-tocopherol acetate per animal per day in pigs fed diets with high levels of fat (100 g/kg rapeseed meal or 200 g/kg full-fat soybeans). This could be explained by increased metabolic demand for vitamin E due to the higher level of PUFAs. Therefore, vitamin E requirement increases when there is an increase in the proportion of PUFAs (Wang *et al.*, 1996). Hoz *et al.* (2003) also reported that 200 mg/kg of α-tocopheryl acetate markedly reduced tenderloin lipid oxidation from pigs fed diets enriched in n-3 fatty acids using linseed, sunflower, and a mixture of linseed with olive oils.

Dietary supplementation of α-tocopherol inhibits the production of cholesterol oxidation products (COPs) in heated and refrigerated pork (Rey *et al.*, 2001). Monahan *et al.* (1992) observed a decrease in total COPs formed in pork from animals whose rations had been supplemented with 200 mg/kg α-tocopherol acetate compared with those consuming unsupplemented rations. Boler *et al.* (2009) concluded that supplementing 200 mg/kg synthetic vitamin E decreased pork lipid oxidation when compared to supplementing 10 mg/kg natural vitamin E. Cardenia *et al.* (2011) evaluated that the supplementation of α-tocopheryl acetate (250 mg/kg), produced pork meat with suitable oxidative stability, which confirmed the antioxidant effect of vitamin E.

The effects of vitamin E in improving muscle antioxidant capacity were evaluated by Jin *et al.* (2018) using pioglitazone hydrochloride (PGZ), a new type of insulin sensitizer that can increase intramuscular fat in pork. However, PGZ reduces oxidative stability due to changes in fatty acid composition, increasing unsaturation. In this experiment, 160 Duroc × Landrace × Large White pigs (75.53±0.04 kg) pigs were randomly divided into a 2 × 2 factorial arrangement with 2 levels of PGZ (0 or 15 mg/kg) and 2 levels of vitamin E (0 or 325 mg/kg) for 28 days. The basal diet already contained 75 mg/kg of vitamin E. No interaction effects were detected, and PGZ increased intramuscular fat. Vitamin E decreased cooking loss from 28.75% in pigs fed the control diet to 25.99% in pigs supplemented with 325 mg/kg. This effect could be due to maintaining the cell membranes' stability and improving the muscle's antioxidant capacity (longissimus toracis), as observed in Figure 5.17.

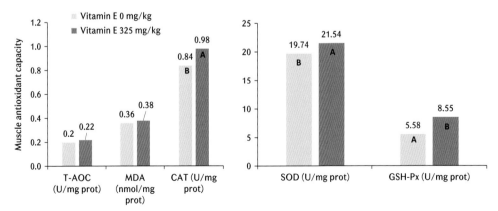

Figure 5.17 Effect of vitamin E supplementation (325 mg/kg; 400 mg/kg total including 75 mg/kg in basal diet) on meat antioxidant capacity of pigs fed the insulin sensitizer pioglitazone hydrochloride (Jin *et al.*, 2018)

Vitamin E and pork color

Meat color is determined mainly by the content and chemical form of the hemin myoglobin pigment. The heme group of myoglobin contains a central atom of iron which can form 6-coordinate bonds, 4 of which occur with N-atoms of the porphyrin ring and a fifth with a hemin apoprotein. The sixth bond, together with hematic iron status, determines meat color. If the unifying molecule is O_2, oxymyoglobin is formed, and bright red color with storage tends to oxidize and form methemoglobin causing dark coloration.

Rhee and Ziprin (1987) found a correlation between raw beef, pork, and chicken meat total pigment, myoglobin content, and lipid peroxidation. Supplementation of animal rations with different quantities of α-tocopherol acetate brought better color stability and a lesser reduction in "*a*" values (directly linked to the color red) than were found in unsupplemented animals. This has also been observed in pigs (Monahan *et al.*, 1994; Asghar *et al.*, 1991; Lanari *et al.*, 1995; Phillips *et al.*, 2001), although data are less conclusive than with cattle (Faustman *et al.*, 1989; Liu *et al.*, 1996) and lambs (López-Bote *et al.*, 2001).

Dietary vitamin E supplementation provides a feasible option to extend the shelf life of meat. According to Sales and Koukolová (2011), the relationship between total dietary vitamin E intake and muscle α-tocopherol concentration reached asymptotic plateau values at 4.83 µg/g. The same study proved that pigs' fractional accumulation rate (per total dietary vitamin E intake) of muscle α-tocopherol concentration was 0.0130.

It has generally been shown that the greater the vitamin E supplementation, the less the color loss (Asghar *et al.*, 1991; Monahan *et al.*, 1994). However, some authors have not found significant differences with higher supplementation levels. Faustman *et al.* (1989) observed that a concentration of 3.0 to 3.7 µg of α-tocopherol/g of tissue was necessary to stabilize the color of beef muscle. In pigs, Asghar *et al.* (1991) determined that when supplementing rations with 0, 100 or 200 mg/kg, deposition in the longissimus dorsi muscle was 0.5 µg of α-tocopherol/g of meat for the unsupplemented group and 2.60 and 4.72 µg of α-tocopherol/g for the groups supplemented with 100 and 200 mg/kg fed respectively, a level that was sufficient to stabilize the color. Peeters *et al.* (2006) reported that pork loins of pigs supplemented with 150 mg of vitamin E/kg of feed for 21 days were redder, less pale, and more yellow than the control. The possible actuating mechanism of α-tocopherol could be related to the inactivation of free radicals, which can oxidize myoglobin, or the systems of reduced metmyoglobin from skeletal muscle (Faustman and Wang, 2000).

Vitamin E and water holding capacity

Tests have shown that it is possible to reduce drip losses by incorporating 100 to 200 mg/kg feed of α-tocopherol acetate in the ration (Trefan *et al.*, 2011). Asghar *et al.* (1991) observed that after 10 days of refrigeration (4°C) under fluorescent light, samples of frozen meat from pigs that had consumed rations supplemented with 200 IU of α-tocopherol acetate/kg of feed had lower drip losses than samples from pigs consuming feeds supplemented with 10 or 100 IU/kg.

Monahan *et al.* (1994) obtained comparable results with fresh muscle. They suggested that this could be explained by the fact that changes in the α-tocopherol content could alter the passage of biomolecules through cell membranes and, therefore, the degree of muscle exudation due to physiochemical interactions of α-tocopherol with molecules in the lipid membrane. Any other change in the lipid microenvironment could affect the ability of membranes to act as a semi-permeable barrier (Monahan *et al.*, 1994). Furthermore, α-tocopherol could preserve the integrity of cellular membranes of the muscle by preventing oxidation of their phospholipids, thereby impeding the passage of sarcoplasmic liquid through them

(Asghar *et al.*, 1991; Monahan *et al.*, 1994). As with color, vitamin E supplementation levels affect this action, although the effect appears less pronounced (Cannon *et al.*, 1996).

Vitamin E and the quality of meat products

The administration of vitamin E in high concentrations to improve meat quality is of particular interest in swine as it has been shown that vitamin E accumulated in tissues remains there during processing, improving the technological properties of the meat (transfer of water) as much as the qualitative attributes of the products (color stability, acceptability, dryness, presence of unpleasant smells and flavors, etc.). It has been possible to observe these effects even in cured products processed for over 10 months (Isabel *et al.*, 1999). In this regard, it is helpful to remember that products from Iberian pigs (one of the best examples of the quality of meat production in swine) show a high α-tocopherol content they acquire from their particular outdoor feeding system (Rey *et al.*, 1997). However, some data indicate that it is possible to reduce the number of certain additives included during processing if the meat contains a good quantity of antioxidants, like α-tocopherol, at the time of slaughter (Dineen *et al.*, 2000), which brings a benefit to public health and the positive commercial implications associated with it.

When the effects of the supply of fatty acids and antioxidants on the quality of these products are considered alongside production costs, the interest in optimizing this supply appears justified. This means matching the feed cost, not the carcass or fresh meat but the end product. This is relevant in Spain, the world leader, where currently around 40 million cured hams are processed, and in Italy, for the typical Parma and San Daniele air-cured ham products.

Dietary lipid peroxidation

Lipid peroxidation in animal feed can negatively affect growth performance and meat quality. Vitamin E can prevent some of these issues, but not when peroxidation has advanced. Song *et al.* (2014) observed that the dietary supplementation of vitamin E (α-tocopheryl acetate) at the NRC (2012) level, or 10 times this level, could not overcome the adverse effects on growth performance and carcass characteristics from feeding weaning pigs with oxidized-distillers dried grains with solubles (DDGS), therefore, making, in this case, the increase in dosage from the NRC (2012) levels unsuccessful. Beneficial effects of high levels of α-tocopherol against lipid oxidation were observed in the subcutaneous fat. Still, it was poorly reflected in the oxidative stability of dry fermented sausages, as it was demonstrated in a study by Vossen *et al.* (2016), with supplementation of 150 mg/kg of α-tocopheryl acetate.

Recommendations and guidelines for administration

Few studies have tried to systematically establish the most appropriate vitamin E intake and administration times for each case. Additionally, the difficulty of analyzing tocopherols in feeds and animal tissues means that the existing data in the literature are very heterogeneous and therefore make comparison difficult.

Roth and Kirchgessner (1975) added tocopherol acetate to the feed in amounts from 5 to 95 mg/kg. They found a linear response to vitamin E incorporation in tissues depending on the amount. Machlin and Gabriel (1982), working with rats, chickens, ducks, and calves, found a logarithmic response between the α-tocopherol supplied in the diet and that analyzed in plasma and various tissues.

In a subsequent study, Hoppe *et al.* (1993) administered 0, 20, 40, 80, and 160 IU of α-tocopherol acetate/kg of feed to groups of 6 animals per treatment. The α-tocopherol analyses were conducted employing saponification of the sample. A fluorescence detector was used in the analysis. According to these authors, there is a logarithmic relationship between the ingestion of vitamin E (expressed in mg of all-*rac*-α-tocopherol acetate/kg of feed) and the content of α-tocopherol in the various tissues (expressed as µg of α-tocopherol/g of fresh tissue). Several equations have been established:

Plasma	$y = -(1.08 \pm 0.27) + (0.89 \pm 0.07) \ln x$ ($r^2 = 0.61$; $p<0.0001$)
Longissimus dorsi	$y = -0.32 + 2.09 \ln x$ ($r^2 = 0.77$; $p<0.0001$)
Liver	$y = -10.2 + 5.54 \ln x$ ($r^2 = 0.62$; $p<0.0001$)
Adipose tissue	$y = -13.9 + 7.63 \ln x$ ($r^2 = 0.63$; $p<0.0001$)

where y = α-tocopherol in the tissues (µg of α-tocopherol/g of fresh tissue) and $\ln x$ = ingestion of vitamin E (mg of all-rac-α-tocopherol acetate/kg feed).

It can be seen that the most significant quantities of vitamin E are found in adipose tissue, followed by the liver and longissimus dorsi muscle. Nevertheless, when the data from these authors are compared with most of the existing literature, it is evident that their values are higher (almost double) than the majority.

A research project (Diet-Ox, 1998) was carried out within several countries of the European Union, which included 14 laboratories that interchange data so that the data were perfectly comparable. If the data supplied by these 14 laboratories only is used (and only in experiments in which feed fortified with vitamin E is given for at least 7 weeks), the dose-response curve obtained is very similar to that of Hoppe *et al.* (1993), but with much lower tissue content. According to data from these 14 research groups, the α-tocopherol concentration in muscle tissue should be between 3.5 and 4 µg/g to have an antioxidant effect. Below this concentration, the effect is marginal. The effective level is equivalent to including 100–200 mg of α-tocopherol acetate per kg feed. These data agree with most existing literature and the most widely used recommendations (Buckley *et al.*, 1995).

Fortification of feed with vitamin E represents an additional cost. Therefore, it is necessary to consider the optimum quantity and the administration period when establishing recommendations for vitamin E supplementation in pig feed. In this case, the work of 2 research groups belonging to the group of 14 constituting the Diet-Ox (1998) project has been selected. First, Morrissey *et al.* (1996) found that supplementation with 200 mg/kg feed for 7 weeks before slaughter produced a concentration of 4 µg/g tissue, only slightly less than in animals receiving feed supplemented with the same concentration throughout the growth phase. According to this investigation, feed fortified for the last 7 weeks increases the α-tocopherol concentration in muscle tissue much more efficiently (around 0.07 µg/g per day) than feed supplemented for a much-extended period (0.03 µg/g per day).

Second, Monahan *et al.* (1994) investigated various administration periods and different quantities. Administering feed with 1,000, 500, or 200 mg/kg of vitamin E produces an average increase of 0.18, 0.10, and 0.04 µg/g of muscle daily. That is to say, approximately 0.20 µg per g tissue per day for each mg of vitamin E above requirements supplied in the feed. This means that if 1,000 mg/kg feed were supplied, the level would reach 3.8 µg/g of tissue in just 1 week. In Monahan's experiment, this muscle concentration was not reached in the 4 weeks of the trial in which 200 mg/kg was supplied. However, a theoretical calculation puts the necessary period at around 6 weeks.

Similarly, in the experiment by Morrissey *et al.* (1996), it took 5 weeks to reach 3.9 µg/g of muscle tissue with a supply of 200 mg of vitamin E/kg of feed. According to these calculations, the same concentration can be achieved in muscle by administering 1,000 mg/kg of vitamin E for 1 week, 500 mg/kg for 2 weeks, or 200 mg/kg for 5–6 weeks. In all cases, the extra consumption is around 20–22 g per pig, and the efficiency of tocopherol accumulation in tissues can be calculated as less than 5% of the total ingested.

The same research group (Wen *et al.*, 1997) reported that vitamin E supplementation in pigs of 1,000 mg/kg α-tocopheryl acetate increased concentrations of α-tocopherol in gluteo biceps muscle, mitochondria, and microsomes by 3.2, 6.1, and 5.6 times more than those fed 30 mg/kg vitamin E. These higher supplementation levels enhanced stability of the membranes to oxidation or reduced muscle lipid oxidation by 59–69%.

Cheah *et al.* (1995) investigated the supplementation of 500 or 1,000 mg vitamin E/kg diet for 46 days in genetic lines prone to pale-soft and exudative (PSE) meat (British Landrace (NN and nn), Landrace × Large White (NN and Nn) and Piétrain (nn) pigs. These authors reported that 500 mg/kg reduced drip loss in unfrozen longissimus thoracic (LT) muscle by 45 and 54% in Nn and NN pigs, respectively. Supplementation of 1,000 mg/kg reduced the excess release of calcium ions and prevented the formation of PSE carcasses by stabilizing membrane integrity, which was associated with inhibiting phospholipase A2 activity (Hamman, 1995).

The research data on optimum amounts and sources of vitamin E to feed before slaughter is still of great interest and debate. Sobotka *et al.* (2012) concluded that the supplementation of grower-finisher pig diets with vitamin E, in a concentration of 100 IU vitamin E/kg, was proven more effective in increasing the level of α-tocopherol in serum and meat and the decrease in pork lipid oxidation, than the use of oat by-products.

Kim *et al.* (2015) estimated that dietary supplementation of vitamin E (700 IU/kg) for 28 days before slaughter is required to maximize muscle vitamin E content (6 mg/kg). At the same time, the backfat thickness was minimized when supplementing at 500 IU/kg (Figure 5.18). Li *et al.* (2015) reported that dietary ferulic acid (100 mg/kg), a natural plant phenolic extract antioxidant, and vitamin E (400 mg/kg) could improve the meat quality and antioxidant capacity of finishing pigs after 28 days of supplementation. These researchers also commented that vitamin E increased the loin eye area.

The efficacy of supplementing vitamins can be due to the form and level used since they can differ in bioavailability for swine. Van Kempen *et al.* (2016) determined that oral dosing of 75 mg/kg of all-*rac*-α-tocopheryl acetate (α-TAc) for piglets (22±1 kg 8-week-old) has a 44%

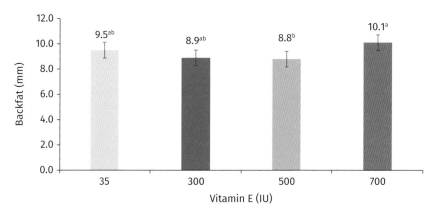

Figure 5.18 Effects of supplemented dietary vitamin E on backfat thickness (Kim *et al.*, 2015). Bars with a different superscript letter (a, b) indicate significant differences (*p*<0.05)

shorter half-life (2.6 hours) than the intravenous doses and lower bioavailability (12.5%). This means that commercial doses of vitamin E are less effective in alleviating oxidative stress than expected, and higher doses could be necessary.

For sows, Liu, Zhou, Duan *et al.* (2017a) demonstrated that supplementation of vitamin E above the recommended doses (95 IU/kg), in combination with other nutrients, reduced the body reserve losses of lactating sows during summer, and therefore, it is recommended to implement during that season.

Vitamin K

The NRC (2012) has established the minimum requirements of vitamin K for swine at 0.5 mg of menadione per kilogram feed for all ages and productive phases (Tables 5.3, 5.4, and 5.5). However, the Brazilian Tables (Rostagno *et al.*, 2017), FEFANA (Tables 5.3, 5.4, and 5.5), DSM Nutritional Products (2022b) OVN™ and the genetic companies (Tables 5.6, 5.7, and 5.8) recommended levels that are 4 to 20 times higher for piglets, 2 to 6 times higher for growing pigs and 2 to 9 times for breeders.

Piglets

It is considered that microbial synthesis of vitamin K in the digestive system is sufficient to meet the needs of these animals. Nevertheless, when animals are produced in confined conditions, with little possibility of contact with feces, mainly when animals are young and the gut microbiota is not well established, vitamin K supplementation is recommended (Campbell and Combs, 1988). Industry surveys (Tables 5.9) indicated that pre-starter diets in Brazil could contain 20 times the NRC (2012) recommended levels; in the USA and China, most producers add up to 8 times. In the nursery phase, the levels supplemented for piglets are 5 to 8 times higher than NRC (2012) levels in all countries. However, the variation between manufacturers of vitamin and mineral premixes for piglets fluctuates between 0 and 10 mg/kg.

Growing pigs

For growing pigs, the levels used in the industry (Table 5.10) are 4 to 5 times more than in NRC (2012). The variability is extensive, with coefficients of variation between 45% and 71%, indicating the diversity in opinions related to vitamin K supplementation and the lack of available research data. The variability in supplementation of this vitamin is among the highest. The Chinese industry tends to use the highest values of vitamin K in grower II and finisher diets.

Breeder pigs

In breeder diets, the dietary levels used by the swine industry worldwide (Table 5.11) are at least 6 times the recommended by NRC (2012). Chinese producers supplement nearly 9 times the NRC (2012) levels in lactation and gestation. The variability in levels used is also very high in breeder diets.

Few studies have been conducted to determine levels or evaluate sources of vitamin K in pigs. One study was conducted by Monegue (2013) to assess the effects of vitamin K in diets with and without mycotoxin-contaminated corn on growth performance, bone characteristics, and related blood metabolites in pigs from weaning to market. They used MSBC (33% vitamin K) as the source of supplemental vitamin K because it is the most common form fed to swine. Vitamin K was tested at 0, 0.5, and 2.0 ppm in a corn-soybean meal-based diet on 2 generations of pigs to evaluate any time and dose responses. The first generation of pigs was subjected to mycotoxin-contaminated corn in the nursery phase to test for any interactions between the toxins and vitamin K. Adding 0.5 ppm of vitamin K reduced ($p<0.001$) prothrombin time. No additional decrease in prothrombin time was detected when increasing vitamin K inclusion from 0.5 to 2.0 ppm. Regarding growth performance, daily gain, feed intake, and feed efficiency were unaffected ($p>0.10$) by supplemental vitamin K. However, pigs fed mycotoxin-contaminated corn ate less ($p = 0.005$) and grew slower ($p = 0.015$) compared to those receiving good corn. The addition of vitamin K did not alleviate the adverse growth effects in response to corn type. Vitamin K did not affect bone characteristics ($p>0.10$), blood calcium ($p>0.05$), or OC ($p>0.10$). Besides blood clotting, dietary vitamin K does not appear to provide additional benefits at these inclusion levels and stages of swine production.

WATER-SOLUBLE VITAMINS

As their name indicates, water-soluble vitamins are soluble in water, so they are present in the plasma, cytoplasm, and cellular organelles. Within this broad group of vitamins, we can further differentiate between the B complex vitamins (which includes thiamine, riboflavin, niacin, pantothenic acid, pyridoxine, cyanocobalamin, folacin, and biotin) and ascorbic acid or vitamin C. Studies to determine optimum levels of the B complex are challenging because the enzymes with which they are involved take an active part in cell metabolism, and they are interrelated in many ways, to the extent that individual recommendations are hard to establish. Water-soluble vitamins are present in many feed ingredients (FEDNA, 2015) (Table 5.15), but their content is variable and unstable during storage and feed processing.

Genetic improvement in recent decades may affect the vitamin levels needed to achieve optimum live performance, carcass traits, meat quality, health status, and reproductive ability. McDowell's review (2006) emphasized the need to use higher vitamin levels due to diverse factors such as the intensification of production, lower use of antimicrobials, the appearance of new diseases, which compromise the animal's immune system, or chronic immune system activation due to stressors that affect efficiency and nutrient needs (Williams *et al.*, 1997; Matte and Lauridsen, 2022), and the need to provide adequate body reserves (Stahly and Cook, 1996b; Heying *et al.*, 2013). Consuming food enriched with these and other nutrients is one of the demands of the 21st-century consumer (Boler *et al.*, 2009; Rosbotham *et al.*, 2021).

Despite this logic and some evidence, the requirements recommended by the NRC (2012) were not substantially modified (Tables 5.3, 5.4, and 5.5) compared to NRC (1998). In contrast, other recommendations like the Brazilian Tables (Rostagno *et al.*, 2017), FEFANA (2015) and DSM Nutritional Products (2022b) OVN™ are generally 2 to 3 times higher (Tables 5.3, 5.4, and 5.5) than the values recommended by the NRC (2012). Also swine genetic companies tend to recommend slightly higher levels (Tables 5.6, 5.7, and 5.8), and the swine industry in Brazil (Dalto and da Silva, 2020), the USA (Flohr *et al.*, 2016; Faccin *et al.*, 2022), and China (Yang *et al.*, 2021b) (Tables 5.9, 5.10 and 5.11) tend to use levels similar to those recommended by the genetic companies or sometimes higher. Recent data reported by Faccin *et al.* (2022) indicated increments in the supplementation of B vitamins for piglet, gilt, gestation, lactation, and boar diets.

In this section, we will conduct a detailed review of each vitamin and then present an overview of requirements, although little information is available.

Table 5.15 Levels of water-soluble vitamins in raw materials commonly used in pig diets (FEDNA, 2015)

Raw materials	Thiamine mg/kg	Riboflavin mg/kg	Niacin mg/kg	Pantothenic acid mg/kg	Vitamin B_6 mg/kg	Vitamin B_{12} µg/kg	Folic acid mg/kg	Biotin mg/kg
Cereals	3–6	1–4	20–60	5–15	3.6	–	0.4	0.2
Cereal by-products	7–20	–	300	18–30	–	–	1.8	0.1
Whole soy	7	2.6	20–60	–	3.5	–	–	0.3
Soy cake	2	3–4		15	0.5	–	–	0.3
Sunflower meal	–	7	200	10	–	–	–	1.6
Peanut meal	–	6	150–220	47	–	–	–	0.4
Peas	2	–	–	5	–	–	–	0.2
Alfalfa	–	15	–	30	–	–	4.5	0.3
Animal proteins (blood, bloodmeal)	–	28	–	–	–	500	1	0.1
Fishmeal	–	5–10	50–150	10–20	4	–	0.2	0.3
Brewer's yeast	33	–	–	–	–	–	–	–
Yeast, fungi and microorganisms	–	28	–	–	–	100–400	–	–
Dairy by-products	–	–	–	20–45	–	–	–	0.4

Vitamin B₁ (thiamine)

Since thiamine is found in almost all feedstuffs, especially cereal grains, pigs are unlikely to suffer thiamine deficiency under practical conditions. According to the NRC (2012), a piglet of between 5 and 7 kg requires 1.5 mg of vitamin B_1 per kilogram feed (Table 5.3). The recommendations for other phases and breeders were set at 1 mg/kg (Tables 5.4 and 5.5). Considering the ready supply and availability of thiamine in almost all the primary materials used in pig nutrition, it may be thought unnecessary to include thiamine in feed for pigs.

The NRC has based these recommendations on studies geared exclusively to production parameters and carried out approximately more than half a century ago (Ellis and Madsen, 1944). It has been suggested that measurement of the activity of certain enzymes linked to oxidative decarboxylation should be used to establish thiamine requirements more precisely, measuring a variation of the enzyme activity. One of the enzymes proposed was erythrocyte transketolase. According to Peng and Heitman (1973), a concentration of approximately 4 times more than the amount proposed by the NRC (2012) is needed to obtain the maximum response in the activity of this enzyme. It has also been shown that a rise in ambient temperature from 20°C to 35°C causes an increase in thiamine requirements. Also, lean growing pigs may have higher requirements (Stahly and Cook, 1996b).

In contrast, the Brazilian Tables (Rostagno *et al.*, 2017) recommended levels 20–60% higher for piglets, while FEFANA (2015) and DSM Nutritional Products (2022b) OVN™ recommended values 3 to 5 times higher (Table 5.3). For growing pigs (Table 5.4), the Brazilian Tables (Rostagno *et al.*, 2017) are 12–27% below NRC (2012), but FEFANA (2015) and DSM Nutritional Products (2022b) OVN™ recommend either similar values or twice the levels recommended by NRC (2012). For breeders, the Brazilian Tables (Rostagno *et al.*, 2017) were 30% higher than NRC (2012), and FEFANA (2015) and DSM Nutritional Products (2022b) OVN™ recommend 2 to 2.5 times more (Table 5.5). Genetic companies recommend nearly 2.5 mg/kg for piglets, and only Topigs recommends 4–5 mg/kg (Table 5.6). The level recommended by genetic companies reduces to 1.5–2 mg/kg in the grower and finisher phases (Table 5.7), and Topigs maintains the recommendation at 2–3 mg/kg. Finally, there is an agreement in all companies for breeder diets with 2–2.2 mg/kg (Table 5.8).

In recent surveys in Brazil (Dalto and da Silva, 2020), the USA (Flohr *et al.*, 2016; Faccin *et al.*, 2022), and China (Yang *et al.*, 2021b) (Tables 5.9, 5.10, 5.11), it was possible to observe that most of the swine industry adds thiamine in vitamin premixes, especially for breeders. Some producers supplement piglets (Table 5.9) up to 8 times higher than the NRC (2012) recommended, and generally keep to the recommended levels for the grower and finisher diets (Table 5.10), and supplement up to 2.6 times the recommended levels for breeders (Table 5.11). The supplementation of thiamine in the USA has increased 2.8 times for nursery I piglets and 21% for nursery II (Faccin *et al.*, 2022).

Piglets and growing animals

A relationship has been established between the thiamine requirement in pigs and the proportion of energy provided by fat and carbohydrates in feed. The higher the fat content of the ration, the less need for thiamine (Ellis and Madsen, 1944). Using different quantities of thiamine between 200% and 720% of the level recommended by the NRC (1998) in feed for piglets weighing between 10–27 kg, Lutz and Stahly (1997) found no significant effect was observed on production parameters or carcass composition. Nevertheless, this figure shows a tendency toward a quadratic response, with a maximum response between 4–5 mg/kg. However, the abnormal behavior of one of the groups did not allow any significant effects to be seen. Woodworth *et al.* (2000) also did not detect any effects of thiamine when comparing groups of piglets fed without added thiamine to others that received feed, including 2.8 and 5.5 mg/kg.

Breeders

In breeders, Faccin *et al.* (2022) reported increments of 18% in thiamine supplementation being given in the USA to sows in gestation and lactation during the past 6 years. For boars, the average weighed supplementation increased by 29%. Audet *et al.* (2004) found a significant increase of motility in seminal cells and a positive tendency in sperm production in boars fed with 20 mg/kg of feed, coupled with higher levels of the remaining B group vitamins, biotin, B_{12}, B_6, folic acid, niacin, riboflavin, pantothenic acid, and choline.

Vitamin B_2 (riboflavin)

The NRC (2012) proposal for the minimum riboflavin requirement of pigs between 5 and 7 kg is 4 mg/kg; between 7 and 11 kg, 3.5 mg; between 11 and 25 kg, 3 mg; between 25 and 50 kg, 2.5 mg (Table 5.3); and growing pigs 2 mg/kg (Table 5.4). In breeders, requirements are 3.75 mg/kg in all cases (Table 5.5). The Brazilian Tables (Rostagno *et al.*, 2017) recommended 68.25% more riboflavin than the NRC (2012). FEFANA (2015) and DSM Nutritional Products (2022b) OVN™ suggested between 2 and 2.5 times higher supplementation for piglets up to 7 kg (Table 5.3). These recommendations increased to almost double or 6 times for bigger piglets. During the growing phases (Table 5.4), the Brazilian Tables (Rostagno *et al.*, 2017) recommended between 58.8% and 64.5% higher levels, FEFANA (2015) and DSM Nutritional Products (2022b) OVN™ between 2.8 and 5 times more riboflavin than the NRC (2012). For breeders (Table 5.5), the Brazilian Tables (Rostagno *et al.*, 2017) proposed vitamin B_2 supplementation at 38.67%. FEFANA (2015) and DSM Nutritional Products (2022b) OVN™ 1.6 to 3 times higher than the NRC (2012).

According to surveys in Brazil (Dalto and da Silva, 2020), the USA (Flohr *et al.*, 2016; Faccin *et al.*, 2022), and China (Yang *et al.*, 2021b) (Tables 5.9, 5.10 and 5.11), the swine industry is using either at least the minimum recommendation of the genetic companies (Tables 5.6, 5.7 and 5.8) or levels higher than the ones recommended for all previous sources of information. In the growing phases (Table 5.7), the swine industry supplements riboflavin between 3.2 and 5 mg/kg. The supplementation for industry breeders (Table 5.8) ranges between 4.66 and 9 mg/kg as a weighted average. The latest report by Faccin *et al.* (2022) indicated an increment between 10% and 14% in the supplementation of vitamin B_2 in USA sows and boars compared to the previous report of Flohr *et al.* (2016).

Breeder sows and piglets

Considering the variability of both content and availability of riboflavin in most feed ingredients, it seems advisable to include a quantity of riboflavin in feed to complement the supply of the feed ingredients, especially for young animals and probably for breeder sows.

Some research groups have found including higher quantities of riboflavin (between 60 and 160 mg/day) in the early stages of gestation to have a positive effect on the number of piglets born (Bazer and Zavy, 1988; Pettigrew *et al.*, 1996), and this effect is most marked in farms with poor reproductive performance. Including higher levels of riboflavin – between 175% and 300% greater than NRC (2012) recommendations – in feed for piglets (between 10 and 27 kg) has also been observed to have a significant effect (Lutz and Stahly, 1998; Matte *et al.*, 1998). Additional weight gain in this period may be calculated as around 6 g per piglet per day per milligram riboflavin included in the feed, with a linear response observed.

Growing pigs

As previously indicated, the NRC (2012) recommendations were established decades ago. Work by Mahan *et al.* (2007) and Cho *et al.* (2017) demonstrated that using levels of riboflavin in conjunction with niacin, pantothenic acid, folic acid, and vitamin B_{12} higher than those recommended by the NRC (2012) produced improvements in the growing performance of pigs. In Mahan *et al.*'s (2007) study with 660 animals, a quadratic response was obtained on the inclusion of levels one, 2, or 4 times as high as those indicated by the NRC (2012). The use of 3 or 4 times NRC levels did not bring a significant response over the addition of double the recommendations estimated by the NRC (2012).

Vitamin B_6 (pyridoxine)

Considering the concentration of pyridoxine in most feedstuffs used commonly for pigs, it is possible to think that supplementation is unnecessary. Indeed, in studies carried out more than 60 years ago, Ritchie *et al.* (1960) did not find an improvement in reproductive indicators or the growth of suckling piglets following the inclusion of 10 mg/kg of vitamin B_6 in breeder sow feed. A couple of decades later, Easter *et al.* (1983) also did not find appreciable benefits of supplementation when they stopped including vitamin B_6 in feed based on soy and corn for piglets, growing or finisher pigs. All this led to the suggestion that this is one of the vitamins for which, in practice, it is least probable that deficiency problems will arise. However, new data has started to show some benefits.

The NRC (2012) suggested that the minimum requirements for vitamin B_6 in pigs weighing between 5 and 11 kg, 11–25 kg, and over 25 kg, including breeders, are 7.0, 3.0, and 1.0 mg/kg, respectively (Tables 5.3, 5.4 and 5.5). The Brazilian Tables (Rostagno *et al.*, 2017) recommended lower supplementation for piglets than the NRC (2012), but FEFANA (2015) and DSM Nutritional Products (2022b) OVN™ proposed similar or slightly higher values to the NRC (Table 5.3). In growing and finisher diets, pyridoxine is 47–313% higher in the Brazilian Tables (Rostagno *et al.*, 2017). FEFANA (2015) and DSM Nutritional Products (2022b) OVN™ are up to 4.5 times higher (Table 5.4). For sows in gestation and lactation, the Brazilian Tables (Rostagno *et al.*, 2017) have recommendations for 95% more vitamin B_6 than the NRC (2012) and both FEFANA (2015) and DSM Nutritional Products (2022b) OVN™ up to 5.5 times more (Table 5.5). The genetic companies recommend around 4 mg/kg for piglets (Table 5.6), around 3 mg/kg for growing pigs (Table 5.7), and 3–4 mg/kg for breeders (Table 5.8).

In commercial practice, vitamin B_6 supplementaiton in feed reflects the discrepancies reported (Tables 5.9, 5.10, and 5.11). In China (Yang *et al.*, 2021b), the weighted average supplementation is only 3.31 mg/kg and reduces to 2.47 mg/kg for piglets up to 20 kg (Table 5.9). The vitamin B_6 supplementation for piglets in the USA is around 7 mg/kg. The USA swine industry is currently using the highest levels. In Brazil (Dalto and da Silva, 2020), the USA (Faccin *et al.*, 2022), and China (Yang *et al.*, 2021b), the supplementation for growing pigs is close to 2 mg/kg (Table 5.10). However, the variability in inclusion levels is very high, and some Chinese producers do not add any vitamin B_6, which indicates the great diversity of opinion. One possible explanation for the discrepancies in current information might be the different effects of vitamin B_6 depending on its quantity and availability in the different feed ingredients used in the formulation. Possible different effects of supplementation depend on the level of protein included in the feed. The benefits of additional vitamin B_6 increase as the protein likely increases above the required level or the imbalance in amino acids (for example, methionine).

Nevertheless, the fact that deficiency symptoms are infrequent does not necessarily mean that including quantities beyond those supplied in ingredients is not helpful. It should not be forgotten that losses of up to 70% in the concentration of this vitamin have been described as a consequence of the handling of feedstuffs during the manufacturing and storage of feeds. Furthermore, information on the availability of this vitamin in different feed ingredients is incomplete, although there is evidence that it is not always equally available. According to a report by Hoffmann-La Roche (1979), the availability of vitamin B_6 in corn and soy is between 45% and 65%.

However, Easter *et al.*'s (1983) experiment showed that supplementing 1 mg/kg pyridoxine in feeds for sows improved litter size at birth and weaning. Russell *et al.* (1985) found significant differences in transaminase enzyme activity in red corpuscles and muscular tissue depending on the level of vitamin B_6 in the feed, such that activity (and therefore transaminase capacity) increased considerably when higher levels were included. These experiments show that the capacity for amino acid interconversion can be modulated according to the level of vitamin B_6 in the feed. It might be helpful to include additional amounts depending on the total quantity of protein in feed and the amino acid imbalance. According to the results of these authors, the minimum requirement for proper transaminase activity in gilts is achieved when feed provides at least 2.1 mg of vitamin B_6 per day.

Piglets

In piglets, weaning brings an abrupt change in the supply and balance of the amino acids they receive. Formulating feeds with an amino acid profile as perfectly balanced in essential and non-essential amino acids as milk is impossible. In humans, it has been shown that weaning involves a considerable increase in vitamin B_6 requirements due to the need to modify amino acids (Bender, 1999). However, the vitamin B_6 concentration in milk (around 0.4 mg/l) is so low (Benedikt *et al.*, 1996) that it can barely meet half of the requirement (Matte *et al.*, 1998; Matte *et al.*, 2001).

Consequently, the vitamin B_6 concentration in weaned piglets is reduced, and the requirement is higher (Kösters and Kirchgessner, 1976; Kirchgessner and Kösters, 1977; Matte *et al.*, 1998). Matte *et al.* (2001) described how administering 7.7 mg/kg vitamin B_6 to piglets weaned at 2 weeks is sufficient to avoid the appearance of deficiency symptoms but not to raise the pyridoxal-5-phosphate concentration in erythrocytes to within the optimum range, suggesting that an even higher supply is necessary, which they calculated as 20 times the recommendation of the NRC. Woodworth *et al.* (2000) also found a positive effect of fortifying feed for piglets with vitamin B_6 (3.9 and 7.7 mg/kg).

Dalto *et al.* (2015) studied the interactive effects of selenium and pyridoxine on the gene expression of blastocysts in gilts. They observed that adding 10 mg/kg of HCl-pyridoxine and selenium considerably maximized mRNA GSH-Px after estrus. This antioxidant capacity is essential in reproduction because ovarian metabolism may produce excess ROS during the peri-estrus period, impairing ovulatory functions and early embryo development.

In piglets, there is an acute 10-fold increase in plasma homocysteine (pHcy), an intermediary metabolite of sulfur amino acids, during the first 2 weeks of life, which may weaken immune competence. Côté-Robitaille *et al.* (2015) described an oral supplementation of pyridoxine in a concentration of 2.6 mg/kg, along with betaine, choline, and creatine, supplied directly to suckling piglets during lactation, reduced the concentration of pHcy.

Another way that vitamin B_6 can influence piglet development is through its effects on intestinal development. Li *et al.* (2019) demonstrated that supplementation of B_6 in concentrations of 4 and 7 mg/kg in weaned piglets affected the intestinal morphology and absorption of protein in a high-protein diet. The diarrhea ratio decreased when 7 mg/kg was

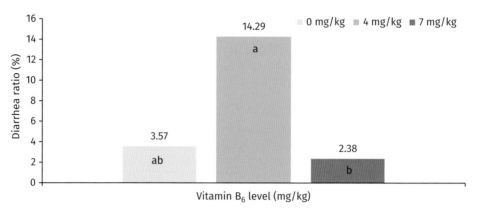

Figure 5.19 Effect of vitamin B₆ on diarrhea ratio (Li *et al.*, 2019). Bars with no-common superscript (a, b) differ significantly (*p*<0.05)

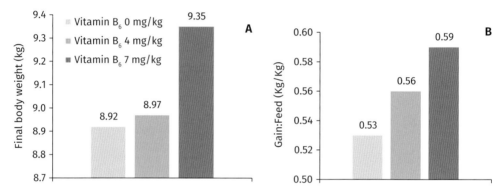

Figure 5.20 Effect of vitamin B₆ levels (0, 4, and 7 mg/kg) on (A) final body weight (kg) and (B) gain: feed ratio (kg: kg) of weaned piglets fed a high protein (22%) diet (Li *et al.*, 2019)

used (Figure 5.19), and the final body weight and feed utilization also improved at this level (Figure 5.20).

Conversely, Yin *et al.* (2020), using weaned piglets fed low-protein diets (18% crude protein), observed that 4 or 7 mg vitamin B₆/kg feed up-regulated inflammatory cytokines (IL-1β, TNF-α, COX-2, IL-10, and TGF-β) and downregulated amino acid transporters (SLC6A20, SLC7A1, SLC7A6, SLC16A14, and SLC38A5)mRNA expression in the ileum. Vitamin B₆ supplementation also decreased villus area and tended to decrease villus height. These findings have implications for the gut health of weaned piglets.

Vitamin B₁₂ (cyanocobalamin)

The NRC (2012) decided that pigs between 5 and 7 kg need at least 20 µg/kg of feed; between 7 and 11 kg, 17.5 µg; between 11 and 25 kg, 15 µg; between 25 and 50 kg, 10 µg (Table 5.3) and only 5 µg/kg above 50 kg body weight (Table 5.4). In breeders (Table 5.5), the NRC requirements are 15 µg/kg in all cases. These recommendations are lower than those made by the Brazilian Tables (Rostagno *et al.*, 2017), FEFANA (2015), DSM Nutritional Products (2022b) OVN™ or the genetic companies (Tables 5.6, 5.7, and 5.8) that propose supplementation levels that are several times higher than the NRC (2012). The swine industry (Tables 5.9, 5.10, and 5.11) has adopted those recommendations and uses between 4 to 6 times the NRC (2012) levels. These surveys indicated that all vitamin and mineral premixes incorporated vitamin B_{12}.

Although there is some evidence that the inclusion of vitamin B_{12} at much higher concentrations than the minimum recommended by the NRC (2012) may be helpful, it is not substantial enough due to the complexity of the processes in which this vitamin is involved, its endogenous production and accumulation in the liver. In this respect, the studies carried out by Teague and Grifo (1966) more than 55 years ago indicated that the inclusion of higher levels of vitamin B_{12} in feed for sows had a positive effect on the number and weight of weaned pigs but that this effect was only appreciable from the third litter onwards if supplementation continued uninterrupted.

Under indoor production conditions, where contact with feces is limited, special attention should be paid to this vitamin because there are few ways of correcting an inadequate supply (Bryant et al., 1981). Considering the enhanced sanitary conditions of operations, it seems advisable to ignore supplies of vitamin B_{12} from pig flora and feces to avoid deficiency. The problem arises precisely when trying to establish these requirements with accuracy. In a study with gilts, Simard et al. (2007) have related the optimization of the reproductive function in sows with concentrations of B_{12} and homocysteine. An optimum maximum of B_{12} is produced by administering 164 µg/kg of feed and a minimum of homocysteine with concentrations of 93 µg of cyanocobalamin/kg of feed.

Furthermore, any aspect that may affect intestinal flora (parasites, antimicrobial agents, etc.) can harm the endogenous production of vitamin B_{12}. Health problems derived from the use of feed of animal origin and their legal and commercial implications mean that it is probably advisable to increase the vitamin B_{12} concentration in feeds in Europe, especially for young animals.

Niacin (vitamin B_3)

The NRC (2012) recommended 30 mg of niacin per kilogram of feed for piglets and growing pigs (Tables 5.3 and 5.4) and 10 mg/kg of feed for breeders in all cases (Table 5.5). These requirements may be considered low compared to the supply usually provided by the ingredients used in feed formulation for pigs and the possibility of obtaining niacin from tryptophan, which suggests that niacin supplementation is unnecessary. Nevertheless, in practice niacin is always included in the vitamin and mineral premix because of the low niacin availability in most feed materials, the low tryptophan content in low crude protein feed (this amino acid may represent a high marginal cost), the fact that these requirements are calculated for low production genotypes with higher consumption than modern ones, and the great variety of factors that can lead to a higher niacin requirement.

Based on this reasoning, the Brazilian Tables (Rostagno et al., 2017) recommended supplementation between 58% and 77.7% higher than the NRC (2012) and both FEFANA (2015) and DSM Nutritional Products (2022b) OVN™ are up to 2.7 times more for piglets (Table 5.3). The recommended levels for growing pigs (Table 5.4) are between the same and 1.5 higher from other sources compared to the NRC (2012). But, for breeders (Table 5.5), all other groups recommend 3 times more niacin than NRC (2012). The genetic companies have suggested supplementation between 23 and 55 mg/kg for piglets (Table 5.6), between 21 and 51 mg/kg for growing pigs (Table 5.7) and for breeders between 15 and 100 mg/kg (Table 5.8).

According to recent surveys, the Chinese swine industry (Yang et al., 2021b) uses the lowest levels of niacin for piglets, 23.2 and 27.1 mg/kg (Table 5.9). In contrast, the US industry (Faccin *et al.*, 2022) currently adds the highest levels (between 50.7 and 36.4 mg/kg). The same tendency is observed for growing pigs (Table 5.10), with Chinese producers supplementing between 15 and 16.7 mg/kg and US producers between 30.1 and 24.6 mg/kg. For breeders (Table 5.11), in China, sows receive diets with niacin between 23 and 24.6 mg/kg, and American sows receive around 44.9 mg/kg. Brazilian levels (Dalto and da Silva, 2020) are intermediate, and the levels increased in the past 6 years in the USA (Flohr *et al.*, 2016; Faccin *et al.*, 2022). All these values are somewhat higher than previously reported surveys (Barroeta *et al.*, 2012), but the variability in the inclusion levels is still very high everywhere.

Gestation and lactation

The supplementation of niacin in sow reproduction and litter performance was investigated by Thaler *et al.* (1987), Weeden *et al.* (1990), Ivers *et al.* (1993), and Goodband *et al.* (1998). All reports agreed that supplemental niacin (reaching 250, 500, or 1,000 mg/d of added niacin) for gilts or gestating sows did not improve reproductive.

Generally, during these studies, the basal diets provided 50 mg/day of niacin during gestation and 100 mg/day of niacin during lactation. In fact, 250 or 500 mg/day of added niacin fed during gestation and lactation actually reduced the number of pigs born (Goodband *et al.*, 1998). All research groups detected effects on fatty acids or glucose metabolism during gestation and lactation (Goodband *et al.*, 1998). These changes in metabolism are reflected in fat accumulation during gestation and backfat loss in lactation (Thaler *et al.*, 1987). Sows supplemented with niacin (250 or 500 mg/day) had more pigs at weaning, better pig survival (Weeden *et al.*, 1990), heavier weanling pigs, and litter weights (Thaler *et al.*, 1987; Goodband *et al.*, 1998).

Piglets

The niacin concentration in piglet feed is approximately twice as much as that in feeds for growing pigs, which is partly explained by the inability of the piglet to convert tryptophan to niacin (Firth and Johnson, 1956; Harmon *et al.*, 1969). Nevertheless, in an experiment, Lutz and Stahly (2000) observed that the inclusion of niacin in feed for piglets (between 10 and 27 kg) at a concentration up to 3 times higher than levels recommended by the NRC (1998), which was similar to NRC (2012), did not have a positive effect on growth, the accumulation of protein or that of fat.

Matte *et al.* (2016) conducted an experiment to determine if tryptophan (Trp) metabolism and growth responses to dietary Trp are modulated by dietary niacin (B$_3$) (15–45 mg/kg) in weanling piglets. The tendencies for vitamin B$_3$ treatment effects on some aspects of growth performance (average daily feed intake and average daily gain) and plasma nicotinamide (Nam) suggested that the 15 mg/kg dietary level was suboptimal and 45 mg/kg may have positive effects in growth (Figure 5.21).

The responses of plasma nicotinamide to both dietary Trp (0 and 1 mg/kg) and B$_3$ suggest that preformed dietary niacin may attenuate Trp oxidation toward niacin metabolites. Plasma nicotinamide concentrations also allowed a novel estimation of the conversion ratio of Trp to niacin in pigs (8–10 weeks of age) of 37:1. Moreover, the postprandial insulinemia suggests a Trp action on insulin clearance rather than on insulin secretion (assessed by C-peptide), without apparent metabolic consequences on glucose utilization.

Recently, Yi *et al.* (2021) illustrated that dietary supplementation with a relatively high level of niacin (45 mg/kg) decreased intestinal villus height and crypt depth but increased mucosal alkaline phosphatase activity and nutrient transporter and tight junction protein expression on day 7. However, on day 14 post-weaning, the high levels of dietary niacin (45–75 mg/kg) increased the jejunal villus height and crypt depth (Figure 5.22). Still, they decreased alkaline

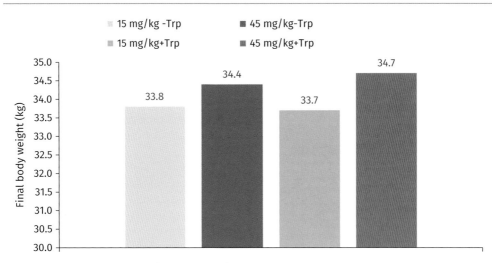

Figure 5.21 Effect of niacin level (15 or 45 mg/kg) on final body weight of weaned piglets at 10 weeks of age fed diets with or without tryptophan (Trp) supplementation (Matte *et al.*, 2016)

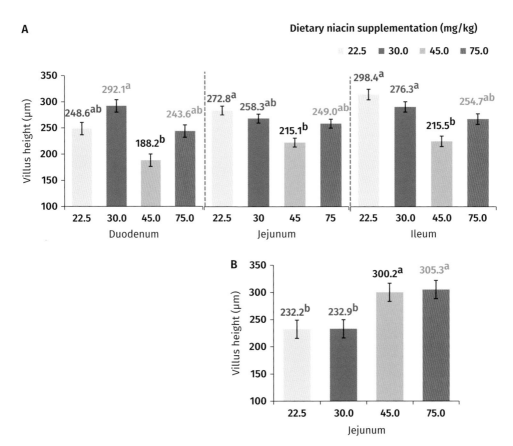

Figure 5.22 Intestinal height of weaned piglet with different niacin supplementation on days 7 (A) and 14 (B), values with no common superscripts differ significantly, *p*<0.05 (Yi *et al.*, 2021)

phosphatase activity, nutrient transporter, and tight junction protein expression compared to diets with lower levels of niacin (22.5–30 mg/kg).

Moreover, dietary supplementation with niacin may affect intestinal morphology and its functions by modulating intestinal cell proliferation. Piglets fed diets with 75 mg/kg niacin had greater diarrhea incidence rates than piglets with 30 and 45 mg/kg niacin-supplemented diets. Therefore, the most suitable dose for weaned piglets is dietary supplementation with 30 to 45 mg/kg niacin on the 7th day after weaning. These results provided novel information on dietary niacin's effects and underlying mechanisms on intestinal morphology and developing weaned piglets.

Niacin may affect intestinal immunity, microbial community, and the intestinal barrier in weaned piglets during starvation. Feng et al. (2021) evaluated the supplementation of 40 mg of niacin in a 10 ml normal saline solution fed once daily for 3 days. The results indicated that niacin attenuated the rate of weight loss and diarrhea in weaned piglets (Figure 5.23). Niacin also enhanced the intestinal epithelial barrier function, improved the expression of antimicrobial peptides, and affected the bacterial community and short-chain fatty acid production in the colon of weaned piglets.

Liu et al. (2021) also reported the protective effect of niacin on improving the growth performance compared to an antagonist for the niacin receptor GPR109A, mepenzolate bromide, and gut health in weaned piglets (Figure 5.24). Niacin supplementation efficiently ensured

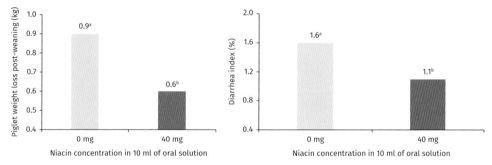

Figure 5.23 Effects of niacin on piglet weight loss (A) and (B) diarrhea index (%), values with no common superscripts differ significantly, p<0.05 (Feng et al., 2021)

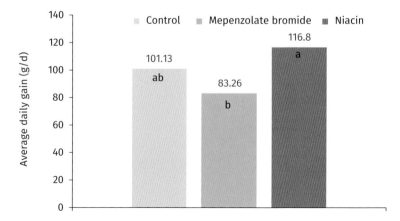

Figure 5.24 Effect of niacin on growth performance in weaned piglet, values with no common superscripts differ significantly, p<0.05 (Liu et al., 2021)

intestinal morphology and attenuated intestinal inflammation of weaned piglets. The protective effects of niacin on gut health may be associated with increased *Lactobacillus* and *Dorea* abundance and butyrate content and decreased abundances of *Peptococcus*.

Growing pigs

Real *et al.* (2002) evaluated niacin supplementation levels that ranged between 13 and 55 mg/kg. They estimated that when feeding practical corn-soybean meal-based diets to finishing pigs in commercial facilities, up to 55 mg/kg of added dietary niacin is required to support maximal growth performance. When evaluating requirements to enhance certain pork quality traits, improvements were observed with up to 110 and 550 mg/kg of added niacin.

Pantothenic acid (vitamin B$_5$)

Pantothenic acid is found in nearly all feeds and is frequently equated with "being very abundant," even in some works on animal nutrition. But this is incorrect because it is frequently found in concentrations inadequate to achieve high production or to avoid deficiency symptoms due to its involvement in various metabolic processes (Stahly and Lutz, 2001).

According to the NRC (2012), the minimum requirement for a piglet of 5–7 kg is 12 mg/kg (Table 5.3), and it reduces progressively up to 8 mg/kg feed for 50 kg body weight; the recommendation for this weight upwards is 7 mg/kg of feed (Table 5.3 and 5.4). For breeders, the established recommendation is 12 mg/kg (Table 5.5). The Brazilian Tables (Rostagno *et al.*, 2017) recommended pantothenic acid for piglets at levels 2.26 to 3 times higher than the NRC (2012), FEFANA (2015) and DSM Nutritional Products (2022b) OVN™ suggested up to 5.6–6 times more (Table 5.3). In the growing phase (Table 5.4), the proposed supplementation levels of the Brazilian Tables (Rostagno *et al.*, 2017) are between 1.57 and 2 times higher than the NRC (2012), FEFANA (2015) and DSM Nutritional Products (2022b) OVN™ suggested between 6.4 and 5.7 times more. For sows, the recommendations are 73.3% and 291% higher than the NRC (2012) in the Brazilian Tables and both FEFANA (2015) and DSM Nutritional Products (2022b) OVN™, respectively (Table 5.5).

Industry surveys (Tables 5.9, 5.10, and 5.11) showed that the weighted average concentration of pantothenic acid provided in the vitamin and mineral premix range between 21.3 and 36.6 mg/kg for piglets up to 5 kg and are gradually reduced to 16.3 and 24.8 mg/kg (Table 5.9). The pantothenic acid supplementation varied between 10.7 and 19.9 mg/kg in growers and finishers (Table 5.10). For breeders, pantothenic acid is added at volumes between 17 and 31.8 mg/kg (Table 5.11). Although there is significant variability, the standard deviations indicated that pantothenic acid was included in all the vitamin and mineral premixes studied by these authors. China always had the lowest supplementation values, while the USA currently presents the highest levels.

Growing pigs and meat quality

Groesbeck *et al.* (2007) and Lo Fiego *et al.* (2009) carried out interesting experiments intended to explain previous findings, which pointed to a relationship between levels of pantothenic acid, body composition, and meat quality (Stahly and Lutz, 2001; Lutz *et al.*, 2004); it also includes ractopamine-HCl showing that the improvements produced by this compound in growth should be associated with higher levels of pantothenic acid in the ration.

The effects of the dietary level of pantothenic acid on the carcass, meat quality traits, and fatty acid composition of thigh subcutaneous adipose tissue in Italian heavy pigs were also

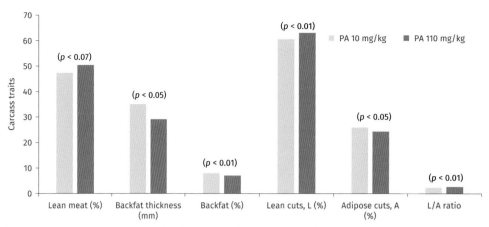

Figure 5.25 Effect of pantothenic acid dietary level (10, or 110 mg/kg) on lean meat, backfat thickness, backfat %, lean cuts L (%), adipose cuts A (%), and L/A ratio of pigs [Duroc × (Landrace × Large White)] fed from 107 to 168 kg live weight (Minelli *et al.*, 2013)

evaluated by Minelli *et al.* (2013). The authors concluded in 2 experiments that were administering super nutritional doses (10 or 110 mg/kg) of pantothenic acid in finishing pigs [Duroc × (Landrace × Large White)] from 107 to 168 kg live weight aid in producing carcasses with lower back fat, more lean cuts, and a lower percentage of fatty cuts without affecting meat quality (Figure 5.25).

In the second experiment, pigs [Dumeco Cofok × (Landrace × Large White)] from 95 to 165 kg live weight were fed 10, 60, and 110 mg/kg of pantothenic acid, confirming the positive effects in carcass quality (Figure 5.26). Vitamin B$_5$ concentrations of 60 mg/kg seem sufficient for its repartitioning action, causing an increase in the degree of unsaturation of the lipids in the subcutaneous adipose tissue, along with increases in the level of linoleic acid and iodine value. The effects detected, though favorable for carcass quality and the characteristics of the lipids from a human nutritional point of view, advise against a generalized over-supplementation to the diets fed to pigs reared for long-seasoned products. The adipose depots are already richer in PUFAs in lean strains and females.

Folic acid (vitamin B$_9$)

Although folacin was discovered in the 1930s, not until very recently has it been considered a vitamin of practical importance in pig nutrition. This is partly because the first studies to evaluate requirements did not establish a minimum (Easter *et al.*, 1983). There is evidence that folic acid is synthesized by the intestinal flora (and its frequent association with coprophagy). However, it has been observed that microbial sources of folate are insufficient to supply the animal (Aufreiter *et al.*, 2011).

The relatively high concentration of folic acid in most pig feed ingredients is sufficient in almost all circumstances to meet these low requirements. However, several factors can increase folic acid needs. Dietary iron levels increase folate needs. O'Connor *et al.* (1989) compared sows fed diets containing 25 or 125 mg iron/kg with diets containing 0.6 mg folic acid/kg throughout gestation and lactation. The progeny was given an intramuscular injection of iron-dextran (100 mg/kg body weight). The sow plasma folate of sows fed 25 mg Fe/kg was 47% and 69% lower than sows fed 125 mg Fe/kg. Milk folate concentration decreased during lactation in sows fed with low levels of iron but not in sows fed diets with 125 mg/kg; consequently, piglets had low liver folate concentration.

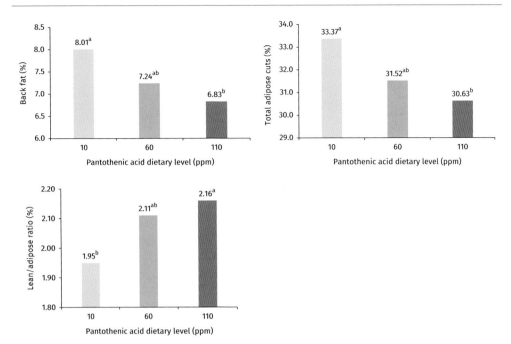

Figure 5.26 Effect of pantothenic acid dietary level (10, 60, and 110 mg/kg) on back fat, total adipose cuts, and lean/adipose ratio of pigs [Dumeco Cofok × (Landrace × Large white)] fed from 95 to 165 kg live weight, values with no common superscripts differ significantly, $p<0.05$ (Minelli *et al.*, 2013)

Even in the 2012 recommendations by the NRC, the level was still only 0.3 mg/kg for piglets and growing pigs (Tables 5.3 and 5.4). The recommended level for breeders was raised to 1.3 mg/kg (Table 5.5). However, the Brazilian Tables (Rostagno *et al.*, 2017) recommended supplementation for piglets 70–91.3% higher than the NRC (2012), and FEFANA (2015) and DSM Nutritional Products (2022b) OVN™ up to 10 times more folic acid (Tables 5.3). The Brazilian Tables (Rostagno *et al.*, 2017) suggested folacin levels similar to the NRC for growing pigs, while FEFANA (2015) and DSM Nutritional Products (2022b) OVN™ proposed levels up to 5 times higher (Tables 5.4). The Brazilian Tables have values similar to the NRC (2012) for breeders, whereas FEFANA (2015) and DSM Nutritional Products (2022b) OVN™ proposed values up to 4.4 times higher (Table 5.5).

The results of industry surveys (Tables 5.9, 5.10, and 5.11) indicated a significant heterogeneity in the implementation of the supplementation of folic acid for pigs. Some vitamin and mineral premixes still do not include folacin, even for sows, in several parts of the world. In piglets, the average weighted values fluctuate between 1.22 and 5.32 mg/kg (Table 5.9). For growing pigs, the levels of supplementation vary between 0.45 and 0.94 mg/kg (Table 5.10). In breeders, feed folic acid levels vary between 1.7 and 2.94 mg/kg (Table 5.11). The highest supplementations were observed in the USA with boars (Faccin *et al.*, 2022).

Sows and piglets

Matte *et al.* (1984b) observed that periodic intramuscular administration of 15 mg of folacin to future breeding sows from weaning up to 60 days after insemination increased the number of piglets born. These same authors also detected increased litter weight gain when supplementing sow diets with 5 and 15 mg folacin/kg during gestation (Matte *et al.*, 1992). The dietary supplementation of folic acid at 6.62 mg/kg of sow diet during gestation and lactation in

2 parities also increased the number of pigs born alive without affecting the conception rate (Thaler *et al.*, 1989). In another study, adding 5.0 mg of folic acid per kilogram of diet improved the survival rate of fetuses during early gestation, 62.2% versus 55.1%, compared to those not receiving folic acid (Tremblay *et al.*, 1989).

It is hard to draw clear conclusions about possible recommendations because of the difficulty of working with animals with such a long production cycle as breeders. They are subject to many factors. It is also difficult to quantify levels of folacin stored in tissues and the levels in the feed before the beginning of the breeding phase. Thus, while in the first experiment, folacin was supplied mainly during the growth phase of the future breeder, in the second, a higher level was given during gestation only.

Others have observed positive effects of folic acid supplementation on the number of piglets per parity. Friendship and Wilson (1991) suggested that folic acid from natural feedstuffs, plus the current low level of supplemental folic acid typically used, may not be sufficient to maximize the reproductive performance of sows. In their experiment, these authors utilized a 400-sow commercial herd experiencing a small litter size. When 25 mg of folic acid was injected at the time of breeding and 1 week later, and if only parities 3 to 5 were analyzed, the litter size was improved by 1 pig per litter over that of the control sows. Lindemann (1993) fed sows during gestation with diets containing 1 mg/kg added folacin, obtaining a mean size of a litter of 10.79 piglets instead of 9.86, which is almost 1 piglet more per litter. Furthermore, the effect was more marked in subsequent parities, reaching a difference of 1.8 piglets in the third litter.

Matte and Girard (1999) calculated folacin requirements of gestating sows by an indirect procedure based on this vitamin's metabolic utilization during different gestation phases. In theory, metabolic utilization is an indicator of current requirements. According to their calculations, folacin requirements are 10 mg/kg feed during gestation (15 mg/kg during the early stages). The same researchers (Matte and Girard, 1989; Matte *et al.*, 1990a,b; Matte *et al.*, 1996) had previously evaluated the effect of folic acid on serum and milk folates in lactating sows as well as on serum folates and growth rate of the piglets. These sows received 15 mg of folic acid intramuscularly from day 2 after parturition to weaning 26 days later. Milk folates decreased from day 7 to 21 of lactation but were higher (11.8±0.7 ng/ml) in folic acid-treated sows than in control sows (7.9±0.4 ng/ml). The same effect was observed in piglet serum, where blood levels increased to 86.3±3.1 ng/ml, but treated sows had piglets with 15% higher folacin. However, the piglet growth rate did not change (Matte *et al.*, 1986).

Despite the evidence provided by Matte *et al.* (1984b), no specific recommendation for folic acid has been indicated for gilts in the NRC. However, Matte *et al.* (1993, 1996) confirmed that adding up to 4 mg/kg folacin in gilt feed increases embryo viability in first parity. The viability was 88.5% in sows receiving feed with a high inclusion level versus 62.9% in control sows.

Furthermore, the benefit produced by administering high dosages of this vitamin differed in the number of piglets born versus the growth rate of the litter (Matte and Girard, 1990). The variability in the effects on the number of piglets and probably their growth potential post-farrow can be explained by the allelic or genetic variation in the expression of the folate-binding protein gene in the uterus reported by Vallet *et al.* (1999, 2005). The effects of higher supplementation of folic acid on the growth of weanlings can be explained by the publication of Wang *et al.* (2011).

In contrast to all previously described research reports, Harper *et al.* (1994) studied a range of between 1 and 4 mg/kg of folacin in feed for sows during all the phases of the breeder's life (including several litters), concluding that there was no additional production benefit with the highest levels of inclusion. Harper *et al.* (2003) evaluated sources of folic acid in gilt gestation (after 105 days), lactation and mating for a second parity. The sources evaluated were oxidized (synthetic pteroylmonoglutamate (MG) form and N5-formyl-5,6,7,8,-tetrahydrofolic acid (THFA), and reduced (bacterial sources) forms of folic acid at 2.1 mg/kg. Supplementing folacin at this low level before farrowing and during lactation did not affect sow and litter performance during the first and second parity. In this study and with this level of supplementation, there was no indication that reduced folate sources were superior to the oxidized pteroylmonoglutamate form as folate supplements for sows.

These findings led the NRC (2012) to recommend in their last report a level of 1.3 mg/kg in feed for sows during gestation and lactation, as well as in feed for boars. But the current information suggests that the recommendation by the NRC in its 2012 report includes only the minimum concentration below which deficiency symptoms can arise, with the apparent result that supplementation improves production indicators, especially those of reproduction and those obtained in young animals.

In an experiment with boars, Audet *et al.* (2004) demonstrated an increase in sperm production when the number of B vitamins in feed was increased; in the case of folic acid, the supplied dose was 40 mg/head day. Owing to practical difficulties, folacin's effects on boars' reproductive parameters have not been studied over multiple parities.

The discrepancies about folic acid supplementation could be solved by studying its effects on embryo development. Liu *et al.* (2012) studied the effects of intrauterine growth retardation and maternal folic acid supplementation on hepatic mitochondrial function and gene expression in piglets. The researchers reported no sign of toxic effects on the reproductive performance of sows or growth performance (Figure 5.27) and the health status of piglets. Therefore, the level of 30 mg folic acid per kilogram diet would be safe for sows and their offspring. The authors concluded that at the peri-weaning stage, piglets with intrauterine growth retardation had impaired mitochondrial respiratory activities, membrane potential, and antioxidant capacity, decreased mitochondrial DNA (mtDNA) biogenesis, and mRNA expression levels of genes related to mitochondrial biogenesis and function. Maternal folic

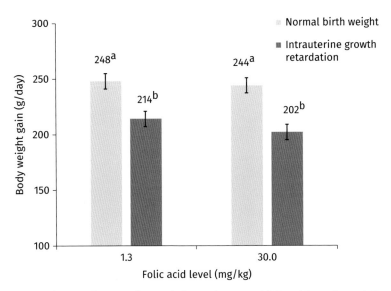

Figure 5.27 Effects of intrauterine growth retardation and maternal folic acid supplementation on piglets' hepatic mitochondrial function and gene expression, values with no common superscripts differ significantly, *p*<0.05 (Liu *et al.*, 2012)

acid supplementation during gestation could ameliorate suppressed antioxidant capacity and change gene expressions.

Other effects of maternal folic acid on embryo development were explored by Li *et al.* (2013). This group worked with sows from a Landrace cross with Laiwu, a Chinese genetic breed with high intramuscular fat content. These sows were fed either a diet with no folic acid supplementation or 1.3 mg/kg, similar to the NRC (2012) recommendation. The folic acid fed to sows during early mid-pregnancy affected piglet body weight, muscle fiber number, and intramuscular triglyceride content. This folic acid supplementation affected the expression of more than 3,154 genes. This indicates that folic acid may be able to have epigenetic effects in genes related to myogenesis and intramuscular fat deposition in piglets.

Folic acid may also affect milk production in sows. Wang *et al.* (2011) evaluated the effects of feeding Landrace × Yorkshire sows during lactation with diets containing 0, 12.5, 50, and 100 mg folic acid/kg feed. Folic acid had a quadratic effect on milk production and was maximized at 60 mg/kg. The ratio of feed intake to milk production had a negative linear effect going from 0.70 to 0.65, which indicates a significant improvement in efficiency. Folic acid at 100 mg/kg increased milk fat, total solids, and non-fat solids. This resulted in a linear increase in average individual piglet weight and total average litter daily gain (Figure 5.28), explaining early observations on litter weight gain during lactation.

In pigs post-weaning, Yu *et al.* (2010) evaluated the effects of folic acid supplementation on growth performance, serum biochemical indicators and hepatic folate metabolism-related gene expression in weaned piglets with an initial body weight of 7.33 kg fed for 28 days. They used a basal diet with 0.5 mg/kg and added folic acid to reach 3.0, 5.5 and 10.5 mg folic acid/kg feed. Pigs fed a basal diet supplemented with 2.5 mg/kg folic acid (3.0 mg/kg) grew faster ($p<0.05$) and consumed more feed ($p<0.01$) than pigs in the other groups during the last 2 weeks of the experiment. The feed efficiency was not affected by dietary treatments. Piglets fed 3.0 mg/kg had greater concentrations of growth hormone, IGF in serum, a greater abundance of folate-binding protein and lower homocysteine concentrations more than piglets fed the basal diet or higher concentrations of folic acid. These results may suggest that a 3.0 mg folic acid/kg diet will be enough for piglets, which is 10 times higher than the NRC (2012) recommendation and very close to other current commercial recommendations.

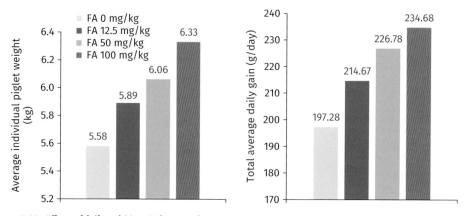

Figure 5.28 Effect of folic acid levels in sow diets on the average individual piglet weight at day 21 (kg) and on the total (21 days) average individual daily gain (g/day) of suckling piglets during lactation (Wang *et al.*, 2011)

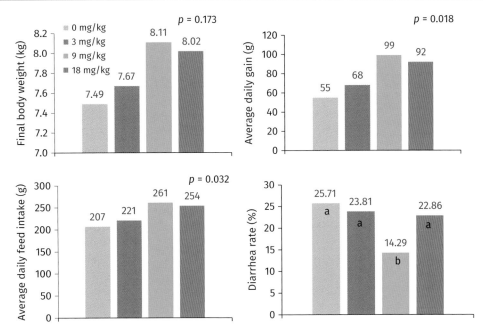

Figure 5.29 Effect of folic acid levels (0, 3, 9, and 18 mg/kg) on nursery pigs' growth performance and diarrhea rate, values with no common superscripts differ significantly, $p<0.05$ (Wang *et al.*, 2021a)

However, a recent report (Wang *et al.*, 2021a) indicated that the weaning stress of piglets could be partially alleviated by dietary folic acid supplementation. Levels up to 18 mg/kg improved the feed intake, gain, and final body weight and reduced the diarrhea rate in nursery pigs at 9 mg/kg (Figure 5.29). The benefits observed in intestinal health could be explained by improved mucosal histomorphology with more significant villus height, surface area, reduced crypt depth, and a bigger villus height to crypt depth ratio. Additionally, folic acid could affect gut microbiota by increasing colon butyric acid and total short-chain fatty acids that could help to inhibit colonization and growth of some pathogens (*E. coli* and *Salmonella*).

In a second paper related to this research, Wang *et al.* (2021b) concluded that folate supplementation (9 and 18 mg/kg) could increase the stomach pH and tend to decrease the cecum pH of weaned piglets. Folate treatment (9 and 18 mg/kg) had a positive effect on the metabolism of short-chain fatty acids in piglets, in particular, compared with the control group, and the content of acetic acid (AA) and valeric acid was markedly increased ($p<0.05$) in the cecum and colon, respectively. These changes in cecum fermentation were related to a higher relative abundance of *Lactobacillus reuteri*, *L. salivarius* and *L. mucosae* in the 9 mg/kg folate supplementation group.

Growing pigs

Lutz and Stahly (1997) found no positive effects on growth and carcass composition in piglets weighing 8 to 23 kg due to folacin inclusion between 200% and 720% of the levels recommended by the NRC (1998), suggesting that the benefit is mainly limited to breeders. In its 2012 report, the NRC gave the same requirements for piglets, growing and finishing pigs as in previous reports (0.3 mg/kg).

Recently, Wang *et al.* (2020) studied the effect of folic acid supplementation and dietary protein level on growth performance, serum chemistry, and immune response in weanling piglets fed differing concentrations of aflatoxins. They found that reducing dietary crude protein levels from 18% to 15% exacerbated the aflatoxicosis effects. However, there were no improvements in growth parameters due to folic acid supplementation. The effects observed by those authors would have presumably been more pronounced if the study had been continued for additional weeks. The aflatoxin effects would have been compounded with time and may affect the practical field responses to aflatoxicosis.

Biotin (vitamin B₇)

For years it was considered that the biotin requirements of pigs could be met by feed ingredients and synthesis by intestinal flora (Bonomi *et al.*, 1996). However, where antimicrobial agents are present in the feed or when the animal has little possibility of contact with feces, the likelihood of insufficient intake increases. According to the NRC (2012), most of the literature agrees that the inclusion of biotin at between 110 and 880 µg/kg does not produce an improvement in production parameters either in piglets weaned between 21 and 28 days or in growers and finishers (Hanke and Meade, 1972; Washam *et al.*, 1975; Simmins and Brooks, 1980; Brooks, 1982; Easter *et al.*, 1983; Bryant *et al.*, 1985a,b,c; Hamilton and Veum, 1986; Kornegay, 1986). The situation is disputed, however, because other authors have observed beneficial effects (Adams *et al.*, 1967; Peo *et al.*, 1970; Partridge and McDonald, 1990; Riveron-Negrete and Fernandez-Mejia, 2017).

Bearing all these inconsistencies in mind, the NRC (2012) recommended only 80 µg/kg for piglets of up to 7 kg and 50 µg/kg for the remaining growth period (Tables 5.3 and 5.4). In breeders, the recommendation is 200 µg/ kg of feed in all cases (Table 5.5). The Brazilian Tables (Rostagno *et al.*, 2017) double or triple these recommendations, and FEFANA (2015) and DSM Nutritional Products (2022b) OVN™ proposed 4 to 10 times more biotin than the NRC (2012) for piglets (Table 5.3). In growing pigs, the Brazilian Tables (Rostagno *et al.*, 2017) are 76% to 214% higher than NRC (2012), while FEFANA (2015) and DSM Nutritional Products (2022b) OVN™ proposed levels are 3 to 6 times higher than the NRC (Table 5.4). In breeder diets, the Brazilian Tables (Rostagno *et al.*, 2017) recommended levels 62.5% higher than the NRC (2012), while FEFANA (2015) and DSM Nutritional Products (2022b) OVN™ recommend 4 times more supplementation than NRC, 2012 (Table 5.5). The genetic companies suggest using 100 to 240 µg/kg for piglets (Table 5.6) and double NRC for growing and gestation diets (Tables 5.7 and 5.8).

The situation in practice (Tables 5.9, 5.10, and 5.11) reflects the confusion resulting from the lack of data or parameters to determine specific values. Thus, the surveys observed that some manufacturers of vitamin and mineral premixes have chosen not to include biotin in any pig production phase, including in Brazil (Dalto and da Silva, 2020), China (Yang *et al.*, 2021b), or the USA (Flohr *et al.*, 2016; Faccin *et al.*, 2022). However, this situation has been changing in the recent years in the USA, and most producers supplement piglets and breeders with biotin (Faccin *et al.*, 2022). Other manufacturers, however, include between 190 and 400 µg/kg for piglets and 70 to 290 µg/kg for growers and finishers (Tables 5.9 and 5.10). Levels between 290 and 430 µg/kg are observed for breeders (Table 5.11). The current supplementation levels are slightly higher than those observed in previous surveys 20 years ago (Barroeta *et al.*, 2012). In previous and recent surveys, the coefficient of variation of biotin supplementation is among the highest for vitamins, indicating the wide variation of values in the market.

Sows and piglets

In sows, biotin inclusion in feed improves hoof resistance or integrity and sometimes reduces the occurrence of toe lesions (Brooks *et al.*, 1977; Brooks and Simmins, 1981; Bryant and Kornegay, 1984; Bryant *et al.*, 1985a). An improvement has also been observed in hair and skin (Misir and Blair, 1986a,b; Bryant *et al.*, 1985c). But, more important, biotin at 440 µg/kg diet improved the conception rate to first estrus postpartum by 9% and reduced the estrus interval from 14.5 to 10.2 days (Bryant *et al.*, 1985b). These results reported by Bryant *et al.* (1985a,b,c) were obtained in sows fed corn or wheat-based diets and collected during 4 parities with 245 litters recorded). Biotin supplementation (440 µg biotin/kg diet) increased ($p<0.001$) the biotin content of sow plasma, milk and liver while sow liver pyruvate carboxylase activity was not altered ($p>0.10$). Pigs farrowed by sows supplemented with biotin had 3 and 5 times higher ($p<0.001$) levels of plasma biotin at birth and 14 days of age, respectively; however, liver biotin levels at birth were not different ($p>0.10$).

However, Lewis *et al.* (1991) found that including 330 µg/kg of biotin in feed for breeders improved the number of pigs weaned, although surprisingly, it did not affect the hoof. These points suggest that a biotin concentration within that range might be advisable. However, there is no agreement on the usefulness of biotin in feed above 200 µg/kg since some authors did not find positive effects (Watkins *et al.*, 1991). In contrast, Hong *et al.* (2012) observed that dietary supplementation of 200 µg/kg to weaning piglets inoculated with porcine circovirus type 2 improved serum IgG and Interferon-gamma (INF-g), indicating better immune response compared to a basal diet containing 50 µg biotin/kg (Figure 5.30).

The variability in results and the consequence of the difficulty in establishing concrete recommendations can be put down to the multiple interactions between different concentrations of vitamins and nutrients and the variability in the concentration and availability of biotin in feed ingredients (Brooks *et al.*, 1977; Bryant *et al.*, 1985b,c; Simmins and Brooks, 1988), with rations based on barley or wheat presenting a biotin deficiency as opposed to the typical American corn-soy diets, the possible effect of the genotype, and even the housing design that affects contact with feces.

Kornegay *et al.* (1989) reported the effects of supplemental biotin (0, 220, 440, and 880 ppb) and copper (0, 200, and 400 ppm) on performance, hemoglobin concentrations, serum, and liver copper levels and immune response (humoral and cell-mediated) of weanling piglets.

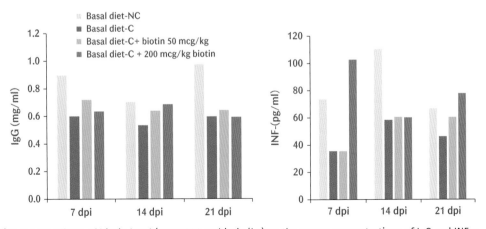

Figure 5.30 Effects of biotin level (50 or 200 µg biotin/kg) on the serum concentrations of IgG and INF-γ of weaned piglets day post-infection (dpi) with porcine circovirus type 2 (PCV2). NC: non-challenged; C: challenged. Basal diet: biotin: 0 mg/kg (Hong *et al.*, 2012)

Supplemental biotin generally did not affect pig performance. However, an interaction ($p<0.01$) during the first 2 weeks was detected; the highest average daily gain and feed intake were observed in piglets fed diets containing 200 and 400 ppm copper combined with the 440 and 880 ppb biotin levels. Although the magnitude of the immune response was small and inconsistent, diets containing 220 and 440 ppb biotin seemed to increase the immune response to sheep red blood cells. However, 880 ppb biotin appeared to depress the response; there was no effect of biotin level on lysozyme titers.

In contrast, the effect of biotin on hoof lesions is difficult to quantify in small populations, as in most experimental situations, since they generally occur in a relatively small proportion of animals. In this context, using large-scale field data obtained in Holland, a marked reduction in limping problems in pigs was observed when biotin was added to feeds systematically, almost halving the number of culled sows. Knauer *et al.* (2007), in a study conducted with culled sows in the US, have related the lesions present in the reproductive system to low biotin provision in the feed.

Hamilton and Veum (2012) evaluated the effects of cecal oxytetracycline infusion and dietary avidin and biotin supplementation on the biotin status of nongravid gilts. They concluded that no gilts in the experiment became biotin deficient because the biotin requirements were met primarily by microbial synthesis and absorption of biotin from the distal small intestine and large intestine, with corn and soybean meal contributing endogenous biotin. Therefore, supplementing diets for gilts entering the breeding herd with 100% of the current NRC biotin requirement for sows was considered adequate.

Evaluations of collective B vitamin level recommendations

Decisions regarding vitamin premixes frequently involve several vitamins. Studies evaluating B complex vitamins at higher levels than the NRC (1998 or 2012) recommended demonstrated potential benefits (Wilson *et al.*, 1991a,b, 1992, 1993; Lindemann *et al.*, 1995; Matte, 1995; Tian *et al.*, 2001; Edmonds and Arentson, 2001; Weiß and Quanz, 2002; Stahly *et al.*, 2007; Mahan *et al.*, 2007; Del Tuffo *et al.*, 2019). These investigations found a higher average daily gain and improvement in production parameters in genotypes with high growth potential. However, another study failed to consistently observe positive effects (Böhmer and Roth-Maier, 2007). This situation caused considerable uncertainty and wide variation in recommendations.

Tian *et al.* (2001) observed that increasing water-soluble vitamins by 200% versus NRC (1998) in growing (20.90±0.44 kg) and finishing (53.55±0.97 kg) pigs (Landrace × Duroc × Yorkshire) improved the overall growth performance and carcass length after 9 weeks of feeding trials. Weiß and Quanz (2002), with a fortification including all vitamins of the B group, supplemented at 8 times the NRC (1998), observed a significant improvement in feed conversion and slightly increased daily gain, fat and muscle area.

Thiamine, riboflavin, pantothenic acid and niacin are directly involved in obtaining energy from carbohydrates via identical biochemical pathways. Therefore, their requirements are pretty likely to be interrelated. Figure 1.3 illustrates the importance of B vitamins to the major metabolic pathways as well as their interrelationships. Chapter 4 provides more detail about the role of individual B vitamins in the metabolism of protein, carbohydrates and fats. The higher need for B vitamins can also be related to the stress level during the experimental period (Blair and Newsome, 1985).

Böhmer and Roth-Maier (2007) observed higher fat accretion without increased protein accretion when feeding 800% of vitamins B_2, B_6 and pantothenic acid or 400 or 800% of biotin, while other vitamins remained at recommended levels, indicating that there was an influence on energy metabolism. The lack of protein accretion could be caused by missed potential of this particular strain of pigs or an insufficient combination of B vitamins, where one crucial ingredient is missing. The same authors verified higher B vitamins in blood, liver, and muscles, which can help pigs regulate potential stress situations or improve meat quality.

A series of studies carried out at the universities of Iowa and Kentucky (USA) supplemented piglets weighing 9 and 28 kg with a blend of B complex vitamins (niacin, vitamin B_2, folacin, pantothenic acid, and vitamin B_{12}). The piglets received 70, 170, 270, 470, and 870% of the levels recommended by the NRC (1998). Results showed a linear and quadratic response which may be adjusted to give an exponential equation such as that shown in Stahly et al. (1995). Surprisingly the response was more pronounced in genotypes with greater productive capacity. Lutz and Stahly (1998) proposed that the quantities of some vitamins (such as riboflavin) required for muscle tissue are up to 5 times higher than those needed for adipose tissue. In the case of growers, Lindemann et al. (1999) observed a quadratic response in the feed conversion rate for the 2 age ranges studied and for the thickness of the loin and the lean meat content of the carcass. This shows that the best response is obtained by supplying approximately 4 times the NRC (1998) recommendation for each of these vitamins.

Cho et al. (2017) supplemented a sow basal diet to provide total dietary bioavailable B vitamins (niacin, riboflavin, folacin, pantothenic acid, and vitamin B_{12}) equivalent to 70 (control), 170, 270, 470, and 870% of the NRC (2012). In the overall period from nursery to finisher (10–104 kg), there was a quadratic effect for body weight and gain-to-feed ratio, with the best result estimated at the 270% level. There was a linear effect on feed intake, and during the growing period, other linear effects were observed in body weight gain. In carcass quality, the loin depth, eye area, and lean gain improved linearly as B vitamin supplementation increased. The plateau was observed at 270% supplementation in a broken line model.

Santos et al. (2020) studied the effects of using either Brazilian Table levels (Rostagno et al., 2011 or OVN™ (DSM Nutritional Products, 2012) for all vitamins during gestation, lactation, nursery, growth, and finishing phases. This study demonstrated that a higher vitamin supplementation of sow proved positive for piglets in the early nursery stage and the sow effect concerning the performance of the litters over the same period. However, it did not lead to greater benefits in the immune response to vaccination against circovirus and mycoplasma or in the performance of pigs during the growing and finishing stages. No positive effect of higher vitamin levels was observed on the reproductive parameters or body condition score of sows during gestation and lactation.

Poulsen and Krogsdahl (2018) in a trial conducted at the Danish Pig Research Centre compared the vitamin supplementation suggested in the official Danish nutrient standards for piglets 6 to 9 kg and 9 to 30 kg (Group 1) and the DSM OVN™ (2016) (Group 2). The OVN™ concept differed from the official Danish vitamin standards by the addition of Hy-D instead of vitamin D, the addition of vitamin C and higher levels of vitamins K and A, and all vitamins in the vitamin B complex. The content of vitamin E was identical in the 2 recommendations. For the entire period (7–30 kg), the results demonstrated significant differences between the 2 groups in all 4 parameters: production value, daily gain, feed intake and feed conversion. The pigs in group 2 have a significantly higher feed intake, daily gain, and production value and a significantly lower feed conversion compared to group 1. However, the authors observed that an unexpected higher aminoacid content in the diet of Group 2 could have influenced part of the improved performance.

Studies that relate the ingestion of vitamin B complex with an improvement in chronic pathological situations have been of great interest due to discoveries made in humans (Andrès et al., 2004). However, pigs may be more responsive to fat-soluble vitamins. Lohakare et al. (2006) evaluated 3 treatments: 100% fat-soluble vitamins (FSV) and water-soluble vitamins (WSV); 150% FSV and 100% WSV at the NRC (1998) level; and 100% FSV and 150% WSV of the NRC (1998) level. Growing pigs were more responsive to additional FSV supplements over the requirements suggested by NRC (1998) than to WSV supplements as measured by growth performance and digestibility of nutrients.

Simard *et al.* (2007) have established the relation between the concentration of B_{12} in plasma and homocysteine as a possible predictor of reproductive status in primiparous sows and their dependence on a greater concentration (close to 200 mg/kg) of cyanocobalamin in the ration. Audet *et al.* (2004) used levels 10 times higher than the NRC (1998) recommendation for boars and obtained improved sperm production. Undoubtedly, the relationship of WSV with reproduction and the prevention of aging will be one of the most exciting lines of study in the near future.

Reduction of vitamin levels has been frequently discussed as an option to reduce feed costs. However, the impacts on performance (Patience and Gillis, 1996; Del Tuffo *et al.*, 2019) or pork nutrient content and fecal excretion (Shaw *et al.*, 2002) should be considered. Hinson *et al.* (2022) evaluated the effects of reducing all vitamins with FSV A, D, and E to the NRC (2012) recommended levels instead of keeping levels similar to the ones used by the USA industry for gestation, lactation, and piglet diets. The levels utilized in this experiment are given in Tables 5.16 and 5.17.

The reduced vitamin premix negatively affected sow lactation feed intake, hepatic vitamin A and serum vitamin D but did not affect sow body weight or litter performance. Regardless of the vitamin level used in the sows, progeny fed reduced levels of vitamins also had lower circulating and stored vitamins that resulted in less average daily feed intake and gain, worst gain:feed ratio and final body weight at the end of the nursery period compared to piglets fed diets containing the industry levels. The reduced levels of vitamins could negatively impact long-term reproductive performance.

Table 5.16 Vitamin premix was used for sows in gestation and lactation in the experiment evaluating either USA swine industry or the NRC (2012) levels (reduced) (Hinson *et al.*, 2022)

Total vitamin content	Gestation		Lactation	
	Industry	Reduced	Industry	Reduced
Vitamin A (IU/kg)	11,332	4,173	11,316	4,156
Vitamin D (IU/kg)	2,213	794	2,213	794
Vitamin E (mg/kg)	75.6	56.2	74.4	51.9
Vitamin K (mg/kg)	1.4	0.51	1.4	0.51
Vitamin B_1 (mg/kg)	3.43	3.28	3.34	3.19
Vitamin B_2 (mg/kg)	8	3.7	8.2	4
Vitamin B_6 (mg/kg)	6.17	6.01	7.16	7.01
Vitamin B_{12} (mg/kg)	0.0309	0.0011	0.0309	0.0011
Niacin (mg/kg)	66	37.7	65.4	37.1
Biotin (mg/kg)	0.53	0.25	0.56	0.27
Pantothenic acid (mg/kg)	30.4	15.3	31.4	16.2
Folic acid (mg/kg)	1.9	0.89	2.1	1
Choline (mg/kg)	1,526	1,528	1,765	1,766

Table 5.17 Vitamin premix was used for suckling piglets in the experiment evaluating either USA swine industry or the NRC (2012) levels (reduced) (Hinson et al., 2022)

Total vitamin content	Phase 1 0.91 kg/pig		Phase 2 1.81 kg/pig		Phase 3 3.63 kg/pig		Phase 4 until week 6	
	Industry	Reduced	Industry	Reduced	Industry	Reduced	Industry	Reduced
Vitamin A (IU/kg)	11,462	2,553	11,222	2,313	11,226	2,315	4,134	1,881
Vitamin D (IU/kg)	2,800	220	2,800	220	2,800	220	946	201
Vitamin E (mg/kg)	135.6	19.3	137	20.7	137.1	20.8	32.4	16.7
Vitamin K (mg/kg)	1.25	0.5	1.25	0.5	1.25	0.5	0.51	0.5
Vitamin B_1 (mg/kg)	5	2.8	6.3	4	6.2	4	4	4
Vitamin B_2 (mg/kg)	8.2	2	8.3	2.1	8.2	2.1	6	2.5
Vitamin B_6 (mg/kg)	7.3	4.1	10	6.8	10.1	6.9	7.1	7.1
Vitamin B_{12} (mg/kg)	0.0331	0.0022	0.0331	0.0022	0.0331	0.0022	0.022	0.0044
Niacin (mg/kg)	102.4	20.5	107	25	106.7	24.8	53.4	26.5
Biotin (mg/kg)	0.08	0.08	0.11	0.11	0.11	0.11	0.11	0.11
Pantothenic acid (mg/kg)	61	10.3	62.7	12	62.5	11.8	26.8	11.8
Folic acid (mg/kg)	0.85	0.37	1.04	0.56	1.04	0.56	0.54	0.52
Choline (mg/kg)	1,286	1,287	1,427	1,427	1,392	1,392	1,316	1,316

Vitamin C

For years it has been assumed that the pig synthesizes an adequate supply of vitamin C. Grollman and Lehninger (1957) estimated production in the liver of pigs of 13,500 μmol of ascorbic acid per day. Nonetheless, under some circumstances, vitamin C supplementation in swine diets has been proposed in the past (Chiang et al., 1985). The NRC different versions of estimated requirements of nutrients for pigs, including the last one published in 2012, have proposed no concrete recommendation.

The same determination was made for the Brazilian Tables (Rostagno et al., 2017). Nevertheless, evidence suggests that, in some circumstances, it is necessary to supplement vitamin C to achieve the maximum productive response. Pigs vary in their capacity for ascorbic acid synthesis, which could occasionally lead to a lack of response. FEFANA (2015) recommended between 100 and 200 mg/kg for piglets and 200 to 300 mg/kg for breeders. DSM Nutritional Products (2022b) OVN™ recommendations are 210 to 260 mg/kg for piglets up to 11 kg, 105–210 mg/kg from 11–50 kg and 210–315 mg/kg for breeders (up to 525 mg/kg for boars) (Tables 5.3, 5.4, and 5.5).

Most genetic companies do not have a recommendation for vitamin C, but 200 mg/kg for piglets and sows is the most common level recommended (Table 5.6, 5.7, and 5.8). However, Brazil's industry (Dalto and da Silva, 2022) reported using around 200 mg/kg for piglets up to 5 kg, around 93 mg/kg up to 15 mg/kg, and 46 mg/kg up to 20 kg (Table 5.9). Finally, vitamin C is added to grower and finisher diets at 122–140 mg/kg in Brazil (Table 5.10). In breeders it is more common to observe American producers using up to 250 mg/kg, and in boars, up to 342 mg/kg (Table 5.11). Brazilian swine producers (Dalto and da Silva, 2022) use vitamin C at 132 mg/kg in gestation and 183 mg/kg in boars.

It has also been confirmed that vitamin C requirements are more significant when the animal suffers pathological processes (parasitic illnesses, infections, tumors, etc.) and in stress (especially heat). In these circumstances, endogenous synthesis cannot meet the elevated demand for ascorbic acid, and the plasma concentration diminishes. Some evidence indicates that calorie supply in carbohydrates or fat could determine the endogenous production of vitamin C.

Piglets and growing pigs

Brown et al. (1970) observed a positive relationship between energy consumption (principally carbohydrates) and the vitamin C concentration in piglet serum, also observing that the addition of vitamin C produced an improvement in production indicators only when piglets received feed with a lower energy concentration (Brown et al., 1975). If feed with a limited supply of carbohydrates is given, the capacity for ascorbic acid synthesis may be reduced. This may be useful if we consider the tendency to increase the level of fat included in the feed to increase its energy concentration, given the high productive potential and the low consumption of modern pig genotypes.

Vitamin C administered to boars at 500 mg per kilogram of diet during the growing period, from 39 to 105 kg body weight, resulted in the straightness of front legs compared to controls (Cleveland et al., 1987a,b). However, Strittmatter (1977) and Strittmatter et al. (1978) could not detect an influence of high levels of dietary ascorbic acid on growth or on reducing the severity and incidence of osteochondrosis in pigs. Additional data by Pointillart et al. (1997) also indicated that high intakes of ascorbic acid have no positive effects on pig bone metabolism and bone characteristics. However, in a separate report, Denis et al. (1997) indicated that high levels of vitamin C had deleterious effects on trabecular bone formation in young pigs but did not alter the overall bone mass.

Conversely, an exogenous supply of vitamin C may cause a negative stimulus on endogenous synthesis (Ching and Mahan, 1998). For all these reasons and other non-controlled variation factors, the literature is complex concerning the possible usefulness of including vitamin C in feeds for piglets or growers (Cleveland *et al.*, 1987b). For example, Jewell *et al.* (1981) observed an improvement in growth when supplementing feed for piglets with vitamin C in one experiment but not in the following one. Yen and Pond (1981) and Mahan *et al.* (1994) also reported a beneficial effect on the weight gain of piglets of 3–4 weeks of age. An improvement was also observed by Cromwell *et al.* (1970) with pigs of up to 90 kg, although these same authors and some others did not find any effect in other experiments (Mahan *et al.*, 1994).

The North Central Region-89 (NCR-89) evaluated the supplementation of vitamin C (0 *vs.* 625 ppm) added to a corn-soybean meal-dried whey diet fed to 1,296 piglets (27 days of age and 6.9 kg) for 28 days. In the environments represented at 11 experiment stations, dietary vitamin C was unnecessary for optimum performance or reduced mortality of weanling pigs. Mahan *et al.* (2004) explain this variability in results by demonstrating how ascorbic acid declines in the adrenal glands under periods of stress. Still, the pig rapidly recovers its resting state once the stressor agent is removed. Consequently, benefits are observed during high environmental stress and early post-weaning, but constant supplementation may not always benefit pig live performance. Nevertheless, the long-term benefits of improving skeletal development, collagen formation, reproduction, immunity and antioxidant capacity should be considered.

In periods of stress, like weaning, dietary supplementation of vitamin C (75 ppm) combined with yeast (*Saccharomyces cerevisiae*, 0.312 g/kg of body weight) enhanced post-weaning growth and reduced inflammatory response in the intestine and liver (Eicher *et al.*, 2006). These results suggested an immunomodulatory role and stress-reducing effect of ascorbic acid supplementation.

Vitamin C's antioxidant properties can aid during incidence of mycotoxicosis and other toxicoses. Shi *et al.* (2017) described the effects of 150 mg/kg of vitamin C on antioxidant markers in the liver of weaning piglets affected by zearalenone-induced oxidative stress (1 mg/kg) during an experimental period of 28 days. The malonyl dialdehyde (MDA), SOD, GSH-Px, and total antioxidant capacity (T-AOC) were enhanced by vitamin C supplementation (Figure 5.31). The liver health measured as relative liver weight was better, and the residues of zearalenone in the liver were reduced in the weaning piglets supplemented with 150 mg/kg vitamin C (Figure 5.32).

Su *et al.* (2018) observed similar effects on the detoxification of zearalenone in female hybrid weaning piglets (Duroc × Landrace × Large White). Four treatments were evaluated with a basal diet supplemented with 150 mg of vitamin C per kilogram of feed, with or without zearalenone contamination (1 mg/kg). Zearalenone induced typical reproductive toxicity signs and caused immunosuppression and hematological toxicity. Vitamin C prevented deformities in the vulva, maintained immunological response almost similar to control, and reduced changes in biochemical and hormonal parameters. Even body weight at the end of the experimental period was improved by vitamin C supplementation (Figure 5.33).

There have been multiple studies demonstrating the different clinical benefits of the usage of vitamin C. For example, Bleilevens *et al.* (2019) found that, in an experimental setting, a bolus administration of 500 mg of vitamin C, followed by a continuous infusion of 60 mg/h, drastically reduced oxidative stress in porcine kidney grafts.

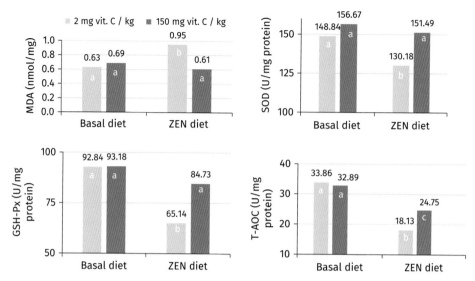

Figure 5.31 Effect of vitamin C supplementation (150 mg/kg) on antioxidant markers in the liver of weaned piglets after zearalenone-induced oxidative stress, values with no common bar labels differ significantly, $p<0.05$ (Shi *et al.*, 2017)

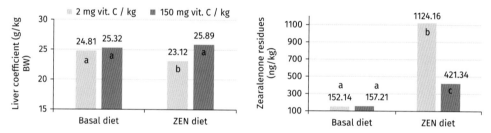

Figure 5.32 Effect of dietary vitamin C supplementation (150 mg/kg) on liver health and zearalenone residues in the liver of weaning piglets after zearalenone-induced oxidative stress, values with no common bar labels differ significantly, $p<0.05$ (Shi *et al.*, 2017)

Breeder pigs

The usefulness of vitamin C in feeds for breeding pigs is even more evident than for piglets. Using *in vitro* reproductive techniques, Huang *et al.* (2011) found that the porcine blastocyst development rate in somatic cell nuclear transfer (SCNT) embryos treated with 50 mg/ml vitamin C, 15 hours after activation (36.0%) was significantly higher than those without treatment. Ascorbate deficiency is involved in embryonic and postnatal development.

In a trial with sows with a genetic defect in vitamin C production (Wegger and Palludan, 1994; Mahan *et al.*, 2004), it was verified that supplementation is necessary to avoid edema problems, blood loss, calcification of the fetal skeleton, etc. Lauridsen and Jensen (2005) conducted a study that points to a close relationship between vitamin E and C levels. They administered 150–250 mg/kg of vitamin C during gestation. They then supplied 500 mg of vitamin C to the weaned piglets, finding higher levels of vitamin E in the tissues and immunoglobulin M (IgM) in the animals' plasma. Pinelli-Saavedra (2003), working with vitamin E and ascorbic

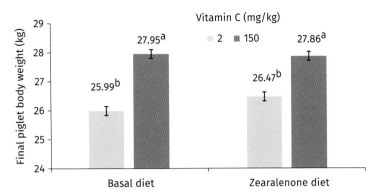

Figure 5.33 Effects of zearalenone with or without vitamin C on growth performance of weaning piglet, values with no common superscripts differ significantly, *p*<0.05 (Su *et al.*, 2018)

acid, found improved immunity in piglets of sows that had received feed with vitamin C levels of 10 g/day and vitamin E of 500 mg/kg.

Evidence from cattle, laboratory rodents and pigs indicates a role for ascorbic acid in diverse female aspects (Yen and Pond, 1984; Wegger, 1994; Wegger and Palludan, 1994) and male reproduction (Yang *et al.*, 2020). Sandholm *et al.* (1979) observed that the umbilical cord ceased bleeding sooner if the mother received an additional supply of 1 g of vitamin C during the last 5 days of gestation and also observed an improvement in the weight of the litter 3 weeks after birth. Other authors have been unable to confirm this response of an increase in the weight of a litter of sows given feed enriched with vitamin C (Lynch and O'Grady, 1981). Positive responses to vitamin C (0.05%) supplementation in sows under heat stress were reported by Feng *et al.* (2017). They observed that supplementation of ascorbic acid together with N-carbamylglutamate improved piglet weight during gestation and lactation.

Solyanik *et al.* (2021) assessed the effects of vitamin C in a concentration of 100 g/kg feed combined with either fumaric acid (4 g/kg) or dipromonium (0.4 g/kg) in primiparous gilt diets from 1 to 20 days of lactation. Fumaric acid is an essential compound of the TCA cycle, producing half its energy. Dipromonium (diisopropylammonia dichloracetate) is a synthetic compound used in medical and veterinary practice to increase antitoxic effects; it is also lipotropic and normalizes liver function. The results indicated that treatments with vitamin C contributed to increments in milk production (21–30%), the viability of piglets, and their growth rate (10.0–27.9%).

Boars

The physiological role of vitamin C in the reproductive male is of great importance because it participates in the development, maturity, and maintenance of semen production, and testosterone synthesis. Experiments have demonstrated that deficient intake of ascorbic acid produces semen of poor quality, including a reduction in fertilization capacity of up to 50% and sperm motility. The testicle, seminal vesicles and prostate may be structurally affected in extreme cases. The supplementation with 500 mg of ascorbic acid daily improved motility and sperm concentration and reduces susceptibility to oxidation (Ford and Whittington, 1998).

These effects were partially explained by Yang *et al.* (2020) with a cell culture that concluded that ascorbic acid promotes the proliferation, suppresses apoptosis and decreases the global nuclei acid methylation levels of porcine immature Sertoli cells through modifications in the expression of several genes. Additionally, ascorbic acid can promote the secretion of the anti-mullerian hormone, inhibin B and lactate, and the activity of lactate dehydrogenase. Additionally, ascorbic acid and other exogenous antioxidants can improve the preservation of pig sperm in liquid and frozen states for artificial insemination (Ribas-Maynou et al., 2021).

Regarding evidence of the efficacy of dietary supplementation, Lin et al. (1985) suggested administering 300 mg daily to boars during summer months, when thermal stress increases vitamin C requirements. It is more likely that the endogenous production is insufficient, producing an increase in sperm concentration and motility with a decrease in the proportion of malformations (Horký et al., 2016).

Independent of stress, it is likely that a situation in which a boar may be subjected frequently to semen collection, unrelated to physiology, could overload the capacity for endogenous synthesis in practice. Other authors have not found any positive effect of including vitamin C in boar feed, probably due to all the previously indicated variable factors, such as inhibition of endogenous synthesis, energy intake from carbohydrates in the ration, etc. (Horký et al., 2016).

In rabbits, Castellini et al. (2000) determined the need to formulate levels of vitamin C in reproductive males in conjunction with an increase of vitamin E and a balance with the rest of the vitamins to prevent adverse effects on reproductive functions. Lechowski et al. (2018) observed improvements in ejaculate volume, sperm cell concentration, and progressive motility of sperm in Durocs, Duroc × Hampshire, and Hampshire boars fed either 2.4 or 1.3 g of vitamin C/100 kg of body weight per day.

Meat quality

Finally, ascorbic acid can affect pork quality, as Wenk et al. (2000) pointed out in their review. One possible explanation is its antioxidant role, although it has not been possible to demonstrate experimentally the existence of a direct relationship between vitamin C intake and the oxidative stability of meat since most mechanisms are indirect. However, ascorbic acid is a precursor of oxalic acid. The sodium salt of this acid (sodium oxalate) is a potent inhibitor of the enzyme pyruvate kinase, essential in the anaerobic metabolism of carbohydrates and, therefore, involved in forming lactic acid, the leading cause of a drop in intramuscular pH after slaughter.

In 1983, Cabadaj et al. proposed vitamin C to prevent PSE and dry, firm, and dark (DFD) meat (Hamman, 1995). Mourot et al. (1992) administered 0, 100, 250, and 500 mg/kg of L-ascorbic acid to pig growers and finishers, observing a higher final pH and a slightly darker coloration of meat from groups with a higher inclusion level. Kremer and Stahly (1999) observed similar results, together with a greater capacity for water retention, which is to be expected, bearing in mind the relationship between the final pH of the meat and water retention.

The possibility of using the antioxidant activity of vitamin C and its possible synergetic use with vitamin E or A is of interest (Osborne et al., 1998). Johnson et al. (2019) evaluated the combined antioxidant effect of vitamins A (200 mg/kg), C (200 mg/kg), AC (100 mg vitamin A + 100 mg vitamin C/kg), AE (100 mg vitamin A + 100 mg vitamin E/kg), and CE (100 mg vitamin C + 100 mg vitamin E) on growing pig performance and pork quality compared to a basal control diet. The experiment was conducted for 4 weeks. All diets with antioxidants promoted better daily gain and feed efficiency than the control diet, but the combination of vitamins C and E had better parameters. In pork quality, a combination of vitamin C with vitamin E and vitamin A with vitamin E had the lowest malondialdehyde (MDA) serum concentrations and the lowest dripping loss with the combination of vitamin A and C (Table 5.18).

Table 5.18 Effects of single and combined antioxidant vitamins on growing pig performance and pork quality (Johnson et al., 2019)

Item	CON	Vitamin A	Vitamin C	Vitamin A + C	Vitamin A + E	Vitamin C + E	SEM	p-value
Performance parameters								
ADFI (g)	357.3	356.8	356	354.7	355.5	355.5	0.95	0.51
ADG (g)	81.17[d]	101.7[c]	101.5[c]	108.3[b]	109.0[b]	116.2[a]	0.43	0.04
FE (g:g)	0.23[d]	0.29[c]	0.29[c]	0.31[b]	0.31[b]	0.33[a]	0.001	0.002
Meat quality parameters								
MDA (nmol/mg)	1.17[a]	0.16[b]	0.16[b]	0.14[c]	0.11[d]	0.11[d]	0.001	0.001
Drip (%)	2.78[a]	1.78[b]	1.76[b]	1.26[c]	1.25[c]	1.13[c]	0.12	0.042

Note: [a-d] Means within a row with unlike superscript letters were significantly different (p<0.05).

Impact on gut microflora

Vitamin C supplementation in the swine diet has been proven to inhibit the growth of pathogenic intestinal flora and reduce pathogenic and relatively pathogenic bacteria in the gastrointestinal tract. Additionally, a concentration of 2.5 g/100 kg body weight/day has been proven to enhance the growth of beneficial bacteria and boost overall health by positively influencing the pig's immunity (Trawińska et al., 2012).

Xu et al. (2014) determined that an antioxidant blend effectively restored gut redox status and microbiota balance after weaning stress, enhancing intestinal health. The antioxidant blend contained 200 mg vitamin C, 100 mg vitamin E, 450 mg tea polyphenols, 1 g lipoic acid, and 5 g microbial antioxidants fermented by *Bacillus*, *Lactobacillus*, photosynthetic bacteria, and beer yeast.

Choline

Choline is a water-soluble vitamin, although the amounts fed exceed the micronutrient category typical of vitamins. In swine diets, it is generally added as choline chloride, which contains 74.6% choline activity. Pigs synthesize choline via methionine metabolism; consequently, a higher dietary intake of methionine may reduce the need for choline (Nesheim et al., 1950; Russett et al., 1979a,b; Simon, 1999). Early studies (North Central Region, 1980) indicated a lack of response to added choline on the performance of corn-soy-lysine diets fed to pigs. However, this practice has changed in commercial swine production, and it is common to observe choline supplementation.

The NRC (2012) recommended 600 mg/kg for piglets up to 7 kg body weight, 500 mg/kg up to 11 kg, 400 mg/kg up to 25 kg, and 300 mg/kg until market age. The recommendation for sows in gestation and boars is 1,250 mg/kg and 1,000 mg/kg for lactation (Table 5.5). The Brazilian Tables (Rostagno et al., 2017) and genetic companies (Tables 5.5 and 5.8) suggested even lower values. FEFANA (2015) and DSM Nutritional Products (2022b) OVN™ recommended similar or slightly lower supplementation than NRC (2012) for all phases (Tables 5.3, 5.4, and 5.5). However, the Brazilian swine industry (Bueno Dalto and da Silva, 2022) uses higher levels for pre-starter pigs and similar values to the NRC (2012) recommendations for piglets (Table 5.9), slightly lower values during growing (Table 5.10), and one-third of the recommendation for gestation and boars, and one-half for lactation (Table 5.11). Some Brazilian producers do not supplement finisher diets. The supplementation in all phases is lower for piglets and growing pigs in China

(Yang et al., 2021b) and the USA (Faccin et al., 2022). However, the highest supplementations in gestation-lactation and boars were reported in the USA, with significant variability among producers, like in other countries.

Reproduction

Mudd et al. (2016a,b), working with sows fed a choline-deficient (483 mg/kg) or choline sufficient (1,591 mg/kg) diet during the last half of the gestational period, observed that limited choline supplementation during the prenatal period profoundly impacts brain maturation. Conversely, choline status during the postnatal period does not appear to have nearly as significant an effect on neurodevelopment. Their data indicated that gestational choline deficiency significantly affects the macrostructural and microstructural development of the piglet brain.

Recently, Zhong et al. (2021) suggested that the dietary choline recommendation of 1,250 mg/kg proposed by NRC (2012) is insufficient for the best reproductive performance of modern hyper prolific sows. In addition, the authors mentioned the potential effects on the plasma metabolome and gut microbiota of sows. They used 260 multiparous sows allocated to 5 dietary treatment groups with increasing choline concentrations (1,050, 1,450, 1,850, 2,250, and 2,650 mg/kg). The sows were fed experimental diets from breeding until farrowing and a standard lactation diet. They concluded that increasing maternal dietary choline levels improved sow backfat gain during gestation (Figure 5.34), the birth weight of piglets, piglets born alive, neonatal piglet weight and uniformity, piglet mortality during lactation (Figure 5.35), and litter performance during lactation.

These results could be associated with better antioxidant capability, metabolic status, and gut microbiota composition of sows during gestation. A quadratic effect of dietary choline level was observed for sows' average daily feed intake during lactation. The feed intake was maximized at 1,910 mg/kg. For the gut microbiota composition, the enhanced dietary choline level decreased the abundance of phylum Proteobacteria and increased the abundance of phylum Actinobacteria at day 30 of gestation. Compared with the 1,050 mg/kg group, the

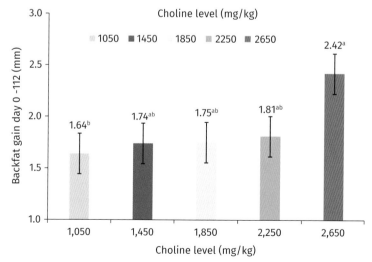

Figure 5.34 Effect of dietary choline level during gestation on sow backfat gain during gestation (A) and (B) on piglet mortality during days 0–18 (Zhong et al., 2021)

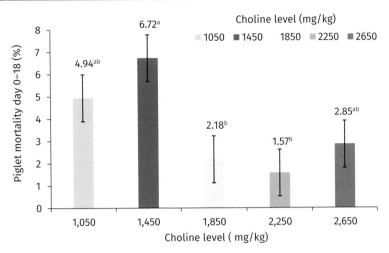

Figure 5.35 Effect of dietary choline level on piglet mortality during days 0–18, values with no common superscripts differ significantly, $p<0.05$ (Zhong et al., 2021)

abundance of the genus *Terrisporobacter* was less in the 1,850 mg/kg group, and the genera *Bacillus* and *Cellulomonas* were greater in the 2,650 mg/kg group.

Piglets

Qiu *et al.* (2021) conducted one experiment to investigate the effects of choline and bile acids on growth performance, lipid use, intestinal immunology, gut microbiota, and bacterial metabolites in weaned piglets. Their results indicated that choline supplementation (597 mg choline/kg, for 28 days) could efficiently improve dietary lipid use and enhance the growth performance and gut health of weaned piglets (21 days of age) by altering the gut microbiota and metabolites. Although no main effect of bile acids on the growth performance of weaned piglets was found, bile acid supplementation exhibited an anti-inflammatory effect via modulation of gut microbiota, microbial butyrate and glycerophospholipids.

Li *et al.* (2018) conducted one study for investigating the effects of dietary choline supplementation on hepatic lipid metabolism and gene expression in finishing pigs with intrauterine growth retardation (IUGR). The levels of choline (average level (NL) and high level (HL)) used by the researchers were (g/kg diet): phase 1 (21–38 days of age) NL: 1.34 HL: 2.68, phase 2 (38–73 days of age) NL: 1.20 HL: 2.40, phase 3 (73–120 days of age) NL: 1.16 HL: 2.32, phase 4 (120–200 days of age) NL: 1.13 HL: 2.26. They concluded that the lipid metabolism was abnormal in IUGR pigs. Still, the IUGR pigs consuming twice the average level of choline had improved circulating lipid parameters, which could be related to the decreased activity of NADP-generating enzymes or the altered expressions of lipid metabolism-related genes.

There is scientific evidence that choline at NRC (2012) levels or slightly higher could have potentially beneficial effects. However, the cost and the multiple dietary factors may not allow us to observe those benefits under commercial conditions.

Bibliography

Adams, C.R. (1973) Effect of environmental conditions on the stability of vitamins in feeds. In "Effect of processing on the nutritional value of feeds". National Academy of Sciences, National Research Council, USA.

Adams, C.R. (1978) Vitamin product forms for animal feeds. In "Vitamin nutrition update-seminar series 2". Hoffman-La Roche Inc., Nutley, NJ, USA. RCD. 5483/1078.

Adams, C.R., Richardson, C.E. and Cunha, T.J. (1967) Supplemental biotin and vitamin B6 for swine. J. Anim. Sci. 26(4):903.

Adams, C.R., Eoff, H.J. and Zimmerman, C.R. (1975) Protecting feeds from vitamin E and A deficits in lightweight moldy and blighted corn. Feedstuffs 47(36):24.

Adenkola, A.Y., Ayo, J.O. and Sackey, A.K.B. (2009) Ascorbic acid-induced modulation of rectal temperature fluctuations in pigs during the harmattan season. J. Therm. Biol. 34(3):152–154. https://doi.org/10.1016/j.jtherbio.2009.01.001.

Adeola, O., Orban, J.I., Ragland, D., Cline, T.R. and Sutton, A.L. (1998) Phytase and cholecalciferol supplementation of low-calcium and low-phosphorus diets for pigs. Can. J. Anim. Sci. 78(3):307–313. https://doi.org/10.4141/A97-124.

Ahmed, F., Jones, D.B. and Jackson, A.A. (1990) The interaction of vitamin A deficiency and rotavirus infection in the mouse. Br. J. Nutr. 63(2):363–373. https://doi.org/10.1079/bjn19900122.

Alhadeff, L., Gualtieri, C.T. and Lipton, M. (1984) Toxic effects of water-soluble vitamins. Nutr. Rev. 42(2): 33–40. https://doi.org/10.1111/j.1753-4887.1984.tb02278.x.

Amavizca-Nazar, A., Montalvo-Corral, M., González-Rios, H. and Pinelli-Saavedra, A. (2019) Hot environment on reproductive performance, immunoglobulins, vitamin E, and vitamin A status in sows and their progeny under commercial husbandry. J. Anim. Sci. Technol. 61(6):340–351. https://doi.org/10.5187/jast.2019.61.6.340.

Amazan, D., Cordero, G., López-Bote, C.J., Lauridsen, C. and Rey, A.I. (2014) Effects of oral micellized natural vitamin E (D-α-tocopherol) v. synthetic vitamin E (DL-α-tocopherol) in feed on α-tocopherol levels, stereoisomer distribution, oxidative stress and the immune response in piglets. Animal 8(3):410–419. https://doi.org/10.1017/S1751731113002401.

Ambrosi, P., Rolland, P.H., Bodard, H., Barlatier, A., Charpiot, P., Guisgand, G., Friggi, A., Ghiringhelli, O., Habib, G., Bouvenot, G., Garçon, D. and Luccioni, R. (1999) Effects of folate supplementation in hyperhomocysteinemic pigs. J. Am. Coll. Cardiol. 34(1): 274–279. https://doi.org/10.1016/S0735-1097(99)00144-8.

An, B.K., Kim, D.H., Joo, W.D., Kang, C.W. and Lee, K.W. (2019) Effects of lycopene and tomato paste on oxidative stability and fatty acid composition of fresh belly meat in finishing pigs. Ital. J. Anim. Sci. 18(1): 630–635. https://doi.org/10.1080/1828051X.2018.1549963.

Anderson, G.C. and Hogan, A.G. (1950) Requirement of the pig for vitamin B12. J. Nutr. 40(2):243–253. https://doi.org/10.1093/jn/40.2.243.

Anderson, L.E., Myer, R.O., Brendemuhl, J.H. and McDowell, L.R. (1995a) The effect of excessive dietary vitamin A on performance and vitamin E status in swine fed diets varying in dietary vitamin E. J. Anim. Sci. 73(4): 1093–1098. https://doi.org/10.2527/1995.7341093x.

Anderson, L.E., Myer, R.O., Brendemuhl, J.H. and McDowell, L.R. (1995b) Bioavailability of various vitamin E compounds for finishing swine. J. Anim. Sci. 73(2):490–495. https://doi.org/10.2527/1995.732490x.

Anderson, L.E., Myer, R.O., Brendemuhl, J.H. and McDowell, L.E. (1997) Effect of injected vitamin A and level of dietary vitamin E on alpha-tocopherol status in gestating swine. Reprod. Nutr. Dev. 37(2):213–220. https://doi.org/10.1051/rnd:19970209.

Anderson, M.D., Speer, V.C., McCall, J.T. and Hays, V.W. (1966) Hypervitaminosis A in the young pig. J. Anim. Sci. 25(4): 1123–1127. https://doi.org/10.2527/jas1966.2541123x.

Andrès, E., Loukili, N.H., Noel, E., Kaltenbach, G., Abdelgheni, M.B., Perrin, A.E., Noblet-Dick, M., Maloisel, F., Schlienger, J.L. and Blicklé, J.F. (2004) Vitamin B12 (cobalamin) deficiency in elderly patients. CMAJ 171(3): 251–259. https://doi.org/10.1503/cmaj.1031155.

Anonymous (1977) Vitamin A and retinol-binding protein in fetal growth and development of the rat. Nutr. Rev. 35(11):305–309. https://doi.org/10.1111/j.1753-4887.1977.tb06506.x.

Apple, J.K. (2007) Effects of nutritional modifications on the water-holding capacity of fresh pork: a review. J. Anim. Breed. Genet. 124 (Suppl 1):43–58. https://doi.org/10.1111/j.1439-0388.2007.00686.x.

Arnold, J., Madson, D.M., Ensley, S.M., Goff, J.P., Sparks, C., Stevenson, G.W., Crenshaw, T., Wang, C. and Horst, R.L. (2015) Survey of serum vitamin D status across stages of swine production and evaluation of supplemental bulk vitamin D premixes used in swine diets. J. Swine Health Prod. 23(1):28–34. https://doi.org/20.500.12876/92104.

Asala, O.O., Ayo, J.O., Rekwot, P.I., Minka, N.S. and Adenkola, A.Y. (2010) Rectal temperature responses of pigs transported by road and administered with ascorbic acid during the hot-dry season. J. Cell Anim. Biol. 4(3):051–057.

Asghar, A., Gray, J.I., Booren, A.M., Gomaa, E.A., Abouzied, M.M., Miller, E.R. and Buckley, D.J. (1991) Effects of supranutritional dietary vitamin E levels on subcellular deposition of α-tocopherol in the muscle and on pork quality. J. Sci. Food Agric. 57(1):31–41. https://doi.org/10.1002/jsfa.2740570104.

Ashoori, M. and Saedisomeolia, A. (2014) Riboflavin (vitamin B$_2$) and oxidative stress: a review. Br. J. Nutr. 111(11):1985–1991. https://doi.org/10.1017/S0007114514000178.

Asrar, F.M. and O'Connor, D.L. (2005) Bacterially synthesized folate and supplemental folic acid are absorbed across the large intestine of piglets. J. Nutr. Biochem. 16(10):587–593. https://doi.org/10.1016/j.jnutbio.2005.02.006.

Asson-Batres, M.A., Smith, W.B. and Clark, G. (2009) Retinoic acid is present in the postnatal rat olfactory organ and persists in vitamin A–depleted neural tissue. J. Nutr. 139(6):1067–1072. https://doi.org/10.3945/jn.108.096040.

Astrup, H.N. and Langebrekke, A. (1985) The effect of a high level of vitamin E and of a ration with hydrogenated free fatty acids upon pork quality. Meld. Nor. Landbrukshogsk. 64(21):6.

Atef, S.H. (2018) Vitamin D assays in clinical laboratory: past, present and future challenges. J. Steroid Biochem. Mol. Biol. 175:136–137. https://doi.org/10.1016/j.jsbmb.2017.02.011.

Audet, I., Laforest, J.P., Martineau, G.P. and Matte, J.J. (2004) Effect of vitamin supplements on some aspects of performance, vitamin status, and semen quality in boars. J. Anim. Sci. 82(2):626–633. https://doi.org/10.2527/2004.822626x.

Aufreiter, S., Kim, J.H. and O'Connor, D.L. (2011) Dietary oligosaccharides increase colonic weight and the amount but not concentration of bacterially synthesized folate in the colon of piglets. J. Nutr. 141(3):366–372. https://doi.org/10.3945/jn.110.135343.

Axelrod, A.E. (1971) Immune processes in vitamin deficiency states. Am. J. Clin. Nutr. 24(2): 265–271. https://doi.org/10.1093/ajcn/24.2.265.

Ayuso, M., Óvilo, C., Fernández, A., Nuñez, Y., Isabel, B., Daza, A., López-Bote, C.J. and Rey, A.I. (2015a) Effects of dietary vitamin A supplementation or restriction and its timing on retinol and α-tocopherol accumulation and gene expression in heavy pigs. Anim. Feed Sci. Technol. 202:62–74. https://doi.org/10.1016/j.anifeedsci.2015.01.014.

Ayuso, M., Óvilo, C., Rodríguez-Bertos, A., Rey, A.I., Daza, A., Fenández, A., González-Bulnes, A., López-Bote, C.J. and Isabel, B. (2015b) Dietary vitamin A restriction affects adipocyte differentiation and fatty acid composition of intramuscular fat in Iberian pigs. Meat Sci. 108:9–16. https://doi.org/10.1016/j.meatsci.2015.04.017.

Bâ, A. (2008) Metabolic and structural role of thiamine in nervous tissues. Cell. Mol. Neurobiol. 28(7):923–931: https://doi.org/10.1007/s10571-008-9297-7.

Babinszky, L., Langhout, D.J., Verstegen, M.W.A., Den Hartog, L.A., Joling, P. and Niewland, N. (1991a) Effect of vitamin E and fat sources in sow's diets on immune response of suckling and weaned piglets. J. Anim. Sci. 69(5): 1833–1842. https://doi.org/10.2527/1991.6951833x.

Babinszky, L., Langhout, D.J., Verstegen, M.W.A., Den Hartog, L.A., Joling, P. and Niewland, N. (1991b) Effect of alpha-tocopherol and dietary fat source on some blood and immunological variables in lactating sows. Anim. Prod. 52(2): 367–375. https://doi.org/10.1017/s0003356100012903.

Babinszky, L., Langhout, D.J., Verstegen, M.W.A., Den Hartog, L.A., Zandstra, T., Bakker, P.L.G. and Verstegen, J.A.A.M. (1992) Dietary vitamin E and fat source and lactating performance of primiparous sows and their piglets. Livest. Prod. Sci. 30(1–2):155–168. https://doi.org/10.1016/S0301-6226(05)80027-2.

Babior, B.M. (1984) The respiratory burst of phagocytes. J. Clin. Invest. 73(3):599–601. https://doi.org/10.1172/JCI111249.

Babu, S. and Srikantia, S.G. (1976) Availability of folates from some foods. Am. J. Clin. Nutr. 29(4):376–379. https://doi.org/10.1093/ajcn/29.4.376.

Bachmann, H., Autzen, S., Frey, U., Wehr, U., Rambeck, W., McCormack, H. and Whitehead, C.C. (2013) The efficacy of a standardized product from dried leaves of *Solanum glaucophyllum* as source of 1,25- dihydroxycholecalciferol for poultry. Br. Poult. Sci. 54(5):642–652. https://doi.org/10.1080/00071668.2013.825692.

Bacou, E., Walk, C., Rider, S., Litta, G. and Perez-Calvo, E. (2021) Dietary oxidative distress: A review of nutritional challenges as models for poultry, swine and fish. Antioxidants (Basel) 10(4):525. https://doi.org/10.3390/antiox10040525.

Badwey, J.A. and Karnovsky, M.L. (1980) Active oxygen species and the functions of phagocytic leukocytes. Annu. Rev. Biochem. 49:695–726. https://doi.org/10.1146/annurev.bi.49.070180.003403.

Bailey, L.B. and Gregory, J.F. (2006) Folate. In "Present knowledge in nutrition" Bowman, B. and Russell, R. (Eds.). International Life Sciences Institute. (pp. 278–301).

Bailey, L.B., Da-Silva, V., West, A.A. and Caudill, M.A. (2013) Folate. In "Handbook of vitamins" 5th edition Zempleni, J., Suttie, J., Gregory, J. and Stover, P.J. (Eds.). CRC Press. (pp. 421–446).

Baker, D.H. and Biehl, R.R. (1996) Phosphorus, trace mineral and amino acid utilization in chickens and pigs fed microbial phytase and 1 a-hydroxycholecalciferol. In Proc. Maryland Nutr. Conf. (pp. 21–26).

Baker, S.S. and Cohen, H.J. (1983) Altered oxidative metabolism in selenium-deficient rat granulocytes. J. Immunol. 130(6):2856–2860. PMID: 6304192.

Balaghi, M. and Wagner, C. (1992) Methyl group metabolism in the pancreas of folate-deficient rats. J. Nutr. 122(7):1391–1396. https://doi.org/10.1093/jn/122.7.1391.

Balaghi, M., Horne, D.W., Woodward, S.C. and Wagner, C. (1993) Pancreatic one-carbon metabolism in early folate deficiency in rats. Am. J. Clin. Nutr. 58(2):198–203. https://doi.org/10.1093/ajcn/58.2.198.

Barash, P.G. (1978) Nutrient toxicities of vitamin K. In "CRC handbook series in nutrition and food, section E: Nutrition disorders" Rechcigl, M., Jr. (Ed.). CRC Press.

Barnhart, C.E., Catron, D.V., Ashton, G.C. and Quinn, L.Y. (1957) Effects of dietary pantothenic acid levels on the weanling pig. J. Anim. Sci. 16(2):396–403. https://doi.org/10.2527/jas1957.162396x.

Barroeta, A.C., Baucells, M.D., Blanco Pérez, A., Calsamiglia, S., Casals, R., Cepero Briz, R., Davin, R., Gonzalez, G., Hernandez, J.M., Isabel, B., Lopez-Bote, C., Rey, I.A., Rodriguez, M., Sanz, J., Soto-Salanova, M.F. and Weber, G. (2012) "Optimum vitamin nutrition in the production of quality animal foods". 5m Publishing, Sheffield.

Barth, C.A., Frigg, M. and Hagemeister, H. (1986) Biotin absorption from the hindgut of the pig. J. Anim. Physiol. Anim. Nutr. 55(1–5):128–134. https://doi.org/10.1111/j.1439-0396.1986.tb00711.x.

Bates, C.J. (2006) Thiamine. In "Present knowledge in nutrition" 9th edition Bowman, B.A. and Russell, R.M. (Eds.). International Life Sciences Institute. (pp. 242–249).

Batra, T.R., Hidiroglou, M. and Menard, L. (1995) Effects of vitamin E injection on body temperature and plasma alpha-tocopherol concentrations in pigs, lambs and calves. Vet. Res. 26(1):68–72.

Bauernfeind, J.C. (1974) Pyridoxine-A use appraisal in animal feeds. Feedstuffs 46(45):30.

Baugh, C.M. and Krumdieck, C.L. (1971) Naturally occurring folates. Ann. N. Y. Acad. Sci. 186:7–28.

Bauriedel, W.R., Hoerlein, A.B., Picken, J.C. and Underkofler, L.A. (1954) Selection of diet for studies of vitamin B12 depletion using unsuckled baby pigs. J. Agric. Food Chem. 2(9):468–472. https://doi.org/10.1021/jf60029a005.

Baustad, B. and Nafstad, I. (1972) Haematological response to vitamin E in piglets. Br. J. Nutr. 28(2):183–190.

Bazer, F.W. and Zavy, M.T. (1988) Supplemental riboflavin and reproductive performance of gilts. J. Anim. Sci. 66(1):324.

Bebiak, D.M. (1977) The influence of vitamin E and selenium on gastric ulcers in swine. Michigan State Univ. Res. Reprod.:(39–41).

Bebravicius, V., Medzevicius, A. and Medzevicius, A. (1987) The dynamics of vitamin A content in the serum of pigs during experimental tricuriosis. Acta Parasitológica Lituanica 22:102.

Beck, M.A. (1997) Increased virulence of coxsackievirus B3 in mice due to vitamin E or selenium deficiency. J. Nutr. 127(5)(Suppl.):966S–970S. https://doi.org/10.1093/jn/127.5.966S.

Beck, M.A. (2007) Selenium and vitamin E status: Impact on viral pathogenicity. J. Nutr. 137(5):1338–1340. https://doi.org/10.1093/jn/137.5.1338.

Beck, M.A., Kolbeck, P.C., Rohr, L.H., Shi, Q., Morris, V.C. and Levander, O.A. (1994) Vitamin E deficiency intensifies the myocardial injury of coxsackievirus B3 infection of mice. J. Nutr. 124(3):345–358. https://doi.org/10.1093/jn/124.3.345.

Becker, E.M., Christensen, J., Frederiksen, C.S. and Haugaard, V.K. (2003) Front-face fluorescence spectroscopy and chemometrics in analysis of yogurt: rapid analysis of riboflavin. J. Dairy Sci. 86(8):2508–2515. https://doi.org/10.3168/jds.S0022-0302(03)73845-4.

Beisel, W.R. (1982) Single nutrients and immunity. Am. J. Clin. Nutr. 35(2)(Suppl.):417–468. https://doi.org/10.1093/ajcn/35.2.417.

Bender, D.A. (1992) "Nutritional biochemistry of the vitamins". Cambridge University Press. https://doi.org/10.1017/CBO9780511615191.

Bender, D.A. (1999) Non-nutritional uses of vitamin B6. Br. J. Nutr. 81(1):7–20. https://doi.org/10.1017/S0007114599000082.

Bendich, A. (1987) Role of antioxidant vitamins on immune function. In Proc. Roche Technical Symp.: "The role of vitamins on animal performance and immune response." RCD 7442. Hoffmann–La Roche Inc.

Benedikt, J., Roth-Maier, D.A. and Kirchgessner, M. (1996) Influence of dietary vitamin B6 supply during gravidity and lactation on total vitamin B6 concentration in blood and milk. Int. J. Vitam. Nutr. Res. 66(2):146–150. PMID: 8843990.

Bengtsson, G., Hakkarainen, J., Jönsson, L., Lannek, N. and Lindberg, P. (1978) Requirement for selenium (as selenite) and vitamin E (as alpha-tocopherol) in weaned pigs. I. The effect of varying alpha-tocopherol levels in a selenium deficient diet on the development of the VESD syndrome. J. Anim. Sci. 46(1):143–152. https://doi.org/10.2527/jas1978.461143x.

Benito, E. and Bosch, M.A. (1997) Impaired phosphatidylcholine biosynthesis and ascorbic acid depletion in lung during lipopolysaccharide-induced endotoxaemia in guinea pigs. Mol. Cell. Biochm 175(1–2): 117–123. https://doi.org/10.1023/a:1006883628365.

Berlin, E., McClure, D., Banks, M.A. and Peters, R.C. (1994) Heart and liver fatty acid composition and vitamin E content in miniature swine fed diets containing corn and menhaden oils. Comp. Biochem. Physiol. Physiol. 109(1):53–61. https://doi.org/10.1016/0300-9629(94)90311-5.

Bettendorff, L. (2013) Vitamin B1. In "Handbook of vitamins" 5th edition Zempleni, J., Suttie, J., Gregory, J. and Stover, P.J. (Eds.). CRC Press. (pp. 267–324).

Bhandari, S.D. and Gregory, J.F. (1992) Folic acid, 5-methyl-tetrahydrofolate and 5-formyl-tetrahydrofolate exhibit equivalent intestinal absorption, metabolism and in vivo kinetics in rats. J. Nutr. 122(9): 1847–1854. https://doi.org/10.1093/jn/122.9.1847.

Bieber-Wlaschny, M. (1988) Vitamin E in swine nutrition. In update of vitamins and nutrition management in swine production technical conference 7776:988.

Biehl, R.R. and Baker, D.H. (1996) Efficacy of supplemental 1 alpha-hydroxycholecalciferol and microbial phytase for young pigs fed phosphorus- or amino acid-deficient corn-soybean meal diets. J. Anim. Sci. 74(12): 2960–2966. https://doi.org/10.2527/1996.74122960x.

Bilodeau, R., Brisson, G.J., Matte, J.J., Passillé, A.M.B. and Girard, C.L. (1989) Effects of floor type on serum folates, serum vitamin B12, plasma biotin and on growth performances of pigs. Can. J. Anim. Sci. 69(3):779–788. https://doi.org/10.4141/cjas89-090.

Binkley, N.C. and Suttie, J.W. (1995) Vitamin K nutrition and osteoporosis. J. Nutr. 125(7): 1812–1821. https://doi.org/10.1093/jn/125.7.1812.

Birdsall, J.J. (1975) "Technology of fortification of foods". Proc. Natl. Acad. Sci. U. S. A.:(126). https://doi.org/10.17226/20201.

Birke, H., Kolb, E., Liebaug, F., Siebert, P., Gollnitz, L., Wahren, M. and Volker, L. (1993) The content of ascorbic acid in tissues of pig fetuses and of newborn piglets as well as that in the blood-plasma and in tissues of pig fetuses and of newborn piglets as well as that in the blood-plasma and in tissues of pigs of different age, with consideration on the influence of the restriction of suckling. Dtsch. Tierarztl Wschr. 100(8):309–313. PMID: 8404518.

Bito, T. and Watanabe, F. (2022) "Seaweeds as a source of vitamin B12. Sustainable global resources of seaweeds volume 2: Food, pharmaceutical and health applications". p. 339. https://doi.org/10.1007/978-3-030-92174-3_18.

Blair, R. and Newsome, F. (1985) Involvement of water-soluble vitamins in diseases of swine. J. Anim. Sci. 60(6): 1508–1517. https://doi.org/10.2527/jas1985.6061508x.

Blair, R., Burton, B.A., Doige, C.E., Halstead, A.C. and Newsome, F.E. (1989) Tolerance of weanling pigs for dietary vitamin A and D. Int. J. Vitam. Nutr. Res. 59(4):329–332. PMID: 2634037.

Blair, R., Aherne, F.X. and Doige, C.E. (1992) Tolerance of growing pigs for dietary vitamin A, with special reference to bone integrity. Int. J. Vitam. Nutr. Res. 62(2):130-133. PMID: 1517034.

Blair, R., Facon, M., Owen, B.D., Jacob, J.P. and Bildfell, R.J. (1996) Tolerance of young pigs for dietary vitamin A and beta-carotene, with special reference to the immune response. Can. J. Anim. Sci. 76(1):121–126. https://doi.org/10.4141/cjas96-016.

Blaxter, K.L. (1962) The significance of selenium and vitamin E in nutrition. Muscular dystrophy in farm animals: Its cause and prevention. Proc. Nutr. Soc. 21(2): 211–216. https://doi.org/10.1079/PNS19620034.

Bleilevens, C., Doorschodt, B.M., Fechter, T., Grzanna, T., Theißen, A., Liehn, E.A., Breuer, T., Tolba, R.H., Rossaint, R., Stoppe, C., Boor, P., Hill, A. and Fabry, G. (2019) Influence of vitamin C on antioxidant capacity of in vitro perfused porcine kidneys. Nutrients 11(8): 1774. https://doi.org/10.3390/nu11081774.

Blomhoff, R., Green, M.H., Green, J.B., Berg, T. and Norum, K.R. (1991) Vitamin A metabolism: New perspectives on absorption, transport, and storage. Physiol. Rev. 71(4):951–990. https://doi.org/10.1152/physrev.1991.71.4.951.

Böhmer, B.M. and Roth-Maier, D.A. (2007) Effects of high-level dietary B-vitamins on performance, body composition and tissue vitamin contents of growing/finishing pigs. J. Anim .Physiol. Anim. Nutr. 91(1–2):6–10. https://doi.org/10.1111/j.1439-0396.2006.00635.x.

Boler, D.D., Gabriel, S.R., Yang, H., Balsbaugh, R., Mahan, D.C., Brewer, M.S., McKeith, F.K. and Killefer, J. (2009) Effect of different dietary levels of natural-source vitamin E in grow-finish pigs on pork quality and shelf life. Meat Sci. 83(4): 723–730. https://doi.org/10.1016/j.meatsci.2009.08.012.

Bonjour, J.P. (1991) Biotin. In "Handbook of vitamins" 2nd edition Machlin, L.J. (Ed.). Marcel Dekker Inc., New York.

Bonnette, E.D., Kornegay, E.T., Lindemann, M.D. and Hammerberg, C. (1990b) Humoral and cell-mediated immune response and performance of weaned pigs fed four supplemental vitamin E levels and housed at two nursery temperatures. J. Anim. Sci. 68(5):1337–1345. https://doi.org/10.2527/1990.6851337x.

Bonnette, E.D., Kornegay, E.T., Lindemann, M.D. and Notter, D.R. (1990a) Influence of two supplemental vitamin E levels and weaning age on performance, humoral antibody production and serum cortisol levels of pigs. J. Anim. Sci. 68(5): 1346–1353. https://doi.org/10.2527/1990.6851346x.

Bonomi, A., Quarantelli, A., Sabbioni, A., Superchi, P. and Bonomi, B.M. (1996) The use of biotin as feed integrator in heavy swine feeding. La Riv. Sci. Aliment. Anno 25(4):399–411.

Booth, S.L. (1997) Skeletal functions of vitamin K-dependent proteins: Not just for clotting anymore. Nutr. Rev. 55(7):282–284. https://doi.org/10.1111/j.1753-4887.1997.tb01619.x.

Bostedt, H. (1980) Nutritional muscular dystrophy of young animals in the first days and weeks of life. Prakt. Tierazt 45(Special Issue 65).

Bourne, F.J., Newby, T.J., Evans, P. and Morgan, K. (1978) The immune requirements of the newborn pig and calf. Ann. Rech. Vet. 9(2):239–244.

Bowland, J.P. and Owen, B.D. (1952) Supplemental pantothenic acid in small grain rations for swine. J. Anim. Sci. 1: 757. https://doi.org/10.5962/bhl.title.142698.

Bowland, J.P., Grummer, R.H., Phillips, P.H. and Bohstedt, G. (1949a) Effect of lactation and ration on the fat and vitamin A level of sow's milk. J. Dairy Sci. 32(1):22–28. https://doi.org/10.3168/jds.S0022-0302(49)92006-8.

Bowland, J.P., Grummer, R.H., Phillips, P.H. and Bohstedt, G. (1949b) The vitamin A and vitamin C content of sows' colostrum and milk. J. Anim. Sci. 8(1):98–106. https://doi.org/10.1093/ansci/8.1.98.

Boyd, R.D., Moser, B.D., Peo, E.R., Lewis, A.J. and Johnson, R.K. (1982) Effect of tallow and choline chloride addition to the diet of sows milk composition, milk yield and preweaning pig performance. J. Anim. Sci. 54(1): 1–7. https://doi.org/10.2527/jas1982.5411.

Brandebourg, T.D. and Hu, C.Y. (2005) Regulation of differentiating pig preadipocytes by retinoic acid. J. Anim. Sci. 83(1): 98–107. https://doi.org/10.2527/2005.83198x.

Brass, E.P. (1993) Hydroxocobalamin [c-lactam] increases total coenzyme A content in primary culture hepatocytes by accelerating coenzyme A biosynthesis secondary to acyl-CoA accumulation. J. Nutr. 123(11):1801–1807. https://doi.org/10.1093/jn/123.11.1801.

Braude, R., Kon, S.K. and White, E.G. (1946) Observations on the nicotinic acid requirements of pigs. Biochem. J. 40(5–6):843–855. PMID: 20277265.

Braude, R., Kon, S.K. and Porter, J.W.G. (1950) Studies in the vitamin C metabolism of the pig. Br. J. Nutr. 4(2–3): 186–199. https://doi.org/10.1079/bjn19500035.

Braun, F. (1986) The effect of bile on intestinal absorption of calcium and vitamin D. Wien. Klin. Wochenschr. 98(166):23. PMID: 3008448.

Bray, D.L. and Briggs, G.M. (1984) Decrease in bone density in young male guinea pigs fed high levels of ascorbic acid. J. Nutr. 114(5):920–928. https://doi.org/10.1093/jn/114.5.920.

Bräunlich, K. (1974) "Vitamin B6". Vol. 1451. F. Hoffmann-La Roche and Co., Ltd.

Bräunlich, K. and Zintzen, H. (1976) "Vitamin B1". Vol. 1593. F. Hoffmann-La Roche and Co. Ltd.

Brezezińska-Slebodzińska, E., Slebodziński, A.B., Pietras, B. and Wieczorek, G. (1995) Antioxidant effect of vitamin E and glutathione on lipid peroxidation in boar semen plasma. Biol. Trace Elem. Res. 47(1–3): 69–74. https://doi.org/10.1007/BF02790102.

Brief, S. and Chew, B.P. (1985) Effects of vitamin A and beta-carotene on reproductive performance in gilts. J. Anim. Sci. 60(4):998–1004. https://doi.org/10.2527/jas1985.604998x.

Brigelius-Flohé, R. (2021) Vitamin E research: Past, now and future. Free Radic. Biol. Med. 177:381–390. https://doi.org/10.1016/j.freeradbiomed.2021.10.029.

Briggs, J.E. and Beeson, W.M. (1951) The supplementary value of riboflavin, calcium pantothenate and niacin in a practical mixed animal and plant protein ration containing B12 and aureomycin for weanling pigs in dry lot. J. Anim. Sci. 10(4): 813–819. https://doi.org/10.2527/jas1951.104813x.

Bronner, F. and Stein, W.D. (1995) Calcium homeostasis – An old problem revisited. J. Nutr. 125(7) (Suppl.):1987S–1995S. https://doi.org/10.1093/jn/125.suppl_7.1987S.

Brooks, C.C., Nakamura, R.M. and Miyahara, A.Y. (1973) Effect of menadione and other factors on sugar-induced heart lesions and hemorrhagic syndrome in the pig. J. Anim. Sci. 37(6):1344–1350. https://doi.org/10.2527/jas1973.3761344x.

Brooks, P.H. (1982) Biotin in pig nutrition. Pig New Inf. 3:29.

Brooks, P.H. and Simmins, P.H. (1981) The effect of supplementing breeding pig diets with biotin on the maintenance of hoof integrity. 4th Int. Conf. Prod. Dis. Farm animals Giesecks, D., Dirksen, G. and Strangassinger, M. (Eds.). West, Munich Germany.

Brooks, P.H., Smith, D.A. and Irwin, V.C. (1977) Biotin supplementation of diets; the incidence of foot lesions and the reproductive performance of sows. Vet. Rec. 101(3):46–50.

Brown, E.S. (1964) Isolation and assay of dipalmityl lecithin in lung extracts. Am. J. Physiol. 207:402-406. https://doi.org/10.1152/ajplegacy.1964.207.2.402.

Brown, G.M. (1962) The biosynthesis of folic acid. J. Biol. Chem. 237(2):536–540. https://doi.org/10.1016/S0021-9258(18)93957-8.

Brown, R.G. (1984) Ascorbic acid nutrition in the domestic pig. In proc. workshop on ascorbic acid in domestic animals Wegger, I., Tagwerker, F.J. and Moustgaard, J. (Eds.). Royal Danish Agricultural Society, Copenhagen.

Brown, R.G. and King, G.J. (1977) Ascorbic acid synthesis in pigs. Can. J. Anim. Sci. 57:831.

Brown, R.G., Sharma, V.D. and Young, L.G. (1970) Ascorbate metabolism in swine. Interrelationships between level of energy and serum ascorbate levels. Can. J. Anim. Sci. 50(3):605–609. https://doi.org/10.4141/cjas70-082.

Brown, R.G., Sharma, V.D., Young, L.G. and Buchanan-Smith, J.G. (1971) Connective tissue metabolism in swine. II. Influence of energy level and ascorbate supplementation on hydroxyproline excretion. Can. J. Anim. Sci. 51(2): 439–444. https://doi.org/10.4141/cjas71-058.

Brown, R.G., Buchanan-Smith, J.G. and Sharma, V.D. (1975) Ascorbic acid metabolism in swine. The effects of frequency of feeding and level of supplementary ascorbic acid on swine fed various energy levels. Can. J. Anim. Sci. 55(3): 353–358. https://doi.org/10.4141/cjas75-043.

Brownlee, N.R., Huttner, J.J., Panganamala, R.V. and Cornwell, D.G. (1977) Role of vitamin E in glutathione-induced oxidant stress: Methemoglobin, lipid peroxidation and hemolysis. J. Lipid Res. 18(5):635–644. https://doi.org/10.1016/S0022-2275(20)41605-0.

Bryant, K.L. and Kornegay, E.T. (1984) Influence of supplemental biotin on growth and development of toes and toe lesions and on hair quality in female swine. In Proc. 8th Int. Pig Vet. Soc. Cong. Belgium.

Bryant, K.L., Combs, G.E. and Wallace, H.D. (1977) Supplemental choline for young and growing-finishing swine. Univ. Florida. (pp. 1–4).

Bryant, K.L., Combs, G.E. and Wallace, H.D. (1981) Influence of supplemental vitamin B12 on performance of barrows and gilts. Univ. Florida. (pp. 4–6).

Bryant, K.L., Kornegay, E.T., Knight, J.W., Webb, K.E. and Notter, D.R. (1985a) Supplemental biotin for swine. I. Influence on feedlot performance, plasma biotin and toe lesions in developing gilts. J. Anim. Sci. 60(1): 136–144. https://doi.org/10.2527/jas1985.601136x.

Bryant, K.L., Kornegay, E.T., Knight, J.W., Webb, K.E. and Notter, D.R. (1985b) Supplemental biotin for swine. II. Influence of supplementation to corn- and wheat-based diets on reproductive performance and various biochemical criteria of sows during four parities. J. Anim. Sci. 60(1):145–153. https://doi.org/10.2527/jas1985.601145x.

Bryant, K.L., Kornegay, E.T., Knight, J.W., Veit, H.P. and Notter, D.R. (1985c) Supplemental biotin for swine. III. Influence of supplementation to corn- and wheat-based diets on the incidence and severity of toe lesions, hair and skin characteristics and structural soundness of sows housed in confinement during four parities. J. Anim. Sci. 60(1):154–162. https://doi.org/10.2527/jas1985.601154x.

Buchet, A., Belloc, C., Leblanc-Maridor, M. and Merlot, E. (2017) Effects of age and weaning conditions on blood indicators of oxidative status in pigs. PLOS ONE 12(5):e0178487. https://doi.org/10.1371/journal.pone.0178487.

Buckley, D.J., Morrissey, P.A. and Gray, J.I. (1995) Influence of dietary vitamin E on the oxidative stability and quality of pig meat. J. Anim. Sci. 73(10):3122–3130. https://doi.org/10.2527/1995.73103122x.

Buckley, J. and Connolly, F. (1980) Influence of alpha-tocopherol (vitamin E) on storage stability of raw pork and bacon. J. Food Prot. 43(4):265–267. https://doi.org/10.4315/0362-028X-43.4.265.

Buhi, W.C. (1981) Further characterization and function of uteroferrin from uterine flushings and allantoic fluid of pigs. Report Univ. Florida. Gainesville, FL, USA.

Burkholder, W.J. and Swecker, W.S. (1990) Nutritional influences on immunity. Semin. Vet. Med. Surg. Small. Anim. 5(3):154–166. PMID: 2236979.

Burroughs, W., Edgington, B.H., Robison, W.L. and Bethke, R.M. (1950) Niacin deficiency and enteritis in growing pigs. J. Nutr. 41(1):51–62. https://doi.org/10.1093/jn/41.1.51.

Butler, J.E. (1984) Immunoglobins of the mammary secretion. In "Lactation: A comprehensive treatise". Vol. III Larson, B.L. and Smith, V.R. (Eds.). Academic Press Inc., New York.

Cabadaj, R., Pleva, J. and Malla, P. (1983) Vitamin C in the prevention of PSE and DFD meat. Folio vet 27(2):81–87.

Cabassi, E., Di Lecce, R., De Angelis, E., Fusari, A., Perillo, A. and Borghetti, P. (2004) Aflatoxicosis and vitamins A and E supplementation in sows: immunological state of their piglets. Vet. Res. Commun. 28(1) Supplement 1:275–277. https://doi.org/10.1023/B:VERC.0000045425.28862.90.

Cadenas, S., Rojas, C. and Barja, G. (1998) Endotoxin increases oxidative injury to proteins in guinea pig liver: protection by dietary vitamin C. Pharmacol. Toxicol. 82(1):11–18. https://doi.org/10.1111/j.1600-0773.1998.tb01391.x.

Cafantaris, B. (1996) "Vitamin Stay C-25 in pigs". Agricultural Univ., Athens.

Calderón-Ospina, C.A. and Nava-Mesa, M.O. (2020) B vitamins in the nervous system: current knowledge of the biochemical modes of action and synergies of thiamine, pyridoxine, and cobalamin. CNS Neurosci. Ther. 26(1): 5–13. https://doi.org/10.1111/cns.13207.

Campbell, D.R. and Combs, G.E. (1988) The influence of supplemental vitamin K on performance of starting pigs. Univ. Florida Res. rep. (pp. 31–32).

Campbell, D.R. and Combs, G.E. (1990a) The influence of excess riboflavin supplementation on performance of growing-finishing pigs. 35. Univ. Florida. (pp. 14–17). Record Number: 19911437490.

Campbell, D.R. and Combs, G.E. (1990b) Effect of excessive niacin supplementation on performance of starting pigs. Univ. Florida 35:9–13.

Campbell, D.R. and Combs, G.E. (1991) Effect of excessive niacin supplementation on performance of starting pigs "Univ. Florida Res". Rep. AL-1991. 1. (pp. 1–4).

Camporeale, G. and Zempleni, J. (2006) Biotin. In "Present knowledge in nutrition" 9th edition Bowman, B.A. and R.M. Russell (Eds.). International Life Sciences Institute. (pp. 250–259).

Canadian Feeds Regulations (1983) https://laws-lois.justice.gc.ca/eng/regulations/sor-83-593/index.html.

Cannon, J.E., Morgan, J.B., Schmidt, G.R., Tatum, J.D., Sofos, J.N., Smith, G.C., Delmore, R.J. and Williams, S.N. (1996) Growth and fresh meat quality characteristics of pigs supplemented with vitamin E. J. Anim. Sci. 74(1): 98–105. https://doi.org/10.2527/1996.74198x.

Cantatore, F.P., Loperfido, M.C., Magli, D.M., Mancini, L. and Carrozzo, M. (1991) The importance of vitamin C for hydroxylation of vitamin D3 to 1,25(OH)2D3 in man. Clin. Rheumatol. 10(2):162–167. https://doi.org/10.1007/BF02207657.

Cao, L., Zhao, J., Ma, L., Chen, J., Xu, J., Rahman, S.U., Feng, S., Li, Y., Wu, J. and Wang, X. (2021) Lycopene attenuates zearalenone-induced oxidative damage of piglet Sertoli cells through the nuclear factor erythroid-2 related factor 2 signaling pathway. Ecotoxicol. Environ. Saf. 225:112737. https://doi.org/10.1016/j.ecoenv.2021.112737.

Cardenia, V., Rodriguez-Estrada, M.T., Cumella, F., Sardi, L., Della Casa, G. and Lercker, G. (2011) Oxidative stability of pork meat lipids as related to high-oleic sunflower oil and vitamin E diet supplementation and storage conditions. Meat Sci. 88(2):271–279. https://doi.org/10.1016/j.meatsci.2010.12.034.

Cargill, C., Judson, G., Cecil, A., Good, A. and Babidge, P. (1994) A survey of vitamin E in pigs and their diets and its effect on selected production indices. In Proceedings of the 13th IPVS Cong. Thailand.

Carmel, R. (1994) In vitro studies of gastric juice in patients with food-cobalamin malabsorption. Dig. Dis. Sci. 39(12): 2516–2522. https://doi.org/10.1007/BF02087684.

Carmona-Garcia, J.B. (1984) Effect of a vitamin C dietary supplement on sow litter size. Nutr. Admin. Rev. 54(10):549.

Carpenter, K.J. (1981) "Pellagra". Hutchinson Ross, Stroudsburg, PA.

Carpenter, K.J., Schelstraete, M., Vilicich, V.C. and Wall, J.S. (1988) Immature corn as a source of niacin for rats. J. Nutr. 118(2):165–169. https://doi.org/10.1093/jn/118.2.165.

Carrion, D., Coma, J. and Ewan, R.C. (1994) Effect of dietary and injectable d-alpha-tocopherol on tocopherol status of sows and pigs over three parities. Iowa State Univ. Swine Res. Rep. (pp. 63–67).

Carson, D.A., Seto, S. and Wasson, D.B. (1987) Pyridine nucleotide cycling and poly (ADP-ribose) synthesis in resting human lymphocytes. J. Immunol. 138(6):1904–1907. https://doi.org/10.4049/jimmunol.138.6.1904.

Carter, E.G. and Carpenter, K.J. (1982) The available niacin values of foods for rats and their relation to analytical values. J. Nutr. 112(11):2091–2103.

Carter, S.D., Cromwell, G.L., Combs, T.R., Colombo, G. and Fanti, P. (1996) The determination of serum concentrations of osteocalcin in growing pigs and its relationship to end-measures of bone mineralization. J. Anim. Sci. 74(11): 2719–2729. https://doi.org/10.2527/1996.74112719x.

Cartwright, G.E. and Wintrobe, M.M. (1948) Studies on free erythrocyte protoporphyrin, plasma copper, and plasma iron in normal and in pyridoxine-deficient swine. J. Biol. Chem. 172(2):557–565. PMID: 18901175.

Cartwright, G.E. and Wintrobe, M.M. (1949) Production of anemia in swine fed purified diets and sulfasuxidine. Proc. Soc. Exp. Biol. Med. 71(1):54–57. https://doi.org/10.3181/00379727-71-17077.

Cartwright, G.E., Wintrobe, M.M. and Humphreys, S. (1944) Studies on anemia in swine due to pyridoxine deficiency, together with data on phenylhydrazine anemia. J. Biol. Chem. 153(1):171–182. https://doi.org/10.1016/S0021-9258(18)51224-2.

Cartwright, G.E., Tatting, B. and Wintrobe, M.M. (1948) Niacin deficiency anemia in swine. Arch. Biochem. 19(1):109–118. PMID: 18884363.

Cartwright, G.E., Palmer, J.G., Tatting, B.S., Ashenbrucker, H. and Wintrobe, M.M. (1950) Experimental production of nutritional macrocytic anemia in swine. III. Further studies on pteroylglutamic acid deficiency. J. Lab. Clin. Med. 36(5): 675–693.

Cartwright, G.E., Tatting, B., Robinson, J., Fellows, N.M., Gunn, F.D. and Wintrobe, M.M. (1951) Hematologic manifestations of vitamin B12 deficiency in swine. Blood 6(10):867–891. https://doi.org/10.1182/blood.V6.10.867.867.

Cartwright, G.E., Tatting, B., Kurth, D. and Wintrobe, M.M. (1952) Experimental production of nutritional macrocytic anemia in swine. V. Hematologic manifestations of a combined deficiency of vitamin B12 and pteroylglutamic acid. Blood 7(10):992–1004. https://doi.org/10.1182/blood.V7.10.992.992.

Cashman, K.D. (2018) Vitamin D requirements for the future—lessons learned and charting a path forward nutrients. Nutrients 10(5):533–545. https://doi.org/10.3390/nu10050533.

Cashman, K.D. and O'Connor, E. (2008) Does high vitamin K1 intake protect against bone loss in later life? Nutr. Rev. 66(9):532–538. https://doi.org/10.1111/j.1753-4887.2008.00086.x.

Castellini, C., Lattaioli, P., Bernardini, M. and Dal Bosco, A. (2000) Effect of dietary α-tocopheryl acetate and ascorbic acid on rabbit semen stored at 5 C. Theriogenology 54(4):523–533. https://doi.org/10.1016/S0093-691X(00)00367-8.

Catani, M.V., Savini, I., Rossi, A., Melino, G. and Avigliano, L. (2005) Biological role of vitamin C in keratinocytes. Nutr. Rev. 63(3):81–90. https://doi.org/10.1111/j.1753-4887.2005.tb00125.x.

Catron, D.V., Richardson, D., Underkofler, L.A., Maddock, H.M. and Friedland, W.C. (1952) Vitamin B12 requirement of weanling pigs: II. Performance on low levels of vitamin B12 and requirement for optimum growth. J. Nutr. 47(3): 461–468. https://doi.org/10.1093/jn/47.3.461.

Cerolini, S., Maldjian, A., Surai, P. and Noble, R. (2000) Viability, susceptibility to peroxidation and fatty acid composition of boar semen during liquid storage. Anim. Reprod. Sci. 58(1–2):99–111. https://doi.org/10.1016/S0378-4320(99)00035-4.

Chan, M.M. (1991) Choline and carnitine. In "Handbook of vitamins" 2nd edition Machlin, L.J. (Ed.). Marcel Dekker. (pp. 537–556).

Chatterjee, G.C. (1967) Effects of ascorbic acid deficiency in animals. In "The enzymes" Vol. I Sebrell W.H. and Harris R.S.(Eds.). Academic Press, Inc., New York.

Chattha, K.S., Kandasamy, S., Vlasova, A.N. and Saif, L.J. (2013) Vitamin A deficiency impairs adaptive B and T cell responses to a prototype monovalent attenuated human rotavirus vaccine and virulent human rotavirus challenge in a gnotobiotic piglet model. PLOS ONE 8(12):e82966. https://doi.org/10.1371/journal.pone.0082966.

Chavez, E.R. (1983) Supplemental value of ascorbic acid during late gestation on piglet survival and early growth. Can. J. Anim. Sci. 63(3):683–687. https://doi.org/10.4141/cjas83-077.

Cheah, K.S., Cheah, A.M. and Krausgrill, D.I. (1995) Effect of dietary supplementation of vitamin E on pig meat quality. Meat Sci. 39(2):255–264. https://doi.org/10.1016/0309-1740(94)p1826-h.

Chen, C., Wang, Z., Li, J., Li, Y., Huang, P., Ding, X., Yin, J., He, S., Yang, H. and Yin, Y. (2019) Dietary vitamin E affects small intestinal histomorphology, digestive enzyme activity, and the expression of nutrient transporters by inhibiting proliferation of intestinal epithelial cells within jejunum in weaned piglets1. J. Anim. Sci. 97(3):1212–1221. https://doi.org/10.1093/jas/skz023.

Chen, J. (1990) "Technical service internal reports". BASF, Corp.

Chen, J., Han, J.H., Guan, W.T., Chen, F., Wang, C.X., Zhang, Y.Z., Lv, Y.T. and Lin, G. (2016) Selenium and vitamin E in sow diets: I. Effect on antioxidant status and reproductive performance in multiparous sows. Anim. Feed Sci. Technol. 221: 111–123. https://doi.org/10.1016/j.anifeedsci.2016.08.022.

Chen, Y.F., Huang, C.F., Liu, L., Lai, C.H. and Wang, F.L. (2019) Concentration of vitamins in the 13 feed ingredients commonly used in pig diets. Anim. Feed Sci. Technol. 247:1–8. https://doi.org/10.1016/j.anifeedsci.2018.10.011.

Chew, B.P. (1993) Effects of supplemental beta-carotene and vitamin A on reproduction in swine. J. Anim. Sci. 71(1): 247–252. https://doi.org/10.2527/1993.711247x.

Chew, B.P. (1995) Antioxidant vitamins affect food animal immunity and health. J. Nutr. 125(6) Supplement: 1804S–1808S.

Chew, B.P. and Park, J.S. (2004) Carotenoid action on the immune response. J. Nutr. 134(1): 257S–261S. https://doi.org/10.1093/jn/134.1.257S.

Chew, B.P., Rasmussen, H., Pubols, M.H. and Preston, R.L. (1982) Effects of vitamin A and beta-carotene on plasma progesterone and uterine protein secretions in gilts. Theriogenology 18(6):643–654. https://doi.org/10.1016/0093-691X(82)90030-9.

Chew, B.P., Holpuch, D.M. and O'Fallon, J.V. (1984) Vitamin A and beta-carotene in bovine and porcine plasma, liver, corpora lutea and follicular fluid. J. Dairy Sci. 67(6):1316–1322. https://doi.org/10.3168/jds.S0022-0302(84)81439-3.

Chew, B.P., Wong, T.S., Michal, J.J., Standaert, F.E. and Heirman, L.R. (1991) Kinetic characteristics of beta-carotene uptake after an injection of β-carotene in pigs. J. Anim. Sci. 69(12):4883–4891. https://doi.org/10.2527/1991.69124883x.

Chiang, S.H., Pettigrew, J.E., Moser, R.L., Cornelius, S.G., Miller, K.P. and Heeg, T.R. (1985) Supplemental vitamin C in swine diets. Nutr. Rep. Int. 31(3):573–581.

Chien, C.T., Chang, W.T., Chen, H.W., Wang, T.D., Liou, S.Y., Chen, T.J., Chang, Y.L., Lee, Y.T. and Hsu, S.M. (2004) Ascorbate supplement reduces oxidative stress in dyslipidemic patients undergoing apheresis. Arterioscler. Thromb. Vasc. Biol. 24(6):1111–1117. https://doi.org/10.1161/01.ATV.0000127620.12310.89.

Ching, S. and Mahan, D.C. (1998) Ascorbic acid synthesis in the fetal, nursing, and weaned pig. J. Anim. Sci. 76(1):33.

Ching, S., Mahan, D.C., Ottobre, J.S. and Dabrowski, K. (2001a) Ascorbic acid synthesis in fetal and neonatal pigs and in pregnant and postpartum sows. J. Nutr. 131(7):1997–2001. https://doi.org/10.1093/jn/131.7.1997.

Ching, S., Mahan, D.C. and Dabrowski, K. (2001b) Liver L-gulonolactone oxidase activity and tissue ascorbic acid concentrations in nursing pigs and the effect of various weaning ages. J. Nutr. 131(7):2002–2006. https://doi.org/10.1093/jn/131.7.2002.

Ching, S., Mahan, D.C., Wiseman, T.G. and Fastinger, N.D. (2002) Evaluating the antioxidant status of weanling pigs fed dietary vitamins A and E. J. Anim. Sci. 80(9):2396–2401. https://doi.org/10.1093/ansci/80.9.2396.

Cho, J.H., Lu, N. and Lindemann, M.D. (2017) Effects of vitamin supplementation on growth performance and carcass characteristics in pigs. Livest. Sci. 204:25–32. https://doi.org/10.1016/j.livsci.2017.08.007.

Chow, C.K. (1979) Nutritional influence on cellular antioxidant defense systems. Am. J. Clin. Nutr. 32(5):1066–1081. https://doi.org/10.1093/ajcn/32.5.1066.

Christensen, K. (1980) Evaluation of the background for the determination of the vitamin requirements of pigs. Livest. Prod. Sci. 7(6):569–590. https://doi.org/10.1016/0301-6226(80)90072-X.

Christensen, K. (1983) Pools of cellular nutrients. In "Dynamic biochemistry of animal production" Riis, P.M. (Ed.) Elsevier. Sci. Pub.

Christensen, N.O., Elkjaer, R., Engelund, A., Munch, T. and Terp, P. (1958) Studies on the absorption of vitamin A. II. Experiments on liver storage in rats and pigs Nord. Vet. Med. 10. (pp. 49–62). Record Number: 19581404943.

Christensen, S. (1973) The biological fate of riboflavin in mammals. A survey of literature and own investigations. Acta Pharmacol. Toxicol. (Copenh) 32(2):3–72. https://doi.org/10.1111/j.1600-0773.1973.tb03313.x.

Chung, T.K. and Baker, D.H. (1990) Riboflavin requirement of chicks fed purified amino acid and conventional corn-soybean meal diets. Poult. Sci. 69(8):1357–1363. https://doi.org/10.3382/ps.0691357.

Clawitter, J.W., Trout, W.E., Burke, M.G., Araghi, S. and Roberts, R.M. (1990) A novel family of progesterone-induced, retinol-binding proteins from uterine secretions of the pig. J. Biol. Chem. 265(6):3248–3255. https://doi.org/10.1016/s0021-9258(19)39760-1.

Cleveland, E.R., Newton, G.L., Mullinix, B.G., Hale, O.M. and Frye, T.M. (1983) Foot-leg and performance traits of boars fed two levels of ascorbic acid. J. Anim. Sci. 57(1):387.

Cleveland, E.R., Bondari, K. and Newton, G.L. (1987a) Effect of ascorbic acid supplementation on performance and foot-leg traits in swine. Livest. Prod. Sci. 17:277–283. https://doi.org/10.1016/0301-6226(87)90072-8.

Cleveland, E.R., Bondari, K. and Newton, G.L. (1987b) Effect of breed and supplemental vitamin C on performance traits and foot-leg scores in growing-finishing boars. Nutr. Rep. Int. 36(4):879–886.

Clifford, A.J., Jones, A.D. and Bills, N.D. (1990) Bioavailability of folates in selected foods incorporated into amino acid-based diets fed to rats. J. Nutr. 120(12):1640–1647. https://doi.org/10.1093/jn/120.12.1640.

Cline, J.H., Mahan, D.C. and Moxon, A.L. (1974) Progeny effects of supplemental vitamin E in sow diets. J. Anim. Sci. 39:974.

Coburn, S.P. (1994) A critical review of minimal B6 requirements for growth in various species with a proposed method of calculation. Vitam. Horm. 48:259–300. https://doi.org/10.1016/s0083-6729(08)60500-2.

Coburn, S.P., Mahuren, J.D., Kennedy, M.S., Schaltenbrand, W.E. and Townsend, D.W. (1992) Metabolism of 14C and 32P pyridoxal 5'-phosphate and 3H pyridoxal administered intravenously to pigs and goats. J. Nutr. 122(2): 393–401. https://doi.org/10.1093/jn/122.2.393.

Coelho, M. (2000) "Update on commercial poultry, swine and dairy vitamin supplement: https://www.feed info.com/home/global-news/update-on-commercial-poultry-swine-and-dairy-vitamin-supplementa tion/52417.

Coelho, M. (2002) Vitamin stability in premixes and feeds: a practical approach in ruminant diets. In Proceedings of the 13th Annual Florida Ruminant Nutrition Symposium, FL, USA. (pp. 127–145).

Coen, G., Ballanti, P., Silvestrini, G., Mantella, D., Manni, M., Di Giulio, S., Pisanò, S., Leopizzi, M., Di Lullo, G. and Bonucci, E. (2009) Immunohistochemical localization and mRNA expression of matrix Gla protein and fetuin-A in bone biopsies of hemodialysis patients. Virchows Arch. 454(3):263–271. https://doi. org/10.1007/s00428-008-0724-4.

Coffey, J.D., Hines, E.A., Starkey, J.D., Starkey, C.W. and Chung, T.K. (2012) Feeding 25-hydroxycholecalciferol improves gilt reproductive performance and fetal vitamin D status. J. Anim. Sci. 90(11):3783–3788. https://doi.org/10.2527/jas.2011-5023.

Coffey, M.T. and Britt, J.H. (1991) "Improvement of embryo and fetal survival through short-term vitamin A therapy in sows (effect of vitamin A injection on sow productivity)". NPPC. (pp. 70–71).

Coffey, M.T. and Britt, J.H. (1993) Enhancement of sow reproductive performance by beta-carotene or vitamin A. J. Anim. Sci. 71(5):1198–1202. https://doi.org/10.2527/1993.7151198x.

Coffey, M.T., Britt, J.H. and Alhusen, H.D. (1989) Effect of beta-carotene injection on reproduction performance of sows. J. Anim. Sci. 67(1):251.

Coffey, M.T., Herman, D.L., Britt, J.H. and Bowie, C.A. (1990) Plasma and tissue response of gestating sow to injection or oral supplementation of beta-carotene. (BC) J. FASEB Bethesda 4:384.

Cohen, N., Scott, C.G., Neukon, C., Lopresti, R.L., Weber, G. and Saucy, G. (1981) Total synthesis of all 8 stereoisomers of alpha-tocopheryl acetate. Analysis of their diastereomeric and enantiomeric purity by gas chromatography. Helv. Chim. Act. 64:1158–1173. https://doi.org/10.1002/hlca.19810640422.

Colby, R.W., Cunha, T.J., Lindley, C.E., Cordy, D.R. and Ensminger, M.E. (1948) Biotin-pantothenic acid interrelationship and enteritis in the pantothenic acid deficient pig. J. Am. Vet. Med. Assoc. 113(861):589–593.

Colby, R.W. and Ensminger, M.E. (1950) Effect of vitamin B12 on the growing pig. J. Anim. Sci. 9(1): 90–93. https://doi.org/10.2527/jas1950.9190.

Colunga Biancatelli, R.M.L., Berrill, M. and Marik, P.E. (2020) The antiviral properties of vitamin C. Expert Rev. Anti. Infect Ther. 18(2):99–101. https://doi.org/10.1080/14787210.2020.1706483.

Combs, Jr., G.F. and McClung, J.P. (2022) "The vitamins. Fundamental aspects in nutrition and health" 6th edition. Elsevier, Amsterdam.

Combs, G.E., Berry, T.H., Wallace, H.D. and Crum, R.C. (1966a) Influence of supplemental vitamin D on gain, nutrient digestibility and tissue composition of young pigs. J. Anim. Sci. 25(1):48–51. https://doi. org/10.2527/jas1966.25148x.

Combs, G.E., Berry, T.H., Wallace, H.D. and Crum, R.C. (1966b) Levels and sources of vitamin D for pigs fed diets containing varying quantities of calcium. J. Anim. Sci. 25(3):827–830. https://doi.org/10.2527/ jas1966.253827x.

Commission on Biochemical Nomenclature of Tocopherols and Related Compounds, Recommendations (IUPAC-IUB) (1973). Eur. J. Biochem. 46:217.

Comunidad profesional porcina (2007). Caso Clin. Carencia Vitamina E y selenio. Sanidad. URL.

Connor, B.J. and Marian, F.J. (1948) Choline deficiency in the baby pig: ten figures. J. Nutr. 36(3): 339–349. https://doi.org/10.1093/jn/36.3.339.

Cooper, D.A., Berry, D.A., Spendel, V.A., Kiorpes, A.L. and Peters, J.C. (1997) The domestic pig as a model for evaluating olestra's nutritional effects. J. Nutr. 127(8) Supplement:1555S–1565S. https://doi.org/10.1093/jn/127.8.1555S.

Cooper, J.R., Roth, R.H. and Kini, M.M. (1963) Biochemical and physiological function of thiamine in nervous tissue. Nature 199:609–610. https://doi.org/10.1038/199609a0.

Cooper, K.M., Kennedy, S., McConnell, S., Kennedy, D.G. and Frigg, M. (1997) An immunohistochemical study of the distribution of biotin in tissues of pigs and chickens. Res. Vet. Sci. 63(3):219–225. https://doi.org/10.1016/S0034-5288(97)90024-2.

Copelin, J.L., Monegue, H. and Combs, G.E. (1980) Niacin levels in growing-finishing swine diets. J. Anim. Sci. 51(1):190.

Corino, C., Oriani, G., Pantaleo, L., Pastorelli, G. and Salvatori, G. (1999) Influence of dietary vitamin E supplementation on "heavy" pig carcass characteristics, meat quality, and vitamin E status. J. Anim. Sci. 77(7): 1755–1761. https://doi.org/10.2527/1999.7771755x.

Côté-Robitaille, M.É., Girard, C.L., Guay, F. and Matte, J.J. (2015) Oral supplementations of betaine, choline, creatine and vitamin B6 and their influence on the development of homocysteinaemia in neonatal piglets. J. Nutr. Sci. 4: e31. https://doi.org/10.1017/jns.2015.19.

Courraud, J., Berger, J., Cristol, J.P. and Avallone, S. (2013) Stability and bioaccessibility of different forms of carotenoids and vitamin A during in vitro digestion. Food Chem. 136(2):871–877. https://doi.org/10.1016/j.foodchem.2012.08.076.

Crenshaw, T.D. (2000) Calcium, phosphorus, vitamin D, and vitamin K in swine nutrition. In "Swine nutrition". CRC Press. (pp. 207–232).

Crenshaw, T.D. (2010) Vitamin D mediated phosphate homeostasis-implications for skeleton growth and mineralization. J. Anim. Sci. 88(2):1. abstr.

Cromwell, G.L., Hays, V.W. and Overfield, J.R. (1969) Effect of dietary ascorbic acid on performance of growing-finishing swine. J. Anim. Sci. 29:23–24.

Cromwell, G.L., Hays, V.W. and Overfield, J.R. (1970) Effect of dietary ascorbic acid on performance and plasma cholesterol levels of growing swine. J. Anim. Sci. 31(1):63–66. https://doi.org/10.2527/jas1970.31163x.

Cromwell, G.L., Coffey, R.D. and Monegue, H.J. (1996) Effects of 1,25-dihydroxycholecalciferol on the utilization of phytate P in low-P, corn-soybean meal diets for pigs. J. Anim. Sci. 74(1):58.

Cromwell, G.L., Hors, R.L., Goff, J.P., Carter, S.D., Lindemann, M.D. and Monegue, H.J. (1997) Inability of 1,25-dihydroxycholecalciferol to improve P utilization in pigs. J. Anim. Sci. 75(1):63.

Csapó, J., Martin, T.G., Csapó-Kiss, Z.S. and Házas, Z. (1996) Protein, fats, vitamin and mineral concentrations in porcine colostrum and milk from parturition to 60 days. Int. Dairy J. 6(8–9):881–902. https://doi.org/10.1016/0958-6946(95)00072-0.

Culbertson, M.S., Herring, W.O., Holl, J.W. and Casey, D. (2017) Genetic improvement and dissemination for the global commercial swine industry. Anim. Prod. Sci. 57(12):2366–2369. https://doi.org/10.1071/AN17317.

Cunha, T.J. (1977) "Swine feeding and nutrition". Academic Press, New York.

Cunha, T.J. (1984) Present status on biotin for pigs. Feed Manag. 35(14):22.

Cunha, T.J. (1985) Nutrition and disease interaction. Feedstuffs 57(41):37.

Cunha, T.J. (1987) Variables in animal nutrition keep shifting the requirements. Feedstuffs 59(42):1.

Cunha, T.J., Lindley, D.C. and Ensminger, M.E. (1946) Biotin deficiency syndrome in pigs fed desiccated egg white. J. Anim. Sci. 5(2):219–225. https://doi.org/10.2527/jas1946.52219x.

Cunha, T.J., Colby, R.W., Bustad, L.K. and Bone, J.F. (1948) The need for and interrelationship of folic acid, anti-pernicious anemia liver extract, and biotin in the pig. J. Nutr. 36(2):215–229.

Da Silveira, P.R.S., Fernandes, L.C.O., De Moraes-Filho, J.C. and Junior, W. (1998) Reproductive performance of sows injected with vitamin A. R. Bras. Zootec. 27(4):743–748.

Dagnelie, P.C., Van Staveren, W.A. and Van den Berg, H. (1991) Vitamin B12 from algae appears not to be bioavailable. Am. J. Clin. Nutr. 53(3):695–697. https://doi.org/10.1093/ajcn/53.3.695.

Daily, J.W. and Sachan, D.S. (1995) Choline supplementation alters carnitine homeostasis in humans and guinea pigs. J. Nutr. 125(7):1938–1944. https://doi.org/10.1093/jn/125.7.1938.

Dakshinamurti, S. and Dakshinamurti, K. (2013) Vitamin B6. In Handbook of vitamins 5th edition Zempleni, J., Suttie, J., Gregory, J. and Stover, P.J. (Eds.). CRC Press. (pp. 351–396).

Dal Jang, Y., Ma, J., Lu, N., Lim, J., Monegue, H.J., Stuart, R.L. and Lindemann, M.D. (2018) Administration of vitamin D3 by injection or drinking water alters serum 25-hydroxycholecalciferol concentrations of nursery pigs. Asian-Australas. J. Anim. Sci. 31(2):278–286. https://doi.org/10.5713/ajas.17.0397.

Dalto, B.D., Tsoi, S., Audet, I., Dyck, M.K., Foxcroft, G.R. and Matte, J.J. (2015) Gene expression of porcine blastocysts from gilts fed organic or inorganic selenium and pyridoxine. Reproduction 149(1):31–42. https://doi.org/10.1530/REP-14-0408.

Dalto, D.B. and da Silva, C.A. (2020) A survey of current levels of trace minerals and vitamins used in commercial diets by the Brazilian pork industry—a comparative study. Transl. Anim. Sci. 4(4):txaa195. https://doi.org/10.1093/tas/txaa195.

Dalto, D.B. and Matte, J.J. (2017) Pyridoxine (vitamin B_6) and the glutathione peroxidase system; a link between one-carbon metabolism and antioxidation. Nutrients 9(3):189. https://doi.org/10.3390/nu9030189.

Dalto, D.B., Roy, M., Audet, I., Palin, M.F., Guay, F., Lapointe, J. and Matte, J.J. (2015) Interaction between vitamin B6 and source of selenium on the response of the selenium-dependent glutathione peroxidase system to oxidative stress induced by oestrus in pubertal pig. J. Trace Elem. Med. Biol. 32:21–29. https://doi.org/10.1016/j.jtemb.2015.05.002.

Danbred (2021) Danbred nutrient specifications. https://danbred-manual.com/en/danbred-nutrient-specifications-uk/.

Darby, W.J., McNutt, K.W. and Todhunter, E.N. (1975) Niacin. Nutr. Rev. 33(10):289–297. https://doi.org/10.1111/j.1753-4887.1975.tb05075.x.

Darlow, B.A., Graham, P.J. and Rojas-Reyes, M.X. (2016) Vitamin A supplementation to prevent mortality and short- and long-term morbidity in very low birth weight infants. Cochrane Database Syst. Rev. 2016(8):CD000501. https://doi.org/10.1002/14651858.CD000501.pub4.

Darr, D., Combs, S., Dunston, S., Manning, T. and Pinnell, S. (1992) Topical vitamin C protects porcine skin from ultraviolet radiation-induced damage. Br. J. Dermatol. 127(3):247–253. https://doi.org/10.1111/j.1365-2133.1992.tb00122.x.

D'Arrigo, M., Hoz, L., Lopez-Bote, C.J., Cambero, I., Pin, C., Rey, A.I. and Ordóñez, J.A. (2002) Effect of dietary linseed oil and α-tocopherol on selected properties of pig fat. Can. J. Anim. Sci. 82(3):339–346. https://doi.org/10.4141/A01-095.

Darroch, C.S. (2000) Vitamin A in swine nutrition. In Swine nutrition. CRC Press. (pp. 283–300).

Darroch, C.S., Chiba, L.I., Lindeman, M.D., Harper, A.F. and Kornegay, E.T. (1998) Effect of injections of high levels of vitamin A on reproductive performance of sows. S-145 Committee on Nutritional Systems for Swine to Increase Reproductive Efficiency.

Dash, S.K. and Mitchell, D.J. (1976) Storage, processing reduce vitamin A. Anim. Nutr. Health 31(7):16.

Davey, R.J. and Stevenson, J.W. (1963) Pantothenic acid requirement of swine for reproduction. J. Anim. Sci. 22(1):9–13. https://doi.org/10.2527/jas1963.2219.

David, V., Dai, B., Martin, A., Huang, J., Han, X. and Quarles, L.D. (2013) Calcium regulates FGF-23 expression in bone. Endocrinology 154(12):4469–4482. https://doi.org/10.1210/en.2013-1627.

Daza, A., Rey, A.I., Ruiz, J. and Lopez-Bote, C.J. (2005) Effects of feeding in free-range conditions or in confinement with different dietary MUFA/PUFA ratios and α-tocopheryl acetate, on antioxidants accumulation and oxidative stability in Iberian pigs. Meat Sci. 69(1):151–163. https://doi.org/10.1016/j.meatsci.2004.06.017.

De Boer-van den Berg, M.A., Verstijnen, C.P. and Vermeer, C. (1986) Vitamin K-dependent carboxylase in skin. J. Invest. Dermatol. 87(3):377–380.

De Jong, M.F. and Sytsema, J.R. (1983) Field experience with d-biotin supplementation to gilt and sow feeds. Vet. Q. 5(2):58–67. https://doi.org/10.1080/01652176.1983.9693873.

De la Huerga, J. and Popper, H. (1952) Factors influencing choline absorption in the intestinal tract. J. Clin. Invest. 31(6):598–603. https://doi.org/10.1172/JCI102646.

De Luca, F., Uyeda, J.A., Mericq, V., Mancilla, E.E., Yanovski, J.A., Barnes, K.M., Zile, M.H. and Baron, J. (2000) Retinoic acid is a potent regulator of growth plate chondrogenesis. Endocrinology 141(1):346–353. https://doi.org/10.1210/endo.141.1.7283.

De Passille, A.M.B., Bilodeau, R.R., Girard, C.L. and Matte, J.J. (1989) A study on the occurrence of coprophagy behavior and its relationship to B-vitamin status in growing-finishing pigs. Can. J. Anim. Sci. 69(2):229. https://doi.org/10.4141/cjas89-033.

De Rodas, B.Z., Maxwell, C.V., Davis, M.E., Mandali, S., Broekman, E. and Stoecker, B.J. (1998) L-ascorbyl-2-polyphosphate as a vitamin C source for segregated and conventionally weaned pigs. J. Anim. Sci. 76(6):1636–1643. https://doi.org/10.2527/1998.7661636x.

Debier, C. and Larondelle, Y. (2005) Vitamins A and E: metabolism, roles and transfer to offspring. Br. J. Nutr. 93(2):153–174. https://doi.org/10.1079/BJN20041308.

Degkwitz, E. (1987) Some effects of vitamin C may be indirect, since it affects the blood levels of cortisol and thyroid hormones. Ann. NY Acad. Sci. 498(1) 470–472 Third Conference on vitamin C. https://doi.org/10.1111/j.1749-6632.1987.tb23786.x.

Del Tuffo, L.D., Tokach, M.D., Jones, C.K., DeRouchey, J.M. and Goodband, R.D. (2019) Evaluation of different vitamin concentrations on grow-finish pig growth and carcass characteristics. J. Anim. Sci. 97(2) (suppl. 2):108–109. https://doi.org/10.1093/jas/skz122.192.

DeLuca, H.F. (2008) Evolution of our understanding of vitamin D. Nutr. Rev. 66(10) (suppl. 2):S73–S87. https://doi.org/10.1111/j.1753-4887.2008.00105.x.

DeLuca, H.F. (2014) History of the discovery of vitamin D and its active metabolites. BoneKEy Rep. 3:479. https://doi.org/10.1038/bonekey.2013.213.

Denis, I., Colin, C., LaCroix, H., Zerath, E. and Pointillart, A. (1997) Vitamin C supplementation and bone metabolism in growing pigs. Journées Rech. Porcine Fr.29:263–268.

Denisova, N.A. and Booth, S.L. (2005) Vitamin K and sphingolipid metabolism: evidence to date. Nutr. Rev. 63(4):111–121. https://doi.org/10.1111/j.1753-4887.2005.tb00129.x.

Dever, J.T., Surles, R.L., Davis, C.R. and Tanumihardjo, S.A. (2011) α-Retinol is distributed through serum retinol-binding protein-independent mechanisms in the lactating sow-nursing piglet dyad. J. Nutr. 141(1):42–47. https://doi.org/10.3945/jn.110.127597.

Dhur, A., Galan, P. and Hercberg, S. (1991) Folate status and the immune system. Prog. Food Nutr. Sci. 15(1–2):43–60. PMID: 1887065.

Diet-Ox (1998). Dietary treatment and quality characteristics of muscle and meat products.

Dinarello, C.A. (1996) Biologic basis for interleukin-1 in disease. Blood 87(6):2095–2147. PMID: 8630372.

Dineen, N.M., Kerry, J.P., Lynch, P.B., Buckley, D.J., Morrissey, P.A. and Arendt, E.K. (2000) Reduced nitrite levels and dietary α-tocopheryl acetate supplementation: effects on the colour and oxidative stability of cooked hams. Meat Sci. 55(4):475–482. https://doi.org/10.1016/S0309-1740(00)00008-5.

Dobson, K.J. (1967) Failure of selenium and vitamin E to prevent gastric ulceration in pigs. Aust. Vet. J. 43(6):219. https://doi.org/10.1111/j.1751-0813.1967.tb15087.x.

Dobson, K.J. (1969) Osteodystrophy associated with hypervitaminosis A in growing pigs. Aust. Vet. J. 45(12):570–573. https://doi.org/10.1111/j.1751-0813.1969.tb16093.x.

Douglass, M., Dikalova, A., Kaplowitz, M.R., Zhang, Y., Cunningham, G., Summar, M. and Fike, C.D. (2021) Folic acid, either solely or combined with L-citrulline, improves NO signaling and ameliorates chronic hypoxia-induced pulmonary hypertension in newborn pigs. Physiol. Rep. 9(21):e15096. https://doi.org/10.14814/phy2.15096.

Dove, C.R. and Cook, D.A. (2000) Water-soluble vitamins in swine nutrition. In Swine nutrition. CRC Press. (pp. 335–376).

Dove, C.R. and Ewan, R.C. (1987) The effect of diet composition on the stability of vitamin E. J. Anim. Sci. 65 (suppl. 1):302 (abstr.).

Dove, C.R. and Ewan, R.C. (1990) Effect of excess dietary copper, iron or zinc on the tocopherol and selenium status of growing pigs. J. Anim. Sci. 68(8):2407–2413. https://doi.org/10.2527/1990.6882407x.

Dove, C.R. and Ewan, R.C. (1991) Effect of trace minerals on the stability of vitamin E in swine grower diets. J. Anim. Sci. 69(5):1994–2000. https://doi.org/10.2527/1991.6951994x.

Driskell, J.A. (1984) Vitamin B6. In Handbook of vitamins Machlin, L.J. (Ed.). Marcel Dekker, Inc., New York.

DSM Nutritional Products (2012) Optimum Vitamin Nutrition® Guidelines.

DSM Nutritional Products (2016) OVN Optimum Vitamin Nutrition® Guidelines.

DSM Nutritional Products (2022a) DSM Product Forms: Quality feed additives for more sustainable farming. https://www.dsm.com/anh/news/downloads/infographics-checklists-and-guides/quality-feed-additives-for-more-sustainable-farming.html.

DSM Nutritional Products (2022b) OVN Optimum Vitamin Nutrition ® guidelines. https://www.dsm.com/anh/products-and-services/tools/ovn.html.

D'Souza, D.N., Pethick, D.W., Dunshea, F.R., Pluske, J.R. and Mullan, B.P. (2003) Nutritional manipulation increases intramuscular fat levels in the longissimus muscle of female finisher pigs. Aust. J. Agric. Res. 54(8):745–749. https://doi.org/10.1071/AR03009.

Duarte, T.L. and Almeida, I.F. (2012) Vitamin C, gene expression and skin health. In "Handbook of diet, nutrition and the skin". Human Health Handbooks no. 1, Vol. 2 Preedy, V.R. (Ed.). Wageningen Academic Publishers:114–127.

DuCoa, L.P. (1994) Choline functions and requirements. DuCoa L.P., a DuPont/ConAgra Co, Higland, Illinois.

Duello, T.J. and Matschiner, J.T. (1971) Characterization of vitamin K from pig liver and dog liver. Arch. Biochem. Biophys. 144(1):330–338. https://doi.org/10.1016/0003-9861(71)90485-1.

Duffy, S.K., Kelly, A.K., Rajauria, G., Clarke, L.C., Gath, V., Monahan, F.J. and O'Doherty, J.V. (2018a) The effect of 25-hydroxyvitamin D3 and phytase inclusion on pig performance, bone parameters and pork quality in finisher pigs. J. Anim. Physiol. Anim. Nutr. (Berl) 102(5):1296–1305. https://doi.org/10.1111/jpn.12939.

Duffy, S.K., Kelly, A.K., Rajauria, G., Jakobsen, J., Clarke, L.C., Monahan, F.J., Dowling, K.G., Hull, G., Galvin, K., Cashman, K.D., Hayes, A. and O'Doherty, J.V. (2018b) The use of synthetic and natural vitamin D sources in pig diets to improve meat quality and vitamin D content. Meat Sci. 143:60–68. https://doi.org/10.1016/j.meatsci.2018.04.014.

Duncan, W.R.H., Garton, G.A., McDonald, I. and Smith, W. (1960) Observations on tocopherol absorption by pigs. Br. J. Nutr. 14(3):371–377. https://doi.org/10.1079/bjn19600048.

Dunnett, C.E. (2003) Antioxidants in physiology and nutrition of exercising horses. In Nutritional biotechnology in the feed and food industries In Lyons, T.P. and Jacques, K.P. (Eds). Nottingham University Press. (pp. 439–448).

Durst, L., Kirchgessner, M. and Roth-Maier, D.A. (1989) Absorption of vitamin B6 in the hindgut of pigs. J. Anim. Physiol. Anim. Nutr. 62(1–2):85–92.

Duthie, G.G., Arthur, J.R., Mills, C.F., Morrice, P. and Nicol, F. (1987) Anomalous tissue vitamin E distribution in stress susceptible pigs after dietary vitamin E supplementation and effects on plasma pyruvate kinase and creatine kinase activities. Livest. Prod. Sci. 17:169–178. https://doi.org/10.1016/0301-6226(87)90062-5.

Duthie, G.G., Arthur, J.R., Nicol, F. and Walker, M.J. (1989) Increased indices of lipid peroxidation in stress susceptible pigs and effects of vitamin E. Res. Vet. Sci. 46(2):226–230. https://doi.org/10.1016/S0034-5288(18)31149-4.

Dutta-Roy, A.K., Gordon, M.J., Campbell, F.M., Duthie, G.G. and James, W.P.T. (1994) Vitamin E requirements, transport, and metabolism: role of α-tocopherol-binding proteins. J. Nutr. Biochem. 5(12):562–570. https://doi.org/10.1016/0955-2863(94)90010-8.

Dvorak, M. (1974a) Levels of vitamin E in the blood plasma of suckling and weaned piglets. Acta Vet. Brno 43(2):103–110.

Dvorak, M. (1974b) Effects of corticotrophin, starvation and glucose on ascorbic acid levels in the blood plasma and liver of piglets. Nutr. Metab. 16(4):215–222. https://doi.org/10.1159/000175492.

Dvorak, M. (1984) Ascorbic acid, stress resistance and reproduction in swine. The Royal Danish Agriculture Society.

Dvorak, M. and Podany, J. (1966) Changes in the ascorbic acid content of testes during the development of boars. Docum Vet. Brno 5:25.

Dvorak, M. and Podany, J. (1971) Ascorbic acid levels in the genital glands of breeding boars and castrates. Acta Vet. 40:397–403.

Easter, R.A., Anderson, P.A., Michel, E.J. and Corley, J.R. (1983) Response of gestating gilts and starter, grower and finisher swine to biotin, pyridoxine, folacin, and thiamine additions to a corn-soybean meal diet. Nutr. Rep. Int. 28:945–954.

Eder, K., Flader, D., Hirche, F. and Brandsch, C. (2002) Excess dietary vitamin E lowers the activities of antioxidative enzymes in erythrocytes of rats fed salmon oil. J. Nutr. 132(11):3400–3404. https://doi.org/10.1093/jn/132.11.3400.

Edmonds, M.S. and Arentson, B.E. (2001) Effect of supplemental vitamins and trace minerals on performance and carcass quality in finishing pigs. J. Anim. Sci. 79(1):141–147. https://doi.org/10.2527/2001.791141x.

EFSA Panel on Additives and Products or Substances used in Animal Feed (FEEDAP) (2014) Scientific opinion on the safety and efficacy of vitamin K3 (menadione sodium bisulphite and menadione nicotinamide bisulphite) as a feed additive for all animal species. EFSA J. 12(1):3532. https://doi.org/10.2903/j.efsa.2014.3532.

Eggersdorfer, M., Laudert, D., Létinois, U., McClymont, T., Medlock, J., Netscher, T. and Bonrath, W. (2012) One hundred years of vitamins a success story of the natural sciences. Angew. Chem. Int. Ed. Engl. 51(52):12960–12990. https://doi.org/10.1002/anie.201205886.

Eichenberger, B., Pfirter, H.P., Wenk, C. and Gebert, S. (2004) Influence of dietary vitamin E and C supplementation on vitamin E and C content and thiobarbituric acid reactive substances (TBARS) in different tissues of growing pigs. Arch. Anim. Nutr. 58(3):195–208. https://doi.org/10.1080/00039420410001701413.

Eicher, S.D., McKee, C.A., Carroll, J.A. and Pajor, E.A. (2006) Supplemental vitamin C and yeast cell wall β-glucan as growth enhancers in newborn pigs and as immunomodulators after an endotoxin challenge after weaning. J. Anim. Sci. 84(9):2352–2360. https://doi.org/10.2527/jas.2005-770.

Ekanayake, A. and Nelson, P.E. (1990) Effect of thermal processing on lima bean vitamin B6 availability. J. Food Sci. 55(1):154–157. https://doi.org/10.1111/j.1365-2621.1990.tb06040.x.

Ellis, N.R. and Madsen, L.L. (1944) The thiamine requirements of pigs as related to the fat content of the diet. J. Nutr. 27(3):253–262. https://doi.org/10.1093/jn/27.3.253.

Ellis, R.P. and Vorhies, M.W. (1976) Effect of supplemental dietary vitamin E on the serologic response of swine to an Escherichia coli bacterin. J. Am. Vet. Med. Assoc. 168(3):231–232. PMID: 765311.

Elvehjem, C. A., Madden, R.J., Strong, F.M. and Wolley, D.W. (1974) The isolation and identification of the anti-black tongue factor. Nutr. Rev. 32(2):48–50. https://doi.org/10.1111/j.1753-4887.1974.tb06263.x.

Emmert, J.L. and Baker, D.H. (1997) A chick bioassay approach for determining the bioavailable choline concentration in normal and overheated soybean meal, canola meal and peanut meal. J. Nutr. 127(5): 745–752. https://doi.org/10.1093/jn/127.5.745.

Emmert, J.L., Garrow, T.A. and Baker, D.H. (1996) Development of an experimental diet for determining bioavailable choline concentration and its application in studies with soybean lecithin. J. Anim. Sci. 74(11):2738–2744. https://doi.org/10.2527/1996.74112738x.

Emmert, J.L., Webel, D.M., Biehl, R.R., Griffiths, M.A., Garrow, L.S., Garrow, T.A. and Baker, D.H. (1998) Hepatic and renal betaine-homocysteine methyltransferase activity in pigs as affected by dietary intakes of sulfur amino acids, choline, and betaine. J. Anim. Sci. 76(2):606–610. https://doi.org/10.2527/1998.762606x.

Engstrom, G.W. and Littledike, E.T. (1986) Vitamin D metabolism in the pig In "swine in biomedical research," Tumbleson, M.E. (Ed.), Vol. 2. Plenum Press, New York.

Engstrom, G.W., Goff, J.P., Horst, R.L. and Reinhardt, T.A. (1987) Regulation of calf renal 25-hydroxyvitamin D- hydroxylase activities by calcium-regulating hormones. J. Dairy Sci. 70(11):2266–2271. https://doi.org/10.3168/jds.S0022-0302(87)80286-2.

Enright, K.L., Anderson, B.K., Ellis, M., McKeith, F.K., Berger, L.L. and Baker, D.H. (1998) The effects of feeding high levels of vitamin D3 on pork quality. J. Anim. Sci. 76(1):149.

Ensminger, A.H., Ensminger, M.E., Konlande, J.E. and Robson, J.R.K. (1983) "Foods and nutrition encyclopedia" In Ensminger, A.H. (Ed.), Ensminger Pub.

Ensminger, M.E., Bowland, J.P. and Cunha, T.J. (1947) Observations on the thiamine, riboflavin, and choline needs of sows for reproduction. J. Anim. Sci. 6(4):409–423. https://doi.org/10.2527/jas1947.64409x.

Ensminger, M.E., Colby, R.W. and Cunha, T.J. (1951) Effect of certain B-complex vitamins on gestation and lactation in swine. Wash. Agric. Exp. Sta. Circ. 134. https://doi.org/10.7273/000002711.

Esch, M.W., Easter, R.A. and Bahr, J.M. (1981) Effect of riboflavin deficiency on estrous cyclicity in pigs. Biol. Reprod. 25(3):659–665. https://doi.org/10.1095/biolreprod25.3.659.

Esmon, C.T., Sadowski, J.A. and Suttie, J.W. (1975) A new carboxylation reaction. The vitamin K-dependent incorporation of H-14-CO3- into prothrombin. J. Biol. Chem. 250(12):4744–4748. PMID: 1141226.

Esteban-Pretel, G., Marín, M.P., Renau-Piqueras, J., Barber, T. and Timoneda, J. (2010) Vitamin A deficiency alters rat lung alveolar basement membrane: reversibility by retinoic acid. J. Nutr. Biochem. 21(3): 227–236. https://doi.org/10.1016/j.jnutbio.2008.12.007.

Ewan, R.C. (1971) Effect of vitamin E and selenium on tissue composition of young pigs. J. Anim. Sci. 32(5): 883–887. https://doi.org/10.2527/jas1971.325883x.

Ewan, R.C., Wastell, M.E., Bicknell, E.J. and Speer, V.C. (1969) Performance and deficiency symptoms of young pigs fed diets low in vitamin E and selenium. J. Anim. Sci. 29(6):912–915. https://doi.org/10.2527/jas1969.296912x.

Eyles, D., Anderson, C., Ko, P., Jones, A., Thomas, A., Burne, T., Mortensen, P.B., Nørgaard-Pedersen, B., Hougaard, D.M. and McGrath, J. (2009) A sensitive LC/MS/MS assay of 25OH vitamin D3 and 25OH vitamin D2 in dried blood spots. Clin. Chim. Acta 403(1–2):145–151. https://doi.org/10.1016/j.cca.2009.02.005.

Faccin, J.E.G., Tokach, M.D., Woodworth, J.C., DeRouchey, J.M., Gebhardt, J.T. and Goodband, R.D. (2022) "A survey of added vitamins and trace minerals in diets utilized in the U.S. swine industry". Kansas Agricultural Experiment Station Research Reports Agricultural Experiment Station, KS 8(10). https://doi.org/10.4148/2378-5977.8388.

Fachinello, M.R., Fernandes, N.L.M., de Souto, E.R., dos Santos, T.C., da Costa, A.E.R. and Pozza, P.C. (2018) Lycopene affects the immune responses of finishing pigs. Ital. J. Anim. Sci. 17(3):666–674. https://doi.org/10.1080/1828051X.2017.1401438.

Fachinello, M.R., Gasparino, E., Monteiro, A.N.T.R., Sangali, C.P., Partyka, A.V.S. and Pozza, P.C. (2020a) Effects of dietary lycopene on the protection against oxidation of muscle and hepatic tissue in finishing pigs. Asian-Australas. J. Anim. Sci. 33(9):1477–1486. https://doi.org/10.5713/ajas.19.0133.

Fachinello, M.R., Gasparino, E., Sturzenegger Partyka, A.V., de Souza Khatlab, A., Castilha, L.D., Diaz Huepa, L.M., Malavazi Ferreira, L.F. and Pozza, P.C. (2020b) Dietary lycopene alters the expression of antioxidant enzymes and modulates the blood lipid profile of pigs. Anim. Prod. Sci. 60(6):806–814. https://doi.org/10.1071/AN18456.

Faustman, C., Cassens, R.G., Schaefer, D.M., Buege, D.R., Williams, S.N. and Scheller, K.K. (1989) Improvement of pigment and lipid stability in Holstein steer beef by dietary supplementation with vitamin E. J. Food Sci. 54(4):858–862. https://doi.org/10.1111/j.1365-2621.1989.tb07899.x.

Faustman, C. and Wang, K. (2000) Vitamin E improves oxidative stability of myoglobin. In Antioxidants in muscle foods: nutritional strategies to improve quality Decker, E.A., Faustman, C. and Lopez-Bote, J. (Ed.). Wiley, Chicter.

FEDNA (Federacion Española Para el Desarrollo Nutricion Animal) (2018) Necesidades nutricionales en avicultura: normas para la formulación de piensos. http://www.fundacionfedna.org/node/75.

FEFANA (2015) Vitamins in animal nutrition. https://fefana.org/app/uploads/2022/06/2015-04-15_booklet_vitamins.pdf.

Feldman, D., Pike, J.W. and Glorieux, F.H. (2003) Vitamin D. Elsevier, Amsterdam.

Feng, J., Wang, L., Chen, Y., Xiong, Y., Wu, Q., Jiang, Z. and Yi, H. (2021) Effects of niacin on intestinal immunity, microbial community and intestinal barrier in weaned piglets during starvation. Int. Immunopharmacol. 95:107584. https://doi.org/10.1016/j.intimp.2021.107584.

Feng, T., Bai, J., Xu, X., Guo, Y., Huang, Z. and Liu, Y. (2018) Supplementation with N-carbamylglutamate and vitamin C: improving gestation and lactation outcomes in sows under heat stress. Anim. Prod. Sci. 58(10):1854–1859. https://doi.org/10.1071/AN15562.

Fenstermacher, D.K. and Rose, R.C. (1986) Absorption of pantothenic acid in rat and chick intestine. Am. J. Physiol. 250(2 Pt 1):G155–G160. https://doi.org/10.1152/ajpgi.1986.250.2.G155.

Ferland, G. (2006) Vitamin K. In Present knowledge in nutrition 9th edition Bowman, B.A. and Russell, R.M. (Eds.). International Life Sciences Institute. (pp. 220–230).

Fichter, S.A. and Mitchell, G.E. (1997) Sheep blood response to orally supplemented vitamin K dissolved in coconut oil. J. Anim. Sci. 72(1):266 (abstr.).

Fidge, N.H., Smith, F.R. and Goodman, D.S. (1969) Vitamin A and carotenoids. The enzymic conversion of beta-carotene into retinal in hog intestinal mucosa. Biochem. J. 114(4):689–694. https://doi.org/10.1042/bj1140689.

Finkelstein, J.D., Martin, J.J., Harris, B.J. and Kyle, W.E. (1982) Regulation of the betaine content of rat liver. Arch. Biochem. Biophys. 218(1):169–173. https://doi.org/10.1016/0003-9861(82)90332-0.

Firth, J. and Johnson, B.C. (1956) Quantitative relationships of tryptophan and nicotinic acid in the baby pig. J. Nutr. 59(2):223–234. https://doi.org/10.1093/jn/59.2.223.

Firth, J., James, M., Chang, S., Mistry, P. and Johnson, B.C. (1953) Vitamin B12 and choline synthesis in the baby pig. J. Anim. Sci. 12:915.

Flachowsky, G., Schöne, F., Schaarmann, G., Lübbe, F. and Böhme, H. (1997) Influence of oilseeds in combination with vitamin E supplementation in the diet on backfat quality of pigs. Anim. Feed Sci. Technol. 64(2–4):91–100. https://doi.org/10.1016/S0377-8401(96)01069-3.

Flohr, J.R., Tokach, M.D., Dritz, S.S., DeRouchey, J.M., Goodband, R.D., Nelssen, J.L. and Bergstrom, J.R. (2014) An evaluation of the effects of added vitamin D3 in maternal diets on sow and pig performance. J. Anim. Sci. 92(2):594–603. https://doi.org/10.2527/jas.2013-6792.

Flohr, J.R., DeRouchey, J.M., Woodworth, J.C., Tokach, M.D., Goodband, R.D. and Dritz, S.S. (2016) A survey of current feeding regimens for vitamins and trace minerals in US swine industry. J. Swine Health Prod. 24(6):290–303.

Follis, R.H. and Wintrobe, M.M. (1945) A comparison of the effects of pyridoxine and pantothenic acid deficiencies on the nervous tissues of swine. J. Exp. Med. 81(6):539–552. https://doi.org/10.1084/jem.81.6.539.

Follis, R.H., Miller, M.H., Wintrobe, M.M. and Stein, H.J. (1943) Development of myocardial necrosis and absence of nerve degeneration in thiamine deficiency in pigs. Am. J. Pathol. 19(2):341–357. PMID: 19970695.

Fonge, J. (1977) Building up biotin beat sagging output. Pig Farming 25(6):61.

Fontaine, M. and Valli, V.E. (1977) Studies on vitamin E and selenium deficiency in young pigs. II. The hydrogen peroxide hemolysis test and the measure of red cell lipid peroxides as indices of vitamin E and selenium status. Can. J. Comp. Med. 41(1):52–56. PMID: 832189.

Fontaine, M., Valli, V.E., Young, L.G. and Lumsden, J.H. (1977a) Studies on vitamin E and selenium deficiency in young pigs. I. Hematological and biochemical changes. Can. J. Comp. Med. 41(1):41–51. PMID: 832188.

Fontaine, M., Valli, V.E. and Young, L.G. (1977b) Studies on vitamin E and selenium deficiency in young pigs. III. Effect on kinetics of erythrocyte production and destruction. Can. J. Comp. Med. 41(1):57–63. PMID: 832190.

Forbes, R.M. and Haines, W.T. (1952) The riboflavin requirement of the baby pig. I. At an environmental temperature of 85 F. and 70% relative humidity. J. Nutr. 47(3):411–424. https://doi.org/10.1093/jn/47.3.411.

Ford, W.C. and Whittington, K. (1998) Antioxidant treatment for male subfertility: a promise that remains unfulfilled. Hum. Reprod. 13(6):1416–1419. https://doi.org/10.1093/oxfordjournals.humrep.a019707.

Fox, H.M. (1991) Pantothenic acid. In Handbook of vitamins 2nd edition Machlin, L.J. (ed.). Marcel Dekker, New York. (pp. 429–451).

Fraga, M.J. and Villamide, M.J. (2000) The composition of vitamin supplements in Spanish pig diets. Pig New Inf. 21:67–72.

Franceschi, R.T. (1992) The role of ascorbic acid in mesenchymal differentiation. Nutr. Rev. 50(3):65–70. https://doi.org/10.1111/j.1753-4887.1992.tb01271.x.

Frank, G.R., Bahr, J.M. and Easter, R.A. (1984) Riboflavin requirement of gestating swine. J. Anim. Sci. 59(6):1567–1572. https://doi.org/10.2527/jas1984.5961567x.

Frank, G.R., Bahr, J.M. and Easter, R.A. (1988) Riboflavin requirement of lactating swine. J. Anim. Sci. 66(1): 47–52. https://doi.org/10.2527/jas1988.66147x.

Frape, D.L., Speer, V.C., Hays, V.W. and Catron, D.V. (1959a) The vitamin A requirement of the young pig. J. Nutr. 68(2):173–187. https://doi.org/10.1093/jn/68.2.173.

Frape, D.L., Speer, V.C., Hays, V.W. and Catron, D.V. (1959b) Thyroid function in the young pig and its relationship with vitamin A. J. Nutr. 68(3):333–341. https://doi.org/10.1093/jn/68.3.333.

Fraser, D.R. (2021) Vitamin D toxicity related to its physiological and unphysiological supply. Trends Endocrinol. Metab. 32(11):929–940. https://doi.org/10.1016/j.tem.2021.08.006.

Frederick, G.L. and Brisson, G.J. (1961) Some observations on the relationship between vitamin B12 and reproduction in swine. Can. J. Anim. Sci. 41(2):212–219. https://doi.org/10.4141/cjas61-029.

Frei, B., England, L. and Ames, B.N. (1989) Ascorbate is an outstanding antioxidant in human blood plasma. Proc. Natl. Acad. Sci. U. S. A. 86(16):6377–6381. https://doi.org/10.1073/pnas.86.16.6377.

Freiser, H. and Jiang, Q. (2009) Optimization of the enzymatic hydrolysis and analysis of plasma conjugated gamma-CEHC and sulfated long-chain carboxychromanols, metabolites of vitamin E. Anal. Biochem. 388(2):260–265. https://doi.org/10.1016/j.ab.2009.02.027.

Friedman, D.I. (2005) Medication-induced intracranial hypertension in dermatology. Am. J. Clin. Dermatol. 6(1):29–37. https://doi.org/10.2165/00128071-200506010-00004.

Friendship, R.M. and Wilson, M.R. (1991) Effects of intramuscular injections of folic acid in sows on subsequent litter size. Can. Vet. J. 32(9):565–566. PMID: 17423862.

Friesecke, H. (1980) Vitamin B12. Vol. 1728. F. Hoffmann-La Roche, and Co. Ltd., Basel.

Frigg, M. (1976) Bio-availability of biotin in cereals. Poult. Sci. 55(6):2310–2318. https://doi.org/10.3382/ps.0552310.

Frigg, M. (1984) Available biotin content of various feed ingredients. Poult. Sci. 63(4):750–753. https://doi.org/10.3382/ps.0630750.

Frigg, M. (1987) Biotin in poultry and swine rations and its significance for optimum performance Proc. Maryland Nutr. Conf. (pp. 101–108).

Frigg, M. and Volker, L. (1994) Biotin inclusion helps optimize animal performance. Feedstuffs 66(1): 12–13.

Fritschen, R.D., Peo, E.R., Lucas, L.E. and Grace, O.D. (1970) Nutritionally induced hemophilia in swine. J. Anim. Sci. 31:199.

Froseth, A.J. (1978) Selenium and Vitamin E: Blood and Tissue Levels in Pigs. Acta Agric. Scand. 28 sup21: 219–231. https://doi.org/10.1080/09064702.1978.11884490.

Frye, T.M. (1994) The performance of vitamins in multicomponent premixes. Proc. Roche Technical Symp.

Fuchs, B., Orda, J. and Wiliczkiewicz, A. (1995) Effect of administering different doses of folic acid to sows on the foetal viability and the number of born piglets. Arch. Vet. Pol. 35(3–4):259–268.

Fuhrmann, H., Sallmann, H.P. and Thesing, E. (1997) Effects of the vitamins A and E on the antioxidative metabolism of weanling pigs given fat of different quality. Dtsch. Tierarztl Wschr. 104(9):387–391. PMID: 9410730.

Funada, U., Wada, M., Kawata, T., Mori, K., Tamai, H., Isshiki, T., Onoda, J., Tanaka, N., Tadokoro, T. and Maekawa, A. (2001) Vitamin B12 deficiency affects immunoglobulin production and cytokine levels in mice. Int. J. Vitam. Nutr. Res. 71(1):60–65. https://doi.org/10.1024/0300-9831.71.1.60.

Funk, C. and Dubin, H.E. (1922) The vitamins. Williams & Wilkins, Co., Baltimore, MD.

Gadient, M. (1986) Effect of pelleting on nutritional quality of feed. Proc. 1986 Maryland Nutrition Conference Feed Manufacturers College Park, Maryland.

Gallop, P.M., Lian, J.B. and Hauschka, P.V. (1980) Carboxylated calcium-binding proteins and vitamin K. N. Engl. J. Med. 302(26):1460–1466. https://doi.org/10.1056/NEJM198006263022608.

Gallo-Torres, H.E. (1970) Obligatory role of bile for the intestinal absorption of vitamin E. Lipids 5(4):379–384. https://doi.org/10.1007/BF02532102.

Gallo-Torres, H.E. (1980) Absorption. In vitamin E: A comprehensive treatise Lawrence, J.M. (Ed.). Marcel Dekker, New York. (pp. 170–193).

Gallo-Torres, H.E., Heimer, E., Scheidl, F., Meienhofer, J. and Miller, O.N. (1980) The gastrointestinal absorption, tissue distribution, urinary excretion and metabolism of N-(2-aminoethyl)-glycine (AEG) in the rat. Life Sci. 27(24):2347–2357. https://doi.org/10.1016/0024-3205(80)90504-4.

Gannon, B., Herrmann, R., Sinha, A., Ghezzi-Kopel, K., Rogers, L., Nieves Garcia-Casal, M.N., Peña-Rosas, J.P. and Mehta, S. (2020) The accuracy of dried blood spots compared to plasma or serum retinol for the diagnosis of vitamin A deficiency: a DTA systematic review and meta-analysis. Curr. Dev. Nutr. 4(2):106. https://doi.org/10.1093/cdn/nzaa041_010.

Gannon, B.M., Davis, C.R., Nair, N., Grahn, M. and Tanumihardjo, S.A. (2017) Single high-dose vitamin A supplementation to neonatal piglets results in a transient dose response in extrahepatic organs and sustained increases in liver stores. J. Nutr. 147(5):798–806. https://doi.org/10.3945/jn.117.247577.

Gardner, H.W. (1989) Oxygen radical chemistry of polyunsaturated fatty acids. Free Radic. Biol. Med. 7(1):65–86. https://doi.org/10.1016/0891-5849(89)90102-0.

Garrow, T.A. (2007) Choline. In Handbook of vitamins 4th edition Zempleni, J., Rucker, R.B., McCormick, D.B. and Suttie, J.W. (ed.). CRC Press, Boca Raton, FL. (pp. 459–487).

Gasperi, V., Sibilano, M., Savini, I. and Catani, M.V. (2019) Niacin in the central nervous system: an update of biological aspects and clinical applications. Int. J. Mol. Sci. 20(4):974. https://doi.org/10.3390/ijms20040974.

Gebert, S., Bee, G., Pfirter, H.P. and Wenk, C. (1999a) Phytase and vitamin E in the feed of growing pigs: 1. Influence on growth, mineral digestibility and fatty acids in digesta. J. Anim. Physiol. Anim. Nutr. 81(1):9–19.

Gebert, S., Bee, G., Pfirter, H.P. and Wenk, C. (1999b) Growth performance and nutrient utilisation as influenced in pigs by microbial phytase and vitamin E supplementation to a diet of high oxidative capacity. Ann. Zootech. 48(2):105–115. https://doi.org/10.1051/animres:19990203.

Gershoff, S.N. (1993) Vitamin C (ascorbic acid): new roles, new requirements? Nutr. Rev. 51(11):313–326. https://doi.org/10.1111/j.1753-4887.1993.tb03757.x.

Ghosh, H.P., Sarkar, P.K. and Guha, B.C. (1963) Distribution of the bound form of nicotinic acid in natural materials. J. Nutr. 79(4):451–453. https://doi.org/10.1093/jn/79.4.451.

Gibson, D.M., Kennelly, J.J. and Aherne, F.X. (1987) The performance and thiamin status of pigs fed sulfur dioxide treated high-moisture barley. Can. J. Anim. Sci. 67(3):841–854. https://doi.org/10.4141/cjas87-087.

Gibson, G.E. and Zhang, H. (2002) Interactions of oxidative stress with thiamine homeostasis promote neurodegeneration. Neurochem. Int. 40(6):493–504. https://doi.org/10.1016/S0197-0186(01)00120-6.

Giguère, A., Matte, J.J. and Girard, C.L. (1998) Characterization of high-affinity folate-binding protein in serum of cow, pig and sheep. J. Anim. Sci. 76(1):184.

Giguère, A., Girard, C.L., Lambert, R., Laforest, J.P. and Matte, J.J. (2000) Reproductive performance and uterine prostaglandin secretion in gilts conditioned with dead semen and receiving dietary supplements of folic acid. Can. J. Anim. Sci. 80(3):467–472. https://doi.org/10.4141/A99-107.

Gipp, W.F., Pond, W.G., Kallfelz, F.A., Tasker, J.B., Van Campen, D.R., Krook, L. and Visek, W.J. (1974) Effect of dietary copper, iron and ascorbic acid levels on hematology, blood and tissue copper, iron and zinc concentrations and 64Cu and 59Fe metabolism in young pigs. J. Nutr. 104(5):532–541. https://doi.org/10.1093/jn/104.5.532.

Glasziou, P.P. and Mackerras, D.E. (1993) Vitamin A supplementation in infectious diseases: a meta-analysis. BMJ 306(6874):366–370. https://doi.org/10.1136/bmj.306.6874.366.

Glättli, H.R., Pohlenz, J., Streiff, K. and Ehrensperger, F. (1975) Clinical and morphologic findings in experimental biotin deficiency. Zentralbl. Veterinarmed. A 22(2):102–116.

Godoy-Parejo, C., Deng, C., Zhang, Y., Liu, W. and Chen, G. (2020) Roles of vitamins in stem cells. Cell. Mol. Life Sci. 77(9):1771–1791. https://https. https://doi.org/10.1007/s00018-019-03352-6.

Goff, J.P., Horst, R.L. and Littledike, E.T. (1984) Effect of sow vitamin D status at parturition on the vitamin D status of neonatal piglets. J. Nutr. 114(1):163–169. https://doi.org/10.1093/jn/114.1.163.

Goff, J.P., Reinhardt, T.A. and Horst, R.L. (1991) Enzymes and factors controlling vitamin D metabolism and action in normal and milk fever cows. J. Dairy Sci. 74(11):4022–4032. https://doi.org/10.3168/jds.S0022-0302(91)78597-4.

Golub, M.S. and Gershwin, M.E. (1985) Stress-induced immunomodulation: what is it, if it is? In Animal stress Moberg, G.P. (ed.). Springer, New York. https://doi.org/10.1007/978-1-4614-7544-6_11.

Gonçalves, A., Roi, S., Nowicki, M., Dhaussy, A., Huertas, A., Amiot, M.J. and Reboul, E. (2015) Fat-soluble vitamin intestinal absorption: absorption sites in the intestine and interactions for absorption. Food Chem. 172:155–160. https://doi.org/10.1016/j.foodchem.2014.09.021.

Goodband, R.D., Nelssen, J.L., Weeden, T.L., Thaler, R.C., Kats, L.J., Blum, S.A., Larsen, L. and Morrow-Tesch, J.L. (1998) The effect of additional niacin during gestation and lactation on sow and litter performance. Prof. Anim. Sci. 14(1):28–35. https://doi.org/10.15232/S1080-7446(15)31787-3.

Goodwin, R.F.W. (1962) Some clinical and experimental observations on naturally-occurring pantothenic-acid deficiency in pigs. J. Comp. Pathol. 72:214–232. https://doi.org/10.1016/S0368-1742(62)80025-3.

Goodwin, R.F.W. and Jennings, A.R. (1958) Mortality of new-born pigs associated with a maternal deficiency of vitamin A. J. Comp. Pathol. 68(1):82–95. https://doi.org/10.1016/S0368-1742(58)80009-0.

Goodwin, T.W. (1984) "The biochemistry of carotenoids. Animals. Chapman & Hall II:(1–21). https://doi.org/10.1007/978-94-009-5542-4_1.

Goss, T. and Bilkei, G. (1994) Influence of vitamin E on the reproduction parameters of the sow. Proceed. 13th IPVS Cong. (p. 274).

Grandhi, R.R. and Strain, J.H. (1980) Effect of biotin supplementation on reproductive performance and foot lesions in swine. Can. J. Anim. Sci. 60(4):961–969. https://doi.org/10.4141/cjas80-114.

Grandhi, R.R., Smith, M.W., Frigg, M. and Thacker, P.A. (1993) Effect of supplemental vitamin E during prepubertal development and early gestation on reproductive performance and nutrient metabolism in gilts. Can. J. Anim. Sci. 73(3):593–603. https://doi.org/10.4141/cjas93-063.

Grant, C.A. (1961) Morphological and etiological studies of dietetic microangiopathy in pigs (mulberry heart). Acta Vet. Scand. 2(3):107.

Gray, J.I. (1990) Vitamin E – its effect on swine growth performance and meat quality. National Feed Ingredients Association (NFIA).

Gray, J.I., Buckley, D.J., Asghar, A., Booren, A.M., Crackel, R.L. and Miller, T.R. (1989) Lipid oxidation in pork products. Nat. Pork Prod. Council Res. Invest. Rep.

Green, R. and Miller, J.W. (2013) Vitamin B12. In Handbook of vitamins 5th edition Zempleni, J., Suttie, J., Gregory, J. and Stover, P.J. (ed.). CRC Press. (pp. 447–490).

Gregoire, F.M., Smas, C.M. and Sul, H.S. (1998) Understanding adipocyte differentiation. Physiol. Rev. 78(3):783–809. https://doi.org/10.1152/physrev.1998.78.3.783.

Gregory, J.F. (1989) Chemical and nutritional aspects of folate research: analytical procedures, methods of folate synthesis, stability and bioavailability of dietary folates. Adv. Food Nutr. Res. 33:1–101. https://doi.org/10.1016/S1043-4526(08)60126-6.

Gregory, J.F. (2001) Case study: folate bioavailability. J. Nutr. 131(4) Supplement:1376S-1382S. https://doi.org/10.1093/jn/131.4.1376S.

Gregory, J.F., Trumbo, P.R., Bailey, L.B., Toth, J.P., Baumgartner, T.G. and Cerda, J.J. (1991a) Bioavailability of pyridoxine-5′-beta-D-glucoside determined in humans by stable-isotopic methods. J. Nutr. 121(2):177–186. https://doi.org/10.1093/jn/121.2.177.

Gregory, J.F., Bhandari, S.D., Bailey, L.B., Toth, J.P., Baumgartner, T.G. and Cerda, J.J. (1991b) Relative bioavailability of deuterium-labeled monoglutamyl and hexaglutamyl folates in human subjects. Am. J. Clin. Nutr. 53(3):736–740. https://doi.org/10.1093/ajcn/53.3.736.

Grela, E. and Jakobsen, K. (1994) Effect of soybean oil and vitamin E on performance and chemical composition of depot fat in growing pigs. Nutr. Admin. Rev. 64(1):49.

Griminger, P. (1984) Vitamin K in animal nutrition: deficiency can be fatal. Part 1. Feedstuffs 56(38):24–25.

Griminger, P. and Donis, O. (1960) Potency of vitamin K1 and two analogues in counteracting the effects of dicumarol and sulfaquinoxaline on the chick. J. Nutr. 70(3):361–368. https://doi.org/10.1093/jn/70.3.361.

Gris, A., Peres-Neto, E., Schimitti da Silva, K., Augusto-Gomes, T.M., Sacco-Surian, S.R., Fronza, N. and Mendes, R.E. (2020) Outbreak of rickets in pigs in the west of Santa Catarina. Acta Sci. Vet. 48. https://doi.org/10.22456/1679-9216.101236.

Groesbeck, C.N., Goodband, R.D., Tokach, M.D., Dritz, S.S., Nelssen, J.L. and DeRouchey, J.M. (2007) Effects of pantothenic acid on growth performance and carcass characteristics of growing-finishing pigs fed diets with or without ractopamine hydrochloride. J. Anim. Sci. 85(10):2492–2497. https://doi.org/10.2527/jas.2005-550.

Grollman, A.P. and Lehninger, A.L. (1957) Enzymic synthesis of L-ascorbic acid in different animal species. Arch. Biochem. Biophys. 69:458–467. https://doi.org/10.1016/0003-9861(57)90510-6.

Grøndalen, T. and Hansen, I. (1981) Effect of megadoses vitamin C on osteochondrosis in pigs. Nord. Vet. Med. 33(9–11):423–426. PMID: 7329783.

Groziak, S.M. and Kirksey, A. (1987) Effects of maternal dietary restriction in vitamin B6 on neocortex development in rats: B6 vitamer concentrations, volume and cell estimates. J. Nutr. 117(6):1045–1052. https://doi.org/10.1093/jn/117.6.1045.

Groziak, S.M. and Kirksey, A. (1990) Effects of maternal dietary restriction in vitamin B6 on neocortex development in rats: neuron differentiation and synaptogenesis. J. Nutr. 120(5):485–492. https://doi.org/10.1093/jn/120.5.485.

Grummer, R.H., Whitehair, C.K., Bohstedt, G. and Phillips, P.H. (1948) Vitamin A, vitamin C and niacin levels in the blood of swine. J. Anim. Sci. 7(2):222–227. https://doi.org/10.2527/jas1948.72222x.

Guay, F., Palin, M.F., Matte, J.J. and Laforest, J.P. (2001) Effects of breed, parity, and folic acid supplement on the expression of leptin and its receptors' genes in embryonic and endometrial tissues from pigs at day 25 of gestation. Biol. Reprod. 65(3):921–927. https://doi.org/10.1095/biolreprod65.3.921.

Guay, F., Matte, J.J., Girad, C.L., Palin, M.F., Giguère, A. and Laforest, J.P. (2002) Effect of folic acid and glycine supplementation on embryo development and folate metabolism during early pregnancy in pigs. J. Anim. Sci. 80(8):2134–2143. https://doi.org/10.1093/ansci/80.8.2134.

Guggenheim, K.Y. (1995) Basic issues of the history of nutrition. Magnes Press, Hebrew University.

Guilarte, T.R. (1993) Vitamin B6 and cognitive development: recent research findings from human and animal studies. Nutr. Rev. 51(7):193–198. https://doi.org/10.1111/j.1753-4887.1993.tb03102.x.

Guilbert, H.R., Miller, R.F. and Hughes, E.H. (1937) The minimum vitamin A and carotene requirement of cattle, sheep and swine. J. Nutr. 13(5):543–564. https://doi.org/10.1093/jn/13.5.543.

Guo, Q., Richert, B.T., Burgess, J.R., Webel, D.M., Orr, D.E., Blair, M., Grant, A.L. and Gerrard, D.E. (2006a) Effect of dietary vitamin E supplementation and feeding period on pork quality. J. Anim. Sci. 84(11):3071–3078. https://doi.org/10.2527/jas.2005-578.

Guo, Q., Richert, B.T., Burgess, J.R., Webel, D.M., Orr, D.E., Blair, M., Fitzner, G.E., Hall, D.D., Grant, A.L. and Gerrard, D.E. (2006b) Effects of dietary vitamin E and fat supplementation on pork quality. J. Anim. Sci. 84(11):3089–3099. https://doi.org/10.2527/jas.2005-456.

Ha, T.Y., Otsuka, M. and Arakawa, N. (1994) Ascorbate indirectly stimulates fatty acid utilization in primary cultured guinea pig hepatocytes by enhancing carnitine synthesis. J. Nutr. 124(5):732–737. https://doi.org/10.1093/jn/124.5.732.

Habibzadeh, N., Schorah, C.J. and Smithells, R.W. (1986) The effects of maternal folic acid and vitamin C nutrition in early pregnancy on reproductive performance in the guinea-pig. Br. J. Nutr. 55(1):23–35. https://doi.org/10.1079/BJN19860006.

Hadden, J.W. (1987) Neuroendocrine modulation of the thymus-dependent immune system. Agonists and mechanisms. Ann. N. Y. Acad. Sci. 496(1):39-–48. https://doi.org/10.1111/j.1749-6632.1987.tb35744.x.

Hakkarainen, J., Lindberg, P., Bengtsson, G. and Jönsson, L. (1978a) Combined therapeutic effect of dietary selenium and vitamin E on manifested VESD syndrome in weaned pigs. Acta Vet. Scand. 19(2):285–297. https://doi.org/10.1186/BF03547633.

Hakkarainen, J., Lindberg, P., Bengtsson, G., Jonsson, L. and Lannek, N. (1978b) Requirement for selenium (as selenite) and vitamin E (as alpha-tocopherol) in weaned pigs. III. The effect on the development of the VESD syndrome of varying selenium levels in a low-tocopherol diet. J. Anim. Sci. 46(4):1001–1008. https://doi.org/10.2527/jas1978.4641001x.

Halama, A.K. (1979) Biotin deficiency in breeding pigs. Wien. Tierätl. Monatsschr. 66:370.

Hale, F. (1935) The Relation of Vitamin a to Anophthalmos in Pigs. Am. J. Ophthalmol. 18(12):1087–1093. https://doi.org/10.1016/S0002-9394(35)90563-3.

Hale, T.W., Rais-Bahrami, K., Montgomery, D.L., Harkey, C. and Habersang, R.W. (1995) Vitamin E toxicity in neonatal piglets. J. Toxicol. Clin. Toxicol. 33(2):123–130. https://doi.org/10.3109/15563659509000461.

Hall, D.D., Cromwell, G.L. and Stahly, T.S. (1985) Hemorrhagic syndrome induced by high dietary calcium levels in growing pigs. J. Anim. Sci. 61(1):319.

Hall, D.D., Cromwell, G.L. and Stahly, T.S. (1986) The vitamin K requirement of the growing pig. J. Anim. Sci. 63(1):268.

Hall, D.D., Cromwell, G.L. and Stahly, T.S. (1991) Effects of dietary calcium, phosphorus, calcium: Phosphorus ratio and vitamin K on performance, bone strength and blood clotting status of pigs. J. Anim. Sci. 69(2):646–655. https://doi.org/10.2527/1991.692646x.

Hamilton, C.R. and Veum, T.L. (1984) Response of sows and litters to added dietary biotin in environmentally regulated facilities. J. Anim. Sci. 59(1):151–157. https://doi.org/10.2527/jas1984.591151x.

Hamilton, C.R. and Veum, T.L. (1986) Effect of biotin and(or) lysine additions to corn-soybean meal diets on the performance and nutrient balance of growing pigs. J. Anim. Sci. 62(1):155–162. https://doi.org/10.2527/jas1986.621155x.

Hamilton, C.R. and Veum, T.L. (2012) Effects of cecal oxytetracycline infusion, and dietary avidin and biotin supplementation on the biotin status of nongravid gilts. J. Anim. Sci. 90(11):3821–3832. https://doi.org/10.2527/jas.2011-4831.

Hamilton, C.R., Veum, T.L., Jewell, D.E. and Siwecki, J.A. (1983) The biotin status of weanling pigs fed semi-purified diets as evaluated by plasma and hepatic parameters. Int. J. Vitam. Nutr. Res. 53(1):44–50. PMID: 6853058.

Hamman, L.L. (1995) Reducing the incidence of low quality (PSE) pork with vitamin/mineral nutritional modulation. Executive Summary. Texas Tech University. http://hdl.handle.net/2346/12343.

Hancock, J.D., Peo, E.R., Lewis, A.J., Crenshaw, T.D. and Moser, B.D. (1986) Vitamin D toxicity in young pigs. J. Anim. Sci. 63(1):268.

Hanke, H.E. and Meade, R.J. (1972) Biotin and pyridoxine additions to diets for pigs weaned at an early age. University of Minnesota Swine Research Report, pp. 18–19.

Hankes, L.V. (1984) Nicotinic acid and nicotinamide. In Handbook of vitamins Machlin, L.J. (ed.). Marcel Dekker Inc., New York.

Hannah, S.S. and Norman, A.W. (1994) 1α,25(OH)2 vitamin D3-regulated expression of the eukaryotic genome. Nutr. Rev. 52(11):376–382. https://doi.org/10.1111/j.1753-4887.1994.tb01368.x.

Harding, J.D.J. (1960) Some observations on the histopathology of mulberry heart disease in pigs. Res. Vet. Sci. 1(2):129–134. https://doi.org/10.1016/S0034-5288(18)35014-8.

Harmon, B.G., Miller, E.R., Hoefer, J.A., Ullrey, D.E. and Luecke, R.W. (1963) Relationship of specific nutrient deficiencies to antibody production in swine. I. Vitamin A. J. Nutr. 79(3):263–268. https://doi.org/10.1093/jn/79.3.263.

Harmon, B.G., Becker, D.E., Jensen, A.H. and Baker, D.H. (1969) Nicotinic acid-tryptophan relationship in the nutrition of the weanling pig. J. Anim. Sci. 28(6):848–852. https://doi.org/10.2527/jas1969.286848x.

Harmon, B.G., Becker, D.E., Jensen, A.H. and Baker, D.H. (1970) Nicotinic acid-tryptophan nutrition and immunologic implications in young swine. J. Anim. Sci. 31(2):339–342. https://doi.org/10.2527/jas1970.312339x.

Harper, A.F., Lindemann, M.D. and Kornegay, E.T. (1989) The effect of supplemental folic acid on ovulation rate and on fetal survival and development at day 45 of gestation in gilts. Virginia Tech livestock res. Rep. 8 19.

Harper, A.F., Lindemann, M.D., Kornegay, E.T. and Knight, J.W. (1991) Diurnal serum folates of gilts fed a single meal containing varying levels of supplemental folic acid. J. Anim. Sci. 69(1):361.

Harper, A.F., Lindemann, M.D., Chiba, L.I., Combs, G.E., Handlin, D.L., Kornegay, E.T. and Southern, L.L. (1994) An assessment of dietary folic acid levels during gestation and lactation on reproductive and lactational performance of sows: a cooperative study. J. Anim. Sci. 72(9):2338–2344. https://doi.org/10.2527/1994.7292338x.

Harper, A.F., Lindemann, M.D. and Kornegay, E.T. (1996) Fetal survival and conceptus development after 42 days of gestation in gilts and sows in response to folic acid supplementation. Can. J. Anim. Sci. 76(1):157–160. https://doi.org/10.4141/cjas96-023.

Harper, A.F., Knight, J.W., Kokue, E. and Usry, J.L. (2003) Plasma reduced folates, reproductive performance, and conceptus development in sows in response to supplementation with oxidized and reduced sources of folic acid. J. Anim. Sci. 81(3):735–744. https://doi.org/10.2527/2003.813735x.

Harris, H.F. (1919). Pellagra. Macmillan Co. New York, New York.

Harrison, E.H. (2012) Mechanisms involved in the intestinal absorption of dietary vitamin A and provitamin A carotenoids Biochim. Biophys. Acta 1821(1):70–77. https://doi.org/10.1016/j.bbalip.2011.06.002.

Harrison, H.E. and Harrison, H.C. (1963) Sodium, potassium, and intestinal transport of glucose, 1-tyrosine, phosphate, and calcium. Am. J. Physiol. 205(1):107–111. https://doi.org/10.1152/ajplegacy.1963.205.1.107.

Harvey, R.B., Kubena, L.F. and Elissalde, M.H. (1995) Effects of aflatoxin on tocopherol and retinol concentrations in growing barrows. Agri-Practice 16(6):12–14. https://doi.org.

Hasan, M., Oster, M., Reyer, H., Wimmers, K. and Fischer, D.C. (2023) Efficacy of dietary vitamin D3 and 25(OH)D3 on reproductive capacities, growth performance, immunity, and bone development in pigs. Br. J. Nutr.:1–10. https://doi.org/10.1017/S0007114523000442.

Hasty, J.L., van Heugten, E.V., See, M.T. and Larick, D.K. (2002) Effect of vitamin E on improving fresh pork quality in Berkshire- and Hampshire-sired pigs. J. Anim. Sci. 80(12):3230–3237. https://doi.org/10.2527/2002.80123230x.

Hayek, M.G., Mitchell, G.E., Harmon, R.J. and Stahly, T.S. (1987) Immunoglobulin transfer to pigs from sows injected with vitamin E and/or selenium. Prog. Rep. Kentucky Agri. Exp. Sta. 299:31.

Hayek, M.G., Mitchell, G.E., Harmon, R.J., Stahly, T.S., Cromwell, G.L., Tucker, R.E. and Barker, K.B. (1989) Porcine immunoglobulin transfer after prepartum treatment with selenium or vitamin E. J. Anim. Sci. 67(5):1299–1306. https://doi.org/10.2527/jas1989.6751299x.

He, C., Deng, J., Hu, X., Zhou, S., Wu, J., Xiao, D., Darko, K.O., Huang, Y., Tao, T., Peng, M., Wang, Z. and Yang, X. (2019) Vitamin A inhibits the action of LPS on the intestinal epithelial barrier function and tight junction proteins. Food Funct. 10(2):1235–1242. https://doi.org/10.1039/c8fo01123k.

Heaney, D.P., Hoefer, J.A., Ullrey, D.E. and Miller, E.R. (1963) Effects of marginal vitamin A intake during gestation in swine. J. Anim. Sci. 22(4):925–928. https://doi.org/10.2527/jas1963.224925x.

Heaney, R.P. and Holick, M.F. (2011) Why the IOM recommendations for vitamin D are deficient. J. Bone Miner. Res. 26(3):455–457. https://doi.org/10.1002/jbmr.328.

Hegazy, E. and Schwenk, M. (1984) Choline uptake by isolated enterocytes of guinea pig. J. Nutr. 114(12):2217–2220. https://doi.org/10.1093/jn/114.12.2217.

Heinemann, W.W., Ensminger, M.E., Cunha, T.J. and McCulloch, E.C. (1946) The relation of the amount of thiamine in the ration of the hog to the thiamine and riboflavin content of the tissue. J. Nutr. 31(1):107–125. https://doi.org/10.1093/jn/31.1.107.

Henderson, L.M. (1984) Vitamin B6. In Nutrition reviews, present knowledge in nutrition 5th edition Olson, R.E., Broquist, H.P., Chichester, O., Darby, W.J., Kolbye, A.C. and Stalvey, R.M. (ed.) The Nutrition Foundation, Inc.

Henderson, L.M. and Gross, C.J. (1979) Metabolism of niacin and niacinamide in perfused rat intestine. J. Nutr. 109(4):654–662. https://doi.org/10.1093/jn/109.4.654.

Hendricks, D.G., Miller, E.R., Ullrey, D.E., Struthers, R.D., Baltzer, B.V., Hoefer, J.A. and Luecke, R.W. (1967) β-carotene vs. retinyl acetate for the baby pig and the effect upon ergocalciferol requirement. J. Nutr. 93(1):37–43. https://doi.org/10.1093/jn/93.1.37.

Henderickx, H.K., Teague, H.S., Redman, D.R. and Grifo, A.P. (1964) Absorption of vitamin B12 from the colon of the pig. J. Anim. Sci. 23(4):1036–1038. https://doi.org/10.2527/jas1964.2341036x.

Hentges, J.F., Grummer, R.H., Phillips, P.H., Bohstedt, G. and Sorensen, D.K. (1952a) Experimental avitaminosis A in young pigs. J. Am. Vet. Med. Assoc. 120(901):213–216. PMID: 14917613.

Hentges, J.F., Grummer, R.H., Phillips, P.H. and Bohstedt, G. (1952b) The minimum requirement of young pigs for a purified source of carotene. J. Anim. Sci. 11(2):266–272. https://doi.org/10.2527/jas1952.112266x.

Herrick, J.B. (1972) The influence of vitamin A on disease states. Vet. Med. Small Anim. Clin. 67(8):906 passim.

Heying, E.K., Grahn, M., Pixley, K.V., Rocheford, T. and Tanumihardjo, S.A. (2013) High-provitamin A carotenoid (Orange) maize increases hepatic vitamin A reserves of offspring in a vitamin A-depleted sow-piglet model during lactation. J. Nutr. 143(7):1141–1146. https://doi.org/10.3945/jn.113.175679.

Hidiroglu, M. (1996) Vitamin A in the tissues of young pigs administered megadoses of vitamin A intramuscularly. J. Anim. Physiol. Anim. Nutr. 75(1–5):257–260. https://doi.org/10.1111/j.1439-0396.1996.tb00489.x.

Hidiroglou, M. and Batra, T.R. (1995) Concentrations of vitamin C in milk of sows and in plasma of piglets. Can. J. Anim. Sci. 75(2):275–277. https://doi.org/10.4141/cjas95-042.

Hidiroglou, M., Farnworth, E. and Butler, G. (1993) Effects of vitamin E and fat supplementation on concentration of vitamin E in plasma and milk of sows and in plasma of piglets. Int. J. Vitam. Nutr. Res. 63(3):180–187. PMID: 8300328.

Hidiroglou, M., Batra, T.R., Farnworth, E.R. and Markham, F. (1995) Effect of vitamin E supplementation on immune status and alpha-tocopherol in plasma of piglets. Reprod. Nutr. Dev. 35(4):443–450. https://doi.org/10.1051/rnd:19950409.

Hidiroglou, N., Madere, R., McDowell, L.R. and Toutain, P.L. (2003) Influence of sources of dietary vitamin E on the maternal transfer of alpha-tocopherol to fetal and neonatal guinea pigs as determined by a stable isotopic technique. Br. J. Nutr. 89(4):455–466. https://doi.org/10.1079/BJN2002788.

Hill, G.M., Link, J.E., Meyer, L. and Fritsche, K.L. (1999) Effect of vitamin E and selenium on iron utilization in neonatal pigs. J. Anim. Sci. 77(7):1762–1768. https://doi.org/10.2527/1999.7771762x.

Hill, K.E., Motley, A.K., Li, X., May, J.M. and Burk, R.F. (2001) Combined selenium and vitamin E deficiency causes fatal myopathy in guinea pigs. J. Nutr. 131(6):1798–1802. https://doi.org/10.1093/jn/131.6.1798.

Hines, E.A., Coffey, J.D., Starkey, C.W., Chung, T.K. and Starkey, J.D. (2013) Improvement of maternal vitamin D status with 25-hydroxycholecalciferol positively impacts porcine fetal skeletal muscle development and myoblast activity. J. Anim. Sci. 91(9):4116–4122. https://doi.org/10.2527/jas.2013-6565.

Hinson, R.B., McCormick, K.A., Moser, R.L., Ackerman, M.A., Main, R.G. and Mahoney, J.A. (2022) Reduced vitamin supplementation with fat-soluble vitamins A, D, and E added at National Research Council requirements may not be adequate for optimal sow and progeny performance. J. Swine Health Prod. 30(2):79–94. https://doi.org/10.54846/jshap/1259.

Hirsch, A. (1982) Vitamin D history, manufacture, analysis and metabolism: An overview. In "Vitamins the life essentials" National Feed Ingredients Association.

Hitchcock, J.P., Miller, E.R., Keahey, K.K. and Ullrey, D.E. (1978) Effects of arsanilic acid and vitamin E upon utilization of natural or supplemental selenium by swine. J. Anim. Sci. 46(2):425–435. https://doi.org/10.2527/jas1978.462425x.

Hjarde, W., Neimann-Sorensen, A., Palludan, B. and Sorensen, P.H. (1961) Investigations concerning vitamin A requirement, utilization and deficiency symptoms in pigs. Acta Agric. Scand. 11(1):13–53. https://doi.org/10.1080/00015126109435653.

Hodges, R.E., Ohlson, M.A. and Bean, W.B. (1958) Pantothenic Acid deficiency in man. J. Clin. Invest. 37(11):1642–1657. https://doi.org/10.1172/JCI103756.

Hoekstra, W.G. (1975) Biochemical function of selenium and its relation to vitamin E. Fed. Proc. 34(11):2083–2089. PMID: 1100437.

Hoffbrand, A.V. (1978) Effects of folate deficiency in man. In Handbook series in nutrition and food, section E: Nutritional disorders Vol. 2 Rechcigl Jr. M. (Ed.). CRC Press Inc. West Palm Beach, Florida.

Hoffmann–La Roche (1979) Rationale for Roche recommended vitamin fortification-swine rations. RCD 5159/979. Hoffmann–La Roche Inc., Nutley, New Jersey.

Hoffmann–La Roche (1984) Roche Technical Bulletin-Vitamin B12. RCD 6723. Hoffmann–La Roche Inc., Nutley, New Jersey.

Hoffmann–La Roche (1991) Vitamin E for swine. RCD 8260/191. Hoffmann–La Roche Inc., Nutley, New Jersey.

Hogan, J.S., Smith, K.L., Weiss, W.P., Todhunter, D.A. and Schockey, W.L. (1990) Relationships among vitamin E, selenium and bovine blood neutrophils. J. Dairy Sci. 73(9):2372–2378. https://doi.org/10.3168/jds.S0022-0302(90)78920-5.

Hogan, J.S., Weiss, W.P., Todhunter, D.A., Smith, K.L. and Schoenberger, P.S. (1992) Bovine neutrophil responses to parenteral vitamin E. J. Dairy Sci. 75(2):399–405. https://doi.org/10.3168/jds.S0022-0302(92)77775-3.

Hogan, J.S., Weiss, W.P., Smith, K.L., Sordillo, L.M. and Williams, S.N. (1996) Alpha-tocopherol concentration in milk and plasma during clinical. J. Dairy Sci. 79(1):71–75. https://doi.org/10.3168/jds.S00220302(96)76335-X.

Holick, M.F. (2007) Vitamin D deficiency. N. Engl. J. Med. 357(3):266–281. https://doi.org/10.1056/NEJMra070553.

Hollander, D. (1973) Vitamin K1 absorption by everted intestinal sacs of the rat. Am. J. Physiol. 225(2):360–364. https://doi.org/10.1152/ajplegacy.1973.225.2.360.

Hong, C., Keying, Z., Xuemei, D. and Daiwen, C. (2012) Biotin affects the immune response of piglets inoculated with porcine circovirus type 2. Turkish Journal of Veterinary & Animal Sciences 36(5):483–490. https://doi.org/10.3906/vet-1007-397.

Hongtrakul, K., Kim, I.H., Loughmiller, J.A., Smith, J.W., Cao, H., Goodband, R.D., Tokach, M.D. and Nelssen, J.L. (1997) Effects of added choline on performance of weanling pigs Kansas state swine research report. Kansas Agricultural Experiment Station Research Reports (10):(70–71). https://doi.org/10.4148/2378-5977.6528.

Hoppe, P.P. (1987) Lethal vitamin K deficiency in weaned piglets. Prakt. Tierarzt 68:32.

Hoppe, P.P., Duthie, G.G., Arthur, J.R., Schoner, F.J. and Wiesche, H. (1989) Vitamin E and vitamin C supplementation and stress-susceptible pigs: Effects of halotthane and pharmacologically induced muscle contractions. Livest. Prod. Sci. 22(3–4):341–350. https://doi.org/10.1016/0301-6226(89)90065-1.

Hoppe, P.P., Schöner, F.J. and Frigg, M. (1992) Effects of dietary retinol on hepatic retinol storage and on plasma and tissue alpha-tocopherol in pigs. Int. J. Vitam. Nutr. Res. 62(2):121–129. PMID: 1517033.

Hoppe, P.P., Schöner, F.J., Wiesche, H., Stahler-Geyer, A., Kammer, J. and Hochadel, H. (1993) Effect of graded dietary alpha-tocopherol supplementation on concentrations in plasma and selected tissues of pigs from weaning to slaughter. Zentralbl. Veterinarmed. A 40(3):219–228. https://doi.org/10.1111/j.1439-0442.1993.tb00620.x.

Horký, P., Zeman, L., Skládanka, J., Nevrkla, P. and Sláma, P. (2016) Effect of selenium, zinc, vitamin C and E on boar ejaculate quality at heat stress. Acta Univ. Agric. Silvic. Mendelianae Brun. 64(4):1167–1172. https://doi.org/10.11118/actaun201664041167.

Hornig, B., Glatthar, B. and Mosw, U. (1984) General aspects of ascorbic acid and metabolism. In Proc. workshop Ascorbic Acid in Domest. Anim. the Royal Danish Agriculture Society Wegger, I., Tagwerker, F.J. and Moustgaard, J. (Eds). Copenhagen, Denmark.

Horst, R.L., Napoli, J.L. and Littledike, E.T. (1982) Discrimination in the metabolism of orally dosed ergocalciferol and cholecalciferol by the pig, rat and chick. Biochem. J. 204(1):185–189. https://doi.org/10.1042/bj2040185.

Hoskinson, C.D., Chew, B.P. and Wong, T.S. (1989) Effects of beta-carotene (BC) and vitamin A (V) on mitogen-induced lymphocyte proliferation in the pig in vivo. FASEB J. 3:A663.

Hoskinson, C.D., Chew, B.P. and Wong, T.S. (1992) Effects of injectable β-carotene and vitamin A on lymphocyte proliferation and polymorphonuclear neutrophil function in piglets. Biol. Neonate 62(5):325–336. https://doi.org/10.1159/000243889.

Hough et al (2021) A summary of evidence for differences in 25(OH)D3 status across different life stages, fortification levels and dietary vitamin D sources. Conference poster presentation.

Hough, S.D., Jennings, S.H. and Almond, G.W. (2015) Thiamine-responsive neurological disorder of swine. J. Swine Health Prod. 23(3):143–151.

Hove, E.L. and Seibold, H.R. (1955) Liver necrosis and altered fat composition in vitamin E-deficient swine. J. Nutr. 56(2):173–186. https://doi.org/10.1093/jn/56.2.173.

Hoving-Bolink, A.H., Eikelenboom, G., Van Diepen, J.T.M., Jongbloed, A.W. and Houben, J.H. (1998) Effect of dietary vitamin E supplementation on pork quality. Meat Sci. 49(2):205–212. https://doi.org/10.1016/S0309-1740(97)00139-3.

Hoz, L., Lopez-Bote, C.J., Cambero, M.I., D'Arrigo, M., Pin, C., Santos, C. and Ordóñez, J.A. (2003) Effect of dietary linseed oil and α-tocopherol on pork tenderloin (psoas major) muscle. Meat Sci. 65(3):1039–1044. https://doi.org/10.1016/S0309-1740(02)00322-4.

Hu, Y., Zhang, L., Zhang, Y., Xiong, H., Wang, F., Wang, Y. and Lu, Z. (2020) Effects of starch and gelatin encapsulated vitamin A on growth performance, immune status and antioxidant capacity in weaned piglets. Anim. Nutr. 6(2):130–133. https://doi.org/10.1016/j.aninu.2020.01.005.

Huang, H.Y. and Appel, L.J. (2003) Supplementation of diets with α-tocopherol reduces serum concentrations of γ- and δ-tocopherol in humans. J. Nutr. 133(10):3137–3140. https://doi.org/10.1093/jn/133.10.3137.

Huang, C., Chiba, L.I., Magee, W.E., Wang, Y., Griffing, D.A., Torres, I.M., Rodning, S.P., Bratcher, C.L., Bergen, W.G. and Spangler, E.A. (2019) Effect of flaxseed oil, animal fat, and vitamin E supplementation on growth performance, serum metabolites, and carcass characteristics of finisher pigs, and physical characteristics of pork. Livest. Sci. 220:143–151. https://doi.org/10.1016/j.livsci.2018.11.011.

Huang, S.W., Frankel, E.N. and German, J.B. (1995) Effects of individual tocopherols and tocopherol mixtures on the oxidative stability of corn oil triglycerides. J. Agric. Food Chem. 43(9):2345–2350. https://doi.org/10.1021/jf00057a006.

Huang, Y., Tang, X., Xie, W., Zhou, Y., Li, D., Zhou, Y., Zhu, J., Yuan, T., Lai, L., Pang, D. and Ouyang, H. (2011) Vitamin C enhances in vitro and in vivo development of porcine somatic cell nuclear transfer embryos. Biochem. Biophys. Res. Commun. 411(2):397–401. https://doi.org/10.1016/j.bbrc.2011.06.160.

Hughes, E.H. (1940) The minimum requirement of riboflavin for the growing pig. J. Nutr. 20(3):233–238. https://doi.org/10.1093/jn/20.3.233.

Hughes, E.H. and Squibb, R.L. (1942) Vitamin B6 (pyridoxine) in the nutrition of the pig. J. Anim. Sci. 1(4):320–325. https://doi.org/10.2527/jas1942.14320x.

Hughes, J.S., Aubel, C.E. and Lienhardt, H.F. (1928) The importance of vitamin A and vitamin C in the ration of swine. Kans. Agric. Exp. Stn. Bull. FAO, Agris.org. 23:1–47.

Hurt, H.D., Hall, R.C., Calhoun, M.C., Rousseau, J.E., Eaton, H.D., Wolke, R.E. and Lucas, J.J. (1966) Chronic hypervitaminosis A in weanling pigs. J. Anim. Sci. 25:891–892.

Hustmyer, F.G., Beitz, D.C., Goff, J.P., Nonnecke, B.J., Horst, R.L. and Reinhardt, T.A. (1994) Effects of in vivo administration of 1,25-dihydroxyvitamin D3 on in vitro proliferation of bovine lymphocytes. J. Dairy Sci. 77(11):3324–3330. https://doi.org/10.3168/jds.S0022-0302(94)77273-8.

Hutagalung, R.I., Chaney, C.H., Wood, R.D. and Waddill, D.G. (1968) Effects of nitrates and nitrites in feed on the utilization of carotene in swine. J. Anim. Sci. 27(1):79–82. https://doi.org/10.2527/jas1968.27179x.

Hutagalung, R.I., Cromwell, G.L., Hays, V.W. and Chaney, C.H. (1969) Effect of dietary fat, protein, cholesterol and ascorbic acid on performance, serum and tissue cholesterol levels and serum lipid levels of swine. J. Anim. Sci. 29(5):700–705. https://doi.org/10.2527/jas1969.295700x.

Huyghebaert, A. (1991) Stability of vitamin K in a mineral premix. World Poult. 7:71.

Hvidsten, J. and Astrup, J.N. (1973) The effect of vitamin E on the keeping quality of pork. Acta Agric. Scand. 13:259–270.

Hypor (2017) Wean to finish feeding guide version 2.0. https://www.hypor.com/en/about/.

Höller, U., Bakker, S.J., Düsterloh, L., Frei, A., Körrle, B., Konz, J., Lietz, T., McCann, G. and Michels, A. (2018) Micronutrient status assessment in humans: Current methods of analysis and future trends. Trends Anal. Chem. 102:110–122. https://doi.org/10.1016/j.trac.2018.02.001.

Ikeda, S., Takasu, M., Matsuda, T., Kakinuma, A. and Horio, F. (1997) Ascorbic acid deficiency decreases the renal level of kidney fatty acid-binding protein by lowering the alpha2u-globulin gene expression in liver in scurvy-prone ods rats. J. Nutr. 127(11):2173–2178. https://doi.org/10.1093/jn/127.11.2173.

Ingram, R.T., Park, Y.K., Clarke, B.L. and Fitzpatrick, L.A. (1994) Age- and gender-related changes in the distribution of osteocalcin in the extracellular matrix of normal male and female bone. Possible involvement of osteocalcin in bone remodeling. J. Clin. Invest. 93(3):989–997. https://doi.org/10.1172/JCI117106.

Isabel, B., J Lopez-Bote, C., Rey, A.I. and Sanz Arias, R. (1999) Influence of dietary α-tocopheryl acetate supplementation of pigs on oxidative deterioration and weight loss in sliced dry-cured ham. Meat Sci. 51(3):227–232. https://doi.org/10.1016/S0309-1740(98)00115-6.

Iskakova, M., Karbyshev, M., Piskunov, A. and Rochette-Egly, C.R. (2015) Nuclear and extranuclear effects of vitamin A. Can. J. Physiol. Pharmacol. 93(12):1065–1075. https://doi.org/10.1139/cjpp-2014-0522.

IUPAC-IUB (1973) Commission on Biochemical Nomenclature. Amendments and corrections (1973) Biochem. J. 135(1):9–10. https://doi.org/10.1042/bj1350009.

Ivers, D.J., Rodhouse, S.L., Ellersieck, M.R. and Veum, T.L. (1993) Effect of supplemental niacin on sow reproduction and sow and litter performance. J. Anim. Sci. 71(3):651–655. https://doi.org/10.2527/1993.713651x.

Ivos, J., Doplihar, C. and Muhaxhiri, G. (1971) Thermic stress as a factor of disturbances in the reproduction of pigs and possibility of prevention of these disturbances by the addition of ascorbic acid. Veteriwarski Arh. Zagreb Knjiga 41(7–8):202–216.

Jacob, R.A. (1995) The integrated antioxidant system. Nutr. Res. 15(5):755–766. https://doi.org/10.1016/0271-5317(95)00041-G.

Jacob, R.A. (2006) Niacin. In "Present knowledge in nutrition" 9th edition Bowman, B.A. and Russell, R.M. (ed.). International Life Sciences Institute. (pp. 261–268).

Jacob, R.A., Wu, M.M., Henning, S.M. and Swendseid, M.E. (1994) Homocysteine increases as folate decreases in plasma of healthy men during short-term dietary folate and methyl group restriction. J. Nutr. 124(7):1072–1080. https://doi.org/10.1093/jn/124.7.1072.

Jang, Y.D., Ma, J.Y., Monegue, J.S., Monegue, H.J., Stuart, R.L. and Lindemann, M.D. (2015) Temporal plasma vitamin concentrations are altered by fat-soluble vitamin administration in suckling pigs. J. Anim. Sci. 93(11):5273–5282. https://doi.org/10.2527/jas.2015-9221.

Jang, Y.D., Rotering, M.J., Isensee, P.K., Rinholen, K.A., Boston-Denton, C.J., Kelley, P.G. and Stuart, R.L. (2020) Distribution of injected fat-soluble vitamins in plasma and tissues of nursery pigs. Asian-Australas J. Anim. Sci. 33(12):1985–1990. https://doi.org/10.5713/ajas.19.0987.

Jensen, C., Guider, J., Skovgaar, I.M., Staun, H., Skibsted, L.H., Jensen, S.K., Møller, A.J., Buckley, J. and Bertelsen, G. (1997) Effects of dietary α-tocopheryl acetate supplementaţion on α-tocopherol deposition in porcine m. Psoas major and m. longissimus dorsi and on drip loss, colour stability and oxidative stability of pork meat. Meat Sci. 45(4):491–500. https://doi.org/10.1016/S0309-1740(96)00130-1.

Jensen, C., Lauridsen, C. and Bertelsen, G. (1998) Dietary vitamin E: quality and storage stability of pork and poultry. Food Sci. Technol. 9(2):62–72. https://doi.org/10.1016/S0924-2244(98)00004-1.

Jensen, M., Fossum, C., Ederoth, M. and Hakkarainen, R.V.J. (1988) The effect of vitamin E on the cell-mediated immune response in pigs. Zentralbl. Veterinarmed. B 35(7):549–555. https://doi.org/10.1111/j.1439-0450.1988.tb00528.x.

Jensen, M., Lindholm, A. and Hakkarainen, J. (1990) The vitamin E distribution in serum, liver, adipose and muscle tissues in the pig during depletion and repletion. Acta Vet. Scand. 31(2):129–136. https://doi.org/10.1186/BF03547553.

Jensen, P.T. and Basse, A. (1984) Inborn ascorbic acid deficiency in pigs. In Proc. Workshop on Ascorbic Acid in Domestic Animals Wegger, I., Tagwerker, F.J. and Moustgaard, J. (Eds.). Royal Danish Agricultural Society.

Jensen, P.T., Basse, A., Nielsen, D.H. and Larsen, H. (1983) Congenital ascorbic acid deficiency in pigs. Acta Vet. Scand. 24(4):392–402. https://doi.org/10.1186/BF03546713.

Jensen, S.K., Nørgaard, J.V. and Lauridsen, C. (2006) Bioavailability of α-tocopherol stereoisomers in rats depends on dietary doses of all-rac- or RRR-α-tocopheryl acetate. Br. J. Nutr. 95(3):477–487. https://doi.org/10.1079/BJN20051667.

Jewell, D.E., Siwecki, J.A. and Veum, T.L. (1981) The effect of dietary vitamin C on performance and tissue vitamin C levels in neonatal pigs. J. Anim. Sci. 53(1):249.

Jiang, X., Yan, J. and Caudill, M.A. (2013) Choline. In "Handbook of vitamins" 5th edition Zempleni, J., Suttie, J., Gregory, J. and Stover, P.J. (ed.). CRC Press. (pp. 491–514).

Jin, C.L., Gao, C.Q., Wang, Q., Zhang, Z.M., Xu, Y.L., Li, H.C., Yan, H.C. and Wang, X.Q. (2018) Effects of pioglitazone hydrochloride and vitamin E on meat quality, antioxidant status and fatty acid profiles in finishing pigs. Meat Sci. 145:340–346. https://doi.org/10.1016/j.meatsci.2018.07.008.

Joachim, A. and Shrestha, A. (2019) Coccidiosis of pigs. In "Coccidiosis in livestock, poultry, companion animals, and humans". CRC Press. (pp. 125–145).

John, A. and Sivakumar, B. (1989) Effect of vitamin A deficiency on nitrogen balance and hepatic urea cycle enzymes and intermediates in rats. J. Nutr. 119(1):29–35. https://doi.org/10.1093/jn/119.1.29.

Johnson, B.C. and James, M.F. (1948) Choline deficiency in the baby pig. J. Nutr. 36(3):339–349. https://doi.org/10.1093/jn/36.3.339.

Johnson, B.C., Neumann, A.L., Nesheim, R.O., James, M.F., Krider, J.L., Dana, A.S. and Thiersch, J.B. (1950) The interrelationship of vitamin B12 and folic acid in the baby pig. J. Lab. Clin. Med. 36(4):537–546.

Johnson, D.W. and Palmer, L.S. (1939) Individual and breed variations in pigs on rations devoid of vitamin D. J. Agric. Res. 58:929–940. naldc.nal.usda.gov.

Johnson, E.J., Qin, J., Krinsky, N.I. and Russell, R.M. (1997) Ingestion by men of a combined dose of beta-carotene and lycopene does not affect the absorption of beta-carotene but improves that of lycopene. J. Nutr. 127(9):1833–1837. https://doi.org/10.1093/jn/127.9.1833.

Johnson, M.A. and Kimlin, M.G. (2006) Vitamin D, aging, and the 2005 dietary guidelines for Americans. Nutr. Rev. 64(9):410–421. https://doi.org/10.1111/j.1753-4887.2006.tb00226.x.

Johnson, N.C., Popoola, S.O. and Owen, O.J. (2019) Effects of single and combined antioxidant vitamins on growing pig performance and pork quality. Inter. J. Adv. Res. Public 3(8):86–89.

Johnson, N.C. and Popoola, S.O. (2020) Dietary effects of single and combined antioxidant vitamins on antioxidant enzymes and oxidants status of growing pigs. Int. J. Adv. Res. Publ. 4(3).

Johnston, C.S. (2006) Vitamin C. In "Present knowledge in nutrition" 9th edition Bowman, B.A. and Russell, R.M. (ed.). agris.fao.org. International Life Sciences Institute, Washington, DC. (pp. 233–241).

Johnston, C.S. and Huang, S.N. (1991) Effect of ascorbic acid nutriture on blood histamine and neutrophil chemotaxis in guinea pigs. J. Nutr. 121(1):126–130. https://doi.org/10.1093/jn/121.1.126.

Johnston, C.S., Steinberg, F.M. and Rucker, R.B. (2013) Ascorbic acid. In "Handbook of vitamins" 5th edition Zempleni, J., Suttie, J., Gregory, J. and Stover, P.J. (ed.). CRC Press, Boca Raton, FL. (pp. 515–550).

Jolly, D.W., Craig, C. and Nelson, T.E. (1977) Estrogen and prothrombin synthesis: effect of estrogen on absorption of vitamin K. Am. J. Physiol. Heart Circ. 232:12. https://doi.org/10.1152/ajpheart.1977.232.1.H12.

Kaempf-Rotzoll, D.E., Traber, M.G. and Arai, H. (2003) Vitamin E and transfer proteins. Curr. Opin. Lipidol. 14(3):249–254. https://doi.org/10.1097/00041433-200306000-00004.

Kallner, A., Hartmann, D. and Hornig, D. (1977) On the absorption of ascorbic acid in man. Int. J. Vitam. Nutr. Res. 47(4):383–388. PMID: 591210.

Kam, K.T., R., Deng, Y., Chen, Y. and Zhao, H. (2012) Retinoic acid synthesis and functions in early embryonic development. Cell Biosci. 2:1–14. https://doi.org/10.1186/2045-3701-2-11.

Kandasamy, S., Chattha, K.S., Vlasova, A.N. and Saif, L.J. (2014) Prenatal vitamin A deficiency impairs adaptive immune responses to pentavalent rotavirus vaccine (RotaTeq®) in a neonatal gnotobiotic pig model. Vaccine 32(7):816–824. https://doi.org/10.1016/j.vaccine.2013.12.039.

Kaneko, K., Kiyose, C., Ueda, T., Ichikawa, H. and Igarashi, O. (2000) Studies of the metabolism of a-tocopherol stereoisomers in rats using [5-methyl-14C] SRR- and RRR-a-tocopherol. J. Lipid Res. 41(3):357–367. https://doi.org/10.1016/S0022-2275(20)34474-6.

Kang, H.G., Lee, S., Jeong, P.S., Kim, M.J., Park, S.H., Joo, Y.E., Park, S.H., Song, B.S., Kim, S.U., Kim, M.K. and Sim, B.W. (2021) Lycopene improves in vitro development of porcine embryos by reducing oxidative stress and apoptosis. Antioxidants (Basel) 10(2):230. https://doi.org/10.3390/antiox10020230.

Kao, C. and Robinson, R.J. (1972) Aspergillus flavus deterioration of grain: its effect on amino acids and vitamins in whole wheat. J. Food Sci. 37(2):261–263. https://doi.org/10.1111/j.1365-2621.1972.tb05831.x.

Käser, T., Gerner, W. and Saalmüller, A. (2011) Porcine regulatory T cells: mechanisms and T-cell targets of suppression. Dev. Comp. Immunol. 35(11):1166–1172. https://doi.org/10.1016/j.dci.2011.04.006.

Kastner, P., Chambon, P. and Leid, M. (1994) "The role of nuclear retinoic acid receptors in the regulation of gene expression in 'vitamin A in health and disease'" Blomhoff, R. (Ed.). Marcel Dekker, New York. (pp. 189–238).

Ke, Z.J. and Gibson, G.E. (2004) Selective response of various brain cell types during neurodegeneration induced by mild impairment of oxidative metabolism. Neurochem. Int. 45(2–3):361–369. https://doi.org/10.1016/j.neuint.2003.09.008.

Kelley, K. and Easter, R. (1987) Nutritional factors can influence immune response of swine. Feedstuffs 59(22):14.

Kerth, C.R., Carr, M.A., Ramsey, C.B., Brooks, J.C., Johnson, R.C., Cannon, J.E. and Miller, M.F. (2001) Vitamin-mineral supplementation and accelerated chilling effects on quality of pork from pigs that are monomutant or noncarriers of the halothane gene. J. Anim. Sci. 79(9):2346–2355. https://doi.org/10.2527/2001.7992346x.

Kesavan, V. and Noronha, J.M. (1983) Folate malabsorption in aged rats related to low levels of pancreatic folyl conjugase. Am. J. Clin. Nutr. 37(2):262–267. https://doi.org/10.1093/ajcn/37.2.262.

Khan, R.U., Rahman, Z.U., Nikousefat, Z., Javdani, M., Tufarelli, V., Dario, C., Selvaggi, M. and Laudadio, V. (2012) Immunomodulating effects of vitamin E in broilers. World's Poultry Science Journal 68(1):31–40. https://doi.org/10.1017/S0043933912000049.

Kilbride, A.L., Gillman, C.E. and Green, L.E. (2009) A cross sectional study of the prevalence, risk factors and population attributable fractions for limb and body lesions in lactating sows on commercial farms in England. BMC Vet. Res. 5:30. https://doi.org/10.1186/1746-6148-5-30.

Kilbride, A.L., Gillman, C.E. and Green, L.E. (2010) A cross-sectional study of prevalence and risk factors for foot lesions and abnormal posture in lactating sows on commercial farms in England. Anim. Welf. 19(4):473–480. https://doi.org/10.1017/S0962728600001950.

Kim, J.C., Jose, C.G., Trezona, M., Moore, K.L., Pluske, J.R. and Mullan, B.P. (2015) Supra-nutritional vitamin E supplementation for 28 days before slaughter maximizes muscle vitamin E concentration in finisher pigs. Meat Sci. 110:270–277. https://doi.org/10.1016/j.meatsci.2015.08.007.

Kim, T.H., Yang, J., Darling, P.B. and O'Connor, D.L. (2004) A Large pool of available folate exists in the large intestine of human infants and piglets. J. Nutr. 134(6):1389–1394. https://doi.org/10.1093/jn/134.6.1389.

Kim, Y.I., Miller, J.W., Da Costa, K.A., Nadeau, M., Smith, D., Selhub, J., Zeisel, S.H. and Mason, J.B. (1994) Severe folate deficiency causes secondary depletion of choline and phosphocholine in rat liver. J. Nutr. 124(11):2197–2203. https://doi.org/10.1093/jn/124.11.2197.

Kirchgessner, M. and Kösters, W.W. (1977) Influence of vitamin B6 deficiency in early weaned piglets on the digestibility and conversion of protein and energy. Arch. Tierernähr. 27(5):299–308. https://doi.org/10.1080/17450397709424583.

Kirkland, J.B. (2013) Niacin. In "Handbook of vitamins" 5th edition Zempleni, J., Suttie, J., Gregory, J. and Stover, P.J. (Eds). Taylor & Francis Group. (pp. 149–190).

Kiyose, C., Muramatsu, R., Ueda, T. and Igarashi, O. (1995) Change in the distribution of alpha-tocopherol stereoisomers in rats after intravenous administration. Biosci. Biotechnol. Biochem. 59(5):791–795. https://doi.org/10.1271/bbb.59.791.

Kliewer, S.A., Umesono, K., Mangelsdorf, D.J. and Evans, R.M. (1992) Retinoid X receptor interacts with nuclear receptors in retinoic acid, thyroid hormone and vitamin D3 signaling. Nature 355(6359):446–449. https://doi.org/10.1038/355446a0.

Kliewer, S.A., Umesono, K., Evans, R.M. and Mangelsdorf, D. (1994) Retinoid X receptor interacts with nuclear receptors in retinoic acid, thyroid hormone and vitamin D3 signaling. In "Vitamin A in health and disease" Blomhoff, R. (Ed.). Marcel Dekker, New York.

Knauer, M., Stalder, K.J., Karriker, L., Baas, T.J., Johnson, C., Serenius, T., Layman, L. and McKean, J.D. (2007) A descriptive survey of lesions from cull sows harvested at two Midwestern US facilities. Prev. Vet. Med. 82(3–4):198–212. https://doi.org/10.1016/j.prevetmed.2007.05.017.

Knap, P.W. (2009) Voluntary feed intake and pig breeding. In "Voluntary feed intake in pigs". Wageningen Academic Publishers, Wageningen, pp. 13–31.

Knights, T.E.N., Grandhi, R.R. and Baidoo, S.K. (1998) Interactive effects of selection for lower backfat and dietary pyridoxine levels on reproduction, and nutrient metabolism during the gestation period in yorkshire and Hampshire sows. Can. J. Anim. Sci. 78(2):167–173. https://doi.org/10.4141/A96-116.

Kodentsova, V.M., Yakusina, L.M., Vrzhesinskaya, O.A., Beketova, N.A. and Sprichev, V.B. (1993) Effect of riboflavin status on pyridoxine metabolism. Vopr.-Pitan. 5:32.

Kodicek, E., Braude, R., Kon, S.K. and Mitchell, K.G. (1956) The effect of alkaline hydrolysis of maize on the availability of its nicotinic acid to the pig. Br. J. Nutr. 10(1):51–67. https://doi.org/10.1079/BJN19560010.

Kodicek, E., Braude, R., Kon, S.K. and Mitchell, K.G. (1959) The availability to pigs of nicotinic acid in tortilla baked from maize treated with limewater. Br. J. Nutr. 13(3):363–384. https://doi.org/10.1079/BJN19590047.

Kodicek, E., Ashby, D.R., Muller, M. and Carpenter, K.J. (1974) The conversion of bound nicotinic acid to free nicotinamide on roasting sweet corn. Proc. Nutr. Soc. 33(3):105A-106A. PMID: 4282141.

Kokue, E., Mizuno, Y. and Shimoda, M. (1998) Synthetic folic acid may interfere with folate bioavailability in pigs. J. Anim. Sci. 76(suppl. 1):184.

Kolb, E. (1984) Metabolism of ascorbic acid in livestock under pathological conditions. In "Ascorbic acid in domestic animals" Wegger, I., Tagwerker, F.J. and Moustgaard, J. (Eds). Workshop. Danish, R. Agr. Soc. Copenhagen. (pp. 162–175).

Kolb, E. and Seehawer, J. (1997) The significance of carotenes and of vitamin A for the reproduction of cattle, of horses, and of pigs – a review. Det. Prakt. Tierarzt 78(9):783–789.

Kominato, T. (1971). Speed of vitamin B 12 turnover and its relation to the intestine in the rat. Bitamin (Vitamins), 44(2), 76–83.

Konowalchuk, J.D., Rieger, A.M., Kiemele, M.D., Ayres, D.C. and Barreda, D.R. (2013) Modulation of weanling pig cellular immunity in response to diet supplementation with 25-hydroxyvitamin D3. Vet. Immunol. Immunopathol. 155(1–2):57–66. https://doi.org/10.1016/j.vetimm.2013.06.002.

Kopinski, J.S. and Leibholz, J. (1985) Post-ileal absorption of biotin in the pig. Proc. Nutr. Soc. Australia 10:170. agris.fao.org.

Kopinski, J.S. and Leibholz, J. (1989) Biotin studies in pigs. 2. The biotin requirement of the growing pig. Br. J. Nutr. 62(3):761–766. https://doi.org/10.1079/bjn19890076.

Kopinski, J.S., Leibholz, J. and Bryden, W.L. (1989a) Biotin studies in pigs. 4. Biotin availability in feedstuffs for pigs and chickens. Br. J. Nutr. 62(3):773–780. https://doi.org/10.1079/bjn19890078.

Kopinski, J.S., Leibholz, J. and Bryden, W.L. (1989b) Biotin studies in pigs. 3. Biotin absorption and synthesis. Br. J. Nutr. 62(3):767–772. https://doi.org/10.1079/bjn19890077.

Kopinski, J.S., Leibholz, J. and Love, R.J. (1989c) Biotin studies in pigs. 5. The post-ileal absorption of biotin. Br. J. Nutr. 62(3):781–789. https://doi.org/10.1079/bjn19890079.

Kopinski, J.S., Leibholz, J., Bryden, W.L. and Fogarty, A.C. (1989d) Biotin studies in pigs. 1. Biotin deficiency in the young pig. Br. J. Nutr. 62(3):751–759. https://doi.org/10.1079/bjn19890075.

Kornegay, E.T. (1986) Biotin in swine production: a review. Livest. Prod. Sci. 14(1):65–89. https://doi.org/10.1016/0301-6226(86)90097-7.

Kornegay, E.T. and Meacham, T.N. (1973) Evaluation of supplemental choline for reproducing sows housed in total confinement on concrete or in dirt lots. J. Anim. Sci. 37(2):506–509. https://doi.org/10.2527/jas1973.372506x.

Kornegay, E.T., Meldrum, J.B., Schurig, G., Lindemann, M.D. and Gwazdauskas, F.C. (1986) Lack of influence of nursery temperature on the response of weanling pigs to supplemental vitamins C and E. J. Anim. Sci. 63(2):484–491. https://doi.org/10.2527/jas1986.632484x.

Kornegay, E.T., Van Heugten, P.H.G., Lindemann, M.D. and Blodgett, D.J. (1989) Effects of biotin and high copper levels on performance and immune response of weanling pigs. J. Anim. Sci. 67(6):1471–1477. https://doi.org/10.2527/jas1989.6761471x.

Kostadinović, L., Teodosin, S., Lević, J., Čolović, R., Banjac, V., Vukmirović, Đ. and Sredanović, S. (2014) Uticaj peletiranja I ekspandiranja na stabilnost vitamin A A u hrani za životinje. J. Process. Energy Agric. 18(1):44–46. 1821–4487.

Kösters, W.W. and Kirchgessner, M. (1976) Change in feed intake of early-weaned piglets in response to different vitamin B6 supply. Z. Tierphysiol. Tierernähr. Futtermittelkd. 37(5):247–254. PMID: 1070212.

Kremer, B.T. and Stahly, T.S. (1999) The effect of dietary vitamin C on meat quality of pork. J. Anim. Sci. 77(1):46.

Krinke, G.J. and Fitzgerald, R.E. (1988) The pattern of pyridoxine-induced lesion: difference between the high and the low toxic level. Toxicology 49(1):171–178. https://doi.org/10.1016/0300-483X(88)90190-4.

Krishnan, S., Bhuyan, U.N., Talwar, G.P. and Ramalingaswami, R. (1974) Effect of vitamin A and protein calorie undernutrition on immune responses. Immunol. 27(3):383–392. PMID: 4213063.

Kristensen, B., Thomsen, P.D., Palludan, B. and Wegger, I. (1986) Mitogen stimulation of lymphocytes in pigs with hereditary vitamin C deficiency. Acta Vet. Scand. 27(4):486–496. https://doi.org/10.1186/BF03548128.

Kroening, G.H. and Pond, W.G. (1967) Methionine, choline and threonine interrelationships for growth and lipotropic action in the baby pig and rat. J. Anim. Sci. 26(2):352–357. https://doi.org/10.2527/jas1967.262352x.

Krumdieck, C.L. (1990) Folic acid. In "Present knowledge in nutrition" 6th edition Int. Brown, M.L. (Ed.) Life Sci. Institute/Nutrition Foundation. (pp. 179–188).

Kumar, S., Pandey, A.K., Rao, M.M. and Razzaque, W.A.A. (2010) Role of β carotene/vitamin A in animal reproduction. Vet. World 3(5):236–237.

Kurnick, A.A., Hanold, F.J. and Stangeland, V.A. (1972) Problems in the use of feed ingredient vitamin values in formulating feeds Proc. 1972 Georgia Nutr. Conf. Feed Ind.

Laenoi, W., Uddin, M.J., Cinar, M.U., Phatsara, C., Tesfaye, D., Scholz, A.M., Tholen, E., Looft, C., Mielenz, M., Sauerwein, H. and Schellander, K. (2010) Molecular characterization and methylation study of matrix gla protein in articular cartilage from pig with osteochondrosis. Gene 459(1–2):24–31. https://doi.org/10.1016/j.gene.2010.03.009.

Lakshmi, A.V., Prasad, R.K. and Bamji, M.S. (1990) Effect of riboflavin deficiency on collagen content of cornea and bone. J. Clin. Biochem. Nutr. 9(2):115–118. https://doi.org/10.3164/jcbn.9.115.

Lakshmi, R., Lakshmi, A.V. and Bamji, M.S. (1989) Skin wound healing in riboflavin deficiency. Biochem. Med. Metab. Biol. 42(3):185–191. https://doi.org/10.1016/0885-4505(89)90054-6.

Lanari, M.C., Schaefer, D.M. and Scheller, K.K. (1995) Dietary vitamin E supplementation and discoloration of pork bone and muscle following modified atmosphere packaging. Meat Sci. 41(3):237–250. https://doi.org/10.1016/0309-1740(95)00006-7.

Langel, S.N., Paim, F.C., Alhamo, M.A., Lager, K.M., Vlasova, A.N. and Saif, L.J. (2019) Oral vitamin A supplementation of porcine epidemic diarrhea virus infected gilts enhances IgA and lactogenic immune protection of nursing piglets. Vet. Res. 50(1):101. https://doi.org/10.1186/s13567-019-0719-y.

Lannek, N., Lindberg, P., Nilsson, G., Nordström, G. and Orstadius, K. (1961) Production of vitamin E deficiency and muscular dystrophy in pigs. Res. Vet. Sci. 2(1):67–72. https://doi.org/10.1016/S0034-5288(18)34980-4.

Larsen, H.J. and Tollersrud, S. (1981) Effect of dietary vitamin E and selenium on the phytohaemagglutinin response of pig lymphocytes. Res. Vet. Sci. 31(3):301–305. https://doi.org/10.1016/S0034-5288(18)32461-5.

Lassaletta, L., Estellés, F., Beusen, A.H.W., Bouwman, L., Calvet, S., Van Grinsven, H.J.M., Doelman, J.C., Stehfest, E., Uwizeye, A. and Westhoek, H. (2019) Future global pig production systems according to the shared socioeconomic pathways. Sci. Total Environ. 665:739–751. https://doi.org/10.1016/j.scitotenv.2019.02.079.

Latshaw, J.D. (1991) Nutrition-mechanisms of immunosuppression. Vet. Immunol. Immunopathol. 30(1):111–120. https://doi.org/10.1016/0165-2427(91)90012-2.

Lauridsen, C. (2014) Triennial Growth Symposium–Establishment of the 2012 vitamin D requirements in swine with focus on dietary forms and levels of vitamin D. J. Anim. Sci. Triennial growth symposium—establishment of the 2012 vitamin D requirements in swine with focus on dietary forms and levels of vitamin D 92(3):910–916. https://doi.org/10.2527/jas.2013-7201.

Lauridsen, C. and Jensen, S.K. (2005) Influence of supplementation of all-rac-α-tocopheryl acetate pre-weaning and vitamin C postweaning on α-tocopherol and immune responses of piglets. J. Anim. Sci. 83(6):1274–1286. https://doi.org/10.2527/2005.8361274x.

Lauridsen, C. and Matte, J.J. (2017) Recent advances in understanding the role of vitamins in pig nutrition. In "Achieving sustainable production of pig meat" Wiseman, J. (Ed.). Burleigh Dodds Science Publishing. https://doi.org/10.1201/9781351114349.

Lauridsen, C., Engel, H., Jensen, S.K., Craig, A.M. and Traber, M.G. (2002) Lactating sows and suckling piglets preferentially incorporate RRR-over all rac-α-tocopherol into milk, plasma, and tissues. J. Nutr. 132(6):1258–1264. https://doi.org/10.1093/jn/132.6.1258.

Lauridsen, C., Halekoh, U., Larsen, T. and Jensen, S.K. (2010) Reproductive performance and bone status markers of gilts and lactating sows supplemented with two different forms of vitamin D. J. Anim. Sci. 88(1):202–213. https://doi.org/10.2527/jas.2009-1976.

Lauridsen, C., Vestergaard, E.M., Højsgaard, S., Jensen, S.K. and Sørensen, M.T. (2011) Inoculation of weaned pigs with E. coli reduces depots of vitamin E. Livest. Sci. 137(1–3):161–167. https://doi.org/10.1016/j.livsci.2010.10.015.

Lauridsen, C., Schönherz, A.A. and Højsgaard, S. (2021a) Effect of maternal dietary redox levels on anti-oxidative status and immunity of the suckling off-spring. Antioxidants (Basel) 10(3):478. https://doi.org/10.3390/antiox10030478.

Lauridsen, C., Matte, J.J., Lessard, M., Celi, P. and Litta, G. (2021b) Role of vitamins for gastro-intestinal functionality and health of pigs. Anim. Feed Sci. Technol. 273:114823. https://doi.org/10.1016/j.anifeedsci.2021.114823.

Lechowski, J. (2009) Effect of vitamin C on semen quality of Duroc breed boars and their crossbreds with Hampshire and Pietrain. Annales UMCS, Zootechnic 27(2):12–18.

Lechowski, J., Kasprzyk, A., Tyra, M. and Trawińska, B. (2016) Effect of ascorbic acid as a feed additive on indicators of the reproductive performance of Pulawska breed gilts. Med. Weter. 72(6):378–382. https://doi.org/10.21521/mw.5518.

Lechowski, J., Kasprzyk, A. and Trawińska, B. (2018) Variability of semen in boars treated with vitamin C in food ration. Med. Weter. 74(1):48–53. https://doi.org/10.21521/mw.5833.

Lee, L.C., Carlson, R.W., Judge, D.L. and Ogawa, M. (1973) The absorption cross sections of N2, O2, CO NO, CO2, N2O, CH4, C2H4, C2H6 and C4H10 from 180 to 700A. Quant, J. Spectrosc. Radiati Transf. 13(10):1023–1031. https://doi.org/10.1016/0022-4073(73)90075-7.

Lee, S.A. and Stein, H.H. (2022) Effects of dietary levels of calcium, phosphorus, and 1-alpha-hydroxycholecalciferol on digestibility, retention of calcium and phosphorus, and concentration of metabolizable energy in diets fed to sows in late-gestation. Can. J. Anim. Sci. 102(1):184–188. https://doi.org/10.1139/cjas-2021-0018.

Le Floc'h, N., Simongiovanni, A., Corrent, E. and Matte J.J. (2017) Comparison of plasma tryptophan-related metabolites in crossbred Piétrain and Duroc pigs J. Anim. Sci. 95(4):1606–1613. https://doi.org/10.2527/jas.2016.1179.

Lehninger, A.L. (1982) "Principles of biochemistry". Worth Publishers, Inc.

Lehrer, W.P. and Wiese, A.C. (1952) Riboflavin deficiency in baby pigs. J. Anim. Sci. 11(2):244–250. https://doi.org/10.2527/jas1952.112244x.

Lehrer, W.P., Wiese, A.C., Moore, P.R. and Ensminger, M.E. (1951) Pyridoxine deficiency in baby pigs. J. Anim. Sci. 10(1):65–72. https://doi.org/10.2527/jas1951.10165x.

Lehrer, W.P., Wiese, A.C. and Moore, P.R. (1952) Biotin deficiency in suckling pigs. J. Nutr. 47(2):203–212. https://doi.org/10.1093/jn/47.2.203.

Leibbrandt, V.D. (1977) Influence of ascorbic acid on suckling pig performance. J. Anim. Sci. 45(suppl. 1):98 (abstr.).

Lemire, J.M. (1992) Immunomodulatory role of 1,25-dihydroxyvitamin D3. J. Cell. Biochem. 49(1):26–31. https://doi.org/10.1002/jcb.240490106.

Leonard, S.W., Terasawa, Y., Farese, R.V. and Traber, M.G. (2002) Incorporation of deuterated RRR- or all-rac-alpha-tocopherol in plasma and tissues of alpha-tocopherol transfer protein–null mice. Am. J. Clin. Nutr. 75(3):555–560. https://doi.org/10.1093/ajcn/75.3.555.

Leskanich, C.O., Matthews, K.R., Warkup, C.C., Noble, R.C. and Hazzledine, M. (1997) The effect of dietary oil containing (n-3) fatty acids on the fatty acid, physicochemical, and organoleptic characteristics of pig meat and fat. J. Anim. Sci. 75(3):673–683. https://doi.org/10.2527/1997.753673x.

Lester, G.E. (1986) Cholecalciferol and placental calcium transport. Fed. Proc. 45(10):2524–2527. PMID: 3017769.

Lewis, A.J., Cromwell, G.L. and Pettigrew, J.E. (1991) Effects of supplemental biotin during gestation and lactation on reproductive performance of sows: a cooperative study. J. Anim. Sci. 69(1):207–214. https://doi.org/10.2527/1991.691207x.

Lewis, L.L., Stark, C.R., Fahrenholz, A.C., Bergstrom, J.R. and Jones, C.K. (2015) Evaluation of conditioning time and temperature on gelatinized starch and vitamin retention in a pelleted swine diet. J. Anim. Sci. 93(2):615–619. https://doi.org/10.2527/jas.2014-8074.

Li, J., Yin, L., Wang, L., Li, J., Huang, P., Yang, H. and Yin, Y. (2019) Effects of vitamin B6 on growth, diarrhea rate, intestinal morphology, function, and inflammatory factors expression in a high-protein diet fed to weaned piglets. J. Anim. Sci. 97(12):4865–4874. https://doi.org/10.1093/jas/skz338.

Li, R., Li, L., Hong, P., Lang, W., Hui, J., Yang, Y. and Zheng, X. (2021) β-carotene prevents weaning-induced intestinal inflammation by modulating gut microbiota in piglets. Anim. Biosci. 34(7):1221–1234. https://doi.org/10.5713/ajas.19.0499.

Li, W., Li, B., Lv, J., Dong, L., Zhang, L. and Wang, T. (2018) Choline supplementation improves the lipid metabolism of intrauterine-growth-restricted pigs. Asian-Australas. J. Anim. Sci. 31(5):686–695. https://doi.org/10.5713/ajas.15.0810.

Li, W., Maeda, N. and Beck, M.A. (2006) Vitamin C deficiency increases the lung pathology of influenza virus-infected gulo-/-mice. J. Nutr. 136(10):2611–2616. https://doi.org/10.1093/jn/136.10.2611.

Li, Y., Zhang, X., Sun, Y., Feng, Q., Li, G., Wang, M., Cui, X., Kang, L. and Jiang, Y. (2013) Folate deficiency during early-mid pregnancy affects the skeletal muscle transcriptome of piglets from a reciprocal cross. PLOS ONE 8(12):e82616. https://doi.org/10.1371/journal.pone.0082616.

Li, Y.J., Li, L.Y., Li, J.L., Zhang, L., Gao, F. and Zhou, G.H. (2015) Effects of dietary supplementation with ferulic acid or vitamin E individually or in combination on meat quality and antioxidant capacity of finishing pigs. Asian-Australas. J. Anim. Sci. 28(3):374–381. https://doi.org/10.5713/ajas.14.0432.

Lima, A.S., Weigel, R.A., Morgado, A.A., Nunes, G.R., Souza, F.N., Moreno, A.M., Della Libera, A.M.M.P. and Sucupira, M.C.A. (2012) Parenteral administration of vitamins A, D and E on the oxidative metabolism and function of polymorphonuclear leukocytes in swine. Pesq. Vet. Bras. 32(8):727–734. https://doi.org/10.1590/S0100-736X2012000800008.

Lin, H.K., Chen, S.Y., Huang, C.Y., Kuo, M.H. and Wung, L.C. (1985) Studies on improving semen quality of working boars fed diets with addition of vitamin C in summer session. Ann. Res. Rep. Anim. Ind. Res. Inst. T.S.C.

Lin, Y., Lv, G., Dong, H., Wu, D., Tao, Z., Xu, S., Che, L., Fang, Z., Bai, S., Feng, B., Li, J. and Xu, X. (2017) Effects of the different levels of dietary vitamin D on boar performance and semen quality. Livestock Science 203:63–68. https://doi.org/10.1016/j.livsci.2017.07.003.

Lindberg, P. (1973) Plasma-tocopherol in pigs. Acta Agric. Scand. (Suppl.9).

Lindemann, M.D. (1988) Further research supports value of folic acid in sow diets. Feedstuffs 60(46):15.

Lindemann, M.D. (1993) Supplemental folic acid: a requirement for optimizing swine reproduction. J. Anim. Sci. 71(1):239–246. https://doi.org/10.2527/1993.711239x.

Lindemann, M.D. and Kornegay, E.T. (1986) Folic acid additions to weanling pig diets. J. Anim. Sci. 63(1):35.

Lindemann, M.D. and Kornegay, E.T. (1989) Folic acid supplementation to diets of gestating-lactating swine over multiple parities. J. Anim. Sci. 67(2):459–464. https://doi.org/10.2527/jas1989.672459x.

Lindemann, M.D., Cromwell, G.L. and Moneque, H.J. (1995) Effects of inadequate and high levels of vitamin fortification on performance of weanling pigs. J. Anim. Sci. 73(1):16.

Lindemann, M.D., Brendemuhl, J.H., Chiba, L.I., Darroch, C.S., Dove, C.R., Estienne, M.J. and Harper, A.F. (2008) A regional evaluation of injections of high levels of vitamin A on reproductive performance of sows. J. Anim. Sci. 86(2):333–338. https://doi.org/10.2527/jas.2007-0153.

Lindemann, M.D., Cromwell, G.L., Van de Ligt, J.L.G. and Monegue, H.J. (1999) Higher levels of selected B-vitamins improve performance and lean deposition in growing/finishing swine. J. Anim. Sci. 77(1):58.

Lindemann, M.D., Stuart, R.L. and Goihl, J. (2013) Oral and injectable fat-soluble vitamin programs for sows, newborn and weaned pigs. American Association of Swine Veterinarians. (pp. 167–170). http://stuart products.com/images/newstouse/Swine/2013_AASV.pdf.

Lindley, D.C. and Cunha, T.J. (1946) Nutritional significance of inositol and biotin for the pig. J. Nutr. 32(1): 47–59. https://doi.org/10.1093/jn/32.1.47.

Lindshield, B.L. and Erdman, J.W. (2006) Carotenoids. In Present knowledge in nutrition 9th ed Bowman, B.A. and Russell, R.M. (Ed.). International Life Sciences Institute. (pp. 184–197).

Lisgara, M., Skampardonis, V., Kouroupides, S. and Leontides, L. (2015) Hoof lesions and lameness in sows in three Greek swine herds. J. Swine Health Prod. 23(5):244–251. aasv.org.

Liu, A., Chen, X., Huang, Z., Chen, D., Yu, B., Chen, H., He, J., Yan, H., Zheng, P., Yu, J. and Luo, Y. (2022) Effects of dietary lycopene supplementation on intestinal morphology, antioxidant capability and inflammatory response in finishing pigs. Anim. Biotechnol. 33(3):563–570. https://doi.org/10.1080/10 495398.2021.2009490.

Liu, F., Cottrell, J.J., Furness, J.B., Rivera, L.R., Kelly, F.W., Wijesiriwardana, U., Pustovit, R.V., Fothergill, L.J., Bravo, D.M., Celi, P., Leury, B.J., Gabler, N.K. and Dunshea, F.R. (2016) Selenium and vitamin E together improve intestinal epithelial barrier function and alleviate oxidative stress in heat-stressed pigs. Exp. Physiol. 101(7):801–810. https://doi.org/10.1113/EP085746.

Liu, F., Cottrell, J.J., Collins, C.L., Henman, D.J., O'Halloran, K.S.B. and Dunshea, F.R. (2017) Supplementation of selenium, vitamin E, chromium and betaine above recommended levels improves lactating performance of sows over summer. Trop. Anim. Health Prod. 49(7):1461–1469. https://doi.org/10.1007/s11250-017-1348-y.

Liu, J., Yu, B., Mao, X., He, J., Yu, J., Zheng, P., Huang, Z. and Chen, D. (2012) Effects of intrauterine growth retardation and maternal folic acid supplementation on hepatic mitochondrial function and gene expression in piglets. Arch. Anim. Nutr. 66(5):357–371. https://doi.org/10.1080/1745039X.2012.710084.

Liu, Q., Scheller, K.K., Arp, S.C., Schaefer, D.M. and Williams, S.N. (1996) Titration of fresh meat color stability and malondialdehyde development with Holstein steers fed vitamin E-supplemented diets. J. Anim. Sci. 74(1):117–126. https://doi.org/10.2527/1996.741117x.

Liu, Q., Zhou, Y., Duan, R., Wei, H., Jiang, S. and Peng, J. (2017a) Lower dietary n-6: n-3 ratio and high-dose vitamin E supplementation improve sperm morphology and oxidative stress in boars. Reprod. Fertil. Dev. 29(5):940–949.

Liu, Q., Zhou, Y.F., Duan, R.J., Wei, H.K., Peng, J. and Jiang, S.W. (2017b) Dietary n-6:n-3 ratio and Vitamin E improve motility characteristics in association with membrane properties of boar spermatozoa. Asian J. Androl. 19(2):223–229. https://doi.org/10.4103/1008-682X.170446.

Liu, S., Zhu, X., Qiu, Y., Wang, L., Shang, X., Gao, K., Yang, X. and Jiang, Z. (2021) Effect of niacin on growth performance, intestinal morphology, mucosal immunity and microbiota composition in weaned piglets. Animals (Basel) 11(8):2186. https://doi.org/10.3390/ani11082186.

Loew, F.M. (1978) Effect of nutrient deficiencies in animals: thiamine. In Handbook series in nutrition and food section E: nutritional disorders, Vol. 2 Rechcigl, Jr., M. (Ed.). CRC Press, Boca Raton, FL.

Lo Fiego, P.D., Macchioni, P., Minelli, G., Cristina Ielo, M. and Santoro, P. (2009) Effect of pantothenic acid level in the diet of the finishing heavy pig on carcass and meat quality traits. Ital. J. Anim. Sci. 8(sup2):504–506. https://doi.org/10.4081/ijas.2009.s2.504.

Lohakare, J.D., Lee, S.H. and Chae, B.J. (2006) Effect of dietary fat-soluble vitamins on growth performance and nutrient digestibility in growing pigs. Asian. Australas J. Anim. Sci. 19(4):563–567. https://doi.org/10.5713/ajas.2006.563.

Long, G.G. (1984) Acute toxicosis in swine associated with excessive dietary intake of vitamin D. J. Am. Vet. Med. Assoc. 184(2):164–170. PMID: 6321415.

Lorenzett, M.P., Armién, A.G., Henker, L.C., Schwertz, C.I., Cruz, R.A.S., Panziera, W., de Barros, C.S.L., Driemeier, D. and Pavarini, S.P. (2023) Motor and somatosensory degenerative myelopathy responsive to pantothenic acid in piglets. Vet. Pathol. 60(1):101–114. https://doi.org/10.1177/03009858221128920.

Lovett, T.D., Coffey, M.T., Miles, R.D. and Combs, G.E. (1986) Methionine, choline and sulfate interrelation-ships in the diet of weanling swine. J. Anim. Sci. 63(2):467–471. https://doi.org/10.2527/jas1986.632467x.

Lozada-Soto, E.A., Lourenco, D., Maltecca, C., Fix, J., Schwab, C., Shull, C. and Tiezzi, F. (2022) Genotyping and phenotyping strategies for genetic improvement of meat quality and carcass composition in swine. Genet. Sel. Evol. 54(1):42. https://doi.org/10.1186/s12711-022-00736-4.

Lucas, R.M., Gorman, S., Geldenhuys, S. and Hart, P.H. (2014) Vitamin D and immunity Rep. 6. F1000Prime Rep. 6:118. https://doi.org/10.12703/P6-118.

Luce, W.G., Peo, E.R. and Hudman, D.B. (1966) Availability of niacin in wheat for swine. J. Nutr. 88(1):39–44. https://doi.org/10.1093/jn/88.1.39.

Luce, W.G., Peo, E.R. and Hudman, D.B. (1967) Availability of niacin in corn and milo for swine. J. Anim. Sci. 26(1):76–84. https://doi.org/10.2527/jas1967.26176x.

Luce, W.G., Buchanan, D.S., Maxwell, C.V., Jordan, H.E. and Bates, R.O. (1985) Effect of supplemental choline and dichlorvos on reproductive performance of gilts. Nutr. Rep. Int. 32(1):245–251.

Luce, W.G., Geisert, R.D., Zavy, M.T., Clutter, A.G., Bazer, F.W., Maxwell, C.V. and Woltmann, M.D. (1990) Effect of riboflavin supplementation on litter parameters of bred sows. J. Anim. Sci. 68(suppl. 1):42.

Luce, W.G., Clutter, A.C., Maxwell, C.V. and Vencl, R. (1995) Supplementation of biotin to hard red winter wheat diets for bred gilts. Oklahoma State University Animal Science Research Report. (pp. 197–200).

Luck, M.R., Jeyaseelan, I. and Scholes, R.A. (1995) Ascorbic acid and fertility. Biol. Reprod. 52(2):262–266. https://doi.org/10.1095/biolreprod52.2.262.

Luecke, R.W. (1955) Antibiotics and vitamins in the treatment of swine enteritis. Ann. N. Y. Acad. Sci. 63(2):195–201. https://doi.org/10.1111/j.1749-6632.1955.tb32087.x.

Luecke, R.W., McMillen, W.N., Thorpe, F. and Tull, C. (1947) The relationship of nicotinic acid, tryptophane and protein in the nutrition of the pig. J. Nutr. 33(3):251–261. https://doi.org/10.1093/jn/33.3.251.

Luecke, R.W., McMillen, W.N., Thorpe, F. and Tull, C. (1948) Further studies on the relationship of nicotinic acid, tryptophane and protein in the nutrition of the pig. J. Nutr. 36(3):417–424. https://doi.org/10.1093/jn/36.3.417.

Luecke, R.W., McMillen, W.N. and Thorp, F. (1950) Further studies of pantothenic acid deficiency in weanling pigs. J. Anim. Sci. 9(1):78–82. https://doi.org/10.2527/jas1950.9178.

Luecke, R.W., Hoefer, J.A. and Thorp, F. (1952) The relationship of protein to pantothenic acid and vitamin B12 in the growing pig. J. Anim. Sci. 11(2):238–243. https://doi.org/10.2527/jas1952.112238x.

Luecke, R.W., Hoefer, J.A. and Thorp, F. (1953) The Supplementary Effects of Calcium Pantothenate and Aureomycin in a Low Protein Ration for Weaning Pigs. J. Anim. Sci. 12(3):605–610. https://doi.org/10.2527/jas1953.123605x.

Lutz, T.L. and Stahly, T.S. (1997) Dietary folic acid needs of high lean growth pigs. Iowa State Univ. Res. Reprod.:(4–6).

Lutz, T.R. and Stahly, T.S. (1998) Dietary riboflavin needs for body maintenance and body protein and fat accretion in pigs. Iowa State University Research Report. (pp. 41–44). http://iastatedigitalpress.com/air/article/id/7622/.

Lutz, T.R. and Stahly, T.S. (2000) Dietary niacin needs of high lean pigs. Iowa State University Animal Industry Report, 1(1). iastatedigitalpress.com.

Lutz, T.R., Autrey, B.A. and Stahly, T.S. (2004) Efficacy of pantothenic acid as a modifier of body composition in pigs. Iowa State University Animal Industry Report, 1(1). dr.lib.iastate.edu.

Lynch, P.B. and O'Grady, J.F. (1981) Effect of vitamin C (ascorbic acid) supplementation on sows in late preg-nancy on piglet mortality. Ir. J. Agric. Res. 20(2–3):217–219. http://jstor.org/stable/25556008.

López-Bote, C.J., Isabel, B. and Flores, J.M. (2001) Effect of dietary linoleic acid concentration and vitamin E supplementation on cell desquamation and susceptibility to oxidative damage of pig jejunal mucosa. J. Anim. Physiol. Anim. Nutr. (Berl) 85(1–2):22–28. https://doi.org/10.1046/j.1439-0396.2001.00298.x.

MacDonald, D.W., Christian, R.G., Whenham, G.R. and Howell, J. (1976) A review of some aspects of vitamin E-selenium responsive diseases with a note on their possible incidence in Alberta. Can. Vet. J. 17(3):61–71.

Machlin, L.J. (1991) Vitamin E. In Handbook of vitamins 2nd ed. Machlin, L.J. (Ed.). Marcel Dekker, New York.

Machlin, L.J. and Gabriel, E. (1982) Kinetics of tissue alpha-tocopherol uptake and depletion following administration of high levels of vitamin E. Ann. N. Y. Acad. Sci. 393:48–60.

Machlin, L.J. and Sauberlich, H.E. (1994) New views on the function and health effects of vitamins. Nutr. Today 29(1):25–29. https://doi.org/10.1097/00017285-199401000-00006.

Mackenzie, A.M., Drennan, M., Rowan, T.G., Dixon, J.B. and Carter, S.D. (1997) Effect of transportation and weaning on humoral immune responses of calves. Res. Vet. Sci. 63(3):227–230. https://doi.org/10.1016/s0034-5288(97)90025-4.

Madsen, A., Mortensen, H.P., Hjarde, W., Leebeck, E. and Leth, T. (1973) Vitamin E in barley treated with propionic acid with special reference to the feeding of bacon pigs. Acta Agric. Scand. 19:169–173.

Madsen, L.L. (1942) "Nutritional diseases of swine". Yearbook of agriculture. (pp. 810–828). http://naldc.nal.usda.gov/download/IND43893881/PDF.

Madsen, P. A., Etheve, S., Heegaard, P. M. H., Skovgaard, K., Mary, A. L., Litta, G, Lauridsen, C. (2023) Influence of vitamin D metabolites on vitamin D status, immunity and gut health of piglets. Vet. Immunol, Immunopath. 257:110557 https://doi.org/10.1016/j.vetimm.2023.110557.

Madson, D.M. and Goff, J. (2012) Vitamin D deficiency syndromes in swine (I). Pig health. http://pig333.com/articles/vitamin-d-deficiency-syndromes-in-swine-i_5470/.

Madson, D.M., Ensley, S.M., Gauger, P.C., Schwartz, K.J., Stevenson, G.W., Cooper, V.L., Janke, B.H., Burrough, E.R., Goff, J.P. and Horst, R.L. (2012) Rickets: case series and diagnostic review of hypovitaminosis D in swine. J. Vet. Diagn. Invest. 24(6):1137–1144. https://doi.org/10.1177/1040638712461487.

Maeda, Y., Kawata, S., Inui, Y., Fukuda, K., Igura, T. and Matsuzawa, Y. (1996) Biotin deficiency decreases ornithine transcarbamylase activity and mRNA in rat liver. J. Nutr. 126(1):61–66. https://doi.org/10.1093/jn/126.1.61.

Mahan, D.C. (1990) Mineral nutrition of the sow: a review. J. Anim. Sci. 68(2):573–582. https://doi.org/10.2527/1990.682573x.

Mahan, D.C. (1991) Assessment of the influence of dietary vitamin E on sows and offspring in three parities: reproductive performance, tissue tocopherol, and effects on progeny. J. Anim. Sci. 69(7):2904–2917. https://doi.org/10.2527/1991.6972904x.

Mahan, D.C. (1993) Supplemental vitamin C for swine–is it essential and if so when are the critical stages? Ohio Swine Research and Industry Report, Animal Science Series 92(2):60–65.

Mahan, D.C. (1994a) Effects of dietary vitamin E on sow reproductive performance over a five-parity period. J. Anim. Sci. 72(11):2870–2879. https://doi.org/10.2527/1994.72112870x.

Mahan, D.C. (1994b) The importance of the antioxidant vitamins in swine nutrition Roche Technical Seminar.

Mahan, D.C. (2000) Selenium and vitamin E in swine nutrition. In Swine nutrition. CRC Press. (pp. 301–334).

Mahan, D.C. and Moxon, A.L. (1980) Effect of dietary selenium and injectable vitamin E-selenium for weanling swine. Nutr. Rep. Int. 21:829–836.

Mahan, D.C. and Saif, L.J. (1983) Efficacy of vitamin C supplementation for weanling swine. J. Anim. Sci. 56(3):631–639. https://doi.org/10.2527/jas1983.563631x.

Mahan, D.C. and Vallet, J.L. (1997) Vitamin and mineral transfer during fetal development and the early postnatal period in pigs. J. Anim. Sci. 75(10):2731–2738. https://doi.org/10.2527/1997.75102731x.

Mahan, D.C., Pickett, R.A., Perry, T.W., Curtin, T.M., Featherston, W.R. and Beeson, W.M. (1966) Influence of various nutritional factors and physical form of feed on esophagogastric ulcers in swine. J. Anim. Sci. 25(4):1019–1023. https://doi.org/10.2527/jas1966.2541019x.

Mahan, D.C., Jones, J.E., Cline, J.H., Cross, R.F., Teague, H.S. and Grifo, A.P. (1973) Efficacy of selenium and vitamin E injections in the prevention of white muscle disease in young swine. J. Anim. Sci. 36(6):1104–1108. https://doi.org/10.2527/jas1973.3661104x.

Mahan, D.C., Lepine, A.J. and Dabrowski, K. (1994) Efficacy of magnesium-L-ascorbyl-2-phosphate as a vitamin C source for weanling and growing-finishing swine. J. Anim. Sci. 72(9):2354–2361. https://doi.org/10.2527/1994.7292354x.

Mahan, D.C., Kim, Y.Y. and Stuart, R.L. (2000) Effect of vitamin E sources (RRR- or all-rac-α-tocopheryl acetate) and levels on sow reproductive performance, serum, tissue, and milk α-tocopherol contents over a five-parity period, and the effects on the progeny. J. Anim. Sci. 78(1):110–119. https://doi.org/10.2527/2000.781110x.

Mahan, D.C., Ching, S. and Dabrowski, K. (2004) Developmental aspects and factors influencing the synthesis and status of ascorbic acid in the pig. Annu. Rev. Nutr. 24:79–103. https://doi.org/10.1146/annurev.nutr.24.012003.132150.

Mahan, D.C., Carter, S.D., Cline, T.R., Hill, G.M., Kim, S.W., Miller, P.S., Nelssen, J.L., Stein, H.H., Veum, T.L. and North Central Coordinating Committee On Swine Nutrition (NCCC-42) (2007) Evaluating the effects of supplemental B vitamins in practical swine diets during the starter and grower-finisher periods—A regional study. J. Anim. Sci. 85(9):2190–2197. https://doi.org/10.2527/jas.2007-0118.

Malm, A., Pond, W.G., Walker, E.F., Homan, M., Aydin, A. and Kirtland, D. (1976a) Effect of polyunsaturated fatty acids and vitamin E level of the sow gestation diet on reproductive performance and on level of alpha-tocopherol in colostrum, milk and dam and progeny blood serum. J. Anim. Sci. 42(2):393–399. https://doi.org/10.2527/jas1976.422393x.

Malm, A., Walker, E.F., Homan, M., Kirtland, D., Aydin, A. and Pond, W.G. (1976b) Glutathione peroxidase and other enzymes in serum of sows and their progeny fed vitamin E-adequate or deficient diets with added Se. Nutr. Rep. Int. 14(2):185–202.

Manolescu, D.C., Sima, A. and Bhat, P.V. (2010) All-trans retinoic acid lowers serum retinol-binding protein concentrations and increases insulin sensitivity in diabetic mice. J. Nutr. 140(2):311–316. https://doi.org/10.3945/jn.109.115147.

Manthey, K.C., Griffin, J.B. and Zempleni, J. (2002) Biotin supply affects expression of biotin transporters, biotinylation of carboxylases and metabolism of interleukin-2 in Jurkat cells. J. Nutr. 132(5):887–892. https://doi.org/10.1093/jn/132.5.887.

Marin-Guzman, J., Mahan, D.C., Jones, L.S. and Pate, J.L. (1989) Effect of dietary vitamin E and selenium on semen quality of boars. Ohio Swine Res. Ind. Rep. The Ohio State Univ., Anim. Sci. Dept. 89(1):20.

Marin-Guzman, J., Mahan, D.C., Chung, Y.K., Pate, J.L. and Pope, W.F. (1997) Effects of dietary selenium and vitamin E on boar performance and tissue responses, semen quality, and subsequent fertilization rates in mature gilts. J. Anim. Sci. 75(11):2994–3003. https://doi.org/10.2527/1997.75112994x.

Marin-Guzman, J., Mahan, D.C. and Whitmoyer, R. (2000) Effect of dietary selenium and vitamin E on the ultrastructure and ATP concentration of boar spermatozoa, and the efficacy of added sodium selenite in extended semen on sperm motility. J. Anim. Sci. 78(6):1544–1550. https://doi.org/10.2527/2000.7861544x.

Marks, J. (1975). In A Guide to the vitamins. Their role in health and disease. Springer, Berlin.

Martin, P.R., Singleton, C.K. and Hiller-Sturmhöfel, S. (2003) The role of thiamine deficiency in alcoholic brain disease. Alcohol Res. Health 27(2):134–142. PMID: 15303623.

Marusich, W.L. (1978) Vitamin E supplementation benefits swine, turkeys and consumer. Feedstuffs 50(50):25.

Matte, J.J. (1995) The importance of some B-complex vitamins in pig nutrition Proc. Eastern Nut. Conf, Longueuil, Quebec. (pp. 61–62).

Matte, J.J. (1997) Optimising pyridoxine for fast-growing pigs. Feed Mix 5(5):9–11.

Matte, J.J. and Audet, I. (2020) Maternal perinatal transfer of vitamins and trace elements to piglets. Animal 14(1):31–38. https://doi.org/10.1017/S175173111900140x.

Matte, J.J. and Girard, C.L. (1989) Effects of intramuscular injections of folic acid and during lactation on folates in serum and milk and performance of sows and piglets. J. Anim. Sci. 67(2):426–431. https://doi.org/10.2527/jas1989.672426x.

Matte, J.J. and Girard, C.L. (1990) The importance of folic acid for the nutrition and reproduction of sows. In Proc. Roche Symposium: Nutrients, the bioavailability factor. Guelph Nutr. Conf., Guelph, Canada.

Matte, J.J. and Girard, C.L. (1999) An estimation of the requirement for folic acid in gestating sows: the metabolic utilization of folates as a criterion of measurement. J. Anim. Sci. 77(1):159–165. https://doi.org/10.2527/1999.771159x.

Matte, J.J. and Lauridsen, C. (2013) Vitamins and vitamin utilization in swine. In "Sustainable swine nutrition" Chiba, L. (Ed.). Wiley-Blackwell. (pp. 139–172).

Matte, J.J., Girard, C.L. and Brisson, G.J. (1984a) Serum folates during the reproductive cycle of sows. J. Anim. Sci. 59(1):158–163. https://doi.org/10.2527/jas1984.591158x.

Matte, J.J., Girard, C.L. and Brisson, G.J. (1984b) Folic acid and reproductive performances of sows. J. Anim. Sci. 59(4):1020–1025. https://doi.org/10.2527/jas1984.5941020x.

Matte, J.J., Girard, C.L. and Brisson, G.J. (1986) Importance of folic acid administered during gestation on hematological status of piglets. Can. J. Anim. Sci. 66(2):523–527. https://doi.org/10.4141/cjas86-054.

Matte, J.J., Girard, C.L. and Brisson, G.J. (1990a) The effect of supplementary folic acid in gestation and lactation diets on folate status and reproductive performances of first parity sows. J. Anim. Sci. 68(suppl. 1):370.

Matte, J.J., Girard, C.L., Bilodeau, R. and Robert, S. (1990b) Effects of intramuscular injections of folic acid on serum folates, haematological status and growth performance of growing-finishing pigs. Reprod. Nutr. Dev. 30(1):103–114. https://doi.org/10.1051/rnd:19900111.

Matte, J.J., Girard, C.L. and Brisson, G.J. (1992) The role of folic acid in the nutrition of gestating and lactating primiparous sows. Livest. Prod. Sci. 32(2):131–148. https://doi.org/10.1016/S0301-6226(12)80032-7.

Matte, J.J., Girard, C.L. and Tremblay, G.F. (1993) Effect of long term addition of folic acid on folate status, growth performance, puberty attainment, and reproductive capacity of gilts. J. Anim. Sci. 71(1):151–157. https://doi.org/10.2527/1993.711151x.

Matte, J.J., Farmer, C., Girard, C.L. and Laforest, J.-P. (1996) Dietary folic acid, uterine function and early embryonic development in sows. Can. J. Anim. Sci. 76(3):427–433. https://doi.org/10.4141/cjas96-062.

Matte, J.J., Ponter, A.A. and Sève, B. (1997a) Effects of chronic parenteral pyridoxine and acute enteric tryptophan on pyridoxine status, glycemia and insulinemia stimulated by enteric glucose in weanling piglets. Can. J. Anim. Sci. 77(4):663–668. https://doi.org/10.4141/A97-013.

Matte, J.J., Ponter, A.A., Girard, C.L. and Seve, B. (1997b) Vitamin B6, its relationship with the metabolism of tryptophan in weanling piglets. In Proc. 7th Intern. Symp. Dig. Physiol. in Pigs, Saint-Malo, France. (pp. 283–287).

Matte, J.J., Girard, C. and Seve, B. (1998) Vitamin B6 (pyridoxine) and B2 (riboflavin): should we revise the requirements for early-weaned piglets? Journees Rech. Porcine Fr. 30:253–257.

Matte, J.J., Girard, C.L. and Sève, B. (2001) Effects of long term parenteral administration of vitamin B6 on B6 status and some aspects of the glucose and protein metabolism of early-weaned piglets. Br. J. Nutr. 85(1):11–21. https://doi.org/10.1079/bjn2000221.

Matte, J.J., Giguère, A. and Girard, C.L. (2005) Some aspects of the pyridoxine (vitamin B6) requirement in weanling piglets. Br. J. Nutr. 93(5):723–730. https://doi.org/10.1079/bjn20051406.

Matte, J.J., Guay, F. and Girard, C.L. (2006) Folic acid and vitamin B12 in reproducing sows: new concepts. Can. J. Anim. Sci. 86(2):197–205. https://doi.org/10.4141/A05-059.

Matte, J.J., Corrent, E., Simongiovanni, A. and Le Floc'h, N. (2016) Tryptophan metabolism, growth responses, and postprandial insulin metabolism in weaned piglets according to the dietary provision of niacin (vitamin B3) and tryptophan. J. Anim. Sci. 94(5):1961–1971. https://doi.org/10.2527/jas.2015-0221.

Matte, J.J. and Lauridsen, C. (2022) Vitamins and vitamin utilization in pigs. In "Sustainable Sswine Nnutrition" (ed. Chiba, L.) (Ed.). Wiley-Blackwell. (pp. 189–227). https://doi.org/10.1002/9781119583998.ch7.

Maurya, V.K. and Aggarwal, M. (2017) Factors influencing the absorption of vitamin D in GIT: an overview. J. Food Sci. Technol. 54(12):3753–3765. https://doi.org/10.1007/s13197-017-2840-0.

Maxwell, C.V., Johnson, R.K. and Luce, W.G. (1987) Effect of level of protein and supplemental choline on reproductive performance of gilts fed sorghum diets. J. Anim. Sci. 64(4):1044–1050. https://doi.org/10.2527/jas1987.6441044x.

Maynard, L.A., Loosli, J.K., Hintz, H.F. and Warner, R.G. (1979) Animal nutrition 7th ed. McGraw-Hill Book Co.

Mbachiantim, J.T., Johnson, N.C. and Ogbamgba, V.M. (2022) Assuaging effects of ingestions of vitamins C and E on the blood parameters of growing pigs fed crude oil-contaminated diets. Eur. J. Sci. Innov. Techn. 2(1):17–21.

McCampbell, H.C., Porter, P.J. and Seerley, R.W. (1974) The effect of ascorbic acid in swine diets. J. Anim. Sci. 38:220.

McCandless, D.W. (2010) "Thiamine deficiency and associated clinical disorders. Humana Press, New York.

McCay, P.B. (1985) Vitamin E: interactions with free radicals and ascorbate. Annu. Rev. Nutr. 5(1):323–340. https://doi.org/10.1146/annurev.nu.05.070185.001543.

McCay, P.B., Gibson, D.D. and Hornbrook, K.R. (1981) Glutathione-dependent inhibition of lipid peroxidation by a soluble, heat-labile factor not glutathione peroxidase. Fed. Proc. 40(2):199–205.

McCollum, E.V. (1957) "A history of nutrition". Houghton Mifflin Co., Boston, MA.

McCormick, C.C. and Parker, R.S. (2004) The cytotoxicity of vitamin E is both vitamer- and cell-specific and involves a selectable trait. J. Nutr. 134(12):3335–3342. https://doi.org/10.1093/jn/134.12.3335.

McCormick, D.B. (1990) "Riboflavin". In "Nutrition reviews, present knowledge in nutrition Brown", M.L. (Ed.), International Life Sci.

McCormick, D.B. (2006) Vitamin B6. In "Present knowledge in nutrition" 9th ed. Bowman, B.A. and Russell, R.M. (Eds). International Life Sciences Institute. (pp. 269–277).

McDowell, L.R. (2000a) "Vitamins in animal and human nutrition". Iowa State University Press, Ames, IA.

McDowell, L.R. (2000b) Reevaluation of the metabolic essentiality of the vitamins – Review –. Asian. Australas J. Anim. Sci. 13(1):115–125. https://doi.org/10.5713/ajas.2000.115.

McDowell, L.R. (2004) Re-evaluation of the essentiality of the vitamins. California Animal Nutrition Conference. (pp. 37–67).

McDowell, L.R. (2006) Vitamins and minerals functioning as antioxidants and vitamin and mineral supplementation considerations. In ARPAS Calif. Chapter Conference Proceedings. (pp. 1–22).

McDowell, L.R. (2013) "Vitamin history, the early years". Design Publishing Inc. Sarasora, FL, USA.

McDowell, L.R. and Ward, N. (2008) Optimum vitamin nutrition for poultry. Int. Poult. Prod. 16(4):27–34.

McDowell, L.R., Froseth, J.A., Kroening, G.H. and Haller, W.A. (1974) Effects of vitamin E and oxidized cottonseed oil of SGOT, erythrocyte hemolysis, testicular fatty acids and testicular selenium in swine fed peas (Pisum sativum). Nutr. Rep. Int. 9:359–369.

McDowell, L.R., Froseth, J.A., Piper, R.C., Dyer, I.A. and Kroening, G.H. (1977) Tissue selenium and serum tocopherol concentrations in selenium-vitamin E deficient pigs fed peas (Pisum sativum). J. Anim. Sci. 45(6):1326–1333. https://doi.org/10.2527/jas1977.4561326x.

McDowell, L.R., Conrad, J.H., Ellis, G.L. and Loosli, J.K. (1983) Minerals for grazing ruminants in tropical regions. Univ. of Florida, Gainesville.

McGhee, J.R., Mestecky, J., Dertzbaugh, M.T., Eldridge, J.H., Hirasawa, M. and Kiyono, H. (1992) The mucosal immune system: from fundamental concepts to vaccine development. Vaccine 10(2):75–88. https://doi.org/10.1016/0264-410x(92)90021-b.

McGinnis, C.H. (1986) Vitamin stability and activity of water-soluble vitamins as influenced by manufacturing processes and recommendations for the water-soluble vitamin. In "Bioavailability of nutrients in feed". National Feed Ingredient Association (NFIA), Des Moines, IA.

McGinnis, C.H. (1988) New concepts in vitamin nutrition. In Proc. 1988 Georgia Nutrition Conference of the Feed Industry.

McIntosh, G.H., Lawson, C.A., Bulman, F.H. and McMurchie, E.J. (1985) Vitamin E status affects platelet aggregation in the pig. Proc. Nutr. Soc. Australia 10:207.

McKigney, J.I., Wallace, H.D. and Cunha, T.J. (1957) The influence of chlortetracycline on the requirement of the young pig for dietary pantothenic acid. J. Anim. Sci. 16(1):35–43. https://doi.org/10.2527/jas1957.16135x.

McMillen, W.N., Luecke, R.W. and Thorp, F. (1948) Pantothenic acid deficiency in swine on diets of natural feedstuffs. J. Anim. Sci. 7:529.

McMillen, W.N., Luecke, R.W. and Thorp, F. (1949) The effect of liberal B-vitamin supplementation on growth of weanling pigs fed rations containing a variety of feedstuffs. J. Anim. Sci. 8(4):518–523. https://doi.org/10.2527/jas1949.84518x.

McMurray, C.H., Rice, D.A. and Blanchflower, W.J. (1980) Changes in plasma levels on linoleic and linolenic acids in calves recently introduced to spring pasture. Proc. Nutr. Soc. 39:65 (abstr.).

Mehansho, H. and Henderson, L.M. (1980) Transport and accumulation of pyridoxine and pyridoxal by erythrocytes. J. Biol. Chem. 255(24):11901–11907. PMID: 7440576.

Mencik, S., Vukovic, V., Spehar, M., Modric, M., Ostovic, M. and Ekert Kabalin, A.E. (2019) Association between ESR1 and RBP4 genes and litter size traits in a hyperprolific line of Landrace × Large White cross sows. Vet. Med. 64(3):109–117. https://doi.org/10.17221/87/2018-VETMED.

Meng, Q., Zhang, Y., Li, J., Shi, B., Ma, Q. and Shan, A. (2022) Lycopene affects intestinal barrier function and the gut microbiota in weaned piglets via antioxidant signaling regulation. J. Nutr. 152(11):2396–2408. https://doi.org/10.1093/jn/nxac208.

Menten, J.F.M., Ku, P.K. and Miller, E.R. (1987) Copper and biotin supplementation to the diets of starter pigs. Michigan State Univ. Agric. exp. Sta. Rep. Swine Res. 487:83.

Meydani, N. and Han, S.N. (2006) Nutrient regulation of the immune response: the case of vitamin E. In "Present knowledge in nutrition" 9th ed. Bowman, B.A. and Russell, R.M. (Eds). International Life Sciences Institute. (pp. 585–603).

Meydani, S.N., Ribaya-Mercado, J.D., Russell, R.M., Sahyoun, N., Morrow, F.D. and Gershoff, S.N. (1991) Vitamin B6 deficiency impairs interleukin 2 production and lymphocyte proliferation in elderly adults. Am. J. Clin. Nutr. 53(5):1275–1280. https://doi.org/10.1093/ajcn/53.5.1275.

Meyer, W.R., Mahan, D.C. and Moxon, A.L. (1981) Value of dietary selenium and vitamin E for weanling swine as measured by performance and tissue selenium and glutathione peroxidase activities. J. Anim. Sci. 52(2):302–311. https://doi.org/10.2527/jas1981.522302x.

Michel, R.L., Whitehair, C.K. and Keahey, K.K. (1969) Dietary hepatic necrosis associated with selenium-vitamin E deficiency in swine. J. Am. Vet. Med. Assoc. 155(1):50–59.

Miller, C.O., Ellis, N.R., Stevenson, J.W. and Davey, R. (1953) The riboflavin requirement of swine for reproduction. J. Nutr. 51(2):163–170.

Miller, E.R. (1971) Copper in growing-finishing rations. In report of swine research 148, Michigan State University, Agricultural Experiment Station, East Lansing. Michigan State University Press. (pp. 52–58).

Miller, E.R. and Kornegay, E.T. (1983) Mineral and vitamin nutrition of swine. J. Anim. Sci. 57(suppl. 2):315–329.

Miller, E.R., Johnston, R.L., Hoefer, J.A. and Luecke, R.W. (1954) The riboflavin requirement of the baby pig. J. Nutr. 52(3):405–413. https://doi.org/10.1093/jn/52.3.405.

Miller, E.R., Schmidt, D.A., Hoefer, J.A. and Luecke, R.W. (1955) The thiamine requirement of the baby pig. J. Nutr. 56(3):423–430. https://doi.org/10.1093/jn/56.3.423.

Miller, E.R., Schmidt, D.A., Hoefer, J.A. and Luecke, R.W. (1957) The pyridoxine requirement of the baby pig. J. Nutr. 62(3):406–419. https://doi.org/10.1093/jn/62.3.407.

Miller, E.R., Ullrey, D.E., Zutaut, C.L., Baltzer, B.V., Schmidt, D.A., Vincent, B.H., Hoefer, J.A. and Luecke, R.W. (1964) Vitamin D2 requirement of the baby pig. J. Nutr. 83(2):140–148. https://doi.org/10.1093/jn/83.2.140.

Miller, E.R., Ullrey, D.E., Zutaut, C.L., Hoefer, J.A. and Luecke, R.L. (1965b) Comparisons of casein and soy proteins upon mineral balance and vitamin D2 requirements of the baby pig. J. Nutr. 85(4):347–354. https://doi.org/10.1093/jn/85.4.347.

Miller, E.R., Ullrey, D.E., Zutaut, C.L., Hoefer, J.A. and Luecke, R.W. (1965a) Mineral balance studies with the baby pig: effects of dietary vitamin D2 level upon calcium, phosphorus and magnesium balance. J. Nutr. 85(3):255–259. https://doi.org/10.1093/jn/85.3.255.

Miller, J.W., Rogerf, L.M. and Rucker, R.B. (2006) Pantothenic acid. In "Present knowledge in nutrition" 9th ed. Bowman, B.A. and Russell, R.M. (Eds). International Life Sciences Institute. (pp. 327–339).

Min, Y.N., Niu, Z.Y., Sun, T.T., Wang, Z.P., Jiao, P.X., Zi, B.B., Chen, P.P., Tian, D.L. and Liu, F.Z. (2018) Vitamin E and vitamin C supplementation improves antioxidant status and immune function in oxidative-stressed breeder roosters by up-regulating expression of GSH-Px gene. Poult. Sci. 97(4):1238–1244.

Minelli, G., Macchioni, P., Ielo, M.C., Santoro, P. and Fiego, D.P.L. (2013) Effects of dietary level of pantothenic acid and sex on carcass, meat quality traits and fatty acid composition of thigh subcutaneous adipose tissue in Italian heavy pigs. Ital. J. Anim. Sci. 12(2):e52. https://doi.org/10.4081/ijas.2013.e52.

Mirvish, S.S. (1986) Effects of vitamins C and E on N-nitroso compound formation, carcinogenesis, and cancer. Cancer 58(suppl. 8):1842–1850. https://doi.org/10.1002/1097-0142(19861015)58:8+<1842::AID-CNCR2820581410>3.0.CO;2-%23.

Misir, R. and Blair, R. (1984) Effect of biotin supplementation on performance of biotin-deficient sows. J. Ani Sci. 59(suppl. 1):254.

Misir, R. and Blair, R. (1986a) Effect of biotin supplementation of a barley-wheat diet on restoration of healthy feet, legs and skin of biotin deficient sows. Res. Vet. Sci. 40(2):212–218. PMID: 3704339.

Misir, R. and Blair, R. (1986b) Reproductive performance of gilts and sows as affected by induced biotin deficiency and subsequent dietary biotin supplementation. J. Anim. Physiol. Anim Nutr. 55(1–5):196–208. https://doi.org/10.1111/j.1439-0396.1986.tb00720.x.

Mitchell, H.H., Johnson, B.C., Hamilton, T.S. and Haines, W.T. (1950) The riboflavin requirement of the growing pig at two environmental temperatures. J. Nutr. 41(2):317–337. https://doi.org/10.1093/jn/41.2.317.

Mock, D.M. (1990) Biotin. In Nutrition reviews, present knowledge in nutrition Olson, R.E. (ed.) Nutritional Foundation.

Mock, D.M. (2013) Biotin. In Handbook of vitamins 5th ed. Zempleni, J., Suttie, J., Gregory, J. and Stover, P.J. (ed.). CRC Press. (pp. 397–420).

Mock, D.M. and Malik, M.I. (1992) Distribution of biotin in human plasma: most of the biotin is not bound to protein. Am. J. Clin. Nutr. 56(2):427–432. https://doi.org/10.1093/ajcn/56.2.427.

Mock, N.I. and Mock, D.M. (1992) Biotin deficiency in rats: disturbances of leucine metabolism are detectable early. J. Nutr. 122(7):1493–1499. https://doi.org/10.1093/jn/122.7.1493.

Moffatt, R.J., Murray, F.A., Grifo, A.P., Haynes, L.W., Kinder, J.E. and Wilson, G.R. (1980) Identification of riboflavin in porcine uterine secretions. Biol. Reprod. 23(2):331–335. https://doi.org/10.1095/biolreprod23.2.331.

Moir, D.C. and Masters, H.G. (1979) Hepatosis dietetica, nutritional myopathy, mulberry heart disease and associated hepatic selenium level in pigs. Aust. Vet. J. 55(8):360–364.

Monahan, F.J., Buckley, D.J., Gray, J.I., Morrissey, P.A., Asghar, A., Hanrahan, T.J. and Lynch, P.B. (1990) Effect of dietary vitamin E on the stability of raw and cooked pork. Meat Sci. 27(2):99–108. https://doi.org/10.1016/0309-1740(90)90058-E.

Monahan, F.J., Buckley, D.J., Morrissey, P.A., Lynch, P.B. and Gray, J.I. (1992) Influence of dietary fat and α-tocopherol supplementation on lipid oxidation in pork. Meat Sci. 31(2):229–241. https://doi.org/10.1016/0309-1740(92)90042-3.

Monahan, F.J., Asghar, A., Gray, J.I., Buckley, D.J. and Morrissey, P.A. (1994) Effect of oxidized dietary lipid and vitamin E on the colour stability of pork chops. Meat Sci. 37(2):205–215. https://doi.org/10.1016/0309-1740(94)90081-7.

Monegue, J.S. (2013) Evaluation of the effects of vitamin K on growth performance and bone health in swine. Doctorate dissertation. https://uknowledge.uky.edu/animalsci_etds/26/.

Moreira, I. and Mahan, D.C. (2002) Effect of dietary levels of vitamin E (all-rac-tocopheryl acetate) with or without added fat on weanling pig performance and tissue α-tocopherol concentration. J. Anim. Sci. 80(3):663–669. https://doi.org/10.2527/2002.803663x.

Morel, P.C.H., Janz, J.A., Zou, M., Purchas, R.W., Hendriks, W.H. and Wilkinson, B.H. (2008) The influence of diets supplemented with conjugated linoleic acid, selenium, and vitamin E, with or without animal protein, on the composition of pork from female pigs. J. Anim. Sci. 86(5):1145–1155. https://doi.org/10.2527/jas.2007-0358.

Morris, M.S., Sakakeeny, L., Jacques, P.F., Picciano, M.F. and Selhub, J. (2010) Vitamin B6 intake is inversely related to, and the requirement is affected by, inflammation status. J. Nutr. 140(1):103–110. https://doi.org/10.3945/jn.109.114397.

Morrissey, P.A. and Sheehy, P.J.A. (1999) Optimal nutrition: vitamin E. Proc. Nutr. Soc. 58(2):459–468. https://doi.org/10.1017/S0029665199000609.

Morrissey, P.A., Buckley, D.J., Sisk, H., Lynch, P.B. and Sheehy, P.J.A. (1996) Uptake of α-tocopherol in porcine plasma and tissues. Meat Sci. 44(4):275–283. https://doi.org/10.1016/S0309-1740(96)00033-2.

Morrissey, P.A., Buckley, D.J. and Galvin, K. (2000) Vitamin E and the oxidative stability of pork and poultry. In "Antioxidants in muscle foods: nutritional strategies to improve quality Decker", E.A., Faustman, C. and Lopez-Bote, J. (Eds). (pp. 263–287).

Morrow, J.L., McGlone, J.J., Tribble, L.F. and Stansbury, W.F. (1987) Effect of dl-alpha-tocopherol injections on piglet performance and immunity. Texas Tech and Univ. Anim Sci. Res. Reprod. 5(233):14.

Mortimer, D.T. (1983) Vitamin E/selenium deficiency syndrome in pigs. Vet. Rec. 112(12):278–279.

Moser, U. and Bendich, A. (1991) Vitamin C. In "Handbook of vitamins" 2nd ed. Machlin, L.J. (Ed.). Marcel Dekker, New York.

Mourot, J., Aumaitre, A. and Wallet, P. (1992) Effect of a dietary supplement of vitamin C on growth and pig meat quality. Proceed. 2nd Symposium ascorbic acid in domestic animals. Kartause Ittingen, Switzerland. (pp. 176–185).

Mozalene, E.E., Medzyavichyus, A.K. and Medzevicius, A. (1991) Effect of vitamin C on serum ceruloplasmin levels in pigs with experimental Trichuris infection. Vet. Bull. 61(3):269.

Mudd, A.T., Alexander, L.S., Johnson, S.K., Getty, C.M., Malysheva, O.V., Caudill, M.A. and Dilger, R.N. (2016a) Perinatal dietary choline deficiency in sows influences concentrations of choline metabolites, fatty acids, and amino acids in milk throughout lactation. J. Nutr. 146(11):2216–2223. https://doi.org/10.3945/jn.116.238832.

Mudd, A.T., Getty, C.M., Sutton, B.P. and Dilger, R.N. (2016b) Perinatal choline deficiency delays brain development and alters metabolite concentrations in the young pig. Nutr. Neurosci. 19(10):425–433. https://doi.org/10.1179/1476830515Y.0000000031.

Mudd, A.T., Getty, C.M. and Dilger, R.N. (2018) Maternal dietary choline status influences brain gray and white matter development in young pigs. Curr. Dev. Nutr. 2(6):nzy015. https://doi.org/10.1093/cdn/nzy015.

Mudron, P., Baumgartner, W., Kovac, G., Bartko, P., Rosival, I. and Zezula, I. (1996) Effects of iron and vitamin E administration on some immunological parameters in pigs. Dtsch Tierarztl. Wochenschr. 103(4):131–133.

Muggli, R. (1994) Physiological requirements of vitamin E as a function of the amount and type of polyunsaturated fatty acid. World Rev. Nutr. Diet. 75:166–168. https://doi.org/10.1159/000423574.

Mujica-Álvarez, J., Gil-Castell, O., Barra, P.A., Ribes-Greus, A., Bustos, R., Faccini, M. and Matiacevich, S. (2020) Encapsulation of vitamins A and E as spray-dried additives for the feed industry. Molecules 25(6):1357. https://doi.org/10.3390/molecules25061357.

Mukhopadhyay, S., Singh, M. and Chatterjee, M. (2000) Vitamin D3 as a modulator of cellular antioxidant defence in murine lymphoma. Nutr. Res. 20(1):91–102. https://doi.org/10.1016/S0271-5317(99)00141-4.

Muralt, A. (1962) The role of thiamine in neurophysiology. Ann. N. Y. Acad. Sci. 98:499.

Muroya, S., Oe, M. and Ojima, K. (2018) Thiamine accumulation and thiamine triphosphate decline occur in parallel with ATP exhaustion during postmortem aging of pork muscles. Meat Sci. 137:228–234. https://doi.org/10.1016/j.meatsci.2017.11.035.

Murray, F.A., Moffatt, R.J. and Grifo, A.P. (1980) Secretion of riboflavin by the porcine uterus. J. Anim. Sci. 50(5):926–929. https://doi.org/10.2527/jas1980.505926x.

Mutetikka, D.B. and Mahan, D.C. (1993) Effect of pasture, confinement, and diet fortification with vitamin E and selenium on reproducing gilts and their progeny. J. Anim. Sci. 71(12):3211–3218. https://doi.org/10.2527/1993.71123211x.

Myer, R.O. (1992) Influence of injecting vitamin E and selenium just before breeding on sow reproductive performance. 5. University of Florida. p. 33.

Myers, G.S., Eaton, H.D. and Rousseau, J.E. (1959) Relative value of carotene from alfalfa and vitamin A from a dry carrier fed to lambs and pigs. J. Anim. Sci. 18(1):288–297. https://doi.org/10.2527/jas1959.181288x.

Nabi, F., Arain, M.A., Rajput, N., Alagawany, M., Soomro, J., Umer, M., Soomro, F., Wang, Z., Ye, R. and Liu, J. (2020) Health benefits of carotenoids and potential application in poultry industry: a review. J. Anim. Physiol. Anim. Nutr. (Berl) 104(6):1809–1818. https://doi.org/10.1111/jpn.13375.

Nabokina, S.M., Kashyap, M.L. and Said, H.M. (2005) Mechanism and regulation of human intestinal niacin uptake. Am. J. Physiol. Cell Physiol. 289(1):C97-C103. https://doi.org/10.1152/ajpcell.00009.2005.

Nafstad, I. (1965) Studies of hematology and bone marrow morphology in vitamin E-deficient pigs. Pathol. Vet. 2(3):277–287. https://doi.org/10.1177/030098586500200305.

Nafstad, I. (1973) Some aspects of vitamin E deficiency in pigs. Acta Agric. Scand. 19:31–34.

Nafstad, I. and Nafstad, H.J. (1968) An electron microscopic study of blood and bone marrow in vitamin E-deficient pigs. Pathol. Vet. 5(6):520–537.

Nafstad, I. and Tollersrud, S. (1970) The vitamin E-deficiency syndrome in pigs. I. Pathological changes. Acta Vet. Scand. 11(3):452–480. https://doi.org/10.1186/BF03547971.

Nagaraj, R.Y., Wu, W.D. and Vesonder, R.F. (1994) Toxicity of corn culture material of Fusarium proliferatum M-7176 and nutritional intervention in chicks. Poult. Sci. 73(5):617–626. https://doi.org/10.3382/ps.0730617.

Nakagawa, K., Shibata, A., Yamashita, S., Tsuzuki, T., Kariya, J., Oikawa, S. and Miyazawa, T. (2007) In vivo angiogenesis is suppressed by unsaturated vitamin E, tocotrienol. J. Nutr. 137(8):1938–1943. https://doi.org/10.1093/jn/137.8.1938.

Nakano, H. and Gregory, J.F. (1995) Pyridoxine and pyridoxine-5'-β-D-glucoside exert different effects on tissue B6 vitamers but similar effects on β-glucosidase activity in rats. J. Nutr. 125(11):2751–2762.

Nakano, H., McMahon, L.G. and Gregory, J.F. (1997) Pyridoxine-5'-beta-glucoside exhibits incomplete bioavailability as a source of vitamin B6 and partially inhibits the utilization of co-ingested pyridoxine in humans. J. Nutr. 127(8):1508–1513. https://doi.org/10.1093/jn/127.8.1508.

Natsuhori, M., Minoru, S. and Kokue, E. (1994) Alteration of plasma folates component during life cycle in pigs. Proceed. 13th IPVS Congress, Bangkok, Thailand. (p. 308).

Nawab, A., Tang s., Liu, W., Wu, J., Ibtisham, F., Kang, K., Ghani, M. W., Birmani, M. W., Li, G., Sun, C., Zhao, Y., Xiao, M. and An, L. (2019) Vitamin E and fertility in the poultry birds; deficiency of vitamin E and its hazardous effects. Approaches Poult Dairy & Vet Sci 6(1). https://doi.org/10.31031/APDV.2019.06.000626.

Nelsestuen, G.L., Zytkovicz, T.H. and Howard, J.B. (1974) The mode of action of vitamin K. Identification of gamma-carboxyglutamic acid as a component of prothrombin. J. Biol. Chem. 249(19):6347–6350. https://doi.org/10.1016/S0021–9258(19)42259-X.

Nelson, E.C., Dehority, B.A., Teague, H.S., Sanger, V.L. and Pounden, W.D. (1962) Effect of vitamin A intake on some biochemical and physiological changes in swine. J. Nutr. 76(4):325–332. https://doi.org/10.1093/jn/76.4.325.

Nelson, E.C., Dehority, B.A., Teague, H.S., Grifo, A.P. and Sanger, V.L. (1964) Effect of vitamin A and vitamin A acid on cerebrospinal fluid pressure and blood and liver vitamin A concentration in the pig. J. Nutr. 82(2):263–268. https://doi.org/10.1093/jn/82.2.263.

Nemec, M., Butler, G., Hidiroglou, M., Farnworth, E.R. and Nielsen, K. (1994) Effect of supplementing gilts' diets with different levels of vitamin E and different fats on the humoral and cellular immunity of gilts and their progeny. J. Anim. Sci. 72(3):665–676. https://doi.org/10.2527/1994.723665x.

Nesheim, R.O. and Johnson, B.C. (1950) Effect of a high level of methionine on the dietary choline requirement of the baby pig. J. Nutr. 41(1):149–152. https://doi.org/10.1093/jn/41.1.149.

Nesheim, R.O., Krider, J.L. and Johnson, B.C. (1950) The quantitative crystalline B12 requirement of the baby pig. Arch. Biochem. 27(1):240–242. PMID: 15419797.

Neumann, A.L., Krider, J.L., James, M.F. and Johnson, B.C. (1949) The choline requirement of the baby pig. J. Nutr. 38(2):195–213. https://doi.org/10.1093/jn/38.2.195.

Neumann, A.L., Johnson, B.C. and Thiersch, J.B. (1950a) Crystalline vitamin B12 in the nutrition of the baby pig. J. Nutr. 40(3):403–414. https://doi.org/10.1093/jn/40.3.403.

Neumann, A.L., Thiersch, J.B., Krider, J.L., James, M.F. and Johnson, B.C. (1950) Requirement of the baby pig for vitamin B12 fed as a concentrate. J. Anim. Sci. 9(1):83–89. https://doi.aorg/10.2527/jas1950.9183.

Newport, M.J. (1981) A note on the effect of low levels of biotin in milk substitutes for neonatal pigs. Anim. Sci. 33(3):333–335. https://doi.org/10.1017/S0003356100031731.

Newsholme, S.J., Cullen, J.S.C., Nel, P.W. and Reyers, F. (1985) A haemorrhagic syndrome in recently weaned pigs ascribed to hypovitaminosis K. J. S. Afr. Vet. Assoc. 56(2):101–102. PMID: 4020809.

Nielsen, H.E., Hojgaard-Olsen, N.J., Hjarde, W. and Leerbeck, E. (1973) Vitamin E content in colostrum and sow's milk yield at two levels of dietary fats. Acta Agric. Scand. suppl. 19:35–38.

Nielsen, H.E., Danielsen, V., Simesen, M.G., Gissel-Nielsen, G., Hjarde, W., Leth, T. and Basse, A. (1979) Selenium and vitamin E deficiency in pigs. I. Influence on growth and reproduction. Acta Vet. Scand. 20(2):276–288. https://doi.org/10.1186/BF03546619.

Nielsen, N.C. and Vinther, K. (1984) Influence of dietary vitamin C supplement on leg-weakness in pigs. In Wegger, I., Tagwerker, F.J. and Moustgaard, J. (Eds) "Proceeding workshop on ascorbic acid in domestic animals" The Royal Danish Agricultural Society. Copenhagen.

Nielsen, T.K., Wolstrup, C., Schirmer, A.L. and Jensen, P.T. (1989) Mulberry heart disease in young pigs without vitamin E and selenium deficiency. Vet. Rec. 124(20):535–537.

Nijhout, H.F., Reed, M.C. and Ulrich, C.M. (2008) Mathematical models of folate-mediated one-carbon metabolism. Vitam. Horm. 79:45–82. https://doi.org/10.1016/S0083-6729(08)00402-0.

Nockels, C.F. (1988) The role of vitamins in modulating disease resistance. Vet. Clin. North Am. Food Anim. Pract. 4(3):531–542. https://doi.org/10.1016/S0749-0720(15)31030-6.

Nockels, C.F. (1990) Mineral alterations associated with stress, trauma and infection and the effect on immunity. Cont. Educ. Pract. Vet. 12(8):1133–1139.

Noel, K. and Brinkhaus, F. (1998) Vitamin A retention of a high pigment broiler growing feed treated with endox or ethoxyquin. Poult. Sci. 77(1):144.

Norman, A.W. (2006) Minireview: Vitamin D receptor: new assignments for an already busy receptor. Endocrinology 147(12):5542–5548. https://doi.org/10.1210/en.2006-0946.

Norman, A.W. and Henry, H.C. (2007) Vitamin D. In Handbook of vitamins 4th ed. Zempleni, J., Rucker, R.B., McCormick, D.B. and Suttle, J.W. (ed.). CRC Press, Boca Raton, FL. (pp. 47–99).

North Central Region (NCR-42) Committee on Swine Nutrition (1976) Effect of supplemental choline on reproductive performance of sows: a cooperative regional study. J. Anim. Sci. 42(5):1211–1216. https://doi.org/10.2527/jas1976.4251211x.

North Central Region-42 (NCR-42) Committee on National Research Council (1998) Nutrient requirements of swine. National Academy of Sciences, Washington, DC. (1980) Effect of supplemental choline on performance of starting, growing, and finishing pigs: a cooperative regional study. J. Anim. Sci. 50(1):99–102. https://doi.org/10.2527/jas1980.50199x.

North Central Region-89 (NCR-89) Committee on Confinement Management of Swine (1989) Effect of vitamin C and space allowance on performance of weanling pigs. J. Anim. Sci. 67(3):624–627. https://doi.org/10.2527/jas1989.673624x.

NRC (1987) "Vitamin tolerance of animals". National Academy of Sciences. National Research Council. https://doi.org/10.17226/949.

NRC (1998) "Nutrient requirements of domestic animals: nutrient requirements of swine" 10th Rev. ed. National Academy Press, Washington, DC http://www.agri.ubu.ac.th/mis/evaluate/assess_learn/upload/67016.pdf.

NRC (2012) "Nutritional requirement of swine" 11th Rev. ed. National Academy Press, Washington, DC.

O'Byrne, S.M. and Blaner, W.S. (2013) Retinol and retinyl esters: biochemistry and physiology. J. Lipid Res. 54(7):1731–1743. https://doi.org/10.1194/jlr.R037648.

O'Connor, D.L., Picciano, M.F., Roos, M.A. and Easter, R.A. (1989) Iron and folate utilization in reproducing swine and their progeny. J. Nutr. 119(12):1984–1991. https://doi.org/10.1093/jn/119.12.1984.

Obel, A.L. (1953) Studies on the morphology and etiology of so-called toxic liver dystrophy (*hepatosis diaetetica*) in swine. Acta Pathol. Microbiol. Scand. Suppl. (1926) 94:1–119. PMID: 13057607.

O'Dell, B.L. and Hogan, A.G. (1943) Additional observations on the chick antianemia vitamin. J. Biol. Chem. 149(2):323–337. https://doi.org/10.1016/S0021-9258(18)72179-0.

Oduho, G.W. and Baker, D.H. (1993) Quantitative efficacy of niacin sources for chicks: nicotinic acid, nicotinamide, NAD and tryptophan. J. Nutr. 123(12):2201–2206.

Okere, C. and Hacker, R.R. (1997) Immunophysiological responses of sows and neonatal pigs to vitamin E and selenium therapy. Ont. Swine Res. Rev.:(87–89).

Oldfield, J.E. (1987) History of nutrition: development of the concept of antimetabolites. Introduction. J. Nutr. 117(7):1322–1323. https://doi.org/10.1093/jn/117.7.1322.

Oldfield, J.E. (2003) Some recollections of early swine research with selenium and vitamin E. J. Anim. Sci. 81 14(2)(suppl.):E145-E148.

Olivares, M., Pizarro, F., Pineda, O., Name, J.J., Hertrampf, E. and Walter, T. (1997) Milk inhibits and ascorbic acid favors ferrous bis-glycine chelate bioavailability in humans. J. Nutr. 127(7):1407–1411. https://doi.org/10.1093/jn/127.7.1407.

Olivares, A., Daza, A., Rey, A.I. and López-Bote, C.J. (2009a) Dietary vitamin A concentration alters fatty acid composition in pigs. Meat Sci. 81(2):295–299. https://doi.org/10.1016/j.meatsci.2008.07.029.

Olivares, A., Rey, A.I., Daza, A. and Lopez-Bote, C.J. (2009b) High dietary vitamin A interferes with tissue α-tocopherol concentrations in fattening pigs: a study that examines administration and withdrawal times. Animal 3(9):1264–1270. https://doi.org/10.1017/S175173110900487X.

Olivares, A., Rey, A.I., Daza, A. and López-Bote, C.J. (2011) Low levels of dietary vitamin A increase intramuscular fat content and polyunsaturated fatty acid proportion in liver from lean pigs. Livest. Sci. 137(1–3):31–36. https://doi.org/10.1016/j.livsci.2010.09.023.

Oloyo, R.A. (1991) Responses of broilers fed guineacorn/palm kernel meal based ration to supplemental biotin. J. Sci. Food Agric. 55(4):539–550. https://doi.org/10.1002/jsfa.2740550406.

Olson, J.A. (1984) Vitamin A. In "Handbook of vitamins" Machlin, L.J. (Ed.). Marcel Dekker, Inc., New York.

Olson, R.E. (1990) Pantothenic acid. In "Nutrition reviews, present knowledge in nutrition" Olson, R.E. (ed.). Nutrition Foundation.

Omelka, R., Martiniaková, M., Peškovičová, D. and Bauerová, M. (2008) Associations between RBP4/MspI polymorphism and reproductive traits in pigs: an application of animal model. J. Agrobiol. 25(1):77–80.

Orstadius, K., Nordstrom, G. and Lannek, N. (1963) Combined therapy with vitamin E and selenite in experimental nutritional muscular dystrophy of pigs. Cornell Vet. 53:60–71.

Osborne, V.R., Hacker, R.R. and Squires, E.J. (1998) The effect of supplementary vitamin E and C on fresh and cooked pork quality. J. Anim. Sci. 76(suppl. 1):253.

Otsuka, M., Matsuzawa, M., Ha, T.Y. and Arakawa, N. (1999) Contribution of a high dose of L-ascorbic acid to carnitine synthesis in guinea pigs fed high-fat diets. J. Nutr. Sci. Vitaminol. (Tokyo) 45(2):163–171. https://doi.org/10.3177/jnsv.45.163.

Padh, H. (1991) Vitamin C: newer insights into its biochemical functions. Nutr. Rev. 49(3):65–70. https://doi.org/10.1111/j.1753-4887.1991.tb07407.x.

Palagina, N.K., Meledina, T.V. and Karpisheva, I.A. (1990) Simplified method for determining pantothenic acid in molasses Applied Biochem. Microbiol. 26. p. 688. Record Number: 19920313555.

Palludan, B. (1961) The teratogenic effect of vitamin A deficiency in pigs. Acta Vet. Scand. 2(1):32–59.

Palludan, B. (1966) Direct effect of vitamin A on Boar testis Nature 211(5049):639–40 10.1038/211639a0.

Palludan, B. and Wegger, I. (1984) Plasma ascorbic acid in calves. In "Ascorbic acid in domestic animals Wegger, I., Tagwerker, F. and Moustgaard, J. (Eds). Royal Danish Agricultural Society, Copenhagen, Denmark. (pp. 131–138).

Palludan, B. and Wegger, I. (1988) The influence of ascorbic acid status on boar performance. Proceed. 10th Congress Inter. Pig. Vet. Soc. Rio de Janeiro. Brazil.

Palm, B.W., Meade, R.J. and Melliere, A.L. (1968) Pantothenic acid requirement of young swine. J. Anim. Sci. 27(6):1596-1601. https://doi.org/10.2527/jas1968.2761596x.

Panagabko, C., Morley, S., Neely, S., Lei, H., Manor, D. and Atkinson, J. (2002) Expression and refolding of recombinant human alpha-tocopherol transfer protein capable of specific alpha-tocopherol binding. Protein Expr. Purif. 24(3):395–403. https://doi.org/10.1006/prep.2001.1576.

Panganamala, R.V. and Cornwell, D.G. (1982) The effects of vitamin E on arachidonic acid metabolism. Ann. N. Y. Acad. Sci. 393:376–391. https://doi.org/10.1111/j.1749-6632.1982.tb31277.x.

Pappu, A.S., Fatterpaker, P. and Sreenivasan, A. (1978) Possible interrelationships between vitamins E and B12 in the disturbance in methylmalonate metabolism in vitamin E deficiency. Biochem. J. 172(1):115–121. https://doi.org/10.1042/bj1720115.

Pardo, D.C. (1995) Vitamin E: pharmacokinetics of parenteral products and its effect on swine reproduction. Iowa State University.

Park, H.D., Zhu, Y.C. and Park, Y.S. (2014) Effects of Vitamin K 1 on the Developmental and Survival Rate of Porcine In Vitro Fertilized Embryos. J. Anim. Reprod. Biotechnol. 29(1):73–81. https://doi.org/10.12750/JET.2014.29.1.73.

Park, T.F. and Harrison, P.C. (1990) Growth performance of nursery-pigs provided tap and carbonated drinking water sources supplemented with monopotassium ascorbate. Univ. of Illinois, Urbana, IL.

Parker, R.S. (1989) Dietary and biochemical aspects of vitamin E. Adv. Food Nutr. Res. 33:157–232. https://doi.org/10.1016/S1043-4526(08)60128-X.

Parrish, D.B., Aubel, C.E., Hughes, J.S. and Wheat, J.D. (1951) Relative value of vitamin A and carotene for supplying the vitamin A requirements of swine during gestation and beginning lactation. J. Anim. Sci. 10(2):551–559. https://doi.org/10.2527/jas1951.102551x.

Parsons, J.L. and Klostermann, H.J. (1967) Dakota scientists report new antibiotic found in flaxseed. Feedstuffs 39(45):74.

Partridge, I.G. and Brown, R.G. (1971) Influence of supplementary ascorbic acid on performance of crowded swine. Can. J. Anim. Sci. 51:824.

Partridge, I.G. and McDonald, M.S. (1990) A note on the response of growing pigs to supplemental biotin. Anim. Sci. 50(1):195–197. https://doi.org/10.1017/S0003356100004608.

Patel, S. and Vajdy, M. (2015) Induction of cellular and molecular immunomodulatory pathways by vitamin A and flavonoids. Expert Opin. Biol. Ther. 15(10):1411–1428. https://doi.org/10.1517/14712598.2015.1066331.

Patience, J.F. and Gillis, D. (1996) Impact of preslaughter withdrawal of vitamin supplements on pig performance and meat quality Prairie Swine Center, Inc. Research Report. (p. 29).

Pearson, P.B., Struglia, L. and Lindahl, I.L. (1953) The fecal and urinary excretion of certain B vitamins by sheep fed hay and semi-synthetic rations. J. Anim. Sci. 12(1):213–218. https://doi.org/10.2527/jas1953.121213x.

Pedersen, O.G. and Udesen, F. (1980) Testing biotin in sows. Communication Nr. 18, Danish Committee on Pig Breeding and Production. Joint Office of Cooperative Slaughterhouses, Copenhagen.

Pedersen, S., Saeed, I., Jensen, S.K., Michaelsen, K.F. and Friis, H. (2001) Marginal vitamin A deficiency in pigs experimentally infected with Trichuris suis: a model for vitamin A inadequacy in children. Trans. R. Soc. Trop. Med. Hyg. 95(5):557–565. https://doi.org/10.1016/S0035-9203(01)90040-9.

Peeters, E., Neyt, A., Beckers, F., De Smet, S., Aubert, A.E. and Geers, R. (2005) Influence of supplemental magnesium, tryptophan, vitamin C, and vitamin E on stress responses of pigs to vibration. J. Anim. Sci. 83(7):1568–1580. https://doi.org/10.2527/2005.8371568x.

Peeters, E., Driessen, B. and Geers, R. (2006) Influence of supplemental magnesium, tryptophan, vitamin C, vitamin E, and herbs on stress responses and pork quality. J. Anim. Sci. 84(7):1827–1838. https://doi.org/10.2527/jas.2005-600.

Peng, C.L. and Heitman, H. (1973) Erythrocyte transketolase activity and the percentage stimulation by thiamin pyrophosphate as criteria of thiamin status in the pig. Br. J. Nutr. 30(3):391–399.

Peng, C.L. and Heitman, H. (1974) The effect of ambient temperature on the thiamin requirement of growing-finishing pigs. Br. J. Nutr. 32(1):1–9. https://doi.org/10.1079/BJN19740053.

Penny, R.H., Cameron, R.D., Johnson, S., Kenyon, P.J., Smith, H.A., Bell, A.W., Cole, J.P. and Taylor, J. (1980) Foot rot of pigs: the influence of biotin supplementation on foot lesions in sows. Vet. Rec. 107(15):350–351.

Penny, R.H.C., Cameron, R.H.A., Johnson, S. Kenyan, P.J. Smith, H.A., Bell, A.W.P., Cole, J.P.L. and Taylor, J. (1981) The influence of biotin supplementation on sow reproductive efficiency. Vet. Rec. 109(4):80–81.

Peo, E.R., Wehrebein, G.F., Mosser, B., Cunningham, P.J. and Vipperman, P.E. (1970) Biotin supplementation of baby pig diets. J. Anim. Sci. 31:209.

Peplowski, M.A., Mahan, D.C., Murray, F.A., Moxon, A.L., Cantor, A.H. and Ekstrom, K.E. (1980) Effect of dietary and injectable vitamin E and selenium in weanling swine antigenically challenged with sheep red blood cells. J. Anim. Sci. 51(2):344–351. https://doi.org/10.2527/jas1980.512344x.

Perks, S.M. and Miller, D.D. (1996) Adding ascorbic acid to iron-fortified cow's milk does not enhance iron bioavailability to piglets. Nutr. Res. 16(6):969–975. https://doi.org/10.1016/0271-5317(96)00096-6.

Perry, S.C. (1978) Vitamin allowances for animal feeds. In Vitamin nutrition update – seminar series 2, RCD 5483/1078. Hoffmann-La Roche.

Petroff, B.K., Ciereszko, R.E., Dabrowski, K., Ottobre, A.C., Pope, W.F. and Ottobre, J.S. (1996) Prostglandin F2a depletes the porcine corpus luteum of vitamin C by inducing secretion of the vitamin into the bloodstream. The Ohio State Res Rev:(321–327).

Pettigrew, J.E., El-Kandelgy, S.M., Johnston, L.J. and Shurson, G.C. (1996) Riboflavin nutrition of sows. J. Anim. Sci. 74(9):2226–2230. https://doi.org/10.2527/1996.7492226x.

Pharazyn, A. and Aherne, F.X. (1987) Folacin requirement of the lactating sow. Univ. of Alberta 66th Ann. Feeders Day Rep. (pp. 16).

Phillips, A.L., Faustman, C., Lynch, M.P., Govoni, K.E., Hoagland, T.A. and Zinn, S.A. (2001) Effect of dietary α-tocopherol supplementation on color and lipid stability in pork. Meat Sci. 58(4):389–393. https://doi.org/10.1016/S0309-1740(01)00039-0.

Piatkowski, T.L., Mahan, D.C., Cantor, A.H., Moxon, A.L., Cline, J.H. and Grifo, A.P. (1979) Selenium and vitamin E in semipurified diets for gravid and non-gravid gilts. J. Anim. Sci. 48(6):1357–1365. https://doi.org/10.2527/jas1979.4861357x.

PIC (2021) Nutrition and feeding guidelines. http://www.pic.com/wp-content/uploads/sites/3/2021/03/PIC-Nutrition-Manual_English-Imperial.pdf.

Pig Champ. https://www.pigchamp.com/news/benchmark-magazine.

Pillai, P.B., Fanatico, A.C., Beers, K.W., Blair, M.E. and Emmert, J.L. (2006a) Homocysteine remethylation in young broilers fed varying levels of methionine, choline and betaine. Poult. Sci. 85(1):90–95. https://doi.org/10.1093/ps/85.1.90.

Pillai, P.B., Fanatico, A.C., Blair, M.E. and Emmert, J.L. (2006b) Homocysteine remethylation in broilers fed surfeit choline or betaine and varying levels and sources of methionine from eight to twenty-two days of age. Poult. Sci. 85(10):1729–1736. https://doi.org/10.1093/ps/85.10.1729.

Pinelli-Saavedra, A. (2003) Vitamin E in immunity and reproductive performance in pigs. Reprod. Nutr. Dev. 43(5):397–408. https://doi.org/10.1051/rnd:2003034.

Pinto, J.T. and Rivlin, R.S. (2013) Riboflavin (vitamin B2). In "Handbook of vitamins" 5th ed. Zempleni, J., Suttie, J., Gregory, J. and Stover, P.J. (Eds). CRC Press. (pp. 191–266).

Pinto, J.T. and Zempleni, J. (2016) Riboflavin. Adv. Nutr. 7(5):973–975. https://doi.org/10.3945/an.116.012716.

Piper, R.C., Froseth, J.A., McDowell, L.R., Kroening, G.H. and Dyer, I.A. (1975) Selenium-vitamin E deficiency in swine fed peas (*Pisum sativum*). Am. J. Vet. Res. 36(3):273–281. PMID: 1115425.

Pluym, L., Van Nuffel, A., Dewulf, J., Cools, A., Vangroenweghe, F., Van Hoorebeke, S. and Maes, D. (2011) Prevalence and risk factors of claw lesions and lameness in pregnant sows in two types of group housing. Vet. Med. 56(3):101–109. https://doi.org/10.17221/3159-VETMED.

Podda, M. and Grundmann-Kollmann, M. (2001) Low molecular weight antioxidants and their role in skin ageing. Clin. Exp. Dermatol. 26(7):578–582. https://doi.org/10.1046/j.1365-2230.2001.00902.x.

Pointillart, A., Denis, I., Colin, C. and Lacroix, H. (1997) Vitamin C supplementation does not modify bone mineral content or mineral absorption in growing pigs. J. Nutr. 127(8):1514–1518. https://doi.org/10.1093/jn/127.8.1514.

Polak, D.M., Elliot, J.M. and Haluska, M. (1979) Vitamin B12 binding proteins in bovine serum. J. Dairy Sci. 62(5):697–701. https://doi.org/10.3168/jds.S0022-0302(79)83312-3.

Polegato, B.F., Pereira, A.G., Azevedo, P.S., Costa, N.A., Zornoff, L.A.M., Paiva, S.A.R. and Minicucci, M.F. (2019) Role of thiamin in health and disease. Nutr. Clin. Pract. 34(4):558–564. https://doi.org/10.1002/ncp.10234.

Polcz, M.E. and Barbul, A. (2019) The role of vitamin A in wound healing. Nutr. Clin. Pract. 34(5):695–700. https://doi.org/10.1002/ncp.10376.

Pond, W.G., Kwong, E. and Loosli, J.K. (1960) Effect of level of dietary fat, pantothenic acid, and protein on performance of growing-fattening swine. J. Anim. Sci. 19(4):1115–1122. https://doi.org/10.2527/jas1960.1941115x.

Poor, C.L., Miller, S.D., Fahey, G.C., Easter, R.A. and Erdman, J.W. (1987) Animal models for carotenoid utilization studies: evaluation of the chick and the pig. Nutr. Rep. Int. 36:229–234.

Poulsen, J. and Krogsdahl, J. (2018) OVN™ Vitamin concept from DSM improves production value in feed for piglets SEGES (Danish Pig Research Centre) Report. https://pigresearchcentre.dk/-/media/PDF/English-site/Research_PDF/Weaners/Meddelelse_1148_UK.ashx.

Powers, H.J., Weaver, L.T., Austin, S., Wright, A.J. and Fairweather-Tait, S.J. (1991) Riboflavin deficiency in the rat: effects on iron utilization and loss. Br. J. Nutr. 65(3):487–496. https://doi.org/10.1079/BJN19910107.

Powers, H.J., Weaver, L.T., Austin, S. and Beresford, J.K. (1993) A proposed intestinal mechanism for the effect of riboflavin deficiency on iron loss in the rat. Br. J. Nutr. 69(2):553–561. https://doi.org/10.1079/bjn19930055.

Powick, W.C., Ellis, N.R. and Dale, C.N. (1947a) Relationship of corn diets to nicotinic acid deficiency in growing pigs. J. Anim. Sci. 6(4):395–400. https://doi.org/10.2527/jas1947.64395x.

Powick, W.C., Ellis, N.R., Madsen, L.L. and Dale, C.N. (1947b) Nicotinic acid deficiency and nicotinic acid requirement of young pigs on a purified diet. J. Anim. Sci. 6(3):310–324.

Powick, W.C., Ellis, N.R. and Dale, C.N. (1948) Relationship of tryptophane to nicotinic acid in the feeding of growing pigs. J. Anim. Sci. 7(2):228–232. https://doi.org/10.2527/jas1948.72228x.

Premkumar, V.G., Yuvaraj, S., Shanthi, P. and Sachdanandam, P. (2008) Co-enzyme Q10, riboflavin and niacin supplementation on alteration of DNA repair enzyme and DNA methylation in breast cancer patients undergoing tamoxifen therapy. Br. J. Nutr. 100(6):1179–1182. https://doi.org/10.1017/S0007114508968276.

Preś, J., Fuchs, B. and Schleicher, A. (1993) The effect of carotene and vitamins A and E supplementation on reproduction of sows. Arch. Vet. Pol. 33(1–2):55–64. PMID: 8055056.

Pryor, W.J., Seawright, A.A. and McCosker, P.J. (1969) Hypervitaminosis A in the pig. Aust. Vet. J. 45(12):563–569. https://doi.org/10.1111/j.1751-0813.1969.tb16092.x.

Pullar, J.M., Carr, A.C. and Vissers, M.C.M. (2017) The roles of vitamin C in skin health. Nutrients 9(8):866–892. https://doi.org/10.3390/nu9080866.

Purser, K. (1981) Folic acid beneficial to young pigs. Anim. Nutr. Health 36(3):38.

Pusateri, A.E., Diekman, M.A. and Singleton, W.L. (1996) Failure of vitamin A results to alter litter size in swine when injected at breeding and various stages of gestation. J. Anim. Sci. 74(suppl. 1):247.

Putnam, M.E. (1984) Vitamin E for pigs. Pig Vet. Soc. Proc. 9:178.

Qiu, Y., Liu, S., Hou, L., Li, K., Wang, L., Gao, K., Yang, X. and Jiang, Z. (2021) Supplemental choline modulates growth performance and gut inflammation by altering the gut microbiota and lipid metabolism in weaned piglets. J. Nutr. 151(1):20–29. https://doi.org/10.1093/jn/nxaa331.

Quackenbush, F.W. (1963) Corn carotenoids: effect of temperature and moisture on losses during storage. Cereal Chem. 40:266.

Quarterman, J., Dalgarno, A.C., Adam, A., Fell, B.F. and Boyne, R. (1964) The distribution of vitamin D between the blood and the liver in the pig and observations on the pathology of vitamin D toxicity. Br. J. Nutr. 18(1):65–77. https://doi.org/10.1079/BJN19640007.

Qureshi, A.A., Salser, W.A., Parmar, R. and Emeson, E.E. (2001) Novel tocotrienols of rice bran inhibit atherosclerotic lesions in C57BL/6 apoE-deficient mice. J. Nutr. 131(10):2606–2618. https://doi.org/10.1093/jn/131.10.2606.

Radhika, M.S., Bhaskaram, P., Balakrishna, N., Ramalakshmi, B.A., Devi, S. and Kumar, B.S. (2002) Effects of vitamin A deficiency during pregnancy on maternal and child health. BJOG 109(6):689–693. https://doi.org/10.1111/j.1471-0528.2002.01010.x.

Raederstorff, D., Wyss, A., Calder, P.C., Weber, P. and Eggersdorfer, M. (2015) Vitamin E function and requirements in relation to PUFA. Br. J. Nutr. 114(8):1113–1122. https://doi.org/10.1017/S000711451500272X.

Rahman, T., Goswami, U.V., Goswami, S. and Baruah, S.N. (1996) Hypovitaminosis – a in piglets in an organised farm. Indian J. Vet. Pathol. 20(2):148–149.

Rajic, I.D. (1971) The effect of ascorbic acid on the prevention of muscle degeneration and pale, soft and exudative meat in swine. Acta Vet. Beograd 21:253–265.

Rajic, I.D., Sevkovic, N., Dakik, M. and Dinic, L. (1977) Effect of vitamin C on the color of hog muscle tissue. Food Sci. Technol. 9(12S):2122.

Rajkhowa, T.K., Katiyar, A.K. and Vegad, J.L. (1996) Effect of ascorbic acid on the inflammatory-reparative response in the punched wounds of the chicken skin. Indian J. Anim. Sci. 66:120–125.

Rammell, C.G., Pearson, A.B. and Bentley, G.R. (1988) Vitamin E, selenium and polyunsaturated fatty acids in clinically normal grower (9–16 weeks old) pigs and their feed: their relationship to the vitamin E/selenium deficiency ("VESD") syndrome. N. Z. Vet. J. 36(3):133–137. https://doi.org/10.1080/00480169.1988.35508.

Rao, C.V., Hirose, Y., Indranie, C. and Reddy, B.S. (2001) Modulation of experimental colon tumorigenesis by types and amounts of dietary fatty acids. Cancer Res. 61(5):1927–1933. PMID: 11280748.

Rawling, J.M., Jackson, T.M., Driscoll, E.R. and Kirkland, J.B. (1994) Dietary niacin deficiency lowers tissue poly (ADP-ribose) and NAD+ concentrations in Fischer-344 rats. J. Nutr. 124(9):1597–1603. https://doi.org/10.1093/jn/124.9.1597.

Real, D.E., Nelssen, J.L., Unruh, J.A., Tokach, M.D., Goodband, R.D., Dritz, S.S., DeRouchey, J.M. and Alonso, E. (2002) Effects of increasing dietary niacin on growth performance and meat quality in finishing pigs reared in two different environments. J. Anim. Sci. 80(12):3203–3210. https://doi.org/10.2527/2002.80123203x.

Reboul, E. and Borel, P. (2011) Proteins involved in uptake, intracellular transport and basolateral secretion of fat-soluble vitamins and carotenoids by mammalian enterocytes. Prog. Lipid Res. 50(4):388–402. https://doi.org/10.1016/j.plipres.2011.07.001.

Reddy, M.U. and Pushpamma, P. (1986) Effect of storage and insect infestation on thiamine and niacin content in different varieties of rice, sorghum, and legumes. Nutr. Rep. Int. 34:393–401.

Regassa, A., Adhikari, R., Nyachoti, C.M. and Kim, W.K. (2015) Effects of 2-(OH)D3 on fecal Ca and P excretion, bone mineralization, Ca and P transporter mRNA expression and performance in growing female pigs. J. Environ. Sci. Health B 50(4):293–299. https://doi.org/10.1080/03601234.2015.999612.

Rehfeldt, C. and Kuhn, G. (2006) Consequences of birth weight for postnatal growth performance and carcass quality in pigs as related to myogenesis. J. Anim. Sci. 84(E)(Suppl.):E113-E123. https://doi.org/10.2527/2006.8413_supple113x.

Rehfeldt, C., Tuchscherer, A., Hartung, M. and Kuhn, G. (2008) A second look at the influence of birth weight on carcass and meat quality in pigs. Meat Sci. 78(3):170–175. https://doi.org/10.1016/j.meatsci.2007.05.029.

Reinhardt, T.A. and Hustmyer, F.G. (1987) Role of vitamin D in the immune system. J. Dairy Sci. 70(5):952–962. https://doi.org/10.3168/jds.S0022-0302(87)80099-1.

Reinisch, F. and Gebhardt, G. (1987) Effect of vitamin B12 on fertility in sows. In Symposium on vitamins Reinhardsbrunn, E. Germany.

Renegar, R.H., Bazer, F.W. and Roberts, R.M. (1981) Endometrial collagenase during early pregnancy and the estrous cycle of gilts. J. Anim. Sci. 53(Suppl. 1):362.

Rey, A.I. and López-Bote, C.J. (2014) Alpha-tocopherol stereoisomer analysis as discriminant method for distinguishing Iberian pig feed intake during the fattening phase. Food Chem. 142:342–348. https://doi.org/10.1016/j.foodchem.2013.07.055.

Rey, A.I., López-Bote, C.J. and Sanz Arias, R.S. (1997) Effect of extensive feeding on α-tocopherol concentration and oxidative stability of muscle microsomes from Iberian pigs. Anim. Sci. 65(3):515–520. https://doi.org/10.1017/S1357729800008729.

Rey, A.I., Kerry, J.P., Lynch, P.B., López-Bote, C.J., Buckley, D.J. and Morrissey, P.A. (2001) Effect of dietary oils and α-tocopheryl acetate supplementation on lipid (TBARS) and cholesterol oxidation in cooked pork. J. Anim. Sci. 79(5):1201–1208. https://doi.org/10.2527/2001.7951201x.

Rey, A.I., Daza, A., López-Carrasco, C. and López-Bote, C.J. (2006) Feeding Iberian pigs with acorns and grass in either free-range or confinement affects the carcass characteristics and fatty acids and tocopherols accumulation in longissimus dorsi muscle and backfat. Meat Sci. 73(1):66–74. https://doi.org/10.1016/j.meatsci.2005.10.018.

Rhee, K.S. and Ziprin, Y.A. (1987) Lipid oxidation in retail beef, pork and chicken muscles as affected by concentrations of heme pigments and nonheme iron and microsomal enzymic lipid peroxidation activity. J. Food Biochemistry 11(1):1–15. https://doi.org/10.1111/j.1745-4514.1987.tb00109.x.

Riabroy, N. and Tanumihardjo, S.A. (2014) Oral doses of α-retinyl ester track chylomicron uptake and distribution of vitamin A in a male piglet model for newborn infants. J. Nutr. 144(8):1188–1195. https://doi.org/10.3945/jn.114.191668.

Ribas-Maynou, J., Mateo-Otero, Y., Delgado-Bermúdez, A., Bucci, D., Tamanini, C., Yeste, M. and Barranco, I. (2021) Role of exogenous antioxidants on the performance and function of pig sperm after preservation in liquid and frozen states: A systematic review. Theriogenology 173:279–294. https://doi.org/10.1016/j.theriogenology.2021.07.023.

Ribeiro, A.M., Estevinho, B.N. and Rocha, F. (2021) The progress and application of vitamin E encapsulation–A review. Food Hydrocoll. 121:106998. https://doi.org/10.1016/j.foodhyd.2021.106998.

Rice, D.A. and Kennedy, S. (1989) Vitamin E, selenium, and polyunsaturated fatty acid concentrations and glutathione peroxidase activity in tissues from pigs with dietetic microangiopathy (mulberry heart disease). Am. J. Vet. Res. 50(12):2101–2104. PMID: 2610435.

Richardson, D., Catron, D.V., Underkofler, L.A., Maddock, H.M. and Friedland, W.C. (1951) Vitamin B12 requirement of male weanling pigs. J. Nutr. 44(3):371–381. https://doi.org/10.1093/jn/44.3.371.

Riedel-Caspari, G., Schmidt, F.W., Gunther, K.D. and Wagner, K. (1986) Influence of oral dosing with vitamin E on the defense mechanisms of pigs at the early fattening stage. J. Vet. Med. 33:650.

Rifici, V.A. and Khachadurian, A.K. (1993) Dietary supplementation with vitamins C and E inhibits in vitro oxidation of lipoproteins. J. Am. Coll. Nutr. 12(6):631–637. https://doi.org/10.1080/07315724.1993.10718353.

Rigotti, A. (2007) Absorption, transport, and tissue delivery of vitamin E. Mol. Aspects Med. 28(5–6):423–436. https://doi.org/10.1016/j.mam.2007.01.002.

Riker, J.T., Perry, T.W., Pickett, R.A. and Heidenreich, C.J. (1967) Influence of controlled temperatures on growth rate and plasma ascorbic acid values in swine. J. Nutr. 92(1):99–103. https://doi.org/10.1093/jn/92.1.99.

Ritchie, H.D., Miller, E.R., Ullrey, D.E., Hoefer, J.A. and Luecke, R.W. (1960) Supplementation of the swine gestation diet with pyridoxine. J. Nutr. 70(4):491–496. https://doi.org/10.1093/jn/70.4.491.

Riveron-Negrete, L. and Fernandez-Mejia, C. (2017) Pharmacological effects of biotin in animals. Mini Rev. Med. Chem. 17(6):529–540. https://doi.org/10.2174/1389557516666160923132611.

Rivlin, R.S. (2006) Riboflavin. In "Present knowledge in nutrition" 9th ed. Bowman, B.A. and Russell, R.M. (Eds.). International Life Sciences Institute. (pp. 250–259).

Roberts, R.M. and Bazer, F.W. (1980) The properties, function and hormonal control of synthesis of uteroferrin, the purple protein of pig uterus. In steroid induced uterine proteins Beato, M. (Ed.). North Holland Biomedical Press. Elsevier, Amsterdam.

Roche (1979) "Optimum vitamin nutrition". Hoffmann-La Roche, Nutley, NJ, USA.

Rodríguez-Meléndez, R. and Zempleni, J. (2003) Regulation of gene expression by biotin [review]. J. Nutr. Biochem. 14(12):680–690. https://doi.org/10.1016/j.jnutbio.2003.07.001.

Rodríguez-Meléndez, R., Cano, S., Méndez, S.T. and Velázquez, A. (2001) Biotin regulates the genetic expression of holocarboxylase synthetase and mitochondrial carboxylases in rats. J. Nutr. 131(7):1909–1913. https://doi.org/10.1093/jn/131.7.1909.

Rojas, C., Cadenas, S., Herrero, A., Méndez, J. and Barja, G. (1996) Endotoxin depletes ascorbate in the guinea pig heart. Protective effects of vitamins C and E against oxidative stress. Life Sci. 59(8):649–657. https://doi.org/10.1016/0024-3205(96)00346-3.

Rosbotham, E.J., Rankin, D., Gill, C.I.R., McDonald, E.J., McRoberts, W.C., Neill, H.R., Boland, R. and Pourshahidi, L.K. (2021) The use of supervised machine learning techniques to identify factors influencing vitamin D bioenrichment of pork. Proc. Nutr. Soc. 80(OCE3):(OCE3). https://doi.org/10.1017/S0029665121002640.

Rose, R. (1990) Vitamin absorption. In "Developments in vitamin nutrition and health applications" Proc. National Feed Ingr. Ass., Nutr. Inst. Kansas City. National Feed Ingredients Association, MO.

Rose, R.C., McCorrmick, D.B., Li, T.K., Lumeng, L., Haddad, J.G. and Spector, R. (1986) Transport and metabolism of vitamins. Fed. Proc. 45(1):30–39. PMID: 3000833.

Rosenberg, I.H. (2012) A history of the isolation and identification of vitamin B6. Ann. Nutr. Metab. 61(3): 236–238. https://doi.org/10.1159/000343113.

Rosenberg, I.H. and Neumann, H. (1974) Multi-step mechanism in the hydrolysis of pteroyl polyglutamates by chicken intestine. J. Biol. Chem. 249(16):5126–5130. https://doi.org/10.1016/S0021-9258(19)42336-3.

Ross, A.C. (1992) Vitamin A status: relationship to immunity and the antibody response. Proc. Soc. Exp. Biol. Med. 200(3):303–320. https://doi.org/10.3181/00379727-200-43436A.

Ross, A.C. (1993) Overview of retinoid metabolism. J. Nutr. 123(2)(Suppl.):346–350. https://doi.org/10.1093/jn/123.suppl_2.346.

Ross, A.C. and Harrison, E.H. (2013) Vitamin A: nutritional aspects of retinoids and carotenoids. In "Handbook of vitamins" 5th ed. Zempleni, J., Suttie, J., Gregory, J. and Stover, P.J. (Eds.). CRC Press. (pp. 1–50).

Rostagno, H.S., Albino, L.F.T., Donzele, J.L., Gomes, P.C., Oliveira, R.F., Lopes, D.C., Ferreira, A.S., Barreto, S.L.T. and Euclides, R.F. (2011) "Tabelas brasileiras para aves e suínos: composição de alimentos e exigências nutricionais" 3rd ed. Universidade Federal de Viçosa, Viçosa, BR.

Rostagno, H.S., Albino, L.F.T., Hannas, M.I., Donzele, J.L., Sakomura, N.K., Perazzo, F.G., Saraiva, A., Abreu, De, M.L.T., Rodrigues, P.B., Oliveira, De, R.F., Barreto, S.L.T. and Brito, C.O. (2017) "Brazilian tables for poultry and swine: composition of feedstuffs and nutritional requirements" 4th ed. Departamento de Zootecnia, Viçosa, Universidade Federal de Vicosa.

Roth, F.X. and Kirchgessner, M. (1975) Vitamin E concentration in blood and tissues of growing pigs fed on varying DL-a-Tocopherylacetate supplements. Int. J. Vitam. Nutr. Res. 45(3):333–341. PMID: 1184299.

Roth-Maier, D.A. and Kirchgessner, M. (1977) Optimal pantothenic acid requirements for market pigs. Z. Tierphysiol. Tierernähr. Futtermittelkd. 38(3):121–131. PMID: 855508.

Roth-Maier, D.A. and Kirchgessner, M. (1993a) The influence of pectin supplementation on the bioavailability of thiamine in a marginal and optimal thiamine supply status of sows. J. Anim. Physiol. Anim. Nutr. (Germany) 69(2–3):162–168.

Roth-Maier, D.A. and Kirchgessner, M. (1993b) Influences of cellulose supplements on vitamin B6 metabolism of sows subjected to dietary suboptimal and optimal vitamin B6 therapy. J. Anim. Physiol. Anim. Nutr. 70(1–5):6–12.

Roth-Maier, V.D., A. and Kirchgessner, M. (1994) Influence of wheat bran and alfalfa meal on the thiamine metabolism of sows provided with a suboptimal thiamine supply. J. Anim. Physiol. Anim. Nutr. 72(2–3):115–122. SSN: 0044-3565.

Roth-Maier, D.A. and Kirchgessner, M. (1997) Influence of wheat bran and alfalfa meal supplements on vitamin B6 metabolism of sows subjected to suboptimal vitamin B6 supply. Arch. Tierernähr. 50(2):155–162. https://doi.org/10.1080/17450399709386127.

Roth-Maier, D.A., Benedikt, J., Stangl, G.I. and Kirchgessner, M. (1996) Effect of feeding various dietary vitamin B6 concentrations during gestation and lactation on vitamin B6 level in liver and carcass of rat dams. Arch. Tierernähr. 49(4):319–324. https://doi.org/10.1080/17450399609381894.

Rothe, S., Gropp, J., Weiser, H. and Rambeck, W.A. (1994) The effect of vitamin C and zinc on the copper-induced increase of cadmium residues in swine. Z. Ernahrungswiss. 33(1):61–67. https://doi.org/10.1007/BF01610579.

Rotruck, J.T., Pope, A.L., Ganther, H.E., Swanson, A.B., Hafeman, D.G. and Hoekstra, W.G. (1973) Selenium: biochemical role as a component of glutathione peroxidase. Science 179(4073):588–590. https://doi.org/10.1126/science.179.4073.588.

Rucker, R.B. and Bauerly, K. (2013) Pantothenic acid. In "Handbook of vitamins" 5th ed. Zempleni, J., Suttie, J., Gregory, J. and Stover, P.J. (Eds.). CRC Press. (pp. 289–313).

Russell, L.E., Bechtel, P.J. and Easter, R.A. (1985) Effect of deficient and excess dietary vitamin B6 on amino transaminase and glycogen phosphorylase activity and pyridoxal phosphate content in two muscles from postpubertal gilts. J. Nutr. 115(9):1124–1135. https://doi.org/10.1093/jn/115.9.1124.

Russett, J.C., Krider, J.L., Cline, T.R. and Underwood, L.B. (1979b) Choline requirement of young swine. J. Anim. Sci. 48(6):1366–1373. https://doi.org/10.2527/jas1979.4861366x.

Russett, J.C., Krider, J.L., Cline, T.R., Thacker, H.L. and Underwood, L.B. (1979a) Choline-methionine interactions in young swine. J. Anim. Sci. 49(3):708–714. https://doi.org/10.2527/jas1979.493708x.

Ruth, G.R. and Van Vleet, J.F. (1974) Experimentally induced selenium-vitamin E deficiency in growing swine: selective destruction of type I skeletal muscle fibers. Am. J. Vet. Res. 35(2):237–244.

Ryu, K.S., Roberson, K.D., Pesti, G.M. and Eitenmiller, R.R. (1995) The folic acid requirements of starting broiler chicks fed diets based on practical ingredients: 1. Interrelationships with dietary choline. Poult. Sci. 74(9):1447–1455. https://doi.org/10.3382/ps.0741447.

Safonova, I., Darimont, C., Amri, E.Z., Grimaldi, P., Ailhaud, G., Reichert, U. and Shroot, B. (1994) Retinoids are positive effectors of adipose cell differentiation. Mol. Cell. Endocrinol. 104(2):201–211. https://doi.org/10.1016/0303-7207(94)90123-6.

Sahin, K., Sahin, N., Onderci, M., Yaralioglu, S. and Kucuk, O. (2001) Protective role of supplemental vitamin E on lipid peroxidation, vitamins E, A and some mineral concentrations of broilers reared under heat stress. Vet. Med. 46(5):140–144. https://doi.org/10.17221/7870-VETMED.

Said, H.M. (2011) Intestinal absorption of water-soluble vitamins in health and disease. Biochem. J. 437(3):357–372. https://doi.org/10.1042/BJ20110326.

Said, H.M. (2012) Biotin: biochemical, physiological and clinical aspects. "Water Soluble Vitamins" Stanger, O. (Eds)Springer, Dordrecht. pp. 1–19. https://doi.org/10.1007/978-94-007-2199-9_1.

Said, H.M. and Derweesh, I. (1991) Carrier-mediated mechanism for biotin transport in rabbit intestine: studies with brush-border membrane vesicles. Am. J. Physiol. 261(1 Pt 2):R94-R97. https://doi.org/10.1152/ajpregu.1991.261.1.R94.

Said, H.M., Hoefs, J., Mohammadkhani, R. and Horne, D.W. (1992) Biotin transport in human liver basolateral membrane vesicles: a carrier-mediated, Na+ gradient-dependent process. Gastroenterology 102(6):2120–2125. https://doi.org/10.1016/0016-5085(92)90341-u.

Said, H.M., Redha, R. and Nylander, W. (1988) Biotin transport in the human intestine: site of maximum transport and effect of pH. Gastroenterology 95(5):1312–1317. https://doi.org/10.1016/0016-5085(88)90366-6.

Sakurai, T., Asakura, T., Mizuno, A. and Matsuda, M. (1992) Absorption and metabolism of pyridoxamine in mice. II. Transformation of pyridoxamine to pyridoxal in intestinal tissues. J. Nutr. Sci. Vitaminol. (Tokyo) 38(3):227–233. https://doi.org/10.3177/jnsv.38.227.

Sales, J. and Koukolová, V. (2011) Dietary vitamin E and lipid and color stability of beef and pork: modeling of relationships. J. Anim. Sci. 89(9):2836–2848. https://doi.org/10.2527/jas.2010-3335.

Sandholm, M., Honkanen-Buzalski, T. and Rasi, V. (1979) Prevention of navel bleeding in piglets by preparturient administration of ascorbic acid. Vet. Rec. 104(15):337–338.

Santos, R.K.S., Novais, A.K., Borges, D.S., Alves, J.B., Dario, J.G.N., Frederico, G., Pierozan, C.R., Batista, J.P., Pereira, M. and Silva, C.A. (2020) Increased vitamin supplement to sows, piglets and finishers and the effect in productivity. Animal 14(1):86–94. https://doi.org/10.1017/S1751731119001927.

Sauberlich, H.E. (1985) Bioavailability of vitamins. Prog. Food Nutr. Sci. 9(1–2):1–33. PMID:3911266.

Sauberlich, H.E. (1999) "Laboratory tests for the assessment of nutritional status" 2nd ed. Routledge. https://doi.org/10.1201/9780203749647.

Sauer, W.C., Mosenthin, R. and Ozimek, L. (1988) The digestibility of biotin in protein supplements and cereal grains for growing pigs. J. Anim. Sci. 66(10):2583–2589. https://doi.org/10.2527/jas1988.66102583x.

Savage, D.G. and Lindenbaum, J. (1995) Folate-cobalamin interactions. In "Folate in health and disease" Bailey, L.B. (Ed.) Marcel Dekker, New York. (pp. 237–285).

Schaffer, S., Müller, W.E. and Eckert, G.P. (2005) Tocotrienols: constitutional effects in aging and disease. J. Nutr. 135(2):151–154. https://doi.org/10.1093/jn/135.2.151.

Schendel, H.E. and Johnson, B.C. (1962) Vitamin K deficiency in the baby pig. J. Nutr. 76(2):124–130. https://doi.org/10.1093/jn/76.2.124.

Scherf, H. (1988) Vitamin for better feed conversion? Pig. Int. 18(9):12–13.

Scherf, H. and Scott, L.J. (1989) How do vitamins affect sow productivity? Pigs-Misset 16:1.

Schneider, J. (1986) Vitamin stability and activity of fat-soluble vitamins as influenced by manufacturing processes. In Proc. 1986 National Feed Ingred. Assoc. Nutr. Inst. "Bioavailability of vitamins in feed ingredients," Chicago, Illinois. National Feed Ingredients Association (NFIA). Des Moines, Iowa.

Schoenbeck, R.A., Thompson, J. and Didion, B.A. (1994) A comparison of vitamin A supplements on reproductive performance of weaned sows. J. Anim. Sci. 77(suppl. 1):375.

Scholtissek, J., Barth, C.A., Hagemeister, H. and Frigg, M. (1990) Biotin supply by large bowel bacteria in minipigs: evidence from intracaecal avidin. Br. J. Nutr. 64(3):715–720. https://doi.org/10.1079/bjn19900073.

Schultze, J. and Willy, V. (1997) Biological efficacy of Rovimix Stay-C 35 as a source of vitamin C for dogs, poultry, calves, growing pigs and horses Roche Vitamins Research Report 167:495.

Schurgers, L.J. and Vermeer, C. (2002) Differential lipoprotein transport pathways of K-vitamins in healthy subjects. Biochim. Biophys. Acta 1570(1):27–32. https://doi.org/10.1016/S0304-4165(02)00147-2.

Schwager, J. and Schulze, J. (1997) Influence of ascorbic acid on the response to mitogens and interleukin production of porcine lymphocytes. Int. J. Vitam. Nutr. Res. 67(1):10–16.

Schwager, J. and Schulze, J. (1998) Dependence of growth, bone metabolism and functions of polymorphonuclear leukocytes on ascorbic acid in pigs. Int. J. Vitam. Nutr. Res. 68(1):48–58.

Schweigert, F.J., Buchholz, I., Schuhmacher, A. and Gropp, J. (2001) Effect of dietary β-carotene on the accumulation of β-carotene and vitamin A in plasma and tissues of gilts. Reprod. Nutr. Dev. 41(1):47–55. https://doi.org/10.1051/rnd:2001111.

Seerley, R.W., Charles, O.W., McCampbell, H.C. and Bertsch, S.P. (1976) Efficacy of menadione dimethylpyrimidinol bisulfite as a source of vitamin K in swine diets. J. Anim. Sci. 42(3):599–607. https://doi.org/10.2527/jas1976.423599x.

Seerley, R.W., Snyder, R.A. and McCampbell, H.C. (1981) The influence of sow dietary lipids and choline on piglet survival, milk and carcass composition. J. Anim. Sci. 52(3):542–550. https://doi.org/10.2527/jas1981.523542x.

Seetharam, B. and Alpers, D.H. (1982) Absorption and transport of cobalamin (vitamin B12). Annu. Rev. Nutr. 2:343–369. https://doi.org/10.1146/annurev.nu.02.070182.002015.

Selke, M.R., Barnhart, C.E. and Chaney, C.H. (1967) Vitamin A requirement of the gestating and lactating sow. J. Anim. Sci. 26(4):759–763. https://doi.org/10.2527/jas1967.264759x.

Seo, E.G., Einhorn, T.A. and Norman, A.W. (1997) 24R,25-dihydroxyvitamin D3: an essential vitamin D3 metabolite for both normal bone integrity and healing of tibial fracture in chicks endocrinology. Endocrinology 138(9):3864–3872. https://doi.org/10.1210/endo.138.9.5398.

Sergeev, I.N., Arkhapchev, Y.P. and Spirichev, V.B. (1990) The role of vitamin E in the metabolism and reception of vitamin E. Biokhimiya-Engl. TR 55(11):1483.

Serman, V. and Mazija, V. (1985) Effects of nutrition on the strength of acquired immunity against Newcastle disease. IV. Role Vitam. Vet. Arch. 55(1):1.

Sevkovic, N., Rajic, I.D. and Murgaski, S. (1976) Effect of vitamin C in preventing PSE meat and muscle degeneration in hogs. Food Sci. Technol. 9(12S):2104.

Sewell, R.F., Cunha, T.J., Shawver, C.B., Ney, W.A. and Wallace, H.D. (1952) Effect of aureomycin on diarrhea and on the vitamin B12 and methionine needs of the pig. Am. J. Vet. Res. 13(47):186–187. PMID: 14924137.

Sewell, R.F., Price, D.G. and Thomas, M.C. (1962) Pantothenic acid requirement of the pig as influenced by dietary fat. Fed. Proc. 21:468.

Sewell, R.F., Nugara, D., Hill, R.L. and Knapp, W.A. (1964) Vitamin B6 requirement of early-weaned pigs. J. Anim. Sci. 23(3):694–699. https://doi.org/10.2527/jas1964.233694x.

Seymour, E.W., Speer, V.C. and Hays, V.W. (1968) Effect of environmental temperature on the riboflavin requirement of young pigs. J. Anim. Sci. 27(2):389–393. https://doi.org/10.2527/jas1968.272389x.

Shanker, A. (2006) Nutritional modulation of immune function and infectious disease. In "Present knowledge in nutrition" 9th ed. Bowman, B.A. and Russell, R.M. (Eds). International Life Sciences Institute. (pp. 604–624).

Shanmugasundaram, R. and Selvaraj, R.K. (2012) Vitamin D-1α-hydroxylase and vitamin D-24-hydroxylase mRNA studies in chickens. Poult. Sci. 91(8):1819–1824. https://doi.org/10.3382/ps.2011-02129.

Sharp, B.A., Van Dreumel, A.A. and Young, L.G. (1972a) Vitamin E, selenium and methionine supplementation of dystrophogenic diets for pigs. Can. J. Comp. Med. 36(4):398–402. PMID: 4263922.

Sharp, B.A., Young, L.G. and Van Dreumel, A.A. (1972b) Dietary induction of mulberry heart and hepatosis dietetica in swine. J. Anim. Sci. 31:210.

Sharp, B.A., Young, L.G. and Van Dreumel, A.A. (1972c) Effect of supplemental vitamin E and selenium in high moisture corn diets on the incidence of mulberry heart disease and hepatosis dietetica in pigs. Can. J. Comp. Med. 36(4):393–397. PMID: 4263921.

Shaw, D.T., Rozeboom, D.W., Hill, G.M., Booren, A.M. and Link, J.E. (2002) Impact of vitamin and mineral supplement withdrawal and wheat middling inclusion on finishing pig growth performance, fecal mineral concentration, carcass characteristics, and the nutrient content and oxidative stability of pork. J. Anim. Sci. 80(11):2920–2930. https://doi.org/10.2527/2002.80112920x.

Shea, M.K. and Booth, S.L. (2008) Update on the role of vitamin K in skeletal health. Nutr. Rev. 66(10): 549–557. https://doi.org/10.1111/j.1753-4887.2008.00106.x.

Shearer, M.J., Barkhan, P. and Webster, G.R. (1970) Absorption and excretion of an oral dose of tritiated vitamin K1 in man. Br. J. Haematol. 18(3):297–308. https://doi.org/10.1111/j.1365-2141.1970.tb01444.x.

Sheffy, B.E. and Schultz, R.D. (1979) Influence of vitamin E and selenium on immune response mechanisms. Fed. Proc. 38(7):2139–2143. PMID: 312742.

Sheffy, B.E., Drouliscos, N., Loosli, J.K. and Willman, J.P. (1954) Vitamin A requirements of baby pigs. J. Anim. Sci. 13:999.

Sheridan, P.A. and Beck, M.A. (2008) The immune response to herpes simplex virus encephalitis in mice is modulated by dietary vitamin E. J. Nutr. 138(1):130–137. https://doi.org/10.1093/jn/138.1.130.

Shi, B., Su, Y., Chang, S., Sun, Y., Meng, X. and Shan, A. (2017) Vitamin C protects the piglet liver against zearalenone-induced oxidative stress by modulating expression of nuclear receptors PXR and CAR and their target genes. Food Funct. 8(10):3675–3687. https://doi.org/10.1039/C7FO01301A.

Shideler, C.E. (1983) Vitamin B6: an overview. Am. J. Med. Technol. 49(1):17–22. PMID: 6342384.

Shields, R.G., Campbell, D.R., Huges, D.M. and Dillingham, D.A. (1982) Researchers study vitamin A stability in feeds. Feedstuffs 54(47):22.

Shin, D.J. and McGrane, M.M. (1997) Vitamin A regulates genes involved in hepatic gluconeogenesis in mice: phosphoenolpyruvate carboxykinase, fructose-1,6-bisphosphatase and 6-phosphofructo-2-kinase/fructose-2,6-bisphosphatase. J. Nutr. 127(7):1274–1278. https://doi.org/10.1093/jn/127.7.1274.

Shojadoost, B., Yitbarek, A., Alizadeh, M., Kulkarni, R.R., Astill, J., Boodhoo, N. and Sharif, S. (2021) Centennial review: effects of vitamins A, D, E, and C on the chicken immune system. Poult. Sci. 100(4):100930. https://doi.org/10.1016/j.psj.2020.12.027.

Shulpekova, Y., Nechaev, V., Kardasheva, S., Sedova, A., Kurbatova, A., Bueverova, E., Kopylov, A., Malsagova, K., Dlamini, J.C. and Ivashkin, V. (2021) The concept of folic acid in health and disease. Molecules 26(12):3731. https://doi.org/10.3390/molecules26123731.

Silva-Guillen, Y., Arellano, C., Martínez, G. and van Heugten, E. (2020) Growth performance, oxidative stress, and antioxidant capacity of newly weaned piglets fed dietary peroxidized lipids with vitamin E or phytogenic compounds in drinking water. Appl. Anim. Sci. 36(3):341–351.

Simard, F., Guay, F., Girard, C.L., Giguère, A., Laforest, J.P. and Matte, J.J. (2007) Effects of concentrations of cyanocobalamin in the gestation diet on some criteria of vitamin B12 metabolism in first-parity sows. J. Anim. Sci. 85(12):3294–3302. https://doi.org/10.2527/jas.2006-523.

Simesen, M.G., Jensen, P.T., Basse, A., Gissel-Nielsen, G., Leth, T., Danielsen, V. and Nielsen, H.E. (1982) Clinico-pathologic findings in young pigs fed different levels of selenium, vitamin E and antioxidant. Acta Vet. Scand. 23(2):295–308. https://doi.org/10.1186/BF03546813.

Simesen, M.G., Nielsen, H.E., Danielsen, V., Gissel-Nielsen, G., Hjarde, W., Leth, T. and Basse, A. (1979) Selenium and vitamin E deficiency in pigs. II. Influence on plasma selenium, vitamin E, ASAT and ALAT and on tissue selenium. Acta Vet. Scand. 20(2):289–305. https://doi.org/10.1186/BF03546620.

Simmins, P.H. (1985) The effect of dietary biotin level on the productivity of the female pig. Ph.D. dissertation. Plymouth Polytechnic in association with Seale-Hayne College, Devon. England.

Simmins, P.H. and Brooks, P.H. (1980) The effect of dietary biotin level on the physical characteristics of pig hoof tissue. Anim. Prod. 30:469.

Simmins, P.H. and Brooks, P.H. (1983) Supplementary biotin for sows: effect on reproductive characteristics. Vet. Rec. 112(18):425–429.

Simmins, P.H. and Brooks, P.H. (1985) Effect of different levels of dietary biotin on the hoof hardness of the gilt. Anim. Prod. 40:544–545.

Simmins, P.H. and Brooks, P.H. (1988) Supplementary biotin for sows: effect on claw integrity. Vet. Rec. 122(18):431–435.

Simon, J. (1999) Choline, betaine and methionine interactions in chickens, pigs and fish (including crustaceans). Worlds Poult. Sci. J. 55(4):353–374. https://doi.org/10.1079/WPS19990025.

Singh, U., Devaraj, S. and Jialal, I. (2005) Vitamin E, oxidative stress, and inflammation. Annu. Rev. Nutr. 25:151–174. https://doi.org/10.1146/annurev.nutr.24.012003.132446.

Sitara, D., Razzaque, M.S., St-Arnaud, R., Huang, W., Taguchi, T., Erben, R.G. and Lanske, B. (2006) Genetic ablation of vitamin D activation pathway reverses biochemical and skeletal anomalies in FGF23-null animals. Am. J. Pathol. 169(6):2161–2170. https://doi.org/10.2353/ajpath.2006.060329.

Sitrin, M.D., Lieberman, F., Jensen, W.E., Noronha, A., Milburn, C. and Addington, W. (1987) Vitamin E deficiency and neurologic disease in adults with cystic fibrosis. Ann. Intern. Med. 107(1):51–54. https://doi.org/10.7326/0003-4819-107-1-51.

Sivertsen, T., Vie, E., Bernhoft, A. and Baustad, B. (2007) Vitamin E and selenium plasma concentrations in weanling pigs under field conditions in Norwegian pig herds. Acta Vet. Scand. 49(1):1. https://doi.org/10.1186/1751-0147-49-1.

Siwecki, J.A. (1985) Dietary ascorbic acid for neonatal pigs reared artificially. Int. J. Vitam. Nutr. Res. 55(4):413–419. https://pubmed.ncbi.nlm.nih.gov/4086211/PMID.

Skliarov, P.M., Fedorenko, S.Y., Naumenko, S.V., Onischenko, O.V. and Holda, K.O. (2020) Retinol deficiency in animals: etiopathogenesis and consequences. Regul. Mech. Biosyst. 11(2):162–169. https://doi.org/10.15421/022024.

Smith, C.M. and Song, W.O. (1996) Comparative nutrition of pantothenic acid. J. Nutr. Biochem. 7(6):312–321. https://doi.org/10.1016/0955-2863(96)00034-4.

Smith, P.J., Tappel, A.L. and Chow, C.K. (1974) Glutathione peroxidase activity as a function of dietary selenomethionine. Nature 247(5440):392–393. https://doi.org/10.1038/247392a0.

Smith, W.J. and Robertson, A.M. (1971) Observations on injuries to sows confined in part slatted stalls. Vet. Rec. 89(20):531–533.

Snow, J.L., Baker, D.H., Parsons, J.H. and Lofton, J.T. (1986) Recent studies on vitamin D and skeletal problems in broilers. In Proc. Maryland Nutr. Conference. (pp. 1–6).

Soares, J.H., Kerr, J.M. and Gray, R.W. (1995) 25-Hydroxycholecalciferol in poultry nutrition. Poult. Sci. 74(12):1919–1919. https://doi.org/10.3382/ps.0741919.

Sobotka, W., Flis, M., Antoszkiewicz, Z., Lipiński, K. and Zduńczyk, Z. (2012) Effect of oat by-product antioxidants and vitamin E on the oxidative stability of pork from pigs fed diets supplemented with linseed oil. Arch. Anim. Nutr. 66(1):27–38. https://doi.org/10.1080/1745039X.2011.647459.

Soleimani, T. and Gilbert, H. (2020) Evaluating environmental impacts of selection for residual feed intake in pigs. Animal 14(12):2598–2608. https://doi.org/10.1017/S175173112000138X.

Solomons, N.W. (2006) Vitamin A. In Present knowledge in nutrition 9th ed. Bowman, B. and Russell, R. (ed.). International Life Sciences Institute. (pp. 157–183).

Solyanik, A.V., Semenov, V.G., Tyurin, V.G., Kuznetsov, A.F., Sofronov, V.G., Volkov, A.K., Solyanik, V.V., Solyanik, S.V. and Solyanik, V.A. (2021) The effect of fumaric acid, dipromonium and vitamin C on the productivity of sows. IOP Conf. Ser.: Earth Environ. Sci. 935(1). https://doi.org/10.1088/1755-1315/935/1/012023.

Song, R., Chen, C., Johnston, L.J., Kerr, B.J., Weber, T.E. and Shurson, G.C. (2014) Effects of feeding diets containing highly peroxidized distillers dried grains with solubles and increasing vitamin E levels to wean–finish pigs on growth performance, carcass characteristics, and pork fat composition. J. Anim. Sci. 92(1):198–210. https://doi.org/10.2527/jas.2013-6334.

Sosnowska, A., Kawęcka, M., Jacyno, E., Kołodziej-Skalska, A., Kamyczek, M. and Matysiak, B. (2011) Effect of dietary vitamins E and C supplementation on performance of sows and piglets. Acta Agric. Scand. A 61(4):196–203. https://doi.org/10.1080/09064702.2012.666560.

Southern, L.L. and Baker, D.H. (1981) Bioavailable pantothenic acid in cereal grains and soybean meal. J. Anim. Sci. 53(2):403–408. https://doi.org/10.2527/jas1981.532403x.

Southern, L.L., Brown, D.R., Werner, D.D. and Fox, M.C. (1986) Excess supplemental choline for swine. J. Anim. Sci. 62(4):992–996. https://doi.org/10.2527/jas1986.624992x.

Sparks, J.C., Wiegand, B.R., Parrish, F.C., Ewan, R.C., Horst, R.L., Tenkle, A.H. and Beitz, D.C. (1998) Effects of short term feeding of vitamin D3 on pork quality. Iowa State Univ. Res. Reprod:(218–220).

Spasevski, N.J., Vukmirovic, D., Levic, J. and Kokic, B. (2015) Influence of pelleting process and material particle size on the stability of retinol acetate. Arch. Zootech. 18(2):67–72.

Spencer, R.P., Purdy, S., Hoeldtke, R., Bow, T.M. and Markulis, M.A. (1963) Studies on intestinal absorption of L-ascorbic acid-1-C14. Gastroenterology 44(6):768–773. https://doi.org/10.1016/S0016-5085(63)80086-4.

Stabler, S.P. (2006) Vitamin B12. In Present knowledge in nutrition 9th ed. Bowman, B.A. and Russell, R.M. (Eds). International Life Sciences Institute. (pp. 302–313).

Stacchiotti, V., Rezzi, S., Eggersdorfer, M. and Galli, F. (2021) Metabolic and functional interplay between gut microbiota and fat-soluble vitamins. Crit. Rev. Food Sci. Nutr. 61(19):3211–3232. https://doi.org/10.1080/10408398.2020.1793728.

Stahl, W., Schwarz, W., Von Laar, J. and Sies, H. (1995) All-trans beta-carotene preferentially accumulates in human chylomicrons and very low density lipoproteins compared with the 9-cis geometrical isomer. J. Nutr. 125(8):2128–2133. https://doi.org/10.1093/jn/125.8.2128.

Stahly, T.S. and Cook, D. (1996a) Dietary B vitamin needs of pigs experiencing a moderate or high level of antigen exposure Iowa State University Research Report. ALS-R1373. (pp. 38–41). http://iastatedigital press.com/air/article/id/7478/.

Stahly, T.S. and Cook, D.R. (1996b) Dietary thiamine needs of high lean growth pigs Iowa State Research Report. (pp. 15–16). http://dr.lib.iastate.edu/handle/20.500.12876/91049.

Stahly, T.S. and Lutz, T.R. (2001) Pantothenic acid needs for specific biological processes in pigs Iowa State University Animal Industry Report 1(1).

Stahly, T.S., Cook, D.R. and Ewan, R.C. (1997) Dietary vitamin A, E, and C needs of pigs experiencing a low or high level of antigen exposure Iowa State University Research Report, ASL-1480. (pp. 9–12). http://dr.lib.iastate.edu/handle/20.500.12876/91083.

Stahly, T.S., Williams, N., Swenson, S.G. and Ewan, R.C. (1995) Dietary B vitamin needs of high and moderate lean growth pigs fed from 20 to 62 pounds body weight Iowa State University Research Report, ALS-R1263. (pp. 15–22).

Stahly, T.S., Williams, N.H., Lutz, T.R., Ewan, R.C. and Swenson, S.G. (2007) Dietary B vitamin needs of strains of pigs with high and moderate lean growth. J. Anim. Sci. 85(1):188–195. https://doi.org/10.2527/jas.2006-086.

Stark, C.R., Hansen, J.A., Goodband, R.D. and Behnke, K.C. (1991) On-farm feed uniformity survey Swine Day Report. Kansas Agricultural Experiment Station Research Reports. Kansas State University (10): (144–145). http://hdl.handle.net/2097/3547.

Steenbock, H. (1924) The induction of growth promoting and calcifying properties in a ration by exposure to light. Science 60(1549):224–225. https://doi.org/10.1126/science.60.1549.224.

Stein, J., Daniel, H., Whang, E., Wenzel, U., Hahn, A. and Rehner, G. (1994) Rapid postabsorptive metabolism of nicotinic acid in rat small intestine may affect transport by metabolic trapping. J. Nutr. 124(1):61–66. https://doi.org/10.1093/jn/124.1.61.

Stender, D., Irvin, R. and Baas, T.J. (1999) Effect of beta-carotene on reproductive performance in swine. Iowa State Univ. swine res (rep.). http://dr.lib.iastate.edu/handle/20.500.12876/91123. (pp. 4–6).

Stephensen, C.B., Moldoveanu, Z. and Gangopadhyay, N.N. (1996) Vitamin A deficiency diminishes the salivary immunoglobulin A response and enhances the serum immunoglobulin G response to influenza A virus infection in BALB/c mice. J. Nutr. 126(1):94–102. https://doi.org/10.1093/jn/126.1.94.

Stockland, W.L. and Blaylock, L.G. (1974) Choline requirement of pregnant sows and gilts under restricted feeding conditions. J. Anim. Sci. 39(6):1113–1116. https://doi.org/10.2527/jas1974.3961113x.

Stothers, S.C., Schmidt, D.A., Johnston, R.L., Hoefer, J.A. and Luecke, R.W. (1955) The pantothenic acid requirement of the baby pig. J. Nutr. 57(1):47–53. https://doi.org/10.1093/jn/57.1.47.

Strittmatter, J.E. (1977) Effect of vitamin C (ascorbic acid) on degenerative arthritis (osteochondrosis) and growth of swine. Res. Rep. Michigan State University, agr. Exp. Stat. East Lansing:(111–115).

Strittmatter, J.E., Ellis, D.J., Hogberg, M.G., Trapp, A.L., Parsons, M.J. and Miller, E.R. (1978) Effects of vitamin C on swine growth and osteochondrosis. J. Anim. Sci. 47(suppl. 1):16.

Su, Y., Sun, Y., Ju, D., Chang, S., Shi, B. and Shan, A. (2018) The detoxification effect of vitamin C on zearalenone toxicity in piglets. Ecotoxicol. Environ. Saf. 158:284–292. https://doi.org/10.1016/j.ecoenv.2018.04.046.

Sun, L.H., Huang, J.Q., Deng, J. and Lei, X.G. (2019) Avian selenogenome: response to dietary Se and vitamin E deficiency and supplementation. Poult. Sci. 98(10):4247–4254. https://doi.org/10.3382/ps/pey408.

Sun, M.K. and Alkon, D.L. (2008) Synergistic effects of chronic bryostatin-1 and α-tocopherol on spatial learning and memory in rats. Eur. J. Pharmacol. 584(2–3):328–337. https://doi.org/10.1016/j.ejphar.2008.02.014.

Sun, S., Meng, Q., Bai, Y., Cao, C., Li, J., Cheng, B., Shi, B. and Shan, A. (2021) Lycopene improves maternal reproductive performance by modulating milk composition and placental antioxidative and immune status. Food Funct. 12(24):12448–12467. https://doi.org/10.1039/D1FO01595H.

Sundeen, G., Richards, J. F. and Bragg D.B. (1980) The Effect of Vitamin A Deficiency on Some Postmortem Parameters of Avian Muscle Poult. Sci. 59(10): 2225–2236 https://doi.org/10.3382/ps.0592225.

Surai, P.F. and Dvorska, J.E. (2005) Effects of mycotoxins on antioxidant status and immunity. In "The mycotoxin blue book" Diaz, D. (Ed.). Nottingham University Press.

Surai, P.F. and Fisinin, V.I. (2015) Antioxidant-prooxidant balance in the intestine: applications in chick placement and pig weaning. Vet, J. Sci. Med. 3(1):66–84.

Surai, P.F., Kochish, I.I., Romanov, M.N. and Griffin, D.K. (2019) Nutritional modulation of the antioxidant capacities in poultry: the case of vitamin E. Poult. Sci. 98(9):4030–4030. https://doi.org/10.3382/ps/pez072.

Surles, R.L., Hutson, P.R., Valentine, A.R., Mills, J.P. and Tanumihardjo, S.A. (2011) 3, 4-Didehydroretinol kinetics differ during lactation in sows on a retinol depletion regimen and the serum:milk 3, 4-Didehydroretinol:Retinol ratios are correlated. J. Nutr. 141(4):554–559. https://doi.org/10.3945/jn.110.131904.

Surles, R.L., Mills, J.P., Valentine, A.R. and Tanumihardjo, S.A. (2007) One-time graded doses of vitamin A to weanling piglets enhance hepatic retinol but do not always prevent vitamin A deficiency. Am. J. Clin. Nutr. 86(4):1045–1053. https://doi.org/10.1093/ajcn/86.4.1045.

Suryawan, A. and Hu, C.Y. (1997) Effect of retinoic acid on differentiation of cultured pig preadipocytes. J. Anim. Sci. 75(1):112–117. https://doi.org/10.2527/1997.751112x.

Suter, C. (1990) Vitamins at the molecular level. In Proc. 'National Feed Ingr. Ass. Nutr. Inst.': "Developments in vitamin nutrition and health applications" Kansas City, Missouri. National Feed Ingredients Association (NFIA), Des Moines, Iowa, USA.

Suttie, J.W. (2007) Vitamin K. In Handbook of vitamins 4th ed. Zempleni, J., Rucker, R.B., McCormick, D.B. and Suttie, J.W. (ed.). CRC Press, Boca Raton, Florida. (pp. 111–139).

Suttie, J.W. (2013) Vitamin K. In Handbook of vitamins 5th ed. Zempleni, J., Suttie, J., Gregory, J. and Stover, P.J. (ed.). CRC Press, Boca Raton, FL. (pp. 89–124).

Suttie, J.W. and Jackson, C.M. (1977) Prothrombin structure, activation, and biosynthesis. Physiol. Rev. 57(1):1–70. https://doi.org/10.1152/physrev.1977.57.1.1.

Suttie, J.W. and Olson, R.E. (1990) Vitamin K. In "Nutrition reviews, present knowledge in nutrition" Olson, R.E. (Ed.). Nutrition Foundation.

Sutton, R.A.L. and Dirks, J.H. (1978) Renal handling of calcium. Fed. Proc. 37(8):2112–2119.

Svihus, B. and Zimonja, O. (2011) Chemical alterations with nutritional consequences due to pelleting animal feeds: a review. Anim. Prod. Sci. 51(7):590–596.

Swanek, S.S., Morgan, J.B., Owens, F.N., Dolezal, H.G. and Gill, D.R. (1997) Effects of vitamin D3 supplementation on longissimus muscle tenderness. J. Anim. Sci. 75:252.

Swanek, S.S., Morgan, J.B., Webb, D.S., Owens, F.N., Gill, D.R. and Dolezal, H.G. (1998) Effects of vitamin D3 supplementation of beef steers on longissimus muscle tenderness. J. Anim. Sci. 76:13 (abstr.).

Sweeny, P.R. and Brown, R.G. (1972) Ultrastructural changes in muscular dystrophy. I. Cardiac tissue of piglets deprived of vitamin E and selenium. Am. J. Pathol. 68(3):479–492. PMID: 5054254.

Szczubiał, M. (2015) Effect of supplementation with vitamins E, C and beta-carotene on antioxidative/oxidative status parameters in sows during the postpartum period. Pol. J. Vet. Sci. 18(2):299–305. https://doi.org/10.1515/pjvs-2015-0039.

Szterk, A., Rogalski, M., Mikiciuk, J., Pakuła, L. and Waszkiewicz-Robak, B. (2016) Effect of Dietary α-Tocopherol on Level of Vitamin E in Pure Polish Landrace and Hybrid Polish Landrace × Duroc Swine Breeds and Processed Meat. J. Food Process. Preserv. 40(6):1270–1279. https://doi.org/10.1111/jfpp.12712.

Tagwerker, F. (1974) Recent research on biotin in the nutrition of pigs and chickens. Roche Information Service Bulletin No. 1494. F. Hoffmann-La Roche & Co. Ltd., Basel, Switzerland.

Tagwerker, F. (1983) New results on the role of biotin in poultry and swine nutrition. Feed Int. 4:22.

Talavera, F. and Chew, B.P. (1988) Comparative role of retinol, retinoic acid and beta-carotene on progesterone secretion by pig corpus luteum in vitro. J. Reprod. Fertil. 82(2):611–615. https://doi.org/10.1530/jrf.0.0820611.

Tanaka, K., Hashimoto, T., Tokumaru, S., Iguchi, H. and Kojo, S. (1997) Interactions between vitamin C and vitamin E are observed in tissues of inherently scorbutic rats. J. Nutr. 127(10):2060–2064. https://doi.org/10.1093/jn/127.10.2060.

Tanumihardjo, S.A. (2013) Vitamin A and bone health: the balancing act. J. Clin. Densitom. 16(4):414–419. https://doi.org/10.1016/j.jocd.2013.08.016.

Tang, F.I. and Wei, I.L. (2004) Vitamin B6 deficiency prolongs the time course of evoked dopamine release from rat striatum. J. Nutr. 134(12):3350–3354. https://doi.org/10.1093/jn/134.12.3350.

Tani, M. and Iwai, K. (1984) Some nutritional effects of folate-binding protein in bovine milk on the bioavailability of folate to rats. J. Nutr. 114(4):778–785. https://doi.org/10.1093/jn/114.4.778.

Tanumihardjo, S.A. and Howe, J.A. (2005) Twice the amount of alpha-carotene isolated from carrots is as effective as beta-carotene in maintaining the vitamin A status of Mongolian gerbils. J. Nutr. 135(11):2622–2626. https://doi.org/10.1093/jn/135.11.2622.

Tanumihardjo, S.A. (2011) Vitamin A: biomarkers of nutrition for development. Am. J. Clin. Nutr. 94(2):658S-665S. https://doi.org/10.3945/ajcn.110.005777.

Tanumihardjo, S.A., Russell, R.M., Stephensen, C.B., Gannon, B.M., Craft, N.E., Haskell, M.J., Lietz, G., Schulze, K. and Raiten, D.J. (2016) Biomarkers of nutrition for development (BOND)—vitamin A review. J. Nutr. 146(9):1816S-1848S. https://doi.org/10.3945/jn.115.229708.

Taylor, T., Hawkins, D.R., Hathway, D.E. and Partington, H. (1972) A new urinary metabolite of pantothenate in dogs. Br. Vet. J. 128(10):500–505.

Teague, H.S. and Grifo, A.P. (1966) Vitamin B12 supplementation of sow rations. J. Anim. Sci. 25:895.

Teague, H.S., Grifo, A.P. and Palmer, A.P. (1971) Pantothenic acid deficiency in the sow. J. Anim. Sci. 33:239.

Teeter, R.G. and Belay, T. (1996) Broiler management during acute heat stress. Anim. Feed Sci. Technol. 58(1–2):127–142. https://doi.org/10.1016/0377-8401(95)00879-9.

Teige, J. (1977) The generalized Schwartzman reaction induced by a single injection of endotoxin in pigs fed a vitamin E deficient commercial diet. Acta Vet. Scand. 18(1):140–142. https://doi.org/10.1186/BF03548475.

Teige, J. and Nafstad, P.H. (1978) Ultrastructure of colonic epithelial cells in vitamin E- and selenium-deficienct pigs. Acta Vet. Scand. 19(4):549–560. https://doi.org/10.1186/BF03547594.

Teige, J., Nordstoga, K. and Aursjo, J. (1977) Influence of diet on experimental swine dysentery. I. Effects of vitamin E- and selenium-deficient diet supplemented with 6.8% cod liver oil. Acta Vet. Scand. 18(3):384–396. https://doi.org/10.1186/BF03548436.

Teige, J., Tollersrud, S., Lund, A. and Larsen, H.J. (1982) Swine dysentery: the influence of dietary vitamin E and selenium on the clinical and pathological effects of Treponema hyodysenteriae infection in pigs. Res. Vet. Sci. 32(1):95–100. PMID: 7089385.

Tengerdy, R.P. (1980) Disease resistance: immune response. In "Vitamin E: a comprehensive treatise" Machlin, L.J. (Ed.). Marcel Dekker Inc.

Terman, A., Kmiec, M., Polasik, D. and Pradziadowicz, K. (2007) Retinol binding protein 4 gene and reproductive traits in pigs. Arch. Tierz. 50. (pp. 181–185).

Terrill, S.W., Ammerman, C.B., Walker, D.E., Edwards, R.M., Norton, H.W. and Becker, D.E. (1955) Riboflavin studies with pigs. J. Anim. Sci. 14(2):593–603. https://doi.org/10.2527/jas1955.142593x.

Thaler, R.C., Turlington, L.M., Allee, G.L., Goodband, R.D. and Nelssen, J.L. (1987) The effects of additional niacin during gestation and lactation on sow and litter performance. J. Anim. Sci. 65(1):138. http://hdl.handle.net/2097/3703.

Thaler, R.C., Nelssen, J.L., Goodband, R.D. and Allee, G.L. (1989) Effect of dietary folic acid supplementation on sow performance through two parities. J. Anim. Sci. 67(12):3360–3369. https://doi.org/10.2527/jas1989.67123360x.

Thayer, M.T., Nelssen, J.L., Langemeier, A.J., Morton, J.M., Gonzalez, J.M., Kruger, S.R., Ou, Z., Makowski, A.J. and Bergstrom, J.R. (2019) The effects of maternal dietary supplementation of cholecalciferol (vitamin D3) and 25(OH)D3 on sow and progeny performance. Transl. Anim. Sci. 3(2):692–708. https://doi.org/10.1093/tas/txz029.

Thierry, M.J., Hermodson, M.A. and Suttie, J.W. (1970) Vitamin K and warfarin distribution and metabolism in the warfarin-resistant rat. Am. J. Physiol. 219(4):854–859. https://doi.org/10.1152/ajplegacy.1970.219.4.854.

Thode Jensen, P., Danielsen, V. and Nielsen, H.E. (1979) Glutathione peroxidase activity and erythrocyte lipid peroxidation as indices of selenium and vitamin E status in young pigs. Acta Vet. Scand. 20:92–101. https://doi.org/10.1186%2FBF03546633.

Thode Jensen, P., Nielsen, H.E., Danielsen, V. and Leth, T. (1983) Effect of dietary fat quality and vitamin E on the antioxidant potential of pigs. Acta Vet. Scand. 24(2):135–147. https://doi.org/10.1186/BF03546742.

Thomas, J.W., Loosli, J.K. and William, J.P. (1947) Placental and mammary transfer of vitamin A in swine and goats as affected by the prepartum diet. J. Anim. Sci. 6(2):141–145. https://doi.org/10.2527/jas1947.62141x.

Tian, J.Z., Lee, J.H., Kim, J.D., Han, Y.K., Park, K.M. and Han, I.K. (2001) Effects of different levels of vitamin-mineral premixes on growth performance, nutrient digestibility, carcass characteristics and meat quality of growing-finishing pigs. Asian. Australas J. Anim. Sci. 14(4):515–524. https://doi.org/10.5713/ajas.2001.515.

Tijburg, L.B., Haddeman, E., Kivits, G.A., Weststrate, J.A. and Brink, E.J. (1997) Dietary linoleic acid at high and reduced dietary fat level decreases the faecal excretion of vitamin E in young rats. Br. J. Nutr. 77(2):327–336. https://doi.org/10.1079/BJN19970033.

Tollersrud, S. (1973) Changes in the enzymatic profile in blood and tissues in preclinical and clinical vitamin E deficiency in pigs. Acta Agric. Scand. suppl. 19:124–129.

Tollersrud, S. and Nafstad, I. (1970) The vitamin E-deficiency syndrome in pigs. II. Investigations on serum and tissue enzyme activity. Acta Vet. Scand. 11(4):495–509. https://doi.org/10.1186/BF03547949.

Tollerz, G. (1973) Vitamin E, selenium and some related compounds and tolerance toward iron in piglets. Acta Agric. Scand. suppl. 19:184–187.

Tollerz, G. and Lannek, N. (1964) Protection against iron toxicity in vitamin E-deficient piglets and mice by vitamin E and synthetic antioxidants. Nature 201:846–847. https://doi.org/10.1038/201846a0.

Topigs Norsvin (2016) Piglet feeding manual. https://topigsnorsvin.com/tn-content/uploads/2020/02/Feeding-Manual-Norsvin-Duroc.pdf.

Tous, N., Lizardo, R., Theil, P.K., Vilà, B., Gispert, M., Font-i-Furnols, M. and Esteve-Garcia, E. (2014) Effect of vitamin A depletion on fat deposition in finishing pigs, intramuscular fat content and gene expression in the longissimus muscle. Livest. Sci. 167:392–399.

Traber, M.G. (2006) Vitamin E. In "Present knowledge in nutrition" 9th ed. Bowman, B. A. and Russell, R. M. (Eds.). Intl. Life Sciences Inst. (pp. 211–219).

Traber, M.G. (2013) Vitamin E. In "Handbook of vitamins" 5th ed. Zempleni, J., Suttie, J., Gregory, J. and Stover, P. J. (Eds.). CRC Press. (pp. 125–148).

Traber, M.G. and Sies, H. (1996) Vitamin E in humans: demand and delivery. Annu. Rev. Nutr. 16:321–347. https://doi.org/10.1146/annurev.nu.16.070196.001541.

Traber, M.G., Rader, D., Acuff, R.V., Ramakrishnan, R., Brewer, H.B. and Kayden, H.J. (1998) Vitamin E dose response studies in humans using deuterated RRR-a-tocopherol. Am. J. Clin. Nutr. 68(4):847–853. https://doi.org/10.1093/ajcn/68.4.847.

Trapp, A.L., Keahey, K.K., Whitenack, D.L. and Whitehair, C.K. (1970) Vitamin E-selenium deficiency in swine: differential diagnosis and nature of field problem. J. Am. Vet. Med. Assoc. 157(3):289–300. PMID: 4915367.

Trawińska, B., Lechowski, J., Polonis, A. and Kowaleczko, M. (2012) Effect of feed supplemented with vitamin C on microbial flora of swine faeces and blood morphology. Bulletin of the Veterinary Institute in Pulawy 56(2):171–175. https://doi.org/10.2478/v10213-012-0031-3.

Trefan, L., Bünger, L., Bloom-Hansen, J., Rooke, J.A., Salmi, B., Larzul, C., Terlouw, C. and Doeschl-Wilson, A. (2011) Meta-analysis of the effects of dietary vitamin E supplementation on α-tocopherol concentration and lipid oxidation in pork. Meat Sci. 87(4):305–314. https://doi.org/10.1016/j.meatsci.2010.11.002.

Tremblay, G.F., Matte, J.J., Lemieux, L. and Brisson, G.J. (1986) Serum folates in gestating swine after folic acid addition to diet. J. Anim. Sci. 63(4):1173–1178. https://doi.org/10.2527/jas1986.6341173x.

Tremblay, G.F., Matte, J.J., Dufour, J.J. and Brisson, G.J. (1989) Survival rate and development of fetuses during the first 30 days of gestation after folic acid addition to a swine diet. J. Anim. Sci. 67(3):724–732. https://doi.org/10.2527/jas1989.673724x.

Tsuchiya, H. and Bates, C.J. (1997) Vitamin C and copper interactions in guinea pigs and a study of collagen cross-links. Br. J. Nutr. 77(2):315–325. https://doi.org/10.1079/bjn19970032.

Turley, C.P. and Brewster, M.A. (1993) α-tocopherol protects against a reduction in adenosylcobalamin in oxidatively stressed human cells. J. Nutr. 123(7):1305–1312. https://doi.org/10.1093/jn/123.7.1305.

Tutt, J.B. and Gale, F.J. (1957) Mulberry heart disease in pigs. Br. Vet. J. 113(5):220–221.

Ullrey, D.E. (1969) Vitamin E and/or selenium deficiency in growing-finishing pigs. Michigan State Univ. Bulletin AH-SW-695.

Ullrey, D.E. (1972) Biological availability of fat-soluble vitamins: vitamin A and carotene. J. Anim. Sci. 35(3):648–657. https://doi.org/10.2527/jas1972.353648x.

Ullrey, D.E. (1981) Vitamin E for swine. J. Anim. Sci. 53(4):1039–1056. https://doi.org/10.2527/jas1981.5341039x.

Ullrey, D.E. (1991) Vitamins A and K in swine nutrition. In "Swine nutrition" Miller, E. R., Ullrey D.E. and Lewis, A.J. (Eds.). Butterworth-Heinemann, Stoneham, MA.

Ullrey, D.E., Becker, D.E., Terrill, S.W. and Notzold, R.A. (1955) Dietary levels of pantothenic acid and reproductive performance of female swine. J. Nutr. 57(3):401–414. https://doi.org/10.1093/jn/57.3.401.

Ullrey, D.E., Miller, E.R., Struthers, R.D., Peterson, R.E., Hoefer, J.A. and Hall, H.H. (1965) Vitamin A activity of fermentation beta-carotene for swine. J. Nutr. 85(4):375–385. https://doi.org/10.1093/jn/85.4.375.

Ullrey, D.E., Miller, E.R., Ellis, D.J., Orr, D.E., Hitchcock, J.P., Keahey, K.K. and Trapp, A.L. (1971) Vitamin E (selenium and choline), Reproduction and MMA. Michigan State Univ. Agr. Exp. Sta Rep. Swine Res. 148. 48–51.

United States Pharmacopeia (1980) 20th edn. Mack Printing Comp., Easton, Pennsylvania.

Upadhaya, S.D., Kim, J.C., Mullan, B.P., Pluske, J.R. and Kim, I.H. (2015) Vitamin E and omega-3 fatty acids independently attenuate plasma concentrations of proinflammatory cytokines and prostaglandin E2 in Escherichia coli lipopolysaccharide-challenged growing–finishing pigs. J. Anim. Sci. 93(6):2926–2934. https://doi.org/10.2527/jas.2014-8330.

Upadhaya, S.D., Chung, T.K., Jung, Y.J. and Kim, I.H. (2022) Dietary 25(OH)D3 supplementation to gestating and lactating sows and their progeny affects growth performance, carcass characteristics, blood profiles and myogenic regulatory factor-related gene expression in wean-finish pigs. Anim. Biosci. 35(3):461–474. https://doi.org/10.5713/ab.21.0304.

Urbanova, J. and Toulova, M. (1975) Lipid peroxidation in vitro and tocopherol levels in the tissues of suckling and weaned piglets. Acta Vet. Brno 44(1–2):17–22.

Vallet, J.L., Christenson, R.K., Klemcke, H.G. and Pearson, P.L. (1999) Effect of intravenous iron and folic acid on uterine protein secretion during early pregnancy. J. Anim. Sci. 77(suppl. 1):50.

Vallet, J.L., Freking, B.A., Leymaster, K.A. and Christenson, R.K. (2005) Allelic variation in the secreted folate binding protein gene is associated with uterine capacity in swine. J. Anim. Sci. 83(8):1860–1867. https://doi.org/10.2527/2005.8381860x.

Van den Ouweland, J.M.W. (2016) Analysis of vitamin D metabolites by liquid chromatography-tandem mass spectrometry, TrAC Trends Anal. Chem. MassSpectrom. Clin. Lab. 84:117.e130.

Van Etten, C., Ellis, N.R. and Madsen, L.L. (1940) Studies on the thiamine requirement of young swine. J. Nutr. 20(6):607–625. https://doi.org/10.1093/jn/22.6.607.

Van Heugten, E. (1999) Potential benefit of using vitmain E in improving pork quality. Carolina Swine Nutrition Conference. (pp. 1–10).

Van Heugten, E., Sweet, L.A., Stumpf, T.T., Risley, C.R. and Schell, T.C. (1997) Effects of water supplementation with selenium and vitamin E on growth performance and blood selenium and serum vitamin E concentrations in weanling pigs. J. Am. Vet. Med. Assoc. 211(8):1039–1042. PMID: 9343551.

Van Heugten, E. (2000) Mycotoxins and other antinutritional factors in swine feeds. In "Swine nutrition" CRC Press. (pp. 583–604).

Van Kempen, T.A.T.G., Reijersen, M.H., de Bruijn, C., De Smet, S., Michiels, J., Traber, M.G. and Lauridsen, C. (2016) Vitamin E plasma kinetics in swine show low bioavailability and short half-life of all-rac-α-tocopheryl acetate. J. Anim. Sci. 94(10):4188–4195. https://doi.org/10.2527/jas.2016-0640.

Van Vleet, J.F. (1975) Retention of selenium in tissues of calves, lambs, and pigs after parenteral injection of a selenium-vitamin E preparation. Am. J. Vet. Res. 36(9):1335–1340. PMID: 1163872.

Van Vleet, J.F. (1976) Induction of lesions of selenium-vitamin E deficiency in pigs fed silver. Am. J. Vet. Res. 37(12):1415–1420. PMID: 999068.

Van Vleet, J.F. (1982) Comparative efficacy of five supplementation procedures to control selenium-vitamin E deficiency in swine. Am. J. Vet. Res. 43(7):1180–1189. PMID: 6213185.

Van Vleet, J.F. (1989) Selenium-vitamin E deficiency in swine. Pract. Vet. Cont (Comp.). Ed. 11:662–668.

Van Vleet, J.F. and Ruth, G.R. (1977) Efficacy of supplements in prevention of selenium-vitamin E deficiency in swine. Am. J. Vet. Res. 38(9):1299–1305. PMID: 921024.

Van Vleet, J.F., Meyer, K.B. and Olander, H.J. (1973) Control of selenium-vitamin E deficiency in growing swine by parenteral administration of selenium-vitamin E preparations to baby pigs or to pregnant sows and their baby pigs. J. Am. Vet. Med. Assoc. 163(5):452–456.

Van Vleet, J.F., Meyer, K.B., Olander, H.J. and Ruth, G.R. (1975) Efficacy and safety of selenium-vitamin E injections in newborn pigs to prevent subclinical deficiency in growing swine. Am. J. Vet. Res. 36(4 Pt.1 Pt. 1):387–393. PMID: 1124875.

Van Vleet, J.F., Ruth, G. and Ferrans, V.J. (1976) Ultrastructural alterations in skeletal muscle of pigs with selenium-vitamin E deficiency. Am. J. Vet. Res. 37(8):911–922. PMID: 949118.

Van Vleet, J.F., Ferrans, V.J. and Ruth, G.R. (1977a) Ultrastructural alterations in nutritional cardiomyopathy of selenium-vitamin E deficient swine. I. Fiber lesions. Lab. Invest. 37(2):188–200. PMID: 881781.

Van Vleet, J.F., Ferrans, V.J. and Ruth, G.R. (1977b) Ultrastructural alterations in nutritional cardiomyopathy of selenium-vitamin E deficient swine. II. Vascular lesions. Lab. Invest. 37(2):201–211. PMID: 881782.

Van Vleet, J.F., Boon, G.D. and Ferrans, V.J. (1981) Induction of lesions of selenium-vitamin E deficiency in weanling swine fed silver, cobalt, tellurium, zinc, cadmium, and vanadium. Am. J. Vet. Res. 42(5):789–799. PMID: 7258798.

Van Vleet, J.F., Runnels, L.J., Cook, J.R. and Scheidt, A.B. (1987) Monensin toxicosis in swine: potentiation by tiamulin administration and ameliorative effect of treatment with selenium and/or vitamin E. Am. J. Vet. Res. 48(10):1520–1524. PMID: 3674564.

Vanderschueren, D., Gevers, G., Raymaekers, G., Devos, P. and Dequeker, J. (1990) Sex- and age-related changes in bone and serum osteocalcin. Calcif. Tissue Int. 46(3):179–182. https://doi.org/10.1007/BF02555041.

Vaxman, F., Olender, S., Lambert, A., Nisand, G., Aprahamian, M., Bruch, J.F., Didier, E., Volkmar, P. and Grenier, J.F. (1995) Effect of pantothenic acid and ascorbic acid supplementation on human skin wound healing process. A double-blind, prospective and randomized trial. Eur. Surg. Res. 27(3):158–166. https://doi.org/10.1159/000129395.

Verbeeck, J. (1975) Vitamin behaivior in premixes. Feedstuffs 47(63):4.

Vermeer, C. (1986) Comparison between hepatic and nonhepatic vitamin K-dependent carboxylase. Haemostasis 16(3–4):239–245. https://doi.org/10.1159/000215296.

Viganò, P., Mangioni, S., Pompei, F. and Chiodo, I. (2003) Maternal conceptus cross talk—a review. Placenta 24(suppl. B):S56-S61. https://doi.org/10.1016/s0143-4004(03)00137-1.

Viganò, P., Mangioni, S., Pompei, F. and Chiodo, I. (2003) Maternal-conceptus cross talk. A review. Placenta 24(suppl. B):S56-S61. https://doi.org/10.1016/s0143-4004(03)00137-1.

Vlasova, A.N., Chattha, K.S., Kandasamy, S., Siegismund, C.S. and Saif, L.J. (2013) Prenatally acquired vitamin A deficiency alters innate immune responses to human rotavirus in a gnotobiotic pig model. J. Immunol. 190(9):4742–4753. https://doi.org/10.4049/jimmunol.1203575.

Voelker, R.W. and Carlton, W.W. (1969) Effect of ascorbic acid on copper deficiency in miniature swine. Am. J. Vet. Res. 30(10): 1825–1830.

Volker, L., Weiser, H., Schulze, J. and Streiff, K. (1984) Ascorbic acid and iron metabolism in pigs. In Proc. workshop on ascorbic acid in domestic animals. I. Wegger, Tagwerker, F.J., and Moustgaard, J. (Eds.). The Royal Danish Agricultural Society, Copenhagen.

Von Rosenberg, S.J., Weber, G.M., Erhardt, A., Höller, U., Wehr, U.A. and Rambeck, W.A. (2016) Tolerance evaluation of overdosed dietary levels of 25-hydroxyvitamin D3 in growing piglets. J. Anim. Physiol. Anim. Nutr. (Berl) 100(2):371–380. https://doi.org/10.1111/jpn.12355.

Vossen, E., Claeys, E., Raes, K., van Mullem, D and De Smet. S. (2016) Supra-nutritional levels of α-tocopherol maintain the oxidative stability of n-3 long-chain fatty acid enriched subcutaneous fat and frozen loin, but not of dry fermented sausage. J. Sci. Food Agric. 96:4523–4530 https://doi.org/10.1002/jsfa.7668.

Wagle, S.R., Mehta, R. and Johnson, B.C. (1958) Vitamin B12 and protein biosynthesis. IV. In vivo and in vitro studies. J. Biol. Chem. 230(1):137–147. PMID: 13502381.

Wagner, C. (2001) Biochemical role of folate in cellular metabolism. Clin. Res. Regul. Aff. 18(3):161–180. https://doi.org/10.1081/CRP-100108171.

Wagner, C., Briggs, W.T. and Cook, R.J. (1984) Covalent binding of folic acid to dimethylglycine dehydrogenase. Arch. Biochem. Biophys. 233(2):457–461. https://doi.org/10.1016/0003-9861(84)90467-3.

Wahlstrom, R.C. and Stolte, D.E. (1958) The effect of supplemental vitamin D in rations for pigs fed in the absence of direct sunlight. J. Anim. Sci. 17(3):699–705. https://doi.org/10.2527/jas1958.173699x.

Wang, D., Lindemann, M.D. and Estienne, M.J. (2020) Effect of folic acid supplementation and dietary protein level on growth performance, serum chemistry and immune response in weanling piglets fed differing concentrations of aflatoxin. Toxins 12(10):651. https://doi.org/10.3390/toxins12100651.

Wang, H., Yang, P., Li, L., Zhang, N. and Ma, Y. (2021) Effects of sources or formulations of vitamin K3 on its stability during extrusion or pelleting in swine feed. Animals (Basel) 11(3):633–640. https://doi.org/10.3390/ani11030633.

Wang, J., Kokinos, B.P., Lang, P.J., Crenshaw, T.D. and Henak, C.R. (2022a) Vitamin D deficiency and anatomical region alters porcine growth plate properties. J. Biomech. 144:111314. https://doi.org/10.1016/j.jbiomech.2022.111314.

Wang, L., Tan, X., Wang, H., Wang, Q., Huang, P., Li, Y., Li, J., Huang, J., Yang, H. and Yin, Y. (2021a) Effects of varying dietary folic acid during weaning stress of piglets. Anim. Nutr. 7(1):101–110. https://doi.org/10.1016/j.aninu.2020.12.002.

Wang, L., Xu, X., Su, G., Shi, B. and Shan, A. (2017) High concentration of vitamin E supplementation in sow diet during the last week of gestation and lactation affects the immunological variables and antioxidative parameters in piglets. J. Dairy Res. 84(1):8–13. https://doi.org/10.1017/S0022029916000650.

Wang, L., Zou, L., Li, J., Yang, H. and Yin, Y. (2021b) Effect of dietary folate level on organ weight, digesta pH, short-chain fatty acid concentration, and intestinal microbiota of weaned piglets. J. Anim. Sci. 99(1):1–9. https://doi.org/10.1093/jas/skab015.

Wang, S.P., Yin, Y.L., Qian, Y., Li, L.L., Li, F.N., Tan, B.E., Tang, X.S. and Huang, R.L. (2011) Effects of folic acid on the performance of suckling piglets and sows during lactation. J. Sci. Food Agric. 91(13):2371–2377. https://doi.org/10.1002/jsfa.4469.

Wang, X., Chen, H., Bühler, K., Chen, Y., Liu, W. and Hu, J. (2022b) Proteomics analysis reveals promotion effect of 1α, 25-dihydroxyvitamin D3 on mammary gland development and lactation of primiparous sows during gestation. J. Proteomics 268:104716. https://doi.org/10.1016/j.jprot.2022.104716.

Wang, Y.H., Leibholz, J., Bryden, W.L. and Fraser, D.R. (1996) Lipid peroxidation status as an index to evaluate the influence of dietary fats on vitamin E requirements of young pigs. Br. J. Nutr. 75(1):81–95. https://doi.org/10.1079/bjn19960112.

Wang, Z., Li, J., Wang, Y., Wang, L., Yin, Y., Yin, L., Yang, H. and Yin, Y. (2020) Dietary vitamin A affects growth performance, intestinal development, and functions in weaned piglets by affecting intestinal stem cells. J. Anim. Sci. 98(2). https://doi.org/10.1093/jas/skaa020.

Wariss, P.D. (1984) Monitoring preslaughter stress in pigs by adrenal ascorbic acid depletion. In "Proc. ascorbic acid in domestic animals" Weger, Copenhagen, Denmark. I. Tagwerker, I., and Moustgaard, J.C. (Eds.). The Royal Danish Agric. (pp. 107–113).

Warriss, P.D. (1979) Adrenal ascorbic acid depletion as an index of preslaughter stress in pigs. Meat Sci. 3(4):281–285. https://doi.org/10.1016/0309-1740(79)90004-4.

Warriss, P.D. (1981) Weight and ascorbic acid content of the adrenal glands in pigs. Res. Vet. Sci. 31(2): 219–223. PMID: 7323467.

Washam, R.D., Sower, J.E. and DeGoey, L.W. (1975) Effect of zinc-proteinate or biotin in swine starter rations. J. Anim. Sci. 40(1):179.

Washington, M.N., Estienne, M.J., Harter-Dennis, J.M. and Hartsock, T.G. (1997) Effect of vitamin A administration on embryo survival in gilts induced to ovulate with exogenous gonadotropins. J. Anim. Sci. 75(suppl. 1):127.

Wasserman, R.H. (1981) Intestinal absorption of calcium and phosphorus. Fed. Proc. 40(1):68–72. PMID: 7192650.

Wastell, M.E., Ewan, R.C., Vorhies, M.W. and Speer, V.C. (1972) Vitamin E and selenium for growing and finishing pigs. J. Anim. Sci. 34(6):969–973. https://doi.org/10.2527/jas1972.346969x.

Watkins, B.A. (1989a) Influence of biotin deficiency and dietary trans-fatty acids on tissue lipids in chickens. Br. J. Nutr. 61(1):99–111. https://doi.org/10.1079/BJN19890096.

Watkins, B.A. (1989b) Levels of dihomo- γ-linoleate are depressed in heart phosphatidylcholine and phosphatidyl-ethanolamine in the biotin-deficient chick. Poult. Sci. 68(5):698–705. https://doi.org/10.3382/ps.0680698.

Watkins, B.A. and Kratzer, F.H. (1987a) Dietary biotin effects on polyunsaturated fatty acids in chick tissue lipids and prostaglandin E2 levels in freeze-clamped hearts. Poult. Sci. 66(11):1818–1828. https://doi.org/10.3382/ps.0661818.

Watkins, B.A. and Kratzer, F.H. (1987b) Effects of dietary biotin and linoleate on polyunsaturated fatty acids in tissue phospholipids. Poult. Sci. 66(12):2024–2031. https://doi.org/10.3382/ps.0662024.

Watkins, B.A. and Kratzer, F.H. (1987c) Tissue lipid fatty acid composition of biotin- adequate and biotin-deficient chicks. Poult. Sci. 66(2):306–313. https://doi.org/10.3382/ps.0660306.

Watkins, K.L., Southern, L.L. and Miller, J.E. (1991) Effect of dietary biotin supplementation on sow reproductive performance and soundness and pig growth and mortality. J. Anim. Sci. 69(1):201–206. https://doi.org/10.2527/1991.691201x.

Weaver, E.M., Libal, G.W., Hamilton, C.R. and Palmer, I.S. (1991) Effects of dietary or injected vitamin E on liver and plasma alpha-tocopherol concentrations in the weaned pig. Nat. Pork Prod. Council Res. Report. (pp. 110–113).

Weaver, E.M., Libal, G.W., Hamilton, C.R. and Parker, I.S. (1989) Relationship between dietary vitamin A and E on performance and vitamin E status of the weaned pig. J. Anim. Sci. 67(suppl. 2):113.

Webb, N.G., Penny, R.H. and Johnston, A.M. (1984) The effect of a dietary supplement of biotin on pig hoof horn strength and hardness. Vet. Rec. 114(8):185–189.

Webel, D.M., Finck, B.N., Baker, D.H. and Johnson, R.W. (1997) Time course of increased plasma cytokines, cortisol, and urea nitrogen in pigs following intraperitoneal injection of lipopolysaccharide. J. Anim. Sci. 75(6):1514–1520. https://doi.org/10.2527/1997.7561514x.

Webel, D.M., Mahan, D.C., Johnson, R.W. and Baker, D.H. (1998) Pretreatment of young pigs with vitamin E attenuates the elevation in plasma interleukin-6 and cortisol caused by a challenge dose of lipopolysaccharide. American Society for Nutritional Sciences. (pp. 16–57).

Weeden, T.L., Li, D.F., Goodband, R.D. and Nelssen, J.L. (1990) The effects of additional niacin during gestation and lactation on sow and litter performance. Swine day, Manhattan, KS, November 15, 1990. (pp. 26–29). http://hdl.handle.net/2097/3591.

Wegger, I. (1994) Ascorbic acid deficiency in sows results in deranged fetal bone composition. Proc. 13th International Pig Vet. Soc. Congress, Bangkok, Thailand.

Wegger, I. and Palludan, B. (1984) Ascorbic acid status of swine. In "Proc. Workshop on Ascorbic Acid Domestic Animals" Weggar, I., Tagwerker, F.J., and Moustgaard, J. (Eds.). The Royal Danish Agricultural Society, Copenhagen.

Wegger, I. and Palludan, B. (1994) Vitamin C deficiency causes hematological and skeletal abnormalities during fetal development in swine. J. Nutr. 124(2):241–248.

Wei, I.L. and Young, T.K. (1994) Vitamin B6 metabolism is altered in chronic renal failure rats. Nutr. Res. 14(2):271–278. https://doi.org/10.1016/S0271-5317(05)80385-9.

Weiser, H. and Vecchi, M. (1982) Stereoisomers of α-tocopheryl acetate. II. Biopotencies of all eight stereoisomers, individually or in mixtures, as deter-mined by rat resorption-gestation tests. Int. J. Vitam. Nutr. Res. 52(3):351–370. PMID: 7174231.

Weiser, H., Schlachter, M., Probst, H.P. and Kormann, A.W. (1990) The relevance of ascorbic acid for bone metabolism. In "Proc. 2nd Symp. Ascorbic Acid in Domestic Animals", Kartause, Switzerland. (pp. 73–95).

Weiß, J. and Quanz, G. (2002) Hat eine erhöhte Versorgung der Mastschweine mit B-Vitaminen einen Effekt auf Leistung und Wirtschaftlichkeit, Vol. 7. Tagung Schweine-und Geflügelernährung, Wittenberg, Germany. (pp. 114–116).

Welch, A.D., Heinle, R.W., Sharpe, G., George, W.L. and Epstein, M. (1947) Chemical antagonism of pteroyl-gutamic acid in a pig: hematopoietic effect of extrinsic and intrinsic factors. Proc. Soc. Exp. Biol. Med. 65(2):364–368. https://doi.org/10.3181/00379727-65-15960.

Wellenreiter, R.H., Ullrey, D.E., Miller, E.R. and Magee, W.T. (1969) Vitamin A activity of corn carotenes for swine. J. Nutr. 99(2):129–136. https://doi.org/10.1093/jn/99.2.129.

Wemheuer, W., Steinbrink, J., Fuhrmann, H., Schmidt, W. and Sallmannn, H.P. (1996) Influence of vitamin A and beta-carotene on vitamin E-status, ejaculate parameter and health of the insemination boar. Dtsch. Tierarztl Wschr. 103(10):431–437. PMID: 9035977.

Wen, J., Morrissey, P.A., Buckley, D.J. and Sheehy, P.J.A. (1997) Supranutritional vitamin E supplementation in pigs: influence on subcellular deposition of α-tocopherol and on oxidative stability by conventional and derivative spectrophotometry. Meat Sci. 47(3–4):301–310. https://doi.org/10.1016/S0309-1740(97)00062-4.

Wen, W., Chen, X., Huang, Z., Chen, D., Yu, B., He, J., Luo, Y., Yan, H., Chen, H., Zheng, P. and Yu, J. (2022) Dietary lycopene supplementation improves meat quality, antioxidant capacity and skeletal muscle fiber type transformation in finishing pigs. Anim. Nutr. 8(1):256–264. https://doi.org/10.1016/j.aninu.2021.06.012.

Wenk, C., Leonhardt, M. and Scheeder, M.R. (2000) Monogastric nutrition and potential for improving muscle quality. In "Antioxidants in muscle foods: nutritional strategies to improve quality" Decker, E.A, Faustman, C. and Lopez-Bote, C.J. (Eds). Wiley Interscience, New York. (pp. 199–228).

Whaley, S.L., Hedgpeth, V.S. and Britt, J.H. (1997) Evidence that injection of vitamin A before mating may improve embryo survival in gilts fed normal or high-energy diets. J. Anim. Sci. 75(4):1071–1077. https://doi.org/10.2527/1997.7541071x.

Whaley, S.L., Hedgpeth, V.S., Farin, C.E., Martus, N.S., Jayes, F.C. and Britt, J.H. (2000) Influence of vitamin A injection before mating on oocyte development, follicular hormones, and ovulation in gilts fed high-energy diets. J. Anim. Sci. 78(6):1598–1607. https://doi.org/10.2527/2000.7861598x.

Whanger, P.D. (1981) Selenium and heavy metal toxicity. In "Selenium in biology and medicine" Spallholz,J.E., Martin, J.L. and Ganther, H.E. (Eds). AVI Publishing Co., Westport, Connecticut.

White, W.S., Peck, K.M., Ulman, E.A. and Erdman, J.W. (1993) The ferret as a model for evaluation of the bioavailabilities of all-trans-beta-carotene and its isomers. J. Nutr. 123(6):1129–1139. PMID: 8505674.

Whitehair, C.K., Miller, E.R., Loudenslager, M. and Hogberg, M.G. (1984) MMA in sows-A vitamin E-selenium deficiency. J. Anim. Sci. 59(suppl. 1):106.

Whitehair, C.K., Vale, O.E., Hogberg, M.G. and Miller, E.R. (1983a) Importance of vitamin E and selenium in high-moisture corn diets of sows on sow productivity. Mich. Swine Research Report.

Whitehair, C.K., Vale, O.E., Loudenslager, M. and Miller, E.R. (1983b) MMA in sows-a vitamin E-selenium deficiency. Michigan State Univ. Agr. Exp. Sta. Res. Swine Report.

Whitehead, C.C., Bannister, D.W. and D'Mello, J.P. (1980) Blood pyruvate carboxylase activity as a criterion of biotin status in young pigs. Res. Vet. Sci. 29(1):126–128. PMID: 7455346.

Whitfield, G.K., Hsieh, J.C., Jurutka, P.W., Selznick, S.H., Haussler, C.A., MacDonald, P.N. and Haussler, M.R. (1995) Genomic acitoins of 1,25-dihydroxyvitamin D3. J. Nutr. 125(6)(suppl.):1690S-1694S.

Whiting, F. and Bezeau, L.M. (1958) The calcium, phosphorus, and zinc balance in pigs as influenced by the weight of pig and the level of calcium, zinc and vitamin D in the ration. Can. J. Anim. Sci. 38(2):109–117. https://doi.org/10.4141/cjas58-016.

Whiting, F. and Loosli, J.K. (1948) The placental and mammary transfer of tocopherols [vitamin E] in sheep, goats and swine. J. Nutr. 36(6):721–726. https://doi.org/10.1093/jn/36.6.721.

Whiting, F., Loosli, J.K. and Willman, J.P. (1949) The influence of tocopherols upon the mammary and placental transfer of vitamin A in the sheep, goat and pig. J. Anim. Sci. 8(1):35–40. https://doi.org/10.1093/ansci/8.1.35.

Wiedermann, U., Hanson, L.A., Kahu, H. and Dahlgren, U.I. (1993) Aberrant T-cell function in vitro and impaired T-cell dependent antibody response in vivo in vitamin A-deficient rats. Immunology 80(4):581–586. PMID: 8307607.

Wiegand, B.R., Sparks, J.C., Beitz, D.C., Parrish, F.C., Horst, R.L., Trenkle, A.H. and Ewan, R.C. (2002) Short-term feeding of vitamin D3 improves color but does not change tenderness of pork-loin chops. J. Anim. Sci. 80(8):2116–2121. https://doi.org/10.1093/ansci/80.8.2116.

Wiese, A.C., Lehrer, W.P., Moore, P.R., Pahnish, O.F. and Hartwell, W.V. (1951) Pantothenic acid deficiency in baby pigs. J. Anim. Sci. 10(1):80–87. https://doi.org/10.2527/jas1951.10180x.

Wilborn, B.S., Kerth, C.R., Owsley, W.F., Jones, W.R. and Frobish, L.T. (2004) Improving pork quality by feeding supranutritional concentrations of vitamin D3. J. Anim. Sci. 82(1):218–224. https://doi.org/10.2527/2004.821218x.

Wilburn, E.E., Mahan, D.C., Hill, D.A., Shipp, T.E. and Yang, H. (2008) An evaluation of natural (RRR-α-tocopheryl acetate) and synthetic (all-rac-α-tocopheryl acetate) vitamin E fortification in the diet or drinking water of weanling pigs. J. Anim. Sci. 86(3):584–591. https://doi.org/10.2527/jas.2007-0377.

Williams, N.H., Stahly, T.S. and Zimmerman, D.R. (1997) Effect of chronic immune system activation on the rate, efficiency, and composition of growth and lysine needs of pigs fed from 6 to 27 kg. J. Anim. Sci. 75(9):2463–2471. https://doi.org/10.2527/1997.7592463x.

Wilson, M.E., Pettigrew, J.E., Johnston, L.J. and Chester-Jones, H. (1992) Effect of B-vitamin supply upon growth of weanling pigs. J. Anim. Sci. 70(suppl. 1):61.

Wilson, M.E., Pettigrew, J.E., Johnston, L.J., Hawton, J.D., Rust, J.W. and Chester-Jones, H. (1991a) Provision of additional B-vitamins improves growth rate of weanling pigs. J. Anim. Sci. 69(suppl. 1):106.

Wilson, M.E., Pettigrew, J.E., Walker, R.D., Chester-Jones, H. and Oeltjenbruns, B. (1991b) Provision of additional vitamin B12 improved growth rate of weanling pigs. J. Anim. Sci. 69(suppl. 1):359.

Wilson, M.E., Tokach, M.D., Walker, R.W., Nelssen, J.L., Goodhand, R.D. and Pettigrew, J.E. (1993) Influence of high levels of individual B vitamins on starter pig performance. J. Anim. Sci. 71(suppl. 1):56.

Wintrobe, M.M., Stein, J.H., Follis, R.H. and Humphreys, S. (1945) Nicotinic acid and the level of protein intake in the nutrition of the pig. J. Nutr. 30(6):395–412. https://doi.org/10.1093/jn/30.6.395.

Witkowska, D., Sedrowicz, L. and Oledzka, R. (1992) Effect of a diet with an increased content of vitamin B6 on the absorption of amino acids in the intestine of rats intoxicated with carbaryl propoxur and thiuram. Methionine. Bromatol. Chem. Toksykoleziczna 25:25.

Witten, S. and Aulrich, K. (2018) Effect of variety and environment on the amount of thiamine and riboflavin in cereals and grain legumes. Anim. Feed Sci. Technol. 238:39–46. https://doi.org/10.1016/j.anifeedsci.2018.01.022.

Wolf, G. (1991) The intracellular vitamin A-binding proteins: an overview of their functions. Nutr. Rev. 49(1):1–12. https://doi.org/10.1111/j.1753-4887.1991.tb07349.x.

Wolf, G. (1993) The newly discovered retinoic acid-X receptors (RXRs). Nutr. Rev. 51(3):81–84. https://doi.org/10.1111/j.1753-4887.1993.tb03075.x.

Wolf, G. (1995) The enzymatic cleavage of beta-carotene: still controversial. Nutr. Rev. 53(5):134–137. https://doi.org/10.1111/j.1753-4887.1995.tb01537.x.

Wolf, G. (2006) How an increased intake of α-tocopherol can suppress the bioavailability of gamma-tocopherol. Nutr. Rev. 64(6):295–299. https://doi.org/10.1111/j.1753-4887.2006.tb00213.x.

Wolf, G. (2007) Identification of a membrane receptor for retinol-binding protein functioning in the cellular uptake of retinol. Nutr. Rev. 66(8):385–388. https://doi.org/10.1111/j.1753-4887.2007.tb00316.x.

Wolf, G. (2010) Retinoic acid activation of peroxisome proliferation-activated receptor δ represses obesity and insulin resistance. Nutr. Rev. 68(1):67–70. https://doi.org/10.1111/j.1753-4887.2009.00261.x.

Wolf, G. and Carpenter, K.J. (1997) Early Research into the vitamins: the work of Wilhelm Stepp. J. Nutr. 127(7):1255–1259. https://doi.org/10.1093/jn/127.7.1255.

Wolke, R.E., Nielsen, S.W. and Rousseau, J.E. (1968) Bone lesions of hypervitaminosis A in the pig. Am. J. Vet. Res. 29(5):1009–1024. PMID: 5689538.

Wood, R.D., Chaney, C.H., Waddill, D.G. and Garrison, G.W. (1967) Effect of adding nitrate or nitrite to drinking water on the utilization of carotene by growing swine. J. Anim. Sci. 26(3):510–513. https://doi.org/10.2527/jas1967.263510x.

Woodworth, J.C., Goodband, R.D., Nelssen, J.L., Tokach, M.D. and Musser, R.E. (2000) Added dietary pyridoxine, but not thiamin, improves weanling pig growth performance. J. Anim. Sci. 78(1):88–93. https://doi.org/10.2527/2000.78188x.

Woolley, D.W. (2012) Antimetabolites of the water-soluble vitamins. In "Metabolic inhibitors". https://dtk.tankonyvtar.hu/xmlui/bitstream/handle/123456789/8939/B9780123956224500173.pdf?sequence=17&isAllowed=y.

Workel, H.A., Keller, T.H., Reeve, A. and Lauwaerts, A. (2002) Choline – the rediscovered vitamin. https://www.thepoultrysite.com/articles/choline-the-rediscovered-vitamin-for-poultry.

Wuryastuti, H., Stowe, H.D., Bull, R.W. and Miller, E.R. (1993) Effects of vitamin E and selenium on immune responses of peripheral blood, colostrum, and milk leukocytes of sows. J. Anim. Sci. 71(9):2464–2472. https://doi.org/10.2527/1993.7192464x.

Wyns, H., Plessers, E., De Backer, P., Meyer, E. and Croubels, S. (2015) In vivo porcine lipopolysaccharide inflammation models to study immunomodulation of drugs. Vet. Immunol. Immunopathol. 166(3–4):58–69. https://doi.org/10.1016/j.vetimm.2015.06.001.

Xu, J., Xu, C., Chen, X., Cai, X., Yang, S., Sheng, Y. and Wang, T. (2014) Regulation of an antioxidant blend on intestinal redox status and major microbiota in early weaned piglets. Nutrition 30(5):584–589. https://doi.org/10.1016/j.nut.2013.10.018.

Xu, Y., Chen, J., Yu, X., Tao, W., Jiang, F., Yin, Z. and Liu, C. (2010) Protective effects of chlorogenic acid on acute hepatotoxicity induced by lipopolysaccharide in mice. Inflamm. Res. 59(10):871–877. https://doi.org/10.1007/s00011-010-0199-z.

Xu, Y., Sladky, J.T. and Brown, M.J. (1989) Dose-dependent expression of neuronopathy after experimental pyridoxine intoxication. Neurology 39(8):1077–1083. https://doi.org/10.1212/WNL.39.8.1077.

Yang, H., Mahan, D.C., Hill, D.A., Shipp, T.E., Radke, T.R. and Cecava, M.J. (2009) Effect of vitamin E source, natural versus synthetic, and quantity on serum and tissue α-tocopherol concentrations in finishing swine. J. Anim. Sci. 87(12):4057–4063. https://doi.org/10.2527/jas.2008-1570.

Yang, J., Tian, G., Chen, D., Zheng, P., Yu, J., Mao, X., He, J., Luo, Y., Luo, J., Huang, Z. and Yu, B. (2019a) Effects of dietary 25-hydroxyvitamin D3 supplementation on growth performance, immune function and antioxidative capacity in weaned piglets. Arch. Anim. Nutr. 73(1):44–51. https://doi.org/10.1080/1745039X.2018.1560113.

Yang, J., Tian, G., Chen, D., Zheng, P., Yu, J., Mao, X., He, J., Luo, Y., Luo, J., Huang, Z., Wu, A. and Yu, B. (2019b) Dietary 25-hydroxyvitamin D3 supplementation alleviates porcine epidemic diarrhea virus infection by improving intestinal structure and immune response in weaned pigs. Animals (Basel) 9(9):627. https://doi.org/10.3390/ani9090627.

Yang, P. and Ma, Y. (2021) Recent advances of vitamin D in immune, reproduction, performance for pig: a review. Anim. Health Res. Rev. 22(1):85–95. https://doi.org/10.1017/S1466252321000049.

Yang, P., Zhao, J., Wang, H., Li, L. and Ma, Y. (2020) Effects of vitamin forms and levels on vitamin bioavailability and growth performance in piglets. Appl. Sci. 10(14):4903. https://doi.org/10.3390/app10144903.

Yang, P., Wang, H., Li, L., Zhang, N. and Ma, Y. (2021a) The stability of vitamin A from different sources in vitamin premixes and vitamin-trace mineral premixes. Appl. Sci. 11(8):3657. https://doi.org/10.3390/app11083657.

Yang, P., Wang, H., Li, L., Zhang, N. and Ma, Y. (2021b) Determination and evaluation of bioavailability of vitamins from different multivitamin supplements using a pig model. Agriculture 11(5):418. https://doi.org/10.3390/agriculture11050418.

Yang, P., Wang, H.K., Li, L.X. and Ma, Y.X. (2021c) The strategies for the supplementation of vitamins and trace minerals in pig production: surveying major producers in China. Anim. Biosci. 34(8):1350–1364. https://doi.org/10.5713/ajas.20.0521.

Yang, P., Wang, H.K., Zhu, M., Li, L.X. and Ma, Y.X. (2021d) Degradation kinetics of vitamins in premixes for pig: effects of choline, high concentrations of copper and zinc, and storage time. Anim. Biosci. 34(4):701–713. https://doi.org/10.5713/ajas.20.0026.

Yang, Y.W., Chen, L., Mou, Q., Liang, H., Du, Z.Q. and Yang, C.X. (2020) Ascorbic acid promotes the reproductive function of porcine immature Sertoli cells through transcriptome reprogramming. Theriogenology 158:309–320. https://doi.org/10.1016/j.theriogenology.2020.09.022.

Yen, J.T. and Pond, W.G. (1981) Effect of dietary vitamin C addition on performance, plasma vitamin C and hematic iron status in weanling pigs. J. Anim. Sci. 53(5):1292–1296. https://doi.org/10.2527/jas1981.5351292x.

Yen, J.T. and Pond, W.G. (1983) Response of swine to periparturient vitamin C supplementation. J. Anim. Sci. 56(3):621–624. https://doi.org/10.2527/jas1983.563621x.

Yen, J.T. and Pond, W.G. (1984) Responses of weanling pigs to dietary supplementation with vitamin C or carbadox. J. Anim. Sci. 58(1):132–137. https://doi.org/10.2527/jas1984.581132x.

Yen, J.T. and Pond, W.G. (1987) Effect of dietary supplementation with vitamin C or carbadox on weanling pigs subjected to crowding stress. J. Anim. Sci. 64(6):1672–1681. https://doi.org/10.2527/jas1987.6461672x.

Yen, J.T. and Pond, W.G. (1988) Response of weanling pigs to dietary supplementation of vitamin C and/or rutin. Nutr. Rep. Int. 38(6):1103–1107.

Yen, J.T., Ku, P.K., Pond, W.G. and Miller, E.R. (1985) Response to dietary supplementation of vitamin C and vitamin E in weanling pigs fed low vitamin E-selenium diets. Nutr. Rep. Int. 31:877–885.

Yen, J.T., Lauxen, R. and Veum, T.L. (1978) Effect of supplemental niacin on finishing pigs fed soybean meal supplemented diets. J. Anim. Sci. 47(suppl. 1):325.

Yi, Z., Tan, X., Wang, Q., Huang, P., Li, Y., Ding, X., Li, J., Huang, J., Yang, H. and Yin, Y. (2021) Dietary niacin affects intestinal morphology and functions via modulating cell proliferation in weaned piglets. Food Funct. 12(16):7402–7414. https://doi.org/10.1039/d0fo03097j.

Yin, L., Li, J., Wang, H., Yi, Z., Wang, L., Zhang, S., Li, X., Wang, Q., Li, J., Yang, H. and Yin, Y. (2020) Effects of vitamin B6 on the growth performance, intestinal morphology, and gene expression in weaned piglets that are fed a low-protein diet. J. Anim. Sci. 98(2). https://doi.org/10.1093/jas/skaa022.

Young, L.G., Lumsden, J.H., Lun, A., Claxton, J. and Edmeades, D.E. (1976) Influence of dietary levels of vitamin E and selenium on tissue and blood parameters in pigs. Can. J. Comp. Med. 40(1):92–97. PMID: 1000383.

Young, L.G., Lun, A., Pos, J., Forshaw, R.P. and Edmeades, D. (1975) Vitamin E stability in corn and mixed feed. J. Anim. Sci. 40(3):495–499. https://doi.org/10.2527/jas1975.403495x.

Young, L.G., Miller, R.B., Edmeades, D.E., Lun, A., Smith, G.C. and King, G.J. (1977) Selenium and vitamin E supplementation of high-moisture corn diets for swine reproduction. J. Anim. Sci. 45(5):1051–1060. https://doi.org/10.2527/jas1977.4551051x.

Young, L.G., Miller, R.B., Edmeades, D.M., Lun, A., Smith, G.C. and King, G.J. (1978) Influence of method of corn storage and vitamin E and selenium supplementation on pig survival and reproduction. J. Anim. Sci. 47(3):639–647. https://doi.org/10.2527/jas1978.473639x.

Yu, B., Yang, G., Liu, J. and Chen, D. (2010) Effects of folic acid supplementation on growth performance and hepatic folate metabolism-related gene expressions in weaned piglets. Front. Agric. China 4(4):494–500. https://doi.org/10.1007/s11703-010-1047-1.

Zee, J.A., Carmichael, L., Codère, D., Poirier, D. and Fournier, M. (1991) Effect of storage conditions on the stability of vitamin C in various fruits and vegetables produced and consumed in Quebec. Journal of Food Composition and Analysis 4(1):77–86. https://doi.org/10.1016/0889-1575(91)90050-G.

Zeisel, S.H. (1990) Choline deficiency. J. Nutr. Biochem. 1(7):332–349. https://doi.org/10.1016/0955-2863(90)90001-2.

Zeisel, S.H. (2006) Choline: critical role during fetal development and dietary requirements in adults. Annu. Rev. Nutr. 26:229–250. https://doi.org/10.1146/annurev.nutr.26.061505.111156.

Zeisel, S.H. and Niculescu, M.D. (2006) Perinatal choline influences brain structure and function. Nutr. Rev. 64(4):197–203. https://doi.org/10.1111/j.1753-4887.2006.tb00202.x.

Zempleni, J., Green, G.M., Spannagel, A.W. and Mock, D.M. (1997) Biliary excretion of biotin metabolites is quantitatively minor in rats and pigs. J. Nutr. 127(8):1496–1500. https://doi.org/10.1093/jn/127.8.1496.

Zhang, J.Z., Henning, S.M. and Swendseid, M.E. (1993) Poly(ADP-ribose) polymerase activity and DNA strand breaks are affected in tissues of niacin-deficient rats. J. Nutr. 123(8):1349–1355.

Zhang, L. and Piao, X. (2021) Use of 25-hydroxyvitamin D3 in diets for sows: a review. Anim. Nutr. 7(3):728–736. https://doi.org/10.1016/j.aninu.2020.11.016.

Zhang, L., Hu, J., Li, M., Shang, Q., Liu, S. and Piao, X. (2019a) Maternal 25-hydroxycholecalciferol during lactation improves intestinal calcium absorption and bone properties in sow-suckling piglet pairs. J. Bone Miner. Metab. 37(6):1083–1094. https://doi.org/10.1007/s00774-019-01020-0.

Zhang, L., Li, M., Shang, Q., Hu, J., Long, S. and Piao, X. (2019b) Effects of maternal 25-hydroxycholecalciferol on nutrient digestibility, milk composition and fatty-acid profile of lactating sows and gut bacterial metabolites in the hindgut of suckling piglets. Arch. Anim. Nutr. 73(4):271–286. https://doi.org/10.1080/1745039X.2019.1620041.

Zhang, Y., Yu, B., Yu, J., Zheng, P., Huang, Z., Luo, Y., Luo, J., Mao, X., Yan, H., He, J. and Chen, D. (2019c) Butyrate promotes slow-twitch myofiber formation and mitochondrial biogenesis in finishing pigs via inducing specific microRNAs and PGC-1α expression. J. Anim. Sci. 97(8):3180–3192. https://doi.org/10.1093/jas/skz187.

Zhang, L., Liu, S., Li, M. and Piao, X. (2020) Effects of maternal 25-hydroxycholecalciferol during the last week of gestation and lactation on serum parameters, intestinal morphology and microbiota in suckling piglets. Arch. Anim. Nutr. 74(6):445–461. https://doi.org/10.1080/1745039X.2020.1822710.

Zhang, L., Yang, M. and Piao, X. (2022) Effects of 25-hydroxyvitamin D3 on growth performance, serum parameters, fecal microbiota, and metabolites in weaned piglets fed diets with low calcium and phosphorus. J. Sci. Food Agric. 102(2):597–606. https://doi.org/10.1002/jsfa.11388.

Zhao, L., Lu, W., Mao, Z., Mou, D., Huang, L., Yang, M., Ding, D., Yan, H., Fang, Z., Che, L., Zhuo, Y., Jiang, X., Xu, S., Lin, Y., Li, J., Huang, C., Zou, Y., Li, L., Wu, D. and Feng, B. (2022) Maternal VD3 supplementation during gestation improves intestinal health and microbial composition of weaning piglets. Food Funct. 13(12):6830–6842. https://doi.org/10.1039/d1fo04303j.

Zhao, Y., Yu, B., Mao, X., He, J., Huang, Z., Zheng, P., Yu, J., Han, G., Liang, X. and Chen, D. (2014) Dietary vitamin D supplementation attenuates immune responses of pigs challenged with rotavirus potentially through the retinoic acid-inducible gene I signaling pathway. Br. J. Nutr. 112(3):381–389. https://doi.org/10.1017/S000711451400097X.

Zhao, Y., Wen, X., Xiao, H., Hou, L., Wang, X., Huang, Y., Lin, Y., Zheng, C., Wang, L. and Jiang, Z. (2022) Effects of phytase and 25-hydroxyvitamin D3 supplementation on growth performance and bone development in weaned piglets in Ca- and P-deficient dietary. J. Sci. Food Agric. 102(3):940–948. https://doi.org/10.1002/jsfa.11426.

Zhao, Z. and Ross, A.C. (1995) Retinoic acid repletion restores the number of leukocytes and their subsets and stimulates natural cytotoxicity in vitamin A-deficient rats. J. Nutr. 125(8):2064–2073. https://doi.org/10.1093/jn/125.8.2064.

Zheng, W. and Teegarden, D. (2013) Vitamin D. In Handbook of vitamins 5th ed. Zempleni, J., Suttie, J., Gregory, J. and Stover, P. J. (Eds.). CRC Press. (pp. 51–88). https://doi.org/10.1201/b15413.

Zhong, W., Hu, L., Zhao, Y., Li, Z., Zhuo, Y., Jiang, X., Li, J., Zhao, X., Che, L., Feng, B., Lin, Y., Xu, S., Fang, Z. and Wu, D. (2021) Effects of dietary choline levels during pregnancy on reproductive performance, plasma metabolome and gut microbiota of sows. Front. Vet. Sci. 8:771228. https://doi.org/10.3389/fvets.2021.771228.

Zhou, H., Chen, Y., Lv, G., Zhuo, Y., Lin, Y., Feng, B., Fang, Z., Che, L., Li, J., Xu, S. and Wu, D. (2016) Improving maternal vitamin D status promotes prenatal and postnatal skeletal muscle development of pig offspring. Nutrition 32(10):1144–1152. https://doi.org/10.1016/j.nut.2016.03.004.

Zhou, H., Chen, Y., Zhuo, Y., Lv, G., Lin, Y., Feng, B., Fang, Z., Che, L., Li, J., Xu, S. and Wu, D. (2017) Effects of 25-hydroxycholecalciferol supplementation in maternal diets on milk quality and serum bone status markers of sows and bone quality of piglets. Anim. Sci. J. 88(3):476–483. https://doi.org/10.1111/asj.12638.

Zhou, H.B., Huang, X.Y., Bi, Z., Hu, Y.H., Wang, F.Q., Wang, X.X., Wang, Y.Z. and Lu, Z.Q. (2021) Vitamin A with L-ascorbic acid sodium salt improves the growth performance, immune function and antioxidant capacity of weaned pigs. Animal 15(2):100133. https://doi.org/10.1016/j.animal.2020.100133.

Zhou, J., Qin, Y., Xiong, X., Wang, Z., Wang, M., Wang, Y., Wang, Q.Y., Yang, H.S. and Yin, Y. (2021) Effects of iron, vitamin A, and the interaction between the two nutrients on intestinal development and cell differentiation in piglets. J. Anim. Sci. 99(10):1–9. https://doi.org/10.1093/jas/skab258.

Zhou, X., Zou, Y., Xu, Y., Zhang, Z., Wu, Y., Cao, J., Qiu, B., Qin, X., Han, D., Piao, X., Wang, J. and Zhao, J. (2022) Dietary supplementation of 25-hydroxyvitamin D3 improves growth performance, antioxidant capacity and immune function in weaned piglets. Antioxidants (Basel) 11(9):1750. https://doi.org/10.3390/antiox11091750.

Zinser, G.M. and Welsh, J. (2004) Accelerated mammary gland development during pregnancy and delayed postlactational involution in vitamin D3 receptor null mice. Mol. Endocrinol. 18(9):2208–2223. https://doi.org/10.1210/me.2003-0469.

Zintzen, H. (1975) A guide to the nutritional management of breeding sows and pigs. Vol. 1465. F. Hoffmann-La Roche & Co. Ltd., Basel, Switzerland.

Zomborszky-Kovács, M., Tuboly, S., Bíró, H., Bárdos, L., Soós, P., Tóth, Á. and Tornyos, G. (1998) The effect of beta-carotene and nucleotide base supplementation on haematological, biochemical and certain immunological parameters in weaned pigs. J. Anim. Feed Sci. 7(suppl. 1):245–251. https://doi.org/10.22358/jafs/69984/1998.

Index